The Complete Book
of Essential Oils *and*
Aromatherapy

Also by Valerie Ann Worwood

The Fragrant Mind:
Aromatherapy for Personality, Mind, Mood, and Emotion

Aromatherapy for the Soul:
Healing the Spirit with Fragrance and Essential Oils

Essential Aromatherapy:
A Pocket Guide to Essential Oils and Aromatherapy

The Endometriosis Natural Treatment Program:
A Complete Self-Help Plan for Improving Health and Well-Being

Aromatherapy for the Healthy Child:
More Than 300 Natural, Nontoxic, and Fragrant Essential Oil Blends

Scents and Scentuality:
Aromatherapy and Essential Oils for Romance, Love, and Sex

Aromatherapy for the Beauty Therapist

The Complete Book of Essential Oils *and* Aromatherapy

— REVISED AND EXPANDED —

Over 800 Natural, Nontoxic, and Fragrant Recipes
to Create Health, Beauty, and Safe Home and Work Environments

VALERIE ANN WORWOOD

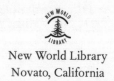

New World Library
Novato, California

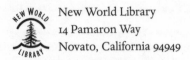

New World Library
14 Pamaron Way
Novato, California 94949

First published in the United Kingdom by Macmillan London Limited, 1990. First published in the United States by New World Library, 1991.

Text design and typography by Tona Pearce Myers and Megan Colman

Library of Congress Cataloging-in-Publication Data
Names: Worwood, Valerie Ann, [date]– author.
Title: The complete book of essential oils and aromatherapy : over 800 natural, nontoxic, and fragrant recipes to create health, beauty, and safe home and work environments / Valerie Ann Worwood.
Description: Revised and updated [edition]. | Novato, California : New World Library, [2016] | Includes bibliographical references and index.
Identifiers: LCCN 2016031708 | ISBN 9781577311393 (paperback) | ISBN 9781608684267 (ebook)
Subjects: LCSH: Aromatherapy. | BISAC: HEALTH & FITNESS / Aromatherapy. | HEALTH & FITNESS / Reference. | REFERENCE / Handbooks & Manuals. | BODY, MIND & SPIRIT / Healing / General.
Classification: LCC RM666.A68 W67 2016 | DDC 615.3/219—dc23
LC record available at https://lccn.loc.gov/2016031708

First printing of revised edition, November 2016

ISBN 978-1-57731-139-3
Ebook ISBN 978-1-60868-426-7
Printed in Canada

New World Library is proud to be a Gold Certified Environmentally Responsible Publisher. Publisher certification awarded by Green Press Initiative.
www.greenpressinitiative.org

10   9   8   7   6

For my mum — Vera Marion Howdown Worwood —
who taught me the true value of unconditional love,
and for my daughter Emma, who uplifts my heart.

Contents

Chapter 1. Medicines Out of the Earth   1

Chapter 2. The Basic Care Kit   27

Chapter 3. The Self-Defense Kit   49

Chapter 4. Occupational Oils for the Working Man and Woman   67

Chapter 5. Emotional Rescue   95

Chapter 6. The Basic Travel Kit   119

Chapter 7. The Gentle Touch for Babies, Children, and Teenagers   137

Chapter 8. A Woman's Natural Choice   191

Chapter 9. The Natural Choice for Men 241

Chapter 10. Essential Help in the Maturing Years   261

Chapter 13. The Fragrant Way to Beauty 351

Chapter 14. The Home Spa — Body Beautiful 399

Chapter 15. Fragrant Care for Your Home 423

Chapter 16. Cooking with Essential Oils   459

Chapter 17. Natural Health for Animals   477

Chapter 18. Gardens for the Future · 495

Chapter 19. Carrier Oils and Hydrolats · 513

Chapter 20. The Essential Oils and Absolutes   533

Melissa • Mimosa • Myrrh • Myrtle • Narcissus • Neem (Margosa Oil) • Neroli • Niaouli • Nutmeg • Orange, Sweet • Oregano • Oregano, Greek • Palmarosa • Patchouli • Peppermint • Petitgrain • Pimento Berry • Pine • Plai • Ravensara • Ravintsara • Rosalina (Swamp Paperbark) • Rose Absolute (Rose de Mai) • Rosemary • Rose Otto (Bulgarian Rose / Turkish Rose) • Rosewood (Bois de Rose) • Sage • Sage, Greek • Sandalwood • Sandalwood, Pacific • Saro (Mandravasarotra) • Savory, Summer • Savory, Winter • Spearmint • Spikenard • Spruce • Spruce, Black • Tagetes • Tangerine • Tarragon • Tea Tree • Thyme Linalol • Tuberose • Turmeric • Valerian • Vanilla • Vetiver • Violet Leaf • Yarrow • Ylang Ylang • Yuzu

Chapter 21. Safety Information   633

Tables

Preface

Botanicals have always been part of my life. As a young child I tended to my own patch of earth in my grandfather's garden, and learned about the symbiotic relationships between plants by getting stung by stinging nettles and finding dock leaves to soothe the sting. I made perfumes out of fragranced petals and extracted juice from wild berries for my toys' tea parties. My grandfather taught me the names of flowers and weeds, while my mother and grandmother taught me how to use herbs for medicine and cooking. My mother made her own remedies and used tried-and-tested herbals before any other medication. When my siblings and I were not feeling well, we'd be given clove oil for toothache, peppermint oil for stomachache, and a sugar cube with a little eucalyptus oil on it for a chesty cough. The pharmacy also supplied something called "horse oil," a blend of wintergreen and birch oils, which Mum rubbed on our legs when we had growing pains. The aroma of essential oils permeated my childhood, along with the smell of delicious food made from fresh vegetables plucked from the garden.

When I worked in Europe and discovered the great healing powers of essential oils, I knew they would form my career path. As the number of my clients grew, so too did their questions and curiosity. I was writing down advice and instructions for them because information about how to use essential oils was simply not otherwise available. My mother noticed that I always seemed to be giving advice and suggested I write a book. That was over twenty-five years ago.

Throughout my career, and to the present day, I've been a "hands-on" practitioner. Although I lecture and research, what gives me the energy to continue is observing the interaction between essential oils and patients, and watching each individual's healing journey. That's the experience that lies at the root of this book, which is a synthesis of experience, practical research, and facts gained from original sources. Invitations to international conferences have given the opportunity to present my work and discuss developments with researchers in both the commercial and academic fields. Traveling as a consultant has offered the chance to visit essential oil producers both large and small. And giving workshops has enabled me to pass on the information gained to a new generation of essential oil therapists.

We've all come a long way, with essential oils now being used in general, maternity, and oncology hospital wards and in care homes, and being studied in research departments of universities. Aromatherapy has become a worldwide movement.

I've been humbled by the positive responses I've received to my books over the years and surprised at how many travelers have carried them in backpacks, along with a basic care kit of oils. Their stories describing how the essential oils have saved many a day have been encouraging. One nurse told me that my book, along with a few essential oils and a small number of medications, was the only help she had when working at a remote location in South Africa. Yet, with this limited resource, she'd managed to solve all manner of health issues and been able to fulfill her role.

It's wonderful to be asked to sign a book that's so dog-eared it's falling to pieces, because it shows that the information in it has been well used. What makes the work worthwhile is to hear from mums and dads about how much essential oils have helped their families, or from a senior now using essential oils in his garden instead of insecticides, or the woman whose aches are relieved enough to allow her to dance a little again. I shall be eternally grateful that I've been able to spread the word about the amazing healing properties of essential oils, and their agent in the world — aromatherapy.

Introduction:
The Fragrant Pharmacy

Nature has blessed us with a treasure trove of sweet-smelling liquid essences, gems with many facets. Hold one to the light and admire its antimicrobial features, turn it again and recognize its anti-inflammatory benefits, turn it again to see how it can positively affect mind, mood, and emotion. Each essential oil, like a prism, contains a rainbow of possibilities.

We cannot but admire the ability of essential oils to operate effectively not only on the biochemical, cellular, physical level, but also in the emotional, intellectual, spiritual, and aesthetic areas of our lives. They provide a system of healing that is in total harmony with people, who are themselves multifaceted. The essential oils have been examined, dissected, and subjected to innumerable analytic processes having to do with their chemistry, weight, light refraction, polarity, and electrical qualities. Science can tell us a great deal about them, but there's still much that remains a mystery.

There's nothing lightweight about essential oils. Although they are sweet smelling, they're powerful. This is recognized by corporations and private institutions that quietly work in laboratories behind the scenes to establish which of the many properties of essential oils they could develop commercially. And they're keeping the patent offices busy. But the benefits of essential oils are already available to you.

The Complete Book of Essential Oils and Aromatherapy offers a thoroughly comprehensive understanding of what essential oils can do in a multitude of different ways. I sincerely hope that this new updated edition will bring much positivity to a new generation of aromatherapy enthusiasts. As well as expanding all subject areas, this edition contains new chapters on self-defense against microbes, emotional rescue, and major health concerns, plus detailed profiles of over 180 essential oils, hydrolats, and carrier oils.

Essential oils are valuable in so many quite different ways that it's hard to find a word or even an expression that fully describes what they can do. They are perhaps best known as a *materia medica* — a system of healing; but essential oils can also be used throughout the home and workplace to enhance well-being and lifestyle. And, as can be seen from the contents of this book, they offer unique assistance to athletes, dancers, travelers, gardeners, animal lovers, and cooks. As well as all this, essential oils are invaluable in beauty and spa treatments.

People who use essential oils on a regular basis say they can't do without them. And newcomers to essential oils will wonder how they got along before. The effectiveness and versatility of essential oils are easy to incorporate into our lives because there are so many different methods of use. The fact that they smell good is just a bonus! There seems no end in sight to the benefits of essential oils, whether newly recognized in a lab or recently experienced in our own homes. As was the case with the first edition of this book, this 25th anniversary edition is intended for use by the home practitioner, as well as by those who are experienced in aromatherapy.

Essential oils may be part of humanity's past, but they're also part of humanity's future. They are an eternal gift from nature, an ongoing adventure of marvels, a friend, a support, and one of the most valuable gifts nature has given us to enjoy.

1

Medicines Out of the Earth

The Lord hath created medicines out of the earth;

and he that is wise will not abhor them.

— Ecclesiasticus 38:4

Essential oils provide us with a fragrant pharmacy full of remedies and delights for all aspects of our lives. This is an extraordinary fact. Already we know the earth provides us with food and water, but to realize as well that nature offers us a huge variety of plant essences capable of solving so many problems, and in addition giving us so much joy — well, that is something to rejoice in.

People have always found around them a number of plants that can heal — medicines out of the earth. But we live in a specially blessed time because we can look around the global village and take from around the world a huge variety of aromatic essential oils distilled from healing plants. This is new. We have a vast selection to choose from, never before available to humankind.

Essential oils are extracted from certain varieties of trees, shrubs, herbs, grasses, roots, fruits,

and flowers. The oil is concentrated in different parts of the plant. Vetiver oil is made from the roots of the grass species *Vetiveria zizanoides*; bay oil is extracted from the leaves of *Laurus nobilis*. Geranium oil comes from the plant's leaves and stalks, cumin oil comes from the seeds, and ginger oil comes from the rhizomes, while rose oil comes from the fragrant petals of the rose flower. Myrrh, frankincense, and benzoin oils are extracted from the resin of their respective trees. Mandarin, lemon, lime, grapefruit, and bergamot oils are extracted from the peel of the fruits, and pine oil comes from the needles and twigs of pine trees, while sandalwood comes from the heartwood of the sandalwood tree.

If you were to look at lavender under a microscope, you'd see the smooth round glands that contain the essential oil, surrounded by a forest of spiky nonsecretory trichomes. Many varieties of plants have similar sessile secretory glands that appear as round, distinct units with a cuticle, or outer membrane, protecting a package of secretory cells. In other species of plants, the essential oil–producing glands look like microscopic stalks. In seeds, the essential oil is stored in vittae, little pockets on the outer surface. In orange and lemon, oil cavities are found in the outer portion of the peel. In clove, a multitude of endogenous oil glands lie just beneath the surface, while in frankincense, resin globules are released from oil ducts. In ginger, the essential oil is found in secretory cells of parenchyma tissue, while in cedarwood the secretory cells line resin ducts.

The oil is extracted from the plant by a variety of means, depending again on the particular species. The most common method is steam distillation; other methods include CO_2 extraction, expression, enfleurage, maceration, and solvent extraction. There are hundreds of species of eucalyptus tree, but they're not all used for the production of essential oils. Likewise, there are innumerable varieties of geranium, most of which are wholly unsuitable for essential oil extraction. Having said that, aromatherapy is a science that's expanding. New plants are being distilled into essential oils, adding to our assets in the fragrant pharmacy.

Each oil has its own medicinal and other properties. Research has confirmed centuries of experience of using the plants from which essential oils are derived. We now know that the fragrant pharmacy contains essential oils that are antiviral, antibacterial, antifungal, antiseptic, anti-inflammatory, antineuralgic, antirheumatic, antispasmodic, antivenomous, antitoxic, antidepressant, sedative, nervine, analgesic, carminative, digestive, decongestive, expectorant, deodorant, restorative, circulatory, diuretic, vulnerary, and much more besides.

There is a wide range of methods of using essential oils for therapeutic purposes, including external application, inhalation, oral ingestion, and suppositories. Their small molecular size means essential oils can be absorbed extremely easily and quickly. Methods used externally include body oils, compresses, gels, lotions, and baths — including hand and foot baths. Inhalation methods include diffusers, room sprays, vaporizers, and a whole range of other environmental methods, as well as simply inhaling directly from the bottle or from a tissue. Although the food and drink and drug industries add essential oils to products that are ingested orally, they are seldom used this way for medicinal purposes in the home unless under the direction of a qualified healthcare practitioner.

The method of use that's chosen will determine both the rate and extent of absorption. Other factors to consider include a person's age, size, diet, and genetics. The rate of healing may differ too if a person has a metabolic disorder or a condition affecting the heart, liver, or kidneys.

Each essential oil has its own story to tell. In the case of jasmine, each flower is picked by hand on the very first day it opens, before the sun becomes hot, whereas the sandalwood tree could be thirty years old and thirty feet high before it's considered ready for distillation. Between these two extremes, a whole range of growing and picking conditions apply to the plants that will ultimately provide the precious essential oils. The price of each oil reflects these conditions; because it takes around 4 million hand-picked jasmine blossoms to produce 1.1 pounds of oil, you can understand why that is one of the most expensive oils on the market. Rose otto essential oil is also costly because it takes around 4,500 pounds of rose flower heads to make 1 pound of oil, while lavender oil is cheaper because it takes only 150 pounds of flower heads to produce the same amount. Obviously, yields vary from location to location, and this too can affect prices.

The trade in essential oils is worldwide, with

consignments passing between the United States, France, China, Brazil, Bulgaria, Turkey, Saudi Arabia, New Zealand, Ethiopia, Indonesia, Réunion, Australia, Argentina, Israel, the United Kingdom, Japan, Thailand, South Africa, Vietnam, Indonesia, Iran, Guatemala, Egypt, Somalia, and Spain, among many other places!

On average, an essential oil contains 100 chemical components. The main components fall within broader groups, such as alcohols, esters, ketones, phenols, terpenes, and aldehydes. But each oil also has a number of smaller trace compounds that even today cannot be identified. It's these mysterious compounds that distinguish essential oils from a simple collection of chemical constituents and gives them their complexity and unique properties. Think of it like this: the human body is 60% to 73% water, having a higher percentage at the obese end of the body mass spectrum — yet when we look in the mirror we don't see a big puddle of water. Likewise, an essential oil could be 30% to 60% linalyl acetate, but that's just the beginning of its story. Some essential oils have as many as 300 components, some as yet unidentified, and the idea that all the known phytochemicals could be put in a pot and made into that essential oil is as presumptuous as thinking a person can be reduced to a number of molecules, starting with the largest in terms of volume, water.

Essential oils are not complex just in terms of their chemistry. They have a whole range of interesting properties that together make them hugely vibrant. In terms of their electromagnetic frequency or vibrational signature, some have a higher megahertz reading than others. The electrical properties of essential oils are defined in terms of positive-negative and polarity. An aroma molecule might be negative and polar, negative and nonpolar, positive and polar, or positive and nonpolar. And even individual components have their own electrical characteristics. Some essential oils have optical activity and rotate light clockwise;

some, counterclockwise — being dextrorotatory and levorotatory, respectively. Their components are crystalline in structure. Put all these things together alongside the body of a human being who also has these properties, and there can be a marriage of harmony and potential.

Essential oils are hugely versatile and also come in the most convenient form to exploit that versatility. A few drops of pure lavender oil applied to a minor burn effects the most remarkable cure as the skin returns to normal within days, whereas without it there could be a blistering patch and, eventually, a scar. You can return to the same small bottle when you have a headache — one drop rubbed on the temples often brings relief. And because lavender is a natural deterrent of mosquitoes and moths, among other insects, it can as easily be dabbed onto a ribbon and hung at the window to deter the former, or put on a cotton ball and placed in the wardrobe to deter the latter. The natural antibiotic and antiseptic qualities of lavender oil make it a highly effective wash for cuts and grazes and also a good addition to the wash water for cleaning tables, tiles, and floors. Its fresh aroma makes lavender a delight to use anywhere and any time, and it's great to include in an air freshener. One little bottle, used with different methods, can attend to issues both physiological and environmental, and just because lavender can be used as an air freshener that's not to say it wouldn't be of huge benefit to burn units in hospitals. Indeed, I can't think of anything that would be more appropriate to use as an air freshener in burn units! That's the thing about essential oils — they can do more than one thing at a time.

Plants are chemical factories inhabiting the interface between light and dark, sun and earth, drawing energy from each and synthesizing this into molecules of carbohydrates, proteins, and fats. They provide our food, and the food of the animals we eat. Plant cells are similar to ours in that they have membranes, DNA, and a range of organelles including Golgi bodies and mitochondria. We're family. We've evolved together. We can't think of plants as inferior to us, because while they can live without us, we can't live without them. That's the relationship between us. So turning to plants for help is like turning to our extended family.

We're all increasingly aware of the number of synthetic chemicals in our lives today, whether we like them or not. They leach from carpets, flooring, and furniture. They're in home cleaning products. They're used in the production of food, in our public water systems, and in the products we put on our faces, hair, and bodies. They're in the very air we breathe. It may seem that escape from this onslaught of synthetic chemicals is impossible. However, for some jobs around the home we can replace the usual shop-bought products with essential oils, and we can make our own entirely natural body, hair, and face products, perfumes, and air fresheners. We can use essential oils in the garden to encourage plant growth and protect our plants from insects. We can use these powerful natural essences on our bodies to alleviate all manner of physical problems, and we can use them for the well-being of our family and friends. You can see from the contents of this book that essential oils are useful and effective in a staggering variety of ways. And each time we use them, we avoid using synthetic chemicals in our lives because we're lucky enough to have been given natural alternatives.

We have been given a huge gift from Mother Nature, and essential oils are something we can feel confident about using if we treat them with the respect they deserve. It might be easy to suppose that because they're so sweet smelling, the value of essential oils is their charm. This would be a mistake. Scientists in labs all over the world are discovering that when they compare the effects of a complete essential oil to those of its main chemical constituents, the essential oils come out on top. They might smell sweet and lovely, but they're potent and work very hard too.

We're All Individuals

In this book, as in the first edition, I very often recommend for particular physical or mental conditions not only specific blends but alternative essential oils, for the very important reason that not everyone is the same. That sounds obvious, but when it comes to using essential oils, although a particular essential oil might suit most people, there are likely to be some for whom that particular essential oil is not so effective. This has nothing to do with the efficacy of that particular essential oil, and possibly has something to do with genetics. Scientists are now realizing that some pharmaceutical drugs simply do not work for everyone, and they're increasingly researching the relationship between those drugs and the genes of these nonresponsive people. For example, a whole range of statin medicines have been examined for causing myotoxicity (a toxic effect on muscle) in some people, who appear to be having these symptoms because they have a certain genetic makeup. In the future, we may all have to accept the need for our medical records to include our full genetic profile. When using essential oils, don't be disheartened if a particular oil isn't as effective for you as it seems to be for others; simply choose another that has similar properties.

Essential Oils — Not So New

Don't think there's anything unusual about essential oils — they've been around a long time. The original recipe for Coca-Cola, invented by John Pemberton in 1886, included the essential oils of orange, lemon, nutmeg, cinnamon, coriander, and neroli. Chewing gum would never have made it off the ground without peppermint and spearmint essential oils. Today, essential oils are widely used in the food and drink industry to give natural flavor and aroma, and they are also used as preservatives. Essential oil components are even put in packaging film to protect food from deterioration. Manufacturers of cosmetics have long appreciated the cell-rejuvenating and beautifying properties of essential oils, and no respectable spa treatment would be without them. Indeed, the essential oil ingredients in products are often their chief selling point. In the past, the entire perfume industry was based on essential oils, although, unfortunately, today they've largely been replaced by synthetic ingredients — which is perhaps why so many people have negative physical reactions to modern fragrance products.

Essential oils are truly holistic in that they affect mind, body, and spirit. The mood-enhancing properties of certain essential oils ensured their inclusion in old-style perfumes. Put simply, they made people feel better. Also aromatics have always been used in spiritual practice — think about the frankincense and myrrh resin burned in huge quantities in certain churches, with great plumes of aromatic smoke engulfing the congregation. Native Americans put fragrant sage and cedar on hot rocks in the sweat lodge for ritual purification and spiritual connection. At the coronation of Britain's Queen Elizabeth II in 1953, the essential oils of neroli, rose, cinnamon, jasmine, and benzoin were included in the coronation oil with which she was anointed, the act that set the seal of God's approval.

Today there are around 300 essential oils easily available, but a well-chosen starting selection of around 10 essential oils will provide enough choice to meet the requirements of most home practitioners. Essential oils should be treated with respect, but also with confidence. Use your common sense, follow the instructions in this book, purchase with care and deliberation, and enjoy!

Synergy

When the combination is more than the sum of the parts, there's a synergistic effect. Mixing together two or more essential oils creates a compound that's different from any of the component parts, and these blends can be very particular and powerful. A blend can increase potency without increasing the dosage. For example, the anti-inflammatory action of chamomile essential oil is greatly increased by adding lavender in the correct proportion. The interaction of particular essential oils with each other gives a vibrancy and dynamism to the whole that might not be achieved by using a single essential oil on its own.

The important point about synergistic blends is that the proportions should be correct, and sometimes it's necessary to prepare more, in volume, than initially needed so that the smallest component oils can be incorporated into the whole in the right proportions. Diluted in a body oil, you may have a component part that is only 0.001% of the whole, and yet that minuscule amount is integral to the whole.

Throughout this book you'll see there are instructions for making blends, and this is best done by mixing the essential oils in a separate bottle. You can use the exact number of drops shown, or multiply *all the components* in the formula by the same rate. In this way you get a larger volume of the synergistic blend for future use.

Adaptogens

Several essential oils act as metabolic regulators. These *adaptogens*, as they're called, will instigate a reaction in the body that is appropriate to achieving a state of homeostasis, or balance. The reactions affect the autonomic nervous system, the endocrine system, and blood pressure, among others. For example, lemon essential oil works on the autonomic nervous system, acting as a sedative when needed, or as a tonic. Peppermint is another oil that might be found on both "relaxant" and "stimulant" lists, and this apparent contradiction can cause confusion unless you understand that these are adaptogens. Interestingly, there are other natural products that fall into this group, including the herb mint and the root ginseng.

Chemotypes

The same species of plant can produce essential oils with different chemical components when grown under different conditions, such as variations in soil type, climate, and altitude. For example, the common herb *Thymus vulgaris* produces several essential oils for medicinal use. Generally, thyme can be a skin irritant and should be used with care, but thyme linalol, which is usually grown at high altitudes, can be used safely in the blends mentioned in this book and is the only chemotype of thyme that can be used in the treatment of children. Because one species of oil-producing plant can break down into several chemotypes, each with different medical potentials, the list of useful plants is more extensive than first appearances might imply.

The Timeless Apothecary

The huge volume of scientific research being carried out all over the world today into the healing properties of essential oils is a revival of work carried out in Europe in the 1880s. The "anti-contagious" properties of distilled plants were of course hugely important when no antibiotics were available. Then, around the turn of the twentieth century, there was a change in attitude, dismissing all things old and becoming excited at all things new — including chemistry and new drugs. We have in a sense come full circle because

we now recognize that the essential oils once dismissed as old-fashioned are, in some cases, more effective for certain conditions than even the newest of drugs. And all the essential oils are being revisited in the hope they can inspire the development of new pharmaceuticals.

In 1888 two doctors from Lyons, France, Célestin Cadéac and Albin Meunier, published a paper in the annals of the Pasteur Institute proving the antibacterial power of the essential oils of cinnamon, clove, and oregano. This was just a few years after another scientist had shown that thyme was, likewise, a powerful antibacterial agent. It's interesting that these men should choose to work with these particular essential oils because we know today that they're among the most powerful antibacterial agents around.

In Germany, essential oils were distilled by apothecaries for their medicinal use, as can be seen in the frontispiece of the 1557 herbal *Kräuterbuch* by doctor of medicine Adam Lonitzer. This work followed an older tradition. For example, Hieronymus Brunschwig's first "small" book of distillation, published in 1500, was followed by his "big" book in 1519 — and that came out in 608 editions, being translated into every European language. The book contained a section advising which essential oils could be used to treat various illnesses, including lavender, rosemary, and pine. His own special recipe, no doubt a powerful one, was a combination of clove, cinnamon, mastic, and frankincense. Glove makers used aromatic oils, probably to prevent mold, and it's reported that only they and others who used fragrant oils and herbs were guaranteed to survive the ravages of the plagues that struck Europe during these centuries.

People throughout time have realized the protective and healing nature of certain plant materials, and they were valued for that as much as for their sweet aromas. It's not just any plant that finds itself in the pages of herbals or in perfume history. For example, stock lists from the Venetian trader Francesco Pegolotti, dated between 1310 and 1340, itemize "spices" any aromatherapist would recognize today, including anise, rose water, cinnamon, cassia, cardamom, cumin, camphor, lemon, clove, fennel, ginger, spikenard, frankincense, mastic, nutmeg, pepper, pine resin, and sandalwood. Another item on his list was the delightful "sugar fragranced with rose and violets."

Venice was a city-state monopolizing trade routes to the East, from where much of the more exotic aromatic material came, and Italy became the first perfume-making center in Europe, especially at Florence. The craft was taken to France by Caterina de' Medici, the pope's niece, when she married the son of King Francois I in 1533, and it was especially promoted by Caterina's personal perfumer, Renato Bianco, after he set up shop in Paris.

One of history's most famous physicians was Ibn Sīnā, who worked in the Persian Empire in the early eleventh century. He wrote over 100 books, the first of which was on the beneficial effects of rose, which he prescribed for digestive problems. Rose had been distilled in Arabic countries from at least the ninth century, and rose water was produced long before that. It was traded into China, as recorded in Chao Ju-Kua's book of 1225 called *Records of Foreign Peoples and Their Trade (Chu Fan Chih)*.

One manufacture process was described in a Chinese book dated 1115: the roses were heated to produce a vapor that condensed and formed a water. From various sources, we can see that rose petals were being processed at this early date to produce rose oil, rose water, and attar of roses. Distinguishing the three products can sometimes be difficult to establish, along with the meaning intended for the terms *rose water* and *rose dew*, but we do know that adulteration was a problem even in these early times. In Chao's book of 1225 he suggests that to distinguish pure rose water from "counterfeited," the liquid should be put in glass bottles and shaken to see if bubbles move up and down — if they do, it's genuine.

Neroli essential oil, so valued today for its exquisite perfume and other valuable properties, is mentioned in a Chinese book dated 1233 by Chang Shih-nan. He says that the perfume exceeds that of all other citrus flowers or fruits, and, interestingly, it's thought he was referring to the same flowers from which neroli is distilled today — *Citrus aurantium*. Chang then goes on to explain how perfumed wood shavings were made: alternate layers of orange blossom petals and wood shavings were placed in a tin steamer, causing "drops of liquid" to collect and be siphoned off to a container; the old flowers were taken out, the distilled liquid was put back onto the wood shavings, and fresh petals were put into the still. The whole process was repeated three or four times. The wood shavings were then dried and put into porcelain vessels, producing a perfume Chang describes as "extraordinarily elegant."

Records of neroli being distilled in tin stills in China go back even further, to Han Yen-Chih's *Orange Record* of 1178, and Wang Shih-Pheng's *Mei-Chhi Shih Chu* of 1140, in which it is recorded that the distilled flowers make a perfume that also keeps insects away from clothes. Although this all sounds very early, records show that steam-distilled peppermint oil was certainly known in China in 982, and even as early as 659, according to a book called the *Hsin Hsiu Pen Tshoo*. The orange tree, still used in Chinese medicine, was carried from China to Europe by Arab traders in the tenth century, while the ninth-century trade between China and Indonesia is known to have included aromatic medicines.

The so-called father of Western medicine, Hippocrates, said in the fourth century BCE that "the way to health is to have an aromatic bath and scented massage every day," and certainly the Greeks, and later the Romans, took this advice to heart. Hippocrates also recognized that burning certain aromatic substances offered protection against contagious diseases. The ancient Greeks had a very high opinion of aromatics, attributing sweet smells to divine origin. In ancient myths, gods descended to earth on scented clouds, wearing robes drenched in aromatic essences. The Greeks believed that after death the virtuous went to Elysium, where the air was permanently filled with a sweet-smelling aroma that rose from perfumed rivers.

The holy anointing oil that God directed Moses to make from "flowing" myrrh, sweet cinnamon, calamus, cassia, and olive oil would have been a powerful antiviral and antibiotic substance, the use of which gave protection and treatment to all those to whom it was administered. Cinnamon is a powerful antiviral and antibacterial agent; myrrh is an effective antiseptic and is cicatrisive — that is, it stimulates cellular growth — and its healing effects on open wounds, ulcers, and boils was legendary even before biblical times.

The ancient Egyptians used aromatics for incense, embalming, and perfume. These included frankincense, myrrh, mastic, cinnamon, juniper berry, mint, and pine resin. Most aromas were of the base note type, thick and cloying, although lotus flower had a much lighter fragrance. The aromatic material was incorporated into different mediums, depending on the purpose. Linseed oil was used in embalming, for example, while honey or honeycomb wax was included into incense, and perfumes were carried in animal fats. The Ebers Papyrus of 1500 BCE described many recipes for health using aromatics and also outlined the earliest known recipe for making a body deodorant. The Egyptians described remedies for mental health issues including manias, depression, and nervousness. Aromatic unguents were stored in fabulous, elaborately carved containers made from alabaster (calcite), often decorated with animals that, curiously, have their tongues poking out of their mouths.

Cuneiform clay tablets from Babylonia dating from around 1800 BCE detail an import order that included the aromatic wood of the cedar tree, myrrh, and cypress — all used as essential oils therapeutically today. Myrtle too was a favorite. The Assyrians also loved aromatics, going so far as to perfume the mortar of their buildings. The first known perfumer was a woman, Tapputi, an overseer at a palace in Mesopotamia in the second millennium BCE. Clay tablets tell us that she used oil, reeds, flowers, resin, and water to make perfumes by a process of distillation and filtration. Throughout the Middle East, perfume was valued and written about by Islamic scholars over hundreds of years, and the appreciation continues today when the walls of mosques and other holy places are washed with rose and oud.

One of the earliest pieces of written evidence that perfume was a commodity commonly available to the man or woman in the street comes from an Indian epic of 2000 BCE, the Ramayana, which includes an episode in which the hero-prince, Rama of Ayodhya, returns after a period of exile to a triumphant homecoming in his village. Everyone, we're told, pours into the street cheering, including the lamp makers, jewelers, potters, bath attendants, wine sellers, weavers, sword millers, perfumers, and incense sellers.

Some people might suppose that perfumes were used in early times to cover up bad smells caused by lack of hygiene, but apart from the fact that nature provided unpolluted rivers and streams long before the Industrial Revolution produced internal plumbing, there's evidence that early civilizations were as concerned with cleanliness as we are. Around 3000 BCE the people in the city of Mohenjo Daro, in modern-day Pakistan, were obsessed with cleanliness according to archaeologists, who found plumbing in every house, a covered municipal drainage system, and a communal bath measuring 39 by 23 feet. Some of the oldest temples in India were built entirely of sandalwood, ensuring an aromatic atmosphere at all times.

The oldest archaeological site of a perfume-making center is at Pyrgos-Mavroraki on the Mediterranean island of Cyprus. Dating back over 4,000 years, a wide range of materials have been discovered there, including stills for distilling plant materials and small perfume bottles made of translucent alabaster. From residues remaining at the site, archaeologists believe that lavender, bay, pine, coriander, rosemary, parsley, myrtle, anise, and cinnamon were processed at the site. All these plant materials are produced as essential oils today. And at that time, like today, fragrant plant material was used not only for cosmetic and pharmaceutical purposes but also in religious ceremony.

The only reason we're here now is because our ancestors survived in conditions far harsher than we will ever have to experience. They had no pharmaceutical drugs and could use only the natural plant materials they found in their environment. Clearly, any useful medicinal plant was remembered because it was so important. In this way, humanity built up knowledge of the medicine chest growing around them. And that chest is remarkably like our own, because even if times change, the healing power of certain plants does not.

Quality Control

The global market in essential oils is pretty much like every other business environment — it's monopolized by a few huge corporations, determined to drive down the prices they have to pay to the producers. They want essential oils to put in food, drink, cosmetics, fragrance, and medications, and they want certainty. Perfume companies need ingredients with aromatic constancy so they can create perfume formulas that always smell the same. Very often they'll incorporate synthetics

to achieve this consistency. The food and drink companies, on the other hand, have to use natural essential oils to comply with the U.S. 1996 Food Chemicals Codex IV. Pharmaceutical companies test essential oils against standards set by the U.S. Pharmacopoeia (USP), the British Pharmacopoeia (BP), the European Pharmacopoeia, or the pharmacopoeia of other nations, including China. Various organizations around the world certify the authenticity of particular essential oils, including the International Organization for Standardization (ISO Standards TC 54) and the Association Française de Normalisation (AFNOR).

Unless you buy an essential oil that specifically states that it complies with these standards, you can't be sure that what you're buying is exactly what it says on the label, and that's because there are many ways in which essential oils can be adulterated. Expensive essential oils may be extended by adding cheaper, but similar smelling, essential oils. Also, an essential oil could be diluted with something that makes no change to the aroma — isopropyl myristate, for example — or in the case of more viscous essential oils such as vetiver, it could be mixed with a little rapeseed oil.

Another issue is that one essential oil might be labeled as another, a practice made possible by the fact that the two essential oils have a similar aroma. Or two essential oils could be blended to create another: for example, black pepper and ylang ylang could be combined to create the aroma of carnation. Another ploy is to bulk out one essential oil by adding to it a particular component extracted from a different essential oil: for example, eucalyptol — pure and natural — could be taken from eucalyptus globulus and added to another essential oil that contains eucalyptol. Once we get to the very rare, precious, and expensive oils and absolutes — rose, jasmine, neroli, gardenia, and so on, some of which are not produced by steam distillation — many devices might be employed to bulk out the oils. These methods include using other essential oils, single or multiple natural components within essential oils, or synthetic chemicals.

If the essential oil is distilled in a country other than the one in which the plant material was grown, the exported material — such as dried herbs, flowers, or resins — may have been irradiated. This is done to eradicate any pests, insects, fungi, or other micro-organisms that might be in the plant material before it crosses the border. But irradiation could change the healing potential of the plant materials. And sometimes an oil advertised as organic is no such thing, just the nonorganic version of the same essential oil.

Now, having read all that, you might think that there are so many issues around buying essential oils that you might just as well give up the whole idea. But forewarned is forearmed. We all need to be aware of the ruses traders get up to so we can recognize those suppliers who genuinely aim to provide us with essential oils that can perform the tasks we expect of them — the tasks that essential oils, if left alone in their entirety, can perform.

Essential oils vary in price for a variety of reasons. For example, even the same oil, lavender, can cost much more if grown in Provence in France than if grown in Bulgaria or Croatia. Also, an absolute flower oil like champaca (*Michelia alba*) could be 35 times the cost of a lovely, perfectly good may chang (*Litsea cubeba*). So the first thing when buying essential oils is to be realistic — you're not going to find a cheap genuine champaca. The more accustomed you become to essential oils, the better feel you will get for those that suit your own personal purpose and preference. Each day there appear to be more essential oil traders stating that they're selling "pure, organic essential oils," and I'm beginning to wonder if there's another planet they're being grown on! The fact is, there simply aren't enough organic

essential oils currently being produced in the world to meet the demand.

And while a particular essential oil company may be good at sourcing some essential oils, that's not to say they're good at sourcing them all. If in doubt, ask advice from a professional aromatherapist who treats people every day, as they'll need to have good essential oils for a successful practice.

Storage is important. All plant-derived raw materials such as herbal extracts, essential oils, and hydrolats should be kept in dark-colored glass bottles or canisters that keep light out and stored in a cool, damp-free area. Keep the tops tightly closed when not in use to prevent oxidization. The therapeutic life of essential oils varies considerably. When oils have been in your cupboard for a couple of years, they're probably still good enough, in terms of their aroma and antiseptic properties, to be utilized in room methods, including as air fresheners, or in kitchen surface wipes, in perfumes, or in making nontherapeutic fragrant gifts. There's no need to waste any essential oil.

In a medical emergency, these elderly essential oils are certainly better than nothing, but if you have a chronic medical condition, seek out the best you can lay your hands on. Get to know the staff of each essential oil company you purchase from; just get a feel for who they are as people. Knowing the true heart of any company is the best route to finding good essential oils, and there are honest and dedicated people out there — you just have to find them. (Also see the section "The Importance of Quality" in chapter 19, regarding carrier oils used to dilute the essential oils; see page 514.)

Quantities to Use and Blending

Throughout this book you will see essential oil formulas that suggest using between, say, 3 and

5 drops per teaspoon (5 mL) of carrier oil. This variation takes into account people's differences in terms of their size, age, medical history, and well-being, and whether a condition is acute or chronic. For a chronic condition, start with the lower number of essential oil drops and adjust upward if necessary; if the condition is acute, start with the higher number of drops.

The expression *dilution percentage* represents the volume of essential oil in relation to the volume of carrier oil. In a clinical setting, essential oils can be used in dilutions upward of 5%, and can even be used undiluted, depending on the health condition being treated. A 5% dilution equates to approximately 5–6 drops per teaspoon (5 mL) of carrier oil, depending on the size of the drop. In a clinical setting the practitioner would understand the client's needs, including any health issues or conditions, and a personal oil would be specifically tailored for that client. In a spa setting, where medical conditions are not treated, a pre-prepared oil for relaxation, for example, might contain 1%–2% of essential oil, although if a personal blend is being made for a specific client that percentage might rise to between 2.5% and 5%.

The order in which ingredients are listed in formulas for blends is not arbitrary. Some might expect that the essential oil with the greatest volume is listed first, running down the formula with the smallest amount at the end. This is not the case. Rather, the essential oils are listed *in the order they should be blended*. Start with the first oil named and continue down the list, adding the number of drops for each as suggested. The sequence has to do both with the intended purpose of the blend and with how particular essential oils interact with each other in that particular formula, which could be to do with their relative weight, physical consistency, chemical constituency, or vibrational frequency.

Because the formulations in this book are professional-style blends, a minute amount of an essential oil might be required to make the whole blend effective. So to introduce this concept in a home setting, sometimes more of the essential oil blend is made than is actually needed at the time. If so, store the blend for future use, or make up a larger diluted amount, following the dilution suggestion accompanying that particular blend.

Some essential oils have a thin consistency, being lighter, while others are more viscous, being thicker and heavier. These differences in consistency among essential oils are known as their *weight* or *specific gravity*. The consistency of an essential oil will determine the rate at which it comes out of the dropper: oil with a thin consistency, such as lavender or rosemary, will come out quickly; viscous oils, such as vetiver or myrrh, will be slow, so be patient with them.

Getting the measurements as accurate as possible is important, so a good set of measuring tools is invaluable to the regular essential oil user. But the one area that can't be controlled is the size of the hole in dropper inserts (sometimes called *orifice reducers*) because they can vary between suppliers. Some drops may seem smaller or larger than average, depending on the size of the hole in the dropper insert. Just be aware of this variability.

Blending is an art — there's no doubt about that. In a carefully considered and calculated essential oil blend, a synergistic effect takes place, making the end result more than the sum of the parts. Blending essential oils for therapeutic applications is an entirely different process than blending for perfumery or fragrance purposes, which is characterized by base, middle, and top notes. For healing purposes, each essential oil is assessed on the therapeutic properties it contains that are applicable to the condition or symptoms the oil is being blended for. The major part of the blend should address the most problematic symptom, and any other essential oils that are added could be those that help — for example, with accompanying psychological issues, or to fight any infection by being antibacterial or antiviral. In other words, there are levels to healing, and the art of blending involves incorporating essential oils that, working synergistically together, address these different levels at the same time.

Volume, in essential oil terms, is unlike many other things, in that it may take just a single drop in a blend to bring it all together and increase the therapeutic potential of the whole blend. Without that one drop a lot could still be accomplished, but with that little drop, an entirely different blend is created. One drop. And that's another thing with essential oils: less is sometimes more. There's no need to apply the "more is best" principle. That's not the case with essential oils. They're way more subtle than that!

Each essential oil has dozens if not hundreds of components. By blending two or more oils, an entirely new compound is being formed. This accounts for the extraordinary potential of aromatherapy. Perhaps one way to understand this is to think of surgery: when surgery is performed, it's a team effort. The surgeon is supported by an anesthetist and a collection of other people who make the operation a success. Or to look at it another way, a band might consist of four members; each member is an artist in their own right, but when they come together, a musical synergy occurs. Essential oils are like this; each one is valuable, but when blended together, sometimes more can be accomplished.

When all the essential oils have been put together in a small bottle, put the top on the bottle and roll it vigorously between the palms of your hands — rather as if creating a vortex in the bottle, allowing all the molecules to be thoroughly blended. When adding the essential oil blend to a carrier oil, do the same thing again — roll the bottle between your hands — but this time follow by shaking the bottle well. If you watch essential oils as they first drop into carrier oil, you can see them

quite distinctly as having a different consistency and, often, a different color. By adding a blend or a single essential oil into the carrier oil (rather than adding the carrier oil to the essential oil), it is easy to judge and control the aromatic strength of your blend and ensure the odor perception is what you wanted to achieve.

How essential oils are handled is important. The healing potential of essential oils is extremely sensitive to electromagnetic frequency and to the positive or negative emotional energy of the person handling or blending them. A blend made in anger may not perform as well as expected. At the very least, try not to let your own personal thoughts or emotions intrude while blending for others. Just focus your mind on the intention or objective in hand — the person for whom the blend is being made, their needs, and the hoped-for outcome.

Conversion Charts

When purchasing essential oils, it's useful to know that, depending upon the essential oils' consistency and the size of the dropper insert, the following are commonly used approximations:

20 drops = $\frac{1}{5}$ teaspoon essential oil = 1 milliliter (mL)

40 drops = $\frac{2}{5}$ teaspoon essential oil = 2 mL

60 drops = $\frac{3}{5}$ teaspoon essential oil = 3 mL

GENERAL DILUTION GUIDE

Because of the variation in dropper insert hole sizes, the following is only a general guide:

TABLE 1. DILUTION GUIDE

MINIMUM–MAXIMUM DROPS OF ESSENTIAL OIL	INTO MILLILITERS OF CARRIER OIL	OR SPOON MEASUREMENTS OF CARRIER OIL
0–1 drop	1	⅕ teaspoon
2–5 drops	5	1 teaspoon
4–10 drops	10	2 teaspoons
6–15 drops	15	1 tablespoon
8–20 drops	20	4 teaspoons
10–25 drops	25	5 teaspoons
12–30 drops	30	2 tablespoons

CONVERSIONS: OUNCES AND MILLILITERS

Very often in this book I suggest blends diluted in 1 fluid ounce (fl. oz.), or 30 mL, of carrier oil. Because of the difficulties of conversion, this is slightly inaccurate; in 1 fl. oz. there are in fact 29.5735296875 mL. If you can, try to measure in milliliters because measuring small quantities is easier in Metric than it is in Imperial. For reference, here are the conversion rates.

To convert volumes in milliliters into fluid ounces:

1 mL = 0.03381 fl. oz.
5 mL = 0.16907 fl. oz.
10 mL = 0.33814 fl. oz.
20 mL = 0.67628 fl. oz.
30 mL = 1.01442 fl. oz.
100 mL = 3.38140 fl. oz.

To convert volumes in fluid ounces into milliliters:

¼ fl. oz. = 7.39338 mL
½ fl. oz. = 14.78676 mL
¾ fl. oz. = 22.18014 mL
1 fl. oz. = 29.57352 mL

I will use approximate equivalences, such as 3½ fl. oz. for 100 mL.

Methods of Use

What follows is an A–Z list of general guidelines for using essential oils with a variety of methods. Some methods for more specific purposes are not listed here but are described throughout the book.

TABLE 2. ESSENTIAL OIL METHODS OF USE: AN A–Z GUIDE

Use the recommended amount of essential oil and methods described throughout this book for more specific purposes, or follow these general guidelines.

METHOD OF USE	AMOUNT TO USE	NOTES
BATHS, GENERAL	Diluted: 3–8 drops Undiluted: 1–4 drops	Run the bath as usual. Keep the door closed to keep the aroma in the room. Essential oils can be used neat — in their concentrated form — or diluted in carrier oil, milk, milk powder, vegetable glycerin, seaweed powder, herbal powders, baking soda, salt, or Epsom salts. To avoid skin sensitivity, dilute the essential oil first in a little carrier oil. Essential oil can also be dropped directly onto the water in the bathtub and dispersed by agitating the water with the hand before getting into the bath.
BATHS, SITZ	2 or 3 drops per sitz bath	A sitz bath is a bath in which you immerse the lower part of your torso in water, from the waist to upper thigh, to treat specific conditions. Run a bath to hip level or use a bowl that is large enough to lower your behind into. Add the essential oil to the water, and then disperse it well with your hand to avoid large globules that may come in contact with delicate mucous membranes.
BATHS, FOOT	5–8 drops in a bowl of water, diluted or undiluted	Fill a large bowl with warm water and add the essential oil, dispersing it well with your hand. For a really relaxing foot bath, place some round, smooth pebbles in the bottom of the bowl and rub the feet gently back and forth over them. Rock or sea salt or Epsom salts can also be added. Soak the feet for a maximum of 20 minutes, adding warm water as needed. If globules of diluted essential oil are floating on the surface of the water, you can gather them in your hands and massage the oil into the feet.

METHOD OF USE	AMOUNT TO USE	NOTES
BATHS, HAND	2–4 drops in a bowl of water	Fill a small bowl with warm water and add the essential oil, diluted in a nourishing carrier oil, and disperse it well with your hand. Leave the hands in the water for a maximum of 10 minutes. If globules of diluted essential oil are floating on the surface of the water, you can massage them into your hands.
BIDETS	1 drop diluted in ½ teaspoon carrier oil	Use warm water. Then add the diluted essential oil and disperse it as well as possible to avoid irritation of mucous membranes.
CLOTHING	1 or 2 drops	Many essential oils can mark clothing, depending upon the material, so use this method only when necessary and on clothes you're prepared to see stained. This method is useful for repelling insects, especially midges and mosquitoes. Put the essential oil neat (undiluted) on socks, on the bottom of shorts or trouser legs, or on the collar, sleeves, or cuffs of shirts. To keep insects away from your head, apply the oil to a hat, hair band, or head scarf.
COMPRESSES	3–10 drops	Compresses can be applied hot or cold. Broadly speaking, hot compresses are used on muscular aches and pains, while cold is used for any inflamed or swollen areas, including sprains and strains. Hot increases circulation to the area, while cold can decrease circulation. Always use 100% natural material, unbleached if possible. There are two methods of applying compresses: 1. Place the essential oil in half a cup of water, and then dampen the material in the cup, collecting the essential oil onto the material. Squeeze out the excess water, and then place over the problematic area. 2. Wet the compress, apply the essential oil directly onto the wet material, rub the material together to disperse the essential oil, and place over the problematic area.

METHOD OF USE	AMOUNT TO USE	NOTES
COTTON PADS OR BALLS	1 or 2 drops	Put undiluted essential oil on the cotton pad or ball, leave to dry, and place in clothes drawers or closets. Infused cotton pads or balls can be placed around the home to deter insects.
COTTON SWABS	1 or 2 drops	Put the undiluted essential oil onto the cotton swab and apply directly to the affected area.
DIFFUSERS	As desired	A wide range of diffusers are available. Some rely on a heat source — a candle or electricity — to heat the essential oil molecules and disperse them into the atmosphere. Other types work in entirely different ways — using a fan, for example, to disperse the molecules. Diffusers are designed for both room and vehicle use. Pottery diffusers should be nonporous to allow cleaning. With diffusers using water, ensure that the water level is maintained so the essential oils don't burn. Nebulizers or oil vaporizers, which issue a fine spray of essential oil into the atmosphere, were designed for clinical use and are often difficult to clean between uses of different blends of essential oil.
DILUTION, HIGH	5 drops of essential oil to 5 drops of carrier oil	This method is used in cases of acute infection, when a higher concentration of essential oil is required but where neat essential oil would not be appropriate. Simply apply to the affected area. Recommendations of essential oils for particular conditions are found throughout the book.
DRESSINGS	1–6 drops applied directly onto a dressing	This method is used to prevent the spread of infection and promote wound healing. Add the essential oil directly onto the dressing that will cover the affected area — such as bandages, lint, cotton, or the fabric part of adhesive bandages. If the area is already dressed, apply the essential oil on the exposed skin around the dressing.

METHOD OF USE	AMOUNT TO USE	NOTES
FACE MASKS	1 or 2 drops per 2 table-spoons (30 mL) of face mask, or use as directed in other sections of the book	Essential oils can be added to any natural face mask. Base your choice of essential oil upon your skin type and the action on the skin you want it to achieve — whether as a treatment for acne, as a general stimulant, as a cleanser, as a purifier, re-juvenator, etc.
FACE OILS	8–15 drops in 1 fl. oz. (30 mL) of carrier oil, or use as directed in other sections of the book	Use the same method as for making a massage oil (see page 19). However, use a more skin-nourishing carrier oil, with additional restorative nut or seed oils, depending on your skin type. Use only a small amount for each application.
FACE TONICS	8–15 drops in 3½ fl. oz. (100 mL) of water or hydrolat, or use as directed in other sections of the book	Use spring or distilled water or hydrolat. Combine the oil and water before filtering through an unbleached paper coffee filter. Hydrolats make excellent face tonics and can be used as purchased, or diluted with 20% water.
FRICTION	20–30 drops to 1 fl. oz. (30 mL) of alcohol, or use as directed in other sections of the book	*Friction* is a term that is often used to describe the action of quickly rubbing a part of the body, a treatment often utilized by sports therapists. For friction, essential oil can be added to ethyl alcohol (also known as *rubbing alcohol*) — which has tradi-tionally been used in sports remedial care. Shake the mixture well before use. An alternative to the alcohol would be a light, easily absorbed carrier oil. This method should not be used on the face or delicate mucous membrane areas.
GARDENING	1 or 2 drops in a gallon (4 liters) of water	Certain essential oils can be very effective as plant misters for microbial infection or to deter insects. Add the essential oil to the water, shake vigor-ously, and leave to blend for 24 hours, before fil-tering through a paper coffee filter. Essential oils should never be combined with chemical garden-ing products, but they can be used with other nat-ural organic methods. See chapter 18, "Gardens for the Future."

METHOD OF USE	AMOUNT TO USE	NOTES
HOT TUBS	Up to 8 drops	Add the essential oil to the water and disperse it well with your hand. Essential oils are not water soluble and may leave a residue in or around pipes.
HUMIDIFIERS	Up to 8 drops per pint (475 mL) of water	Add the essential oil to the water in the humidifier. For humidifiers that hang over radiators, just add the essential oil to the water. More complex machines, however, may be damaged by sticky residue, so assess each humidifier to make sure it can be used in conjunction with essential oils.
INHALATION (as a vapor from a bowl)	3–5 drops per bowl of water, or use as directed in other sections of the book	Put steaming hot water in a bowl and add the essential oil. Cover the head with a towel, which should be large enough to reach over the sides of the bowl. Keep the face 12 inches (30 cm) away from the water and shut both eyes. Inhale the steam through the nose, with each inhalation lasting around 2–3 seconds. Repeat as needed but for no more than 5–10 minutes per session.
INHALATION (from a tissue or handkerchief)	1 or 2 drops	Simply put the essential oil onto a tissue or handkerchief and inhale through the nose when required.
JACUZZIS	Up to 8 drops	Add the essential oil to the Jacuzzi water, then disperse it with the hand. Essential oils are not water soluble and may leave a residue in or on the pipes.
LOTIONS AND CREAMS (for body)	5–20 drops to each 1 fl. oz. (30 mL) of natural, unfragranced lotion or cream, or use as directed in other sections of the book	Use an unscented lotion or cream, made of organic natural ingredients. Add the required number of essential oil drops and mix in well. Use as you would a normal body cream.

METHOD OF USE	AMOUNT TO USE	NOTES
MASSAGE OIL (for body)	10–30 drops to each 1 fl. oz. (30 mL) of carrier oil, or use as directed in other sections of the book	Use a dark-colored glass bottle. Measure the carrier oil. If using a single essential oil or a pre-prepared blend, add it to the carrier oil. If making your own blend of essential oils, first combine them, then add the required number of drops to the carrier oil. Use no more than the amount required to cover the area being massaged.
NEAT APPLICATION (undiluted)	1 or 2 drops, or use as directed in other sections of the book	In some conditions certain essential oils can be used undiluted on the skin due to the nature of that condition. But some essential oils are not suitable for this method due to potential skin irritation. Use this method only with the essential oils suggested for this purpose throughout the book.
PERFUMES	Between 15% and 30% of the total perfume	Absolutes and essential oils are the original perfume materials. To create a natural perfume they can be blended together and incorporated into a carrier oil, liquid wax base, or alcohol. (See the section "Making Your Own Perfumes and Eau de Cologne" in chapter 15.)
PILLOWS	1–3 drops	Essential oils can be applied on pillows to assist breathing in cases of respiratory infection or sleeping problems. Simply place 1–3 drops of essential oil on the corner or underside of a pillow, away from the eyes. Alternatively, put the essential oil on a cotton ball or tissue and tuck it under the corner of the pillow or inside the pillowcase — behind the pillow. Ensure that the essential oil is located in an area away from the face, especially the eyes.
POTPOURRIS	As desired	Add the essential oils to the potpourri in the same way as you would add a commercial synthetic potpourri-refresher product. Single essential oils or blends can be used. Essential oils may cause color changes to potpourri material that has been colored.

METHOD OF USE	AMOUNT TO USE	NOTES
ROOM SPRAYS	As room purifier: 10–20 drops per pint (475 mL) of water As general fragrance: 8–10 drops per pint (475 mL) of water	The quick and easy method is to use a new plant mister. Add the essential oil to about a pint of warm water in the mister, avoiding the thicker viscous types of essential oil as these may accumulate around the nozzle. Shake vigorously each time it's used, as essential oils are not water soluble. Avoid spraying over fine furniture, wood, fabrics, and anything that could be damaged by water.
SAUNAS	2–5 drops per 2 pints (950 mL) of water	Only use this method if the sauna uses water to induce heat. Add the essential oil to the water, mixing as best as you can, and filter the mixture through a paper coffee filter before placing on the hot coals or rocks. Use essential oils of juniper, cypress, pine, or eucalyptus. Essential oils are flammable and should never be placed on a heat source unless diluted in water and filtered.
SCALP TREATMENTS	5–10 drops in ½ fl. oz. (15 mL) of carrier, or use as directed in other sections of the book	A variety of base carriers can be used for scalp treatments. These can include natural (botanical), ready-made scalp treatments, to which the essential oil can be added. Or the essential oil can be added to aloe vera gel, water, or jojoba oil, and massaged into the scalp. Use 2–3 drops of your prepared mix for each application. Alternatively, simply add the essential oil to a bowl of final rinse water after washing the hair.
SHAMPOOS	5–10 drops in 3½ fl. oz. (100 mL), or use as directed in other sections of the book	Essential oils can be added to any unscented shampoo that is composed of organic natural ingredients. Ensure the essential oils are well distributed. Choose essential oils that can be used on sensitive skin.

METHOD OF USE	AMOUNT TO USE	NOTES
SHOWERS	1–5 drops	Wash as usual. Then drop the essential oil onto a washcloth or sponge and rub it briskly over the body as you continue to stand under the running water. Breathe in the aromatic steam through your nose. Avoid the face and delicate membrane areas.
SILK (FAUX) FLOWERS	As desired	Open the flower completely and place the essential oil right at the center. Close the flower again if desired. Remember that essential oils may cause discoloration, so try this on one flower before proceeding with the others. Essential oils can also be placed on paper that is put in the bottom of the vase.

SPRAYS AND MISTS FOR FACE AND BODY	For body: 10–20 drops to each pint (475 mL) of water
	
	For face: 2–5 drops to each half pint (240 mL) of water
	
	Or use as directed in other sections of the book.
		Add the essential oils to warm water or a hydrolat, shake thoroughly, pour through an unbleached paper coffee filter, and place in a spray container. Cool before using.
		    Shake before each use.
		    This method is useful for body or face. Keep the eyes closed when spraying the face.

WASHES	15–32 drops in ½ pint (240 mL) of warm water. Or use as directed in other sections of the book.	A *wash* is a prepared mixture for washing infected areas, such as wounds, grazes, and cuts. Mix the essential oils and water together in a bottle and shake well. Keep stored in the fridge for no longer than 14 days, and shake before each use.
WATER BOWL (room diffuser)	2–10 drops per pint (475 mL)	Boil a pint (475 mL) of water and put the steaming water in a heatproof bowl, then add the essential oil. Place on the floor or on a heatproof surface, ensuring that it's not within reach of children or pets. Close doors and windows to keep the aroma molecules inside.

TABLE 3. SPECIAL SITUATIONS TO CONSIDER

SPECIAL SITUATION	GENERAL DOSAGE RULES	NOTES
CHRONIC PAIN	For a body oil: 30 drops to 1 fl. oz. (30 mL) of oil Other methods: Up to maximum dosage	Certain essential oils have analgesic properties. See table 22, "Quick Reference Chart," in chapter 20 (page 534).
WITH MEDICATION	For all methods, use up to half the recommended dosages. If using essential oils as therapeutic treatments, inform your physician or healthcare provider.	If using homeopathy, inform the homeopath that you intend to use essential oils because it's thought that the strong aromas of some essential oils may negate the effect of homeopathy.
PRE- AND POSTOPERATIVE USE	In the preoperative period: Dosages should be half the suggested amounts, and the physician should be informed if using essential oils for therapeutic purposes. In the postoperative period: Essential oils can be used at maximum dosage if necessary to help lessen the risk of infection. If you are on medication, inform your physician that you intend to use essential oils.	Certain essential oils can considerably lessen the risk of infection. They can be used postoperatively on the body and dropped directly onto the bedclothes. If diffused, stronger essential oils such as oregano, cinnamon leaf, and thyme can be used for infection control.
WITH RADIATION THERAPY	While undergoing radiation therapy, avoid essential oil use during the treatment itself. Essential oil preparations can be used in between sessions to help alleviate soreness and radiation burns. Dosages should be half the maximum general dosage.	Only organic essential oils should be used at this time until the treatments are completed.

SPECIAL SITUATION	GENERAL DOSAGE RULES	NOTES
ADDICTION: PRESCRIPTION DRUG ADDICTION	During addiction to prescription drugs, your physician should be informed that you intend to use essential oils. Use no more than half the recommended amount, unless otherwise directed in this book.	While reducing the dosage of prescribed medication, essential oils that have a calming effect upon the nervous system could be used.
ADDICTION: SUBSTANCE ADDICTION	Follow the general guidelines for dosages and use essential oils to help ease the specific withdrawal symptoms being experienced.	While reducing the use of any substance, essential oils that have an anti-anxiety or stress-relieving effect on the nervous system could be used.
ADDICTION: ALCOHOLISM	When using alcohol to excess, all essential oil dosages should be half the general suggested amounts.	Essential oils that have an effect on the digestive and nervous systems may be helpful.
TERMINAL ILLNESS	During the various stages of terminal illness, dosages should be adjusted according to the medications being given. Use aromas that the person enjoys and that are relevant to the symptoms they are experiencing.	Room fragrances are very comforting at this time — both for the person concerned and for their carers. See the "Palliative Care" section in chapter 12, page 332.

Methods of Use to Be Avoided by the Home Practitioner

Professional aromatherapists and healthcare providers use several methods that may not be appropriate for use by the home practitioner. Professional medical practitioners might suggest the use of essential oils orally, for example, but always in extremely low and precise dosages, because ingesting essential oils involves the rigors of the digestive system. Home practitioners should avoid the oral use of essential oils unless under the direction of a professional healthcare provider.

On the very rare occasions when this method is suggested, the directions must be followed exactly. For example, a single drop of an essential oil — usually one that's found in food products, such as peppermint — might be recommended, given on a sugar lump or in a spoonful of honey and then diluted again in some form of liquid to avoid irritation of the membranous lining of the esophagus.

It's increasingly being recognized that taking anything orally may have its disadvantages, and skin patches and inhalation methods have been developed to avoid the oral route. For example, nasal sprays are now employed to deliver inoculation against influenza in children, and insulin in a crystallized form can be inhaled by diabetics.

Environmental Issues

Many health conditions are caused by environmental issues, either at work or at home or because of a problem in the neighborhood. The following examples are taken from my case files to illustrate that there are times when a person's ill health is caused not by a physical or mental disorder but by an environmental imbalance.

A woman brought her teenage daughter to the clinic because she thought the girl might have a hormonal problem, causing her to be constantly on edge. Once in the consulting room, away from her mother, the girl identified the problem herself — she had no peace at home. Her mother always had the TV on, even when no one was watching it, while her brother played his favorite music loudly in his room. To cut these sounds out, the girl played music she liked in her room. She was exhausted and just wanted to be somewhere else — anywhere that was peaceful. I called her mother in and explained the situation. The music problem was easily solved with earphones — the brother wore them from that point on — and the girl could then turn her own music off. Her mother agreed to turn off the TV when no one was watching it. This story tells us two things. Before launching into a course of medication, ask yourself, "Am I feeling like this because I have no peace or control over my home environment?" In today's noise-polluted world, I wonder how many people simply need some peace and quiet.

A man visited the clinic because his legs, from the knees down, had stopped working. He had to roll out of bed, crawl into another room, and wait a few hours for the power of movement to come back. His doctors, completely bewildered, suggested he had some kind of mental disorder bordering on hysteria. It was all very mysterious. During the consultation we discussed his home situation, and he said something interesting: his neighbors had relocated their boiler and it was now on the wall adjacent to where he slept. I asked if he could hear the boiler, as it could be emitting low-frequency noise. He said that yes, he could hear it. But more than that, he could feel it inside his spine. He could actually feel the vibrations made by the boiler inside his spinal cord. And, yes, his mobility troubles had progressed from the time the boiler was relocated. He went home and moved his bed into another room. Two weeks later he called to say that he felt much better and his mobility problems had gone.

An artist named Richard Box, working with the chemistry department of Bristol University in the UK, placed 1,300 fluorescent lighting tubes in an upright position in the ground, beneath and to the sides of high-voltage cables between electricity pylons. The tubes all lit up like a Christmas tree, without any electricity supply other than what was in the air. The lights were powered by the electromagnetic field created by the 400,000-volt cables suspended above.

The research chemist Professor Dennis Henshaw suggests that electromagnetism splits molecules in the air to form charged particles, called *corona ions*, which attach to tiny pollutants in the air and get carried on the wind, perhaps several hundred meters, where they can be inhaled. Because the pollutant is now electrically charged, it more easily attaches to the lung and gets carried into the bloodstream. If you have any serious health problem and live close to high-voltage cables, I suggest you research this subject.

The National Aeronautics and Space Administration (NASA) has looked at space stations, the home environment of their astronauts, and considered what could be done to improve the air quality inside them. Their research found a solution that can be applied to all home environments and involves the fact that all plants absorb carbon dioxide and release oxygen. But some, additionally, can help clear the air of traces of chemicals routinely used in plastics and furniture. Some plants are more effective than others at clearing benzene, formaldehyde, trichloroethylene, xylene, toluene, and ammonia from the atmosphere, although the plants most effective in reducing formaldehyde or trichloroethylene are unfortunately toxic if ingested by either children or pets: golden pothos / devil's ivy (*Scindapsus aureus / Epipremnum aureum*), peace lily (*Spathiphyllum wallisii*), red-edged dracaena (*Dracaena marginata*), snake plant / mother-in-law's tongue (*Sansevieria trifasciata*), gerbera / barberton daisy (*Gerbera jamesonii*), and pot mum / florist's chrysanthemum (*Chrysanthemum morifolium*). All these plants are also helpful in cleaning traces of benzene, which is found in plastics and synthetic fibers, among other things. Other helpful plants include bamboo palm / reed palm (*Chamaedorea sefritzii*), which helps clear formaldehyde, xylene, and toluene, found in some home-maintenance products, and the very effective air-filtering plant English ivy (*Hedera helix*).

2

The Basic Care Kit

Lavender (*Lavandula angustifolia*) • Geranium (*Pelargonium graveolens*)

Thyme linalol (*Thymus vulgaris ct. linalool*) • Chamomile roman (*Anthemis nobilis*)

Rosemary (*Rosmarinus officinalis*) • Peppermint (*Mentha piperita*) • Cardamom (*Elettaria cardamomum*)

Lemon (*Citrus limon*) • Eucalyptus radiata (*Eucalyptus radiata*) • Tea tree (*Melaleuca alternifolia*)

Essential oils are versatile — each one can perform a variety of functions. There are 10 essential oils in the Basic Care Kit, which between them will manage a huge number of problems. The short profile of each of these oils that follows may help you decide which to include in your kit, and which to add as time goes on. The choice will very much depend on your own requirements. Have a look also at "The Basic Care Kit Applications" section in this chapter to see which conditions affect you or your family. In this chapter you're given the tools to quickly and efficiently address on a practical level many of the common health issues and situations that can occur.

The suggestions outlined in this chapter are fairly concise, yet effective. Some of the conditions listed here are discussed in more detail in other chapters. So please do refer to the index.

This Basic Care Kit chapter is like a first aid section, but there are also chapters specifically for men, women, children, seniors, travel, and sports, which may have information and advice more specific to your needs.

The 10 essential oils in this Basic Care Kit also feature strongly throughout this book and have useful applications for a wide diversity of purposes — from health care to well-being to the enhancement of mind, mood, and emotion, from skin care to gardening, and from home care to celebrations. So on all counts these oils make a hugely helpful contribution to any household.

In addition to these 10 oils, other useful additions to your care kit would be aloe vera gel, witch hazel water, rose water, and lavender and chamomile hydrolat. Aloe vera comes from the leaf of the aloe vera succulent plant (*Aloe barbadensis*) and is a fine healing agent for cuts, inflammation, and.

burns, as well as being a good carrying agent for the essential oils. It can be bought in gel or liquid form, or try growing your own plant so you can cut a leaf and squeeze out the gel whenever you need it. Witch hazel, extracted from the shrub *Hamamelis virginiana*, is known for its astringent and anti-inflammatory properties. Rose hydrolat is a by-product of the distillation of the various varieties of rose essential oil and is used for its mild antiseptic and soothing properties. You will also need a neutral carrier oil or two to dilute the essential oils, such as sweet almond. Clove bud essential oil is another very useful essential oil to add to your Basic Care Kit for its analgesic and other properties.

The 10 essential oils I have chosen for the Basic Care Kit are versatile, easy to use, and readily available. Compared to many other essential oils, they are reasonably priced, so it should be possible for you to purchase oils of good quality. Let us now have a brief look at the 10 essential oils that comprise the Basic Care Kit.

The Basic Care Kit Oils

LAVENDER (*Lavandula angustifolia*)

Lavender is an indispensable essential oil — it's not only useful to have at home but many people won't leave home without it. In a sense, it's the mother of all essential oils: incredibly versatile, yet powerful. The aroma doesn't suit all tastes, but when someone suffers a minor burn or scald, a cut or graze, an insect bite or a headache, a tooth abscess or sleeplessness, it's lavender they call for.

Not only is lavender a spectacular healer that also prevents scarring, it's a mood tonic that brings calm, relaxation, and stress relief. Lavender oil is a natural antiseptic, antibiotic, and slightly antifungal agent that's also a sedative and antidepressant. Although not known specifically as a circulatory stimulant, lavender oil certainly seems

to allay the effects of clinical shock. Lavender is one of the few essential oils that could be applied undiluted to the skin in certain acute conditions.

GERANIUM (*Pelargonium graveolens*)

Geranium is deceptively charming. If the quality is good, the aroma of geranium essential oil is clean and floral and enjoyed by most everyone, including children and teenagers. The sweet aroma of geranium masks the fact that this is an antiseptic and antibacterial oil, making it a good choice to include in anti-infective blends, while also being an analgesic. Geranium is indispensable in the treatment of circulatory and blood disorders; it will help chilblains to disappear and help alleviate the effects of frostbite. Geranium brings hormonal balance and is a vital component in addressing female reproductive conditions, including menstrual and menopausal problems and infertility.

Geranium oil is excellent in body care and brings a radiant glow when used in skin care. Its astringent properties contribute to its general usefulness. It also works profoundly on the emotions, serving as a nerve tonic and as a sedative. It's fantastic in blends because just one drop used as a back note will mask a healing aroma that might otherwise be too medicinal. Aromatically, geranium is an equalizer, making everything smell a bit better, and as such it is a great all-rounder in room fragrances.

THYME LINALOL (*Thymus vulgaris ct. linalool*)

There are several types of *Thymus vulgaris* essential oil available, but the chemotype (ct.) *linalool* is preferred because it's versatile, has a long history of use in clinical aromatherapy, and is more compatible with skin applications because it's considered nonirritating.

Thyme linalol is like a valued warrior, having powerful antiseptic, antiviral, antibacterial, and antifungal properties. Few oils are as useful as thyme linalol when there's an internal infection of some sort, or when "flu" or other contagious conditions are a threat. Even one or two drops of thyme linalol used in a room diffuser mix of, for example, geranium, lemon, and cardamom will add purifying anti-infectious protection.

The antimicrobial aspects of thyme linalol are enhanced by other properties attributed to this oil, such as its immune stimulant and diuretic properties. Thyme linalol is excellent in the treatment of soft tissue and joint conditions, including rheumatism. It's also used in cases of neuralgia and fatigue and in hair- and skin-care regimes, including those for acne. In addition, thyme linalol is a good brain stimulant, boosting the capacity for analytical thought.

CHAMOMILE ROMAN (Anthemis nobilis)

There are several essential oil–producing plants called *chamomile*, but the two most·commonly used in aromatherapy and known as the true chamomiles are chamomile roman, which is included here, and chamomile german (*Matricaria recutita*), which is distinguished by its beautiful deep-blue color, due to a high azulene content.

Chamomile roman is an excellent anti-inflammatory oil, which makes it valuable in a wide range of conditions. It is also antiseptic, antibacterial, and when combined with other oils, analgesic, and it is used in recovery from burns, including sunburn, as well as for asthma, sprains, strains, diarrhea, nausea, and fever. It is also used for a variety of skin care issues, including in rejuvenation treatments. Chamomile roman is calming and sedative — particularly effective in the treatment of nervous conditions, depressive states, and insomnia. It has a balancing effect in blends.

Chamomile is a strong but humble oil that works on the mind, body, and spirit, the psychological as well as the physical. As it's essentially a soothing oil, chamomile roman is good to use with children, and also with the inner child in adults. This is an oil with many subtle levels.

ROSEMARY (Rosmarinus officinalis)

Rosemary is a good analgesic essential oil, useful in the treatment of all muscular problems, as well as joint conditions such as arthritis and rheumatism. It's used both for respiratory tract issues and, in small amounts, for conditions of the liver and kidneys. Rosemary is a very stimulating essential oil, having an effect on both the physical body and the analytical mind. All these attributes make rosemary energizing when facing an exhausting, mentally challenging day, or following a physically stressful one.

Rosemary is an aid to memory — whether required for enhancing the ability of the brain to function well or exploring long-term emotional memory. It's also used in the treatment of depression, migraine, headaches, anxiety, and stress. Rosemary is helpful in a variety of beauty treatments, including those for cellulite, acne, and hair care. For the sportsperson, cook, or gardener, rosemary is invaluable.

PEPPERMINT (Mentha piperita)

Peppermint is hugely helpful in all problems of the digestive tract, including indigestion, flatulence, irritable bowel syndrome, and stomach-derived halitosis. It's also useful in certain conditions of the respiratory and circulatory systems and as an all-round tonic. Peppermint is an analgesic, antiseptic, cooling, anti-inflammatory oil with some antifungal properties. It has a place in the treatment of catarrh, headaches, migraines, skin irritations, rheumatism, toothache, and fatigue. In small amounts, it can be incorporated into complex perfumes or room blends, providing a subtle back note. It has a unique place in cookery, while also being able to keep ants, fleas, and mice away. Peppermint is a multipurpose oil, and a useful addition to the Basic Care Kit.

CARDAMOM *(Elettaria cardamomum)*

Cardamom has layers of healing ability, starting with its calming effect on the digestive system, making it a good choice when dealing with flatulence, stomach or abdominal cramps, irritable bowel syndrome, or Crohn's disease. Cardamom is antibacterial and antifungal, as well as analgesic and anti-inflammatory. It helps ease muscular cramps and spasm and, as an adaptogen, has a calming yet stimulating effect. Cardamom can also be used for most types of coughs and is useful for respiratory problems, as well as for certain types of food-related infection.

As if all this were not enough, cardamom can be used in cases of exhaustion — whether physical, mental, or emotional. It's stimulating in cases of tiredness or fatigue, yet has a calming effect on the mind and nerves during times of stress. Cardamom has a balancing and harmonizing effect on the body and mind. It's also a gentle ingredient in skin preparations and can be used in cooking.

LEMON *(Citrus limon)* Adaptogen

Lemon essential oil has a tonic action on the lymphatic system and a stimulating action on the digestive system. It can be used to alleviate bilious attacks, and when combined with other essential oils, it can contribute to the treatment of verrucas, insect bites, and tension headaches. Lemon can assist the metabolic function and is useful in skin care. Although slightly sedative and calming, lemon essential oil greatly aids focus and concentration, especially when part of a blend. The fresh, clean aroma of lemon is universally liked, making it highly useful as a synergistic addition to room fragrances and perfuming blends. This antiseptic and uplifting essential oil has a place in household care and, of course, is invaluable as a flavoring agent. Lemon essential oil can be used for so many things — as a water purifier, in skin care and body treatments — it is a true all-rounder.

EUCALYPTUS RADIATA *(Eucalyptus radiata)*

Eucalyptus radiata has been chosen for the Basic Care Kit because it's the species of the genus *Eucalyptus* that can safely be used on those with long-term chronic conditions, while also being a strong and effective essential oil.

Eucalyptus radiata is perhaps best known for its effectiveness against respiratory tract infections, but it has many other uses too. This is an antiseptic, antibiotic, antiviral, and analgesic essential oil, with anti-inflammatory, diuretic, and deodorizing properties. As part of complex blends, eucalyptus radiata can also be helpful in the treatment of cystitis and candida. It cools the body in summer, while also treating sunburn and deterring insects, and it is warming in the winter, while keeping infection at bay.

TEA TREE *(Melaleuca alternifolia)*

Tea tree essential oil is antiseptic, antibiotic, antiviral, and antifungal — making it useful for a wide range of conditions. It's used in the treatment of various infections, including candida, ringworm, and athlete's foot, as well as for toothache, sunburn, cuts and grazes, and various skin conditions, including acne. It could also be incorporated into mouthwashes and hair shampoos. Tea tree oil is widely used as an insect repellent and to treat insect stings. Although the aroma is not to everyone's taste, it can easily be disguised with other essential oils for use in room diffusion methods when someone in the household has a contagious airborne infection.

The Basic Care Kit Applications: An A–Z Guide

This section provides an alphabetical list of conditions in which the Basic Care Kit oils could be used. Where you see reference to "carrier oil," choose one from the "Carrier Oils" section in chapter 19 or use sweet almond oil, which can be used on all skins and is well tolerated by most people.

At the end of each condition, you'll find a section called "Other Essential Oils That Could Be Used to Treat This Condition." The essential oils preceded by asterisks are not in the Basic Care Kit but have been included here for your information.

Throughout this section of the chapter, certain methods of treatment are referred to, such as compresses, steam inhalations, and ice treatments. For details of these methods please refer to table 2, "Essential Oil Methods of Use: An A–Z Guide," in chapter 1.

The dosages are indicated in drops — often as a range from minimum to maximum; for example, 3–5 drops. This variability reflects the fact that people come in different sizes, and their condition can be mild, acute, or chronic. The ratio of essential oil(s) to carrier oil should be maintained when making larger quantities.

ABDOMINAL PAIN

Any abdominal pain that persists and increases in intensity should be checked by a doctor because it could be appendicitis or another condition that needs to be properly diagnosed.

Abdominal Pain — Lower Area

Apply the following oil over the painful area in a clockwise direction:

BASIC CARE KIT BLEND

Thyme linalol	2 drops
Eucalyptus radiata	3 drops
Cardamom	3 drops

Blend together and then dilute by adding 3–5 drops to each teaspoon (5 mL) of carrier oil.

ALTERNATIVE BLEND

Geranium	3 drops
Ginger	2 drops

Blend together and then dilute by adding 3–5 drops to each teaspoon (5 mL) of carrier oil.

Other Essential Oils That Could Be Used to Treat This Condition: geranium, peppermint, rosemary, *patchouli (Pogostemon cablin), *ginger (Zingiber officinale), *immortelle (Helichrysum italicum), *basil linalol (Ocimum basilicum ct. linalool), *clove bud (Syzygium aromaticum), *marjoram, sweet (Origanum majorana)

Abdominal Pain — Upper Area

Apply the following oil over the painful area in a clockwise direction:

BASIC CARE KIT BLEND

Peppermint	1 drop
Cardamom	3 drops
Chamomile roman	2 drops

Blend the essential oils together and then dilute by adding 3–5 drops to each teaspoon (5 mL) of carrier oil.

ALTERNATIVE BLEND

Coriander seed	3 drops
Peppermint	1 drop
Cardamom	1 drop

Blend together and then dilute by adding 3–5 drops to each teaspoon (5 mL) of carrier oil.

Other Essential Oils That Could Be Used to Treat This Condition: eucalyptus radiata, rosemary, *basil linalol (Ocimum basilicum ct. linalool), *chamomile german (Matricaria recutita), *marjoram, sweet (Origanum majorana), *coriander seed (Coriandrum sativum), *spearmint (Mentha spicata)

ABRASIONS

Clean the area well with 5 drops of lavender oil diluted in a bowl of warm water. Apply 1 undiluted drop of lavender *around* (not on) the abrasion.

Or clean the area using 5 drops of thyme linalol diluted in a bowl of warm water. Apply 1 drop of chamomile roman *around* the abrasion and leave to heal.

Other Essential Oils That Could Be Used to Treat This Condition: tea tree, thyme linalol, chamomile roman, *frankincense (*Boswellia carterii*), *myrrh (*Commiphora myrrha*), *manuka (*Leptospermum scoparium*)

ABSCESSES

Make a cold compress using one of the following blends and apply it to the area of swelling twice a day:

Basic Care Kit Blend 1
Lavender	2 drops
Tea tree	2 drops
Chamomile roman	3 drops

Basic Care Kit Blend 2
Thyme linalol	2 drops
Eucalyptus radiata	2 drops
Lavender	3 drops

Other Essential Oils That Could Be Used to Treat This Condition: lemon, *juniper berry (*Juniperus communis*), *sandalwood (*Santalum album*), *palmarosa, (*Cymbopogon martinii*), *ravensara (*Ravensara aromatica*), *ravintsara (*Cinnamomum camphora ct. cineole*), *bergamot (*Citrus bergamia*), *oregano (*Origanum vulgare*)

ANAL FISSURES

Bathe the area with warm water to which you have added 5 drops of lavender and 2 drops of lemon oil. Also gently apply around the anal area with the following oil:

Basic Care Kit Blend
Chamomile roman	2 drops
Geranium	1 drop
Lavender	3 drops

Blend together and then dilute by adding 3–5 drops to each teaspoon (5 mL) of carrier oil.

Alternative Blend
Tea tree	1 drop
Geranium	2 drops
Lavender	1 drop
Myrrh	1 drop

Blend together and then dilute by adding 3–5 drops to each teaspoon (5 mL) of carrier oil.

Other Essential Oils That Could Be Used to Treat This Condition: eucalyptus radiata, thyme linalol, *chamomile german (*Matricaria recutita*), *manuka (*Leptospermum scoparium*), *cypress (*Cupressus sempervirens*), *myrrh (*Commiphora myrrha*), *mastic (*Pistacia lentiscus*), *fragonia (*Agonis fragrans*)

ATHLETE'S FOOT

Make up a mixture of 2 drops of tea tree and 1 drop of lavender, dip a cotton ball into the undiluted essential oil and wipe it between the toes and around the nails. Also make up one of the following blends and rub it over the feet, paying special attention to the toes. The essential oils could also be diluted in cider vinegar.

Basic Care Kit Blend
Tea tree	5 drops
Lemon	1 drop

Blend together and then dilute by adding 4–5 drops to each teaspoon (5 mL) of carrier oil.

Alternative Blend
Manuka	5 drops
Lemongrass	5 drops

Blend together and then dilute by adding 3–5 drops to each teaspoon (5 mL) of carrier oil.

Other Essential Oils That Could Be Used to Treat This Condition: thyme linalol, *frankincense (*Boswellia carterii*), *manuka (*Leptospermum scoparium*), *lemongrass (*Cymbopogon citratus/flexuosus*), *eucalyptus lemon (*Eucalyptus citriodora*), *patchouli (*Pogostemon cablin*)

BILIOUS ATTACKS

Inhale from a tissue on which you've placed 1 drop of peppermint and 1 drop of lemon oil. And also add 2 drops of peppermint or 2 drops of cardamom to 1 teaspoon (5 mL) of carrier oil and apply over the stomach and gall bladder area (around the right, lower rib cage).

Alternatively, inhale from a tissue onto which you've put 1 drop of ginger oil.

Other Essential Oils That Could Be Used to Treat This Condition: rosemary, *ginger (*Zingiber officinale*), *clove bud (*Syzygium aromaticum*), *basil linalol (*Ocimum basilicum ct. linalool*), *grapefruit (*Citrus paradisi*), *coriander seed (*coriandrum sativum*)

BLACK EYES

Dilute 1 drop of geranium and 1 drop of chamomile roman in 2 teaspoons (10 mL) of witch hazel and blend well together. Now add this to 1 tablespoon (15 mL) of ice-cold water, mix well, and strain through a paper coffee filter or clean muslin cloth. Then soak some cotton-wool pads in the mixture, and keep them in the fridge. As needed, gently squeeze out the excess liquid, close your eye, and apply a pad to the eyelid and surrounding area. You could blend witch hazel with a chamomile roman or geranium hydrolat and use in the same way.

Other Essential Oils That Could Be Used to Treat This Condition: lavender, *immortelle (*Helichrysum italicum*), *chamomile german (*Matricaria recutita*)

BLEEDING

Clean and soothe areas of minor bleeding by using a cold compress. Add one of the following

blends to a bowl of cold water, and swish the water around to help disperse the essential oil before soaking the compress. Apply the compress over the area before applying a dressing.

BASIC CARE KIT BLEND

Geranium	1 drop
Lemon	1 drop
Chamomile roman	1 drop

ALTERNATIVE BLEND

Lavender	1 drop
Tea tree	1 drop
Chamomile german	1 drop

Other Essential Oils That Could Be Used to Treat This Condition: *cistus (*Cistus ladaniferus*), *immortelle (*Helichrysum italicum*), *cypress (*Cupressus sempervirens*), *palmarosa (*Cymbopogon martinii*), *chamomile german (*Matricaria recutita*)

BLEEDING, NOSE

Pinch the nostrils, then inhale the following essential oils from a tissue:

BASIC CARE KIT BLEND

Lemon	3 drops
Lavender	1 drop

Other Essential Oils That Could Be Used to Treat This Condition: rosemary, chamomile roman, *cistus (*Cistus ladaniferus*), *immortelle (*Helichrysum italicum*), *cypress (*Cupressus sempervirens*), *palmarosa (*Cymbopogon martinii*)

BLEPHARITIS (inflammation of the eyelids)

See **Conjunctivitis**.

BLISTERS

Apply 1 drop of undiluted lavender and 1 drop of undiluted chamomile roman to the blister. Apply gently and thoroughly but carefully, so as not to break the surface of the blister.

Other Essential Oils That Could Be Used to Treat This Condition: tea tree, lemon, *frankincense (*Boswellia carterii*), *myrrh (*Commiphora myrrha*)

BOILS

Bathe the area with 2 drops of lavender and 2 drops of thyme linalol diluted in a small bowl of hot water. If the inflammation is severe, add 1 drop of chamomile roman. Then put 1 drop of either undiluted lavender or undiluted chamomile roman directly onto the boil. If the boil has burst and is open, apply 1 drop each of lavender and thyme linalol *around* the boil. Alternatively, use 1 drop of thyme linalol combined with 1 drop of lemon and apply as above.

Hot compresses can be applied to draw out the pus from a boil. Put 1 drop of thyme linalol and 1 drop of lavender onto a hot compress and apply twice a day. After the pus has been dispelled, apply a little of the following oil *around* the affected area, twice a day:

BASIC CARE KIT BLEND

Lavender	3 drops
Thyme linalol	2 drops
Tea tree	2 drops

Blend together and then dilute by adding 4–5 drops to 1 teaspoon (5 mL) of aloe vera gel.

Other Essential Oils That Could Be Used to Treat This Condition: *chamomile german (*Matricaria recutita*), *oregano (*Origanum vulgare*), *frankincense (*Boswellia carterii*), *fragonia (*Agonis fragrans*)

BRUISES

Make up 2 bowls of water, 1 hot and 1 cold, and add the following to both:

BASIC CARE KIT BLEND

Lavender	2 drops
Rosemary	3 drops
Geranium	1 drop

Soak a washcloth in each bowl and apply them alternately to the bruise and the surrounding area.

Then apply a small amount of the following oil:

Geranium	2 drops
Rosemary	2 drops
Lavender	1 drop

Blend together and then dilute by adding 4–5 drops to each teaspoon (5 mL) of carrier oil or aloe vera gel.

ALTERNATIVE BLEND

Immortelle	3 drops
Lavender	2 drops

Blend together and then dilute by adding 4–5 drops to each teaspoon (5 mL) of carrier oil or aloe vera gel.

Other Essential Oils That Could Be Used to Treat This Condition: *chamomile german (*Matricaria recutita*), *cypress (*Cupressus sempervirens*), *immortelle (*Helichrysum italicum*)

BUMPS (accidental)

Treat as for **bruises**.

Other Essential Oils That Could Be Used to Treat This Condition: *niaouli (*Melaleuca quinquenervia*), *basil linalol (*Ocimum basilicum ct. linalool*), *ginger (*Zingiber officinale*), *immortelle (*Helichrysum italicum*)

BURNS

For minor burns apply ice-cold water for at least 10 minutes. Then put 2 drops of undiluted lavender oil directly onto the affected area. Put 5 drops of lavender onto a dry, cool compress and cover the area. Repeat as needed.

Cigarette Burns

Cool by running the area under a cold-water tap, dry, and then apply 1 drop of undiluted lavender to the burn.

Other Essential Oils That Could Be Used to Treat This Condition: *chamomile german (*Matricaria recutita*)

Blisters from Burns and Scalds

Do not pierce the blister. Put 1 drop of undiluted lavender oil onto the blister and then hold an ice-cold compress over the area for at least 10 minutes. Cover with a piece of dry, clean gauze. Repeat up to three times a day.

Other Essential Oils That Could Be Used to Treat This Condition: geranium, tea tree, eucalyptus radiata, *chamomile german (*Matricaria recutita*), *palmarosa (*Cymbopogon martinii*)

CATARRH (sinus congestion)

Firstly use the bowl method of steam inhalation: blend the following essential oils together and use 3–4 drops in a bowl of hot water and inhale the steam for at least 10 minutes. Keep your eyes tightly closed.

Basic Care Kit Blend — Steam Inhalation

Rosemary	2 drops
Peppermint	1 drop
Tea tree	1 drop
Eucalyptus radiata	1 drop
Cardamom	2 drops

When it's convenient also rub your chest and back with the following oil:

Basic Care Kit Blend — Chest and Back Rub

Tea tree	2 drops
Rosemary	2 drops
Eucalyptus radiata	5 drops
Thyme linalol	1 drop

Blend together and dilute by adding 3–5 drops to each teaspoon (5 mL) of carrier oil or aloe vera gel.

Also, put 2 drops of any of the catarrh essential oil blends, undiluted, on a paper tissue and inhale when needed.

Alternative Blend

Eucalyptus radiata	5 drops
Niaouli	3 drops
Cajuput	3 drops
Frankincense	2 drops

Mix together well and use 3–4 drops in the bowl method of steam inhalation.

A chest rub can also be made by mixing together the essential oils in this alternative blend. Dilute the blend by adding 3–5 drops to each teaspoon (5 mL) of carrier oil or aloe vera gel.

Other Essential Oils That Could Be Used to Treat This Condition: lavender, *pine (*Pinus sylvestris*), *frankincense (*Boswellia carterii*), *niaouli (*Melaleuca quinquenervia*), *cajuput (*Melaleuca cajuputi*), *ravensara (*Ravensara aromatica*), *ravintsara (*Cinnamomum camphora ct. cineole*), *basil linalol (*Ocimum basilicum ct. linalool*)

CHAPPED LIPS

Apply to the lips:

Basic Care Kit Blend

Chamomile roman	2 drops
Geranium	2 drops

Mix well with 2 teaspoons (10 mL) of aloe vera gel or basic balm. Use a small amount for each application.

Other Essential Oils That Could Be Used to Treat This Condition: eucalyptus radiata, *rose otto (*Rosa damascena*), *sandalwood (*Santalum album*), *neroli (*Citrus aurantium*)

CHAPPED SKIN

Make up the following oil and gently massage over the chapped area, including the face if affected:

BASIC CARE KIT BLEND

Geranium	2 drops
Chamomile roman	2 drops
Lemon	1 drop
Lavender	1 drop

Blend together and then dilute by adding 3–4 drops to each teaspoon (5 mL) of carrier oil. Use a small amount each time.

Other Essential Oils That Could Be Used to Treat This Condition: *rose otto (*Rosa damascena*), *sandalwood (*Santalum album*), *carrot seed (*Daucus carota*), *neroli (*Citrus aurantium*)

CHILBLAINS

Apply 1 drop of undiluted geranium oil to the affected area, usually the toes or fingers. Do this for two days, then apply a little of the following oil:

BASIC CARE KIT BLEND

Geranium	5 drops
Lavender	1 drop
Rosemary	1 drop

Blend together and then dilute by adding 3–5 drops to each teaspoon (5 mL) of carrier oil or aloe vera gel.

ALTERNATIVE BLEND

Chamomile german	5 drops
Lemon	5 drops
Geranium	5 drops

Blend together and then dilute by adding 3–5 drops to each teaspoon (5 mL) of carrier oil, or add to aloe vera gel.

Other Essential Oils That Could Be Used to Treat This Condition: tea tree, lemon, chamomile roman, *chamomile german (*Matricaria recutita*), *ginger (*Zingiber officinale*), *black pepper (*Piper nigrum*)

COLD SORES / FEVER BLISTERS
(herpes simplex virus)

If you have a cold sore around your mouth or feel that one might be coming, put 1 drop of geranium oil on a cotton swab and apply it directly onto the sore. Repeat several times a day. Also, apply the following body oil over the whole torso, including the neck:

BASIC CARE KIT BLEND

Geranium	10 drops
Lavender	10 drops
Thyme linalol	2 drops
Lemon	8 drops

Dilute the above essential oils in 2 tablespoons (30 mL) of carrier oil, and use about 2 teaspoons (10 mL) of the blend per application.

ALTERNATIVE BLEND

Eucalyptus radiata	8 drops
Tea tree	2 drops
Geranium	10 drops
Ravensara	8 drops

Dilute the above essential oils in 2 tablespoons (30 mL) of carrier oil, and use about 2 teaspoons (10 mL) of the blend per application.

Although pure melissa essential oil is very expensive, it's extremely effective against herpes simplex and is prescribed widely in Europe for this purpose. It can be applied directly to the affected site and may assist in reducing the severity of the outbreak.

Other Essential Oils That Could Be Used to Treat This Condition: *melissa (*Melissa officinalis*), *chamomile german (*Matricaria recutita*), *rose otto (*Rosa damascena*), *cedarwood atlas (*Cedrus atlantica*), *ho wood (*Cinnamomum camphora ct. linalool*), *hyssop decumbens (*Hyssopus officinalis var. decumbens*), *palmarosa (*Cymbopogon martinii*), *fragonia (*Agonis fragrans*)

COMMON COLD

Blend the following essential oils together and use 3–4 drops in a hot bath, first diluted in a little carrier oil. Lie back and deeply inhale the aroma:

BASIC CARE KIT BLEND — BATH

Thyme linalol	2 drops
Tea tree	2 drops
Eucalyptus radiata	1 drop
Geranium	3 drops
Cardamom	3 drops

For the steam inhalation method, use 1 drop each of the following: thyme linalol, lavender, and geranium.

Also, combine 2 drops each of thyme linalol, peppermint, eucalyptus radiata, and 1 drop of cardamom in a bottle and use 1 drop of this blend on a tissue to inhale whenever needed.

Another method involves massaging around the chest, neck, and sinus area (forehead, nose, and cheekbones — keeping the eyes tightly closed) with the following:

BASIC CARE KIT BLEND — MASSAGE

Lemon	1 drop
Eucalyptus radiata	2 drops
Rosemary	2 drops

Dilute the blend in 2 teaspoons (10 mL) of carrier oil or aloe vera gel and use a tiny amount for each application.

ALTERNATIVE BLEND — MASSAGE

Niaouli	2 drops
Ravensara	2 drops
Eucalyptus radiata	5 drops
Thyme linalol	1 drop

Blend the essential oils together and then dilute by adding 5 drops to each teaspoon (5 mL) of carrier oil or aloe vera gel, and massage over the chest and back.

Other Essential Oils That Could Be Used to Treat This Condition: *oregano (*Origanum vulgare*), *cinnamon leaf (*Cinnamomum zeylanicum*), *clove bud (*Syzygium aromaticum*), *basil linalol (*Ocimum basilicum ct. linalool*), *ravensara (*Ravensara aromatica*), *frankincense (*Boswellia carterii*), *niaouli (*Melaleuca viridiflora*)

CONJUNCTIVITIS (pink eye)

Add 1 drop of chamomile roman to 1 teaspoon (5 mL) witch hazel and mix as well as possible. Then add to 2 tablespoons (30 mL) of rose water and leave for at least seven hours. Strain through a paper coffee filter and use with a cold compress on the eyelids (keeping eyes tightly closed).

CONSTIPATION

Constipation can have underlying causes — check dietary habits and fluid intake.

In some cases, massage can help. Always massage in a clockwise direction over the lower abdomen. Make up the following oil and use a small amount three times a day:

BASIC CARE KIT BLEND

Rosemary	15 drops
Lemon	10 drops
Peppermint	5 drops

Blend together and then dilute by adding 3–5 drops to each teaspoon (5 mL) of carrier oil or aloe vera gel.

ALTERNATIVE BLEND

Black pepper	3 drops
Sweet orange	10 drops
Coriander seed	3 drops
Cardamom	2 drops

Blend together and then dilute by adding 3–5 drops to each teaspoon (5 mL) of carrier oil or aloe vera gel.

Other Essential Oils That Could Be Used to Treat This Condition: *patchouli (*Pogostemon cablin*), *cedarwood atlas (*Cedrus atlantica*), *orange, sweet (*Citrus sinensis*), *black pepper (*Piper nigrum*), *coriander seed (*Coriandrum sativum*), *grapefruit (*Citrus paradisi*), *bergamot (*Citrus bergamia*)

CONVALESCENCE

If you have a convalescent at home it may well be worth investing in essential oils that are not included in the Basic Care Kit. The following oils, which are in the kit, are all helpful and can be used in body oils, in the bath, or in a room diffuser and other room methods: geranium, lemon, lavender, rosemary, chamomile roman.

Any blends used during convalescence should be ones that the patient really likes and enjoys. Lavender has universal appeal, as does geranium. Add in lemon and you have a gentle blend to start off the process of recovery. Always start with the lowest suggested amount of dilution. If a blend says to use between 3 and 5 drops, use 3.

Other Essential Oils That Could Be Used: *mandarin (*Citrus reticulata*), *palmarosa (*Cymbopogon martinii*), *rose otto (*Rosa damascena*), *rosewood (*Aniba rosaeodora*), *ginger (*Zingiber officinale*), *sandalwood (*Santalum album*), *frankincense (*Boswellia carterii*), *orange, sweet (*Citrus sinensis*)

COUGHS

Dry Coughs

BASIC CARE KIT BLEND

Eucalyptus radiata	3 drops
Thyme linalol	2 drops

Blend together and then dilute by adding 4–5 drops to each teaspoon (5 mL) of carrier oil. Apply a small amount over the back and chest at least twice a day.

For the steam inhalation method, use 3 drops of lavender and 3 drops of eucalyptus radiata.

ALTERNATIVE BLEND

Frankincense	5 drops
Ginger	5 drops
Niaouli	5 drops

Blend together and then dilute by adding 4–5 drops to each teaspoon (5 mL) of carrier oil, and rub a small amount onto the chest and back every night.

Other Essential Oils That Could Be Used to Treat This Condition: chamomile roman, tea tree, *oregano (*Origanum vulgare*), *sandalwood (*Santalum album*), *frankincense (*Boswellia carterii*), *ginger (*Zingiber officinale*), *niaouli (*Melaleuca quinquenervia*), *elemi (*Canarium luzonicum*), *cajuput (*Melaleuca cajuputi*), *ravensara (*Ravensara aromatica*)

Coughs with Mucus

Follow the steam inhalation treatment outlined above, in dry coughs.

BASIC CARE KIT BLEND

Eucalyptus radiata	2 drops
Thyme linalol	2 drops
Tea tree	1 drop
Geranium	1 drop

Blend together and then dilute by adding 6 drops to each teaspoon (5 mL) of carrier oil. Massage a small amount over the back and chest at least twice a day.

ALTERNATIVE BLEND

Niaouli	5 drops
Frankincense	5 drops

Blend together and then dilute by adding 5 drops to each teaspoon (5 mL) of carrier oil, and rub a small amount onto the chest and back every night.

Other Essential Oils That Could Be Used to Treat This Condition: *niaouli (*Melaleuca quinquenervia*), *frankincense (*Boswellia carterii*), *cajuput (*Melaleuca cajuputi*), *elemi (*Canarium luzonicum*), *ravensara (*Ravensara aromatica*), *palmarosa (*Cymbopogon martinii*), *cypress (*Cupressus sempervirens*), *ho wood (*Cinnamomum camphora ct. linalool), *basil linalol (*Ocimum basilicum ct. linalool*)

CUTS AND WOUNDS

Bathe the affected area using 3½ fl. oz. (100 mL) of warm water to which the following essential oils have been added, ensuring the water is agitated to avoid globules:

BASIC CARE KIT BLEND 1
Lavender   5 drops
Tea tree   2 drops

BASIC CARE KIT BLEND 2
Chamomile roman   5 drops
Lavender   5 drops

Also, place 3 drops of lavender on a piece of gauze and place it over the area. Renew it twice a day and expose the injury to air on the third day if possible.

Other Essential Oils That Could Be Used to Treat This Condition: *cypress (*Cupressus sempervirens*), *myrrh (*Commiphora myrrha*), *palmarosa (*Cymbopogon martinii*), *manuka (*Leptospermum scoparium*), *fragonia (*Agonis fragrans*), *lemongrass (*Cymbopogon citratus/ flexuosus*)

DENTAL ABSCESS

Put 1 drop of chamomile roman on a cotton ball and apply directly to the abscess. Also, rub the following oil around the external jaw and cheek area:

BASIC CARE KIT BLEND
Lavender   3 drops
Tea tree   2 drops

Blend together and then dilute by adding 3–5 drops to each teaspoon (5 mL) of carrier oil. If you don't want to use a carrier oil, the essential oils can be diluted in aloe vera gel.

Other Essential Oils That Could Be Used to Treat This Condition: lemon, geranium, chamomile roman, thyme linalol, *bergamot (*Citrus bergamia*), *myrrh (*Commiphora myrrha*), *chamomile german (*Matricaria recutita*), *basil linalol (*Ocimum basilicum ct. linalool*), *clove bud (*Syzygium aromaticum*)

DIARRHEA

Diarrhea may be caused by a whole range of conditions that generally fall into three categories: food-related, nerve-related, and viral-related. In all cases, drink large quantities of water and take a rehydration solution to help prevent dehydration and balance the body. (See also chapter 6, "The Basic Travel Kit," page 127.)

Whatever the cause, follow the same treatment methods but use the oils that are appropriate to your particular condition. Choose from the oils below to make a body oil, or use one of the following blends. Dilute 5 drops of essential oil in 1 teaspoon (5 mL) of carrier oil. Massage a small amount over the whole of the abdominal area three times a day.

Essential Oils for Diarrhea Due to Food
Peppermint   Eucalyptus radiata
Thyme linalol   Chamomile roman
Tea tree   Cardamom

Essential Oils for Diarrhea Due to Nerves
Lavender   Geranium
Lemon   Chamomile roman
Peppermint   Cardamom

Essential Oils for Diarrhea Due to Viral Infection
Tea tree   Thyme linalol
Lemon   Lavender
Eucalyptus radiata

Blend for Diarrhea Due to Food

Chamomile roman	1 drop
Peppermint	3 drops
Cardamom	2 drops

Blend for Diarrhea Due to Nerves

Chamomile roman	1 drop
Lemon	2 drops
Lavender	3 drops

Blend for Diarrhea Due to Viral Infection

Thyme linalol	3 drops
Lavender	2 drops
Cardamom	1 drop

A drink can be made by adding 1 drop each of peppermint and cardamom essential oil to a teaspoon of honey, and diluting it in 3½ fl. oz. (100 mL) of warm water, then filtering it through an unbleached paper coffee filter. Then, take a tablespoon of the filtered mixture and add to a small glass of warm water, and sip slowly. Other essential oils should not be substituted in this method.

Ginger essential oil, although not in the Basic Care Kit, can be diluted — 5 drops in 1 teaspoon (5 mL) of carrier oil — and massaged all over the abdominal area. Store the mixture in the fridge, ready for other occasions.

DIVERTICULOSIS

The inflammation, pain, flatulence, and discomfort of this condition are effectively eased by using essential oils. Rub a small amount of the following oil over the abdomen twice a day:

Basic Care Kit Blend

Peppermint	2 drops
Chamomile roman	1 drop

Rosemary	3 drops
Cardamom	2 drops

Blend together and then dilute by adding 3–5 drops to each teaspoon (5 mL) of carrier oil.

An infusion can be made by adding 1 drop of peppermint essential oil to a teaspoon of honey, and diluting it in 3½ fl. oz. (100 mL) of warm water, then filtering it through an unbleached paper coffee filter. Then, take a tablespoon of the filtered mixture and add to a small glass of warm water, and sip slowly. Other essential oils should not be substituted in this method. Store the mixture in the fridge, ready for other occasions.

Other Essential Oils That Could Be Used to Treat This Condition: *basil linalol (*Ocimum basilicum ct. linalool*), *marjoram, sweet (*Origanum majorana*), *spearmint (*Mentha spicata*), *clary sage (*Salvia sclarea*), *coriander seed (*Coriandrum sativum*), *ginger (*Zingiber officinale*)

EARACHE

Persistent pain and earache could indicate a perforated eardrum or an infection, and you should seek a medical diagnosis.

General Earache

For general earache that could be due to hardened wax buildup, warm a teaspoon of olive oil and add to it 1 drop of lavender and 1 drop of chamomile roman, and blend well. Soak a piece of cotton wool in this mixture, wring out any excess oil, and gently place in the ear.

Also use the following oil to massage *around* the ear area, up the neck, and across the cheekbone:

Basic Care Kit Blend

Chamomile roman	2 drops
Lavender	1 drop
Tea tree	1 drop
Geranium	1 drop

Blend together and then dilute by adding 3–5 drops to each teaspoon (5 mL) of carrier oil.

Applying a warm compress to the cheek and ear area after massaging also helps to ease the pain.

Other Essential Oils That Could Be Used to Treat This Condition: eucalyptus radiata, *chamomile german (*Matricaria recutita*), *manuka (*Leptospermum scoparium*), *frankincense (*Boswellia carterii*)

Ear Infections

Treat as for **general earache** (see above), but use different essential oils: warm a teaspoon of olive oil and add to it 3 drops of tea tree and 2 drops of lavender, and blend well. Soak a piece of cotton wool in this mixture, wring out any excess oil, and gently place in the ear.

Also use the following oil to massage around the ear area, up the neck, and across the cheekbone:

BASIC CARE KIT BLEND

Tea tree	2 drops
Thyme linalol	2 drops
Lavender	2 drops

Blend together and then dilute by adding 4–5 drops to each teaspoon (5 mL) of carrier oil.

Other Essential Oils That Could Be Used to Treat This Condition: chamomile roman, eucalyptus radiata, *chamomile german (*Matricaria recutita*), *niaouli (*Melaleuca quinquenervia*), *marjoram, sweet (*Origanum majorana*), *juniper berry (*Juniperus communis*)

FAINTING

Untie any tight clothing and raise the legs slightly higher than the head. Hold an open bottle of essential oil under the patient's nose: use lavender, rosemary, or peppermint. Or put 2 drops of any of these essential oils onto a tissue.

Fainting from Exhaustion or Fatigue

Treat as above, followed by a warm bath to which you have added the following blend. Only do this if the person is not left alone. If a shower is preferred, the essential oils can be added to a washcloth and used to rub on the body. Bed rest should follow immediately.

BASIC CARE KIT BLEND

Chamomile roman	2 drops
Lavender	1 drop
Geranium	1 drop

FEVERS

See the section on fevers in chapter 6, "The Basic Travel Kit," page 129.

FIBROSITIS AKA Fibromyalgia

Massage the following blend gently but thoroughly into the affected area:

BASIC CARE KIT BLEND

Rosemary	2 drops
Lavender	1 drop
Chamomile roman	1 drop
Cardamom	1 drop

Blend together and then dilute by adding 3–5 drops to each teaspoon (5 mL) of carrier oil.

It's helpful to apply this body oil after a cabbage compress has been applied: iron a large outer leaf from a green cabbage (see page 304) to release the enzymes and apply to the affected area while still warm. Leave on the area for 15 minutes.

Also use the combination of essential oils above diluted in a little carrier oil in warm baths, using 4 drops per bath.

ALTERNATIVE BLEND

Marjoram	10 drops
Black pepper	3 drops
Clary sage	3 drops
Frankincense	3 drops
Lavender	10 drops
Plai	3 drops

Blend together and then dilute by adding 3–5 drops to each teaspoon (5 mL) of carrier oil.

Other Essential Oils That Could Be Used to Treat This Condition: chamomile roman, thyme linalol, *clary sage (Salvia sclarea)*, *marjoram, sweet (Origanum majorana)*, *ginger (Zingiber officinale)*, *black pepper (Piper nigrum)*, *frankincense (Boswellia carterii)*, *plai (Zingiber cassumunar)*

FLU

See **Influenza**.

FROSTBITE

Massage up to 3 drops of undiluted geranium into the affected area. When the person is warm, massage the area with the following oil:

BASIC CARE KIT BLEND

Geranium	4 drops
Thyme linalol	2 drops

Dilute in 1 teaspoon (5 mL) of carrier oil.

Other Essential Oils That Could Be Used to Treat This Condition: *hyssop decumbens (Hyssopus officinalis var. decumbens)*, *ginger (Zingiber officinale)*, *clove bud (Syzygium aromaticum)*, *black pepper (Piper nigrum)*

FROZEN SHOULDER

Frozen shoulder can often be eased by using the same treatment as for **fibrositis**. Gently massage the following oil onto the affected area:

BASIC CARE KIT BLEND

Cardamom	3 drops
Chamomile roman	3 drops
Thyme linalol	3 drops

Blend together and then dilute by adding 3–5 drops to each teaspoon (5 mL) of carrier oil.

ALTERNATIVE BLEND

Immortelle	10 drops
Ginger	10 drops
Black pepper	5 drops
Plai	5 drops

Blend together and then dilute by adding 3–5 drops to each teaspoon (5 mL) of carrier oil.

Other Essential Oils That Could Be Used to Treat This Condition: rosemary, lavender, *black pepper (Piper nigrum)*, *ginger (Zingiber officinale)*, *clove bud (Syzygium aromaticum)*, *immortelle (Helichrysum italicum)*, *plai (Zingiber cassumunar)*

GRAZES

See **Abrasions**.

HAY FEVER

Put 1 drop each of chamomile roman and lemon essential oils onto a tissue and inhale. Also add the following combination to baths, diluted first in a little carrier oil:

BASIC CARE KIT BLEND — BATHS

Chamomile roman	2 drops
Lemon	2 drops
Lavender	1 drop

The neck, chest, and back can be massaged with the following oil:

BASIC CARE KIT BLEND — MASSAGE

Chamomile roman	2 drops
Geranium	1 drop
Lemon	1 drop

Blend together and then dilute by adding 3–5 drops to each teaspoon (5 mL) of carrier oil.

Because hay fever affects people in different ways, it can take trial and error to find an effective treatment. Experiment with the essential oils.

Other Essential Oils That Could Be Used to Treat This Condition: peppermint, rosemary, geranium, *immortelle (*Helichrysum italicum*), *spearmint (*Mentha spicata*), *cajuput (*Melaleuca cajuputi*), *niaouli (*Melaleuca quinquenervia*)

HEADACHES

Several essential oils in the Basic Care Kit can ease headaches, but since headaches arise from a variety of causes, refer to all the sub-sections here before deciding which treatment is most appropriate.

General Headache, with No Apparent Cause

Massage around the temples and the base of the skull, along the hairline, with 1 drop of the following combination of oils, diluted with 1 drop of carrier oil:

BASIC CARE KIT BLEND

Lavender	3 drops
Peppermint	1 drop

Other Essential Oils That Could Be Used to Treat This Condition: rosemary, chamomile roman, *rose otto (*Rosa damascena*), *marjoram, sweet (*Origanum majorana*), *coriander seed (*Coriandrum sativum*)

Gastric Headache

This is often caused by eating the wrong foods. Mix 1 drop of cardamom oil with 1 teaspoon of honey dissolved in 3½ fl. oz. (100 mL) of warm water and filter through an unbleached paper coffee filter. Then add 2 teaspoons (10 mL) of the mixture to 1 small glass of warm water and sip.

Also, make up the following combination of essential oils to be used in several ways:

BASIC CARE KIT BLEND

Rosemary	1 drop
Peppermint	2 drops
Lavender	1 drop

Use 1 drop of the essential oil blend, diluted in 1 drop of carrier oil, to massage the back of the neck. Also, apply a further 1 drop of essential oil diluted in 1 drop of carrier oil over the upper abdomen. You could also either inhale 1 drop of the essential oil blend on a tissue, or use 3 drops in a steam inhalation.

Other Essential Oils That Could Be Used to Treat This Condition: chamomile roman, *ginger (*Zingiber officinale*), *coriander seed (*Coriandrum sativum*), *spearmint (*Mentha spicata*), *basil linalol (*Ocimum basilicum ct. linalool*)

Nervous Headache/Tension Headache

Massage around the base of the skull, along the hairline, with 1 drop of the following combination of essential oils, diluted with 1 drop of carrier oil:

BASIC CARE KIT BLEND

Lavender	3 drops
Chamomile roman	1 drop

Also massage over the solar plexus (upper abdomen) in a clockwise direction using the following oil:

BASIC CARE KIT BLEND — MASSAGE

Geranium	1 drop
Lemon	2 drops
Lavender	3 drops

Blend together and then dilute by adding 3–5 drops to each teaspoon (5 mL) of carrier oil.

Other Essential Oils That Could Be Used to Treat This Condition: rosemary, cardamom, *ginger (*Zingiber officinale*)

Sinus Headache
See **Sinusitis**.

HEARTBURN

Rub a little of the following oil over the upper abdomen:

Basic Care Kit Blend

Cardamom	3 drops
Peppermint	2 drops

Dilute 3–5 drops in 1 teaspoon (5 mL) of carrier oil.

Other Essential Oils That Could Be Used to Treat This Condition: lavender, geranium, *clove bud (*Syzygium aromaticum*), *fennel, sweet (*Foeniculum vulgare var. dulce*), *coriander seed (*Coriandrum sativum*), *basil linalol (*Ocimum basilicum ct. linalool*), *marjoram, sweet (*Origanum majorana*), *spearmint (*Mentha spicata*)

HERPES

See **Cold Sores / Fever Blisters**. (Also see chapter 3, "The Self-Defense Kit," pages 58–60.)

HICCUPS

Put 1 drop of chamomile roman oil in a brown paper bag and hold it over the nose and mouth. Breathe in deeply and slowly through the nose.

Other Essential Oils That Could Be Used to Treat This Condition: lavender, lemon, cardamom, *ginger (*Zingiber officinale*)

INFLUENZA

There are many viruses, identified and unidentified, that are responsible for "flu." Viral attacks that involve fever, tiredness, coughs, colds, muscular pain, and exhaustion are all likely to be given this label.

Treatment needs to be quick and aimed at raising immunity levels, as well as combating the virus. Depending on the severity of the attack it could be advisable to consult chapter 3, "The Self-Defense Kit." In the Basic Care Kit there are several oils that have a profound effect on such viral infections. Using essential oils may lessen the symptoms of the viral attack.

If you are shivery and cold, take a warm bath to which the following essential oils have been added after being diluted in a small amount of carrier oil:

Basic Care Kit Blend — Baths

Tea tree	5 drops
Lavender	2 drops
Thyme linalol	2 drops

Then massage your whole body with the following essential oils, diluted in 1 teaspoon (5 mL) of carrier oil. And then go to bed.

Basic Care Kit Blend — Massage

Tea tree	2 drops
Eucalyptus radiata	3 drops
Thyme linalol	1 drop

Try to drink plenty of plain water or fruit juice. Use a diffuser method to circulate the essential oils throughout your living area, using them singly or in combinations of your choice, or trying the blend below:

Alternative Blend to Diffuse throughout the Home

Cinnamon leaf	2 drops
Clove bud	2 drops
Ravensara	5 drops
Eucalyptus radiata	5 drops
Oregano	5 drops

See other sections in this book for more specific advice on how to treat the symptoms. However, bear in mind that flu-like symptoms accompany many conditions, and awareness and vigilance should be maintained.

Other Essential Oils That Could Be Used to Treat This Condition: chamomile roman, eucalyptus radiata, *oregano (*Origanum vulgare*), *cinnamon leaf (*Cinnamomum zeylanicum*), *ravensara (*Ravensara aromatica*), *ravintsara (*Cinnamomum camphora ct. cineole*), *niaouli (*Melaleuca quinquenervia), *cajuput (*Melaleuca cajuputi*), *clove bud (*Syzygium aromaticum*), *hyssop decumbens (*Hyssopus officinalis var. decumbens*)

INSECT BITES

Remove the stinger if there is one, and apply undiluted lavender to the site. See the subsection on insects, "Little Things That Bite," in chapter 6, "The Basic Travel Kit" (see page 127).

Other Essential Oils That Could Be Used to Treat This Condition: chamomile roman, *chamomile german (*Matricaria recutita*)

LARYNGITIS

Blend the following essential oils together:

BASIC CARE KIT BLEND — INHALATION
Chamomile roman	2 drops
Lavender	3 drops
Thyme linalol	2 drops

Use 3–4 drops of this blend in the inhalation water bowl method. Inhale the steam through the nose, keeping the eyes tightly shut.

Also, apply a small amount of the following oil over the throat area and behind the ears:

BASIC CARE KIT BLEND — THROAT APPLICATION
Chamomile roman	5 drops
Thyme linalol	1 drop
Lemon	2 drops

Blend together and then dilute by adding 3–5 drops to each teaspoon (5 mL) of carrier oil.

Other Essential Oils That Could Be Used to Treat This Condition: geranium, *ravensara (*Ravensara aromatica*), *ravintsara (*Cinnamomum camphora ct. cineole*), *cajuput (*Melaleuca cajuputi*), *niaouli (*Melaleuca quinquenervia*), *ho wood (*Cinnamomum camphora ct. linalool*), *palmarosa (*Cymbopogon martinii*), *ginger (*Zingiber officinale*), *sage (*Salvia officinalis*), *pine (*Pinus sylvestris*), *fragonia (*Agonis fragrans*)

LUMBAGO (lower back pain)

Combine the following essential oils:

BASIC CARE KIT BLEND — COMPRESS
Rosemary	4 drops
Eucalyptus radiata	4 drops
Geranium	1 drop
Thyme linalol	2 drops

Place 3 drops of the blend above on a hot compress and apply to the lower back. When the compress becomes cold, replace it with another hot compress. Do this at least three times a day.

BASIC CARE KIT BLEND — MASSAGE
Peppermint	2 drops
Rosemary	5 drops
Chamomile roman	2 drops
Lavender	3 drops

Blend together, then dilute in 2 teaspoons (10 mL) of carrier oil. Use a small amount to massage the lower back and into the crevice of the buttocks, but not as far as the anus.

The following blend can be used in both compress and massage methods and is particularly helpful if the painful area feels cold:

ALTERNATIVE BLEND
Immortelle	10 drops
Ginger	3 drops
Clove bud	2 drops

For massage, dilute in 4 teaspoons (20 mL) of carrier oil and use a small amount for each application. Or for hot compresses use 3 drops of the essential oil blend.

Other Essential Oils That Could Be Used to Treat This Condition: lavender, *ginger (*Zingiber officinale*), *black pepper (*Piper nigrum*), *sage (*Salvia officinalis*), *plai (*Zingiber cassumunar*), *immortelle (*Helichrysum italicum*), *clove bud (*Syzygium aromaticum*), *clary sage (*Salvia sclarea*), *marjoram, sweet (*Origanum majorana*), *bay laurel (*Laurus nobilis*)

NETTLE RASH (urticaria)

Apply up to 2 undiluted drops of lavender over the stung area as soon as possible.

As soon as you can, make up the following mixture and smooth it over any rash:

BASIC CARE KIT BLEND

Lavender	5 drops
Chamomile roman	5 drops

Blend in 1 tablespoon (15 mL) of aloe vera gel or aloe vera liquid. Use enough to cover the affected area. Taking warm baths to which 1 handful of Epsom salts and 4 drops of chamomile roman have been added can calm any persistent rash.

NEURALGIA

Numbing the area with ice often relieves the pain initially, so use a cold compress or ice treatment over the affected part. To help relieve any inflammation, gently apply the following oil:

BASIC CARE KIT BLEND

Lavender	5 drops
Chamomile roman	5 drops
Eucalyptus radiata	2 drops
Cardamom	2 drops

Blend together and then dilute by adding 3–5 drops to each teaspoon (5 mL) of carrier oil.

ALTERNATIVE BLEND

Immortelle	10 drops
Geranium	10 drops
Chamomile roman	5 drops
Rosemary	1 drop

Blend together and then dilute by adding 3–4 drops into each teaspoon (5 mL) of carrier oil. Gently massage a tiny amount into the area and repeat after five minutes.

Other Essential Oils That Could Be Used to Treat This Condition: peppermint, eucalyptus radiata, thyme linalol, *marjoram, sweet (*Origanum majorana*), *juniper berry (*Juniperus communis*), *immortelle (*Helichrysum italicum*)

NOSE BLEEDS

See **Bleeding, Nose**.

PALPITATIONS

If someone is experiencing palpitations, medical advice should be sought at the earliest opportunity. Inform the physician if you intend using essential oils to support any treatment given for palpitations.

BASIC CARE KIT BLEND — INHALATION

Lavender	2 drops
Chamomile roman	1 drop
Geranium	2 drops

Blend the essential oils together and put 1 drop on a tissue and inhale as needed.

BASIC CARE KIT BLEND — MASSAGE

Lavender	8 drops
Chamomile roman	5 drops
Lemon	7 drops

Dilute in 1 fl. oz. (30 mL) of carrier oil, or use 2–3 drops of the essential oil blend in 1 teaspoon (5 mL) of carrier oil, and use half a teaspoon per application.

Other Essential Oils That Could Be Used to Treat This Condition: *valerian (*Valeriana officinalis*), *neroli (*Citrus aurantium*), *rose otto (*Rosa damascena*), *petitgrain (*Citrus aurantium*), *vetiver (*Vetiveria zizanoides*), *marjoram, sweet (*Origanum majorana*), *spikenard (*Nardostachys jatamansi*), *jasmine (*Jasminum grandiflorum/officinale*)

PINK EYE

See **Conjunctivitis**.

SCALDS

See **Burns**.

SHOCK

See **Fainting**.

Shock can be treated as for fainting. Massage the body before sleep with the following:

BASIC CARE KIT BLEND

Lemon	3 drops
Geranium	2 drops
Lavender	1 drop

Dilute 3–4 drops in 1 teaspoon (5 mL) of carrier oil.

Other Essential Oils That Could Be Used to Treat This Condition: chamomile roman, peppermint, rosemary, *valerian (*Valeriana officinalis*), *rose otto (*Rosa damascena*), *neroli (*Citrus aurantium*), *palmarosa (*Cymbopogon martinii*), *basil linalol (*Ocimum basilicum ct. linalool*), *orange, sweet (*Citrus sinensis*)

SINUSITIS

There are three methods that could be used. For the steam inhalation method, use the following combination of essential oils:

BASIC CARE KIT BLEND — STEAM INHALATION

Rosemary	3 drops
Thyme linalol	1 drop
Peppermint	1 drop
Geranium	1 drop

Blend the essential oils together, place 3 drops in a bowl of hot water, and inhale the steam through the nose. Keep the eyes tightly closed.

BASIC CARE KIT BLEND — TISSUE INHALATION

Rosemary	2 drops
Geranium	1 drop
Eucalyptus radiata	1 drop

Blend the essential oils using these proportions, put 1 drop of the blend on a tissue, and inhale as needed.

BASIC CARE KIT BLEND — MASSAGE

Rosemary	5 drops
Geranium	5 drops
Eucalyptus radiata	2 drops
Peppermint	1 drop

Blend the oils together, then dilute 3–5 drops to each teaspoon (5 mL) of carrier oil. Massage starting around the neck and moving behind and in front of the ears. Then, using no more than 1 drop of the blend, massage over the cheekbone, the nose, and the forehead. Be very careful to avoid the eye area. Remove any excess with a tissue.

Other Essential Oils That Could Be Used to Treat This Condition: tea tree, *basil linalol (*Ocimum basilicum ct. linalool*), *juniper berry (*Juniperus communis*), *benzoin (*Styrax benzoin*), *niaouli (*Melaleuca quinquenervia*), *pine (*Pinus sylvestris*), *cajuput (*Melaleuca cajuputi*), *ravintsara (*Cinnamomum camphora ct. cineole*)

SORE THROATS

See **Laryngitis**.

SPLINTERS

Remove the splinter with a sterilized needle or pair of tweezers. When the whole splinter has been removed, apply 1 undiluted drop of lavender.

Other Essential Oils That Could Be Used to Treat This Condition: tea tree, *myrrh (*Commiphora myrrha*), *frankincense (*Boswellia carterii*)

STIES

First prepare the liquid needed for a warm compress. Heat 2 tablespoons of rose water and add to it 1 drop of chamomile roman essential oil. Strain this liquid through an unbleached paper coffee filter and leave to cool. Then soak a cotton ball in the rose water and chamomile mix, squeeze to remove any excess liquid, and then place over your closed eyelid, being very careful not to get any liquid into the eye. Repeat the whole procedure twice a day for three days. Also use the massage treatment given above for **sinusitis**.

SYNOVITIS

Massage the inflamed joint with a small amount of the following oil:

BASIC CARE KIT BLEND

Chamomile roman	10 drops
Eucalyptus radiata	5 drops
Rosemary	2 drops
Lavender	3 drops
Peppermint	2 drops

Blend together and then dilute by adding 3–5 drops to each teaspoon (5 mL) of carrier oil.

Other Essential Oils That Could Be Used to Treat This Condition: tea tree, *juniper berry (Juniperus communis), *cajuput (Melaleuca cajuputi), *plai (Zingiber cassumunar), *ginger (Zingiber officinale), *immortelle (Helichrysum italicum)

WHITLOWS

Although whitlows seem a minor thing, they can be extremely painful and sore and can reappear during stressful times when immunity is low. Make up the following combination of oils:

BASIC CARE KIT BLENDS

Thyme linalol	2 drops
Lemon	3 drops
Geranium	1 drop

Apply 1 undiluted drop around the affected area three times a day.

Once any pus has been dispersed, follow the same procedure three times per day but using 1 drop of the following combination:

Lavender	2 drops
Chamomile roman	2 drops

Other Essential Oils That Could Be Used to Treat This Condition: tea tree, *manuka (Leptospermum scoparium), *chamomile german (Matricaria recutita), *benzoin (Styrax benzoin), *myrrh (Commiphora myrrha)

3

The Self-Defense Kit

Bacteria and viruses are smart. When they realize that an antibacterial or antiviral is being used to wipe them out, they mutate. It's evolution at work, in super-quick time. But they're not only smart, they also work together. Through a process known as *bacterial conjugation*, bacteria under threat can swap DNA with other nearby bacteria species and essentially become a new organism, resistant to antibacterial pharmaceuticals.

Once, very few bacteria came into contact with antibacterial drugs because their use was not widespread. People used them when they got sick, and that was it. Nowadays, antimicrobials are routinely given to animals not only when they're ill but as preventatives or as growth promoters. These animals excrete the antimicrobials, as indeed do we, and the sewage ends up in the environment somewhere. More antimicrobials are used in fish farming, plant agriculture, industrial paints, and even for the maintenance of oil pipelines. In other words, our whole planet is awash with antimicrobials, and the microbes are aware of this and are mutating to escape them. The end result is that the once-effective drugs are effective no longer.

This is where we are today, in an international crisis of antimicrobial resistance, known as AMR.

In 2013, the National Institutes of Health reported that each year 1.7 million Americans get an infection in the hospital, of whom about 99,000 will die as a result. Of the bugs responsible for hospital infections in the United States, around 70% are resistant to one or more drugs that would have dispatched them a few years ago.

In 2013, the chief medical officer of the UK, Professor Dame Sally Davies, asked the British government to recognize antibiotic resistance as a national catastrophe. The World Health Organization made AMR the theme for World Health Day in 2011, recognizing the huge potential for death on a worldwide scale. Globally, each year about 440,000 people are struck down with multidrug-resistant tuberculosis, of whom approximately 150,000 die. Many conditions that we once felt confident we could treat are now a major worry again. With infections that are more difficult to treat, such as methicillin-resistant *Staphylococcus aureus* (MRSA) and *Clostridium difficile*, on the loose in hospitals, routine surgery suddenly looks a lot more risky.

Scientific journals today are bursting with new research into the antibacterial and antiviral potential of essential oils or their components, and the efficacy of essential oils is not in doubt. The research being carried out is not only to find solutions to human health problems but to counter microbial problems prevalent in veterinary practice, in the food and drink industry, and in farming. Commercial crops are, like us, susceptible to bacteria, viruses, and fungi, and it is precisely because plants have always had to fight these pesky micro-organisms that some of them developed a defense mechanism — essential oil.

There's no longer any doubt that sweet-scented essential oils have an important part to play in the fight against the toughest microbes. Countless tests have been carried out in university research labs all over the world, using a huge variety of essential oils against a long and varied list of micro-organisms. Clearly, certain essential oils are effective against some bacteria, while others are not. The same can be said for viruses and fungi.

This section is not intended as a replacement for allopathic treatment. What essential oils could do for you is act as a preventative when other people around you have infections, provide an emergency self-defense kit, and act as a backup therapeutic option. Generally, essential oils can be used alongside most other preparations and medications you may be using.

The successful transmission of micro-organisms is largely due to the close proximity of people in crowded commuter trains, schools, supermarkets, movie theaters, and so on. In many Asian countries, it's common practice to wear a face mask if you have an airborne infection to protect others. Essential oils can easily be incorporated into masks, to give us double protection. This is just one of the many methods we can use to protect ourselves and our families.

I travel a great deal and prepare special blends before I go, in case of emergencies, and I consider the person next to me on a long-haul flight sneezing and coughing to be an emergency. Whatever they have, I don't want it! The beauty of essential oils is that they are small and easy to transport, versatile, and can be used in different ways.

I know several people — including medics — who never go into a hospital without smearing a dab of essential oil gel under their noses. It may sting, but they think it's worth it. One or two drops of essential oil on a tissue can be inhaled during flu season as you shop in crowds or travel by train or bus. At the workplace, various environmental methods of dispersing the essential oils can be used, and in higher doses. Of course, you will need to consult with your work colleagues and check that they don't find the aroma unpleasant. If they do, it's easy to find an equally effective alternative they will like.

This chapter starts with the Self-Defense Kit of essential oils, which is followed by a chart showing some essential oils with antibacterial, antiviral, and antifungal properties. After considering the best methods to use to prevent microbial infection, we take a closer look at essential oils that are particularly effective against bacteria, then those pertinent to viral infection, including postviral fatigue. Broad-spectrum blends and oils for fungal infection follow, before turning to the hospital and nursing home environments. Please look through this whole chapter before deciding which essential oils to use. You may also want to refer to other sections within this book that address microbial self-defense, such as chapters 6 and 7, on travel and children. If working in a hospital or nursing home, please see the section on hospitals in chapter 4 (page 70).

The Self-Defense Kit

All essential oils are antiseptic to some degree, and in the lists of essential oils that follow you'll find those that are known to have an inhibiting effect on bacteria, viruses, or fungi — or all three. With these, we can create blends that are effective in doing the job of protecting health.

In the world of microbes, there are two groups — the Gram-positive type and the Gram-negative type. This is a complex subject, but put simply, the distinction is based on whether the cell wall has a single or a double layer. In the world of pharmaceutical antibiotics, whether an organism is Gram-positive or Gram-negative will very strongly determine whether a particular antibiotic will be effective against it. Also, there are a multitude of micro-organisms, and, as we know, a particular pharmaceutical drug may be effective against some, but not others. The same is true of essential oils.

What this means is that although an essential oil is listed as "antibacterial," that is not to say it will be effective against *all* bacteria. This is not a big concern for us because essential oils — unlike pharmaceuticals — can be used in blends. We can use a number of essential oils with antibacterial qualities, mix them together, and attack the microbe on all fronts. The complexity of the compounds in each and every essential oil is an advantage, while a blend provides an enhanced complexity of compounds. Indeed, synergistic blends of essential oils have been tested against microbes and found to be extremely effective. The Self-Defense Kit provides a huge armory, and because we can modify our ingredients quickly, we can outwit most microbes.

At present essential oils can be analyzed only to a certain extent. Although many chemical components can be ascertained by gas chromatography, there are always trace elements that remain a mystery. Yet, it is *all* the elements of an essential oil, including its trace elements, that make it so effective. Researchers are keen to identify the effective antibacterial chemical in the particular oil they're working on, in the hope that it will provide a step toward solving the problem of bacterial resistance and can be synthetically reproduced. But it's not that simple. Research shows that it is the complete essential oil — rather than any of its isolated chemicals — that is more effective, and it's also less toxic to the rodents this research is usually carried out on.

Trace elements are important in the human body too. We have only about 0.000002% of

cobalt and chromium in our bodies, but without them we may have trouble forming proteins and regulating DNA and insulin. Nobody denies that trace elements are important in humans, and I maintain they're important in essential oils too.

In an ideal world, we would all know the precise name of the microbe that's causing us or our family harm. Sometimes our health professional will do a test and determine that for us, but most of the time that exact information simply isn't available. And when someone at work has an infection, we certainly are not privy to their medical records. If you have a bacterial infection, use blends of essential oils with antibacterial properties, or if you think it's a virus, use a blend of essential oils with antiviral action. If you have no idea whatever, use one of the "broad spectrum" blends I suggest later in this chapter. Above all, be prepared to move as quickly as our little microbe enemies do. We can evolve too, and with essential oils on hand, we have a choice in how to approach the problem of unwelcome bacteria, viruses, and fungi.

10 SELF-DEFENSE KIT ESSENTIAL OILS

As so many essential oils have antimicrobial properties, I am suggesting here the 10 essential oils that would be most useful in protecting us against a range of microbes. All these are readily available and can multitask — having more than one defensive property.

Eucalyptus radiata (*Eucalyptus radiata*)
Ho wood (*Cinnamomum camphora ct. linalool*)
Lavender (*Lavandula angustifolia*)
Manuka (*Leptospermum scoparium*)
May chang (*Litsea cubeba*)
Niaouli (*Melaleuca quinquenervia*)
Oregano (*Origanum vulgare*)
Palmarosa (*Cymbopogon martinii*)
Ravensara (*Ravensara aromatica*)
Thyme linalol (*Thymus vulgaris ct. linalool*)

Other useful additions to the Self-Defense Kit would be clove bud (*Syzygium aromaticum*), fragonia (*Agonis fragrans*), and rosalina (*Melaleuca ericifolia*).

TABLE 4. GUIDELINES TO THE ANTIBACTERIAL, ANTIVIRAL, AND ANTIFUNGAL PROPERTIES OF ESSENTIAL OILS

ESSENTIAL OIL	PROPERTY		
	Antibacterial	Antiviral	Antifungal
Bay laurel (*Laurus nobilis*)	*	*	*
Bay, West Indian (*Pimenta racemosa*)	*	*	
Benzoin (*Styrax benzoin*)	*		
Bergamot (*Citrus bergamia*)	*		
Caraway seed (*Carum carvi*)	*		*
Cardamom (*Elettaria cardamomum*)	*		*
Chamomile german (*Matricaria recutita*)	*		
Chamomile roman (*Anthemis nobilis*)	*		
Cinnamon leaf (*Cinnamomum zeylanicum*)	*	*	*
Citronella (*Cymbopogon nardus*)	*	*	*
Clove bud (*Syzygium aromaticum*)	*	*	*
Coriander seed (*Coriandrum sativum*)	*		*
Elemi (*Canarium luzonicum*)	*		
Eucalyptus globulus (*Eucalyptus globulus*)	*	*	
Eucalyptus lemon (*Eucalyptus citriodora*)	*		*
Eucalyptus radiata (*Eucalyptus radiata*)	*	*	

ESSENTIAL OIL	PROPERTY		
	Antibacterial	Antiviral	Antifungal
Fennel, sweet (*Foeniculum vulgare var. dulce*)			*
Fragonia (*Agonis fragrans*)	*	*	*
Frankincense (*Boswellia carterii*)	*		
Geranium (*Pelargonium graveolens*)	*	*	
Ginger (*Zingiber officinale*)	*		
Ho wood (*Cinnamomum camphora ct. linalool*)	*	*	*
Hyssop decumbens (*Hyssopus officinalis var. decumbens*)	*	*	
Kanuka (*Kunzea ericoides*)	*	*	*
Lavender (*Lavandula angustifolia*)	*		
Lavender, spike (*Lavandula latifolia*)	*		*
Lemon (*Citrus limon*)	*		
Lemongrass (*Cymbopogon citratus/flexuosus*)	*		*
Lemon tea tree (*Leptospermum petersonii*)	*		
Manuka (*Leptospermum scoparium*)	*	*	*
Marjoram, sweet (*Origanum majorana*)	*		*
May chang (*Litsea cubeba*)	*	*	*
Melissa (*Melissa officinalis*)	*	*	*
Neroli (*Citrus aurantium*)	*		
Niaouli (*Melaleuca quinquenervia*)	*	*	*
Orange, sweet (*Citrus sinensis*)	*		
Oregano (*Origanum vulgare*)	*	*	*

ESSENTIAL OIL	PROPERTY		
	Antibacterial	Antiviral	Antifungal
Palmarosa (*Cymbopogon martinii*)	*	*	*
Patchouli (*Pogostemon cablin*)			*
Peppermint (*Mentha piperita*)	*		*
Petitgrain (*Citrus aurantium*)	*		
Pine (*Pinus sylvestris*)	*		
Ravensara (*Ravensara aromatica*)	*	*	
Ravintsara (*Cinnamomum camphora ct. cineole*)	*	*	
Rosalina (*Melaleuca ericifolia*)	*	*	*
Rosemary (*Rosmarinus officinalis*)	*		*
Rose otto (*Rosa damascena*)	*		
Rosewood (*Aniba rosaeodora*)	*		*
Sage (*Salvia officinalis*)	*	*	*
Sandalwood (*Santalum album*)	*		
Savory, winter (*Satureja montana*)	*	*	*
Spearmint (*Mentha spicata*)	*		
Tea tree (*Melaleuca alternifolia*)	*	*	*
Thyme (*Thymus vulgaris*)	*	*	*
Thyme linalol (*Thymus vulgaris ct. linalool*)	*	*	*
Vetiver (*Vetiveria zizanoides*)	*		*

In addition to the pure essential oils in table 4, cold-pressed black cumin seed oil (*Nigella sativa*) is a useful addition to a Self-Defense Kit, with antibacterial, antiviral, and antifungal properties. This oil cannot be used in a room diffuser.

How to Use Essential Oils to Help Protect Against Bacterial and Viral Infections

There are two basic ways to use the essential oils: in the environment around you, and on your physical body.

ENVIRONMENTAL METHODS

Diffusers

Room diffusers can be electric or designed around a simple tea light candle. Follow the instructions that come with the product. If you don't possess a diffuser, the essential oil molecules can be dispersed by using a glass bowl or cup filled with steaming hot water, with the essential oils dropped on the water. The steam will rise and circulate the essential oils around the room.

If there's a lot of infection around, use 5–10 drops of essential oil per use with your diffuser. In clinical settings, equipment that emits a fine mist of pure essential oil is sometimes used to treat cases of severe infection. These include cold air nebulizers, oil vaporizers, and cold or fan diffusers.

Sprays

A simple anti-infectious room spray can easily be made using water and essential oil. As water and oil don't mix, add the essential oils to a little colorless alcohol or vegetable glycerin to help emulsify them before adding to the water, and shake before each use. If you don't have any emulsifier, just shake more vigorously before spraying the room. Spray high into the air, and avoid letting the water fall on wood, velvet, silk, or other delicate furniture and materials. Use a minimum of 20 drops of essential oil to each 3½ tablespoons (50 mL) of water — with or without 1 teaspoon (5 mL) of emulsifier. Use a clean, preferably new sprayer; plant misters are ideal.

PHYSICAL METHODS

Body Sprays

Body sprays are easy to make and versatile, as they can be made small enough to carry around, even when traveling. Combine your chosen essential oils, then add to water or hydrolat (use a small amount of emulsifier if you have one handy). Hydrolats often have antibacterial properties of their own, depending on the material they were distilled from. Shake very well and leave for 24 hours, shaking occasionally. Then filter through an unbleached paper coffee filter and bottle. Use the spray in the atmosphere and around your body.

Baths

Aromatic baths are very good for helping relieve the symptoms of colds and flu. However, many essential oils that treat flu cannot be used undiluted, or even diluted, in baths, as they could be irritating to the skin. So take care in your choice of oils. I've suggested several bath blends in this chapter. Choose oils that are specific to your particular symptoms — aching muscles or headache, for example. Use a maximum of 8 drops per bath, diluted in the medium of your choice before adding to the water.

Body Oils

Use no more than 30 drops of essential oil to each fluid ounce (30 mL) of carrier oil, unless otherwise directed. Choose the oils that are specific to your symptoms. Be aware that some essential oils, such as cinnamon and clove, can be skin irritants. The most effective time for application is before retiring to bed. This allows the essential oils to do their work as you sleep. A body oil can also be applied before taking a bath, when the body absorbs the essential oil by osmosis and inhalation.

Inhalation

Paper tissues: Use 1 or 2 drops of your chosen essential oil or blend on a paper tissue and inhale as needed.

Disposable face masks: Adding liquid to any protective paper face mask can nullify the effects of the mask, depending upon the type of face mask used. I generally apply 1 drop of essential oil to a small piece of tissue and put that inside my face mask when traveling on planes and trains during an epidemic, such as swine or bird flu. Essential oils can irritate your nose, so always apply the oil to the tissue before use so it has a chance to soak into the paper. Good choices for this method would be tea tree, fragonia, thyme linalol, manuka, eucalyptus radiata, niaouli, frankincense, ravensara, and ravintsara.

Honey Paste

Some wounds seem very resistant to healing and can easily become inflamed. In these cases it's worth trying a honey wash. Add 1 drop of manuka essential oil to 1 teaspoon of good-quality organic manuka honey (active 24+). Although there's a difference between the manuka pollen collected by bees to make the honey and the essential oil distilled from the shrub-like manuka tree, they seem to complement each other therapeutically. Other essential oils can be added to this basic paste. Put the honey paste around the wound, not directly on it, as often as needed.

Bacterial Infection

The essential oils can be used in various methods, so the best way to approach self-defense is to make up a blend of essential oils in a bottle, and then take the drops you need for each method of use when required. Kept undiluted in this way, they will remain active for a much longer time

than if diluted. You can multiply the number of drops, but keep the proportions the same:

ANTIBACTERIAL BLEND 1

Ravensara	10 drops
Eucalyptus radiata	8 drops
Niaouli	5 drops
Ginger	10 drops
Thyme	4 drops
Lemongrass	3 drops

ANTIBACTERIAL BLEND 2

Frankincense	5 drops
Ho wood	6 drops
Eucalyptus radiata	8 drops
Lemon	5 drops
Palmarosa	6 drops

ANTIBACTERIAL BLEND 3

Rosalina	10 drops
Lavender	8 drops
Geranium	4 drops
Lemon	6 drops
Palmarosa	6 drops
Ravintsara	10 drops

Blends 2 and 3 could be added to unscented shower or bath products made using natural ingredients. For baths, add 4 drops of the blend to 1 teaspoon of carrier oil and 1 teaspoon of salt before adding to the water and dispersing well with your hand.

MRSA

Methicillin-resistant *Staphylococcus aureus* (MRSA) is a bug that has taken control all over the world. Signs of a staph infection — whether in the hospital or at home — can include skin infections that appear as a rash, spots, or pimples, and swelling in the glands. Dealing with the infection early is always the best option.

The following blend is designed to give protection and, if no other help is available, can be used in cases where infection has already taken hold. There are 46 drops in the blend — the largest ingredient contributing 10 drops, and the smallest just 2 drops. You can double or triple the whole recipe, but always stick with the essential oil proportions.

MRSA Blend

Geranium	10 drops
Manuka	10 drops
Thyme linalol	5 drops
Clove bud	3 drops
Lavender	5 drops
Lemongrass	5 drops
Tea tree	3 drops
Oregano	2 drops
Cinnamon leaf	3 drops

Mix the essential oils together in a small bottle. From this bottle, take 30 drops and add to 1 fl. oz. (30 mL) of carrier oil or an alternative carrier of your choice such as aloe vera or silica gel, for example. Massage both feet, using ½–1 teaspoon of the diluted blend, depending on the size of the feet.

In severe cases, a stronger dilution can be used. This should be used only in tiny amounts, and when needed: dilute the essential oil blend in 1 fl. oz. (30 mL) of a carrier oil of your choice. It's not advisable to use these blends during pregnancy or on children.

HELICOBACTER PYLORI

Helicobacter pylori is one of those Gram-negative bacteria that are often resistant to pharmaceutical antibiotics. Although it can be found in various parts of the body, *Helicobacter pylori* is usually found in the stomach, and for this reason, the first method involves making an infusion.

Take 1 tablespoon of organic manuka honey (active 24+) and mix with 1 drop of organic manuka essential oil. Once a day from this mix take

½ teaspoon, and stir it into a 5 fl. oz. (150 mL) mug of warm water and sip. It's best to do this before going to sleep. Repeat for no longer than four days, then leave it for two days, and then repeat for a further four days. Only use this method if you are not taking antibiotics or when the course has finished.

Also, make an upper abdominal rub using the following essential oils:

Orange, sweet	3 drops
Black pepper	1 drop
Cardamom	1 drop

Dilute into 1 teaspoon (5 mL) of carrier oil and apply a small amount — enough to cover the upper abdomen — every night until the infection eases.

Viral Infection

There are many essential oils with some antiviral qualities, but quite a few of them are not widely available. The most easily obtained antiviral essential oils for home use are the following:

Bay laurel (*Laurus nobilis*)
Bay, West Indian (*Pimenta racemosa*)
Cinnamon leaf (*Cinnamomum zeylanicum*)
Citronella (*Cymbopogon nardus*)
Clove bud (*Syzygium aromaticum*)
Eucalyptus radiata (*Eucalyptus radiata*)
Fragonia (*Agonis fragrans*)
Geranium (*Pelargonium graveolens*)
Ho wood (*Cinnamomum camphora* ct. linalool)
Hyssop decumbens (*Hyssopus officinalis* var. decumbens)
Kanuka (*Kunzea ericoides*)
Manuka (*Leptospermum scoparium*)
May chang (*Litsea cubeba*)
Melissa (*Melissa officinalis*)
Niaouli (*Melaleuca quinquenervia*)
Oregano (*Origanum vulgare*)
Palmarosa (*Cymbopogon martinii*)
Ravensara (*Ravensara aromatica*)

Ravintsara (*Cinnamomum camphora ct. cineole*)
Rosalina (*Melaleuca ericifolia*)
Savory, winter (*Satureja montana*)
Tea tree (*Melaleuca alternifolia*)
Thyme (*Thymus vulgaris*)
Thyme linalol (*Thymus vulgaris ct. linalool*)

GENERAL ANTIVIRAL BLENDS

The following three antiviral blends should not be used in body oils or baths but can be used in diffusers, room sprays, or for inhalation — use 1 drop on a tissue. Blend the essential oils together using these proportions, and use as required.

Antiviral Blend 1

Clove bud	5 drops
Cinnamon leaf	5 drops
Thyme linalol	7 drops

Antiviral Blend 2

Oregano	9 drops
Hyssop decumbens	5 drops
Thyme linalol	10 drops

Antiviral Blend 3

Hyssop decumbens	5 drops
Cinnamon leaf	7 drops
Oregano	8 drops
Clove bud	4 drops
Thyme linalol	6 drops
Ravensara	10 drops

FLU-LIKE SYMPTOMS

If you think you might be coming down with flu, or if you already have it, try using the essential oils below, either on their own or in a blend, in any method that suits you. If using in the bath, first dilute in ½ teaspoon of carrier. It's often the case that we can recognize the early symptoms of flu before it strikes us down, and that is the time

to start using the essential oils and hopefully ward off the flu.

Essential Oils for Flu Symptoms
Eucalyptus radiata (*Eucalyptus radiata*)
Geranium (*Pelargonium graveolens*)
Niaouli (*Melaleuca quinquenervia*)
Palmarosa (*Cymbopogon martinii*)
Ravensara (*Ravensara aromatica*)
Ravintsara (*Cinnamomum camphora ct. cineole*)

VIRAL-INDUCED COLD SORES ON THE MOUTH: HSV-1

Herpes simplex virus 1 (HSV-1) is part of the Herpesviridae family that includes HSV-2, genital herpes. See "Viral-Induced Genital Sores: HSV-2" below.

Cold sores on the lips can be painful and annoying because they're so visible, and it can feel as if your life is on hold until they're gone. The virus lies dormant and can manifest at the most inconvenient time, especially during times of stress. Even on a relaxing holiday the sores can erupt because of prolonged exposure to the sun. Each person's symptoms are unique, but there's usually a warning itching or tingling sensation, redness, or swelling at the site where the sore will appear, and even before that there can be flu-type symptoms including headache, tiredness, or muscle pain. Using the essential oils at these early stages may help prevent or lessen the effects of the outbreak.

Essential Oils for Herpes Virus (HSV-1)
Clove bud (*Syzygium aromaticum*)
Eucalyptus radiata (*Eucalyptus radiata*)
Manuka (*Leptospermum scoparium*)
Melissa (*Melissa officinalis*)
Oregano (*Origanum vulgare*)
Sage (*Salvia officinalis*)
Sandalwood (*Santalum album*)
Star anise (*Illicium verum*)

Tea tree (*Melaleuca alternifolia*)
Thyme linalol (*Thymus vulgaris ct. linalool*)

HSV-1 PREVENTATIVE BLEND 1

Coriander seed	1 drop
Sandalwood	2 drops
Melissa	2 drops

When you notice the first signs that an outbreak is likely to occur, apply a small amount of this blend directly to the usual site with a disposable cotton swab. This is used undiluted, so prepare a small bottle using these proportions. If you're going to be in the sun, avoid using melissa and use manuka instead. This will help lessen the sensation, reduce the likelihood of a sore breaking out, and over time the number of outbreaks will hopefully reduce.

The alternative blend below provides a strong-acting synergistic blend in these proportions:

HSV-1 PREVENTATIVE BLEND 2

Tea tree	10 drops
Eucalyptus radiata	10 drops
Eucalyptus lemon	5 drops
Thyme linalol	8 drops
Manuka	15 drops
Clove bud	3 drops
Melissa	4 drops
Oregano	3 drops
Geranium	3 drops
Chamomile german	5 drops

Blend the essential oils together in a bottle. Shake well. Then dilute when needed with jojoba oil in a 1-to-1 drop proportion. Mix well and apply with a disposable cotton swab directly to the affected area twice a day.

Honey and Aloe Vera HSV-1 Healing Gel

The preparation of this healing gel has several stages. First, combine 1 drop of pure melissa essential oil or manuka essential oil with 2 teaspoons (10 mL) of a good locally sourced honey. Add this to 1 fl. oz. of pure aloe vera gel, and blend well. Then mix together 1 teaspoon of tamanu oil (*Calophyllum inophyllum*) and 1 teaspoon of chaulmoogra oil (*Hydnocarpus laurifolia*), before adding to the honey and aloe vera mix. These two seed extracts are effective at healing sores, reducing skin infection, and reducing inflammation. If you do not have these last two seed oils, then substitute 2 teaspoons of whatever good carrier oil you do have — jojoba (*Simmondsia chinensis*), for example. (Another alternative would be neem oil, although the aroma is not very appealing.) To this healing gel, add 25 drops of the HSV-1 Preventative Blend 2 above, and mix as thoroughly as possible. The healing gel can be used wherever the HSV-1 is found. (Surprisingly perhaps, it is not just found on the lips; the blisters can appear anywhere on the body.)

VIRAL-INDUCED GENITAL SORES: HSV-2

The following gel is not a treatment as such but a soothing method that may have beneficial overall effects. It could be used by women on the outer labia, but not the inner labia, and by men on the shaft of the penis, but not the tip.

HSV-2 BLEND

Geranium	5 drops
Lavender	6 drops
Chamomile german	10 drops
Manuka	7 drops
Melissa	8 drops
Eucalyptus radiata	2 drops

First blend the essential oils in a bottle. Then prepare the base: To 1 fl. oz. of organic aloe vera gel add 1 teaspoon of tamanu oil (*Calophyllum inophyllum*), 1 teaspoon of chaulmoogra oil (*Hydnocarpus laurifolia*), and 1 teaspoon of jojoba oil (*Simmondsia chinensis*). Blend well. Then add 10 drops of the essential oil blend above. Apply a small amount to the affected area with a cotton swab. If you can't obtain the tamanu or chaulmoogra, substitute those 2 teaspoons with jojoba.

The base healing gel above (that is, before adding the essential oils) has a cooling and soothing effect and once made up is a useful base for adding appropriate essential oils for treating all manner of skin infections.

POSTVIRAL RECOVERY

Viruses can be extremely debilitating. Some people never recover and instead slide into a life of fatigue and medical problems that go by the names of *chronic fatigue syndrome* and *chronic fatigue immune dysfunction syndrome*. (This subject is discussed further in chapter 12, "Major Health Concerns," under "Chronic Fatigue Syndrome"; see page 347). Symptoms vary from person to person, which can make diagnosis difficult, and include extreme and constant fatigue, exhaustion after short periods of activity, insomnia, sleeping too long and waking more tired, inability to concentrate, memory loss, feeling something is wrong all the time, irritability, anxiety, depression, muscle pain — myalgia, aching limbs, and tired legs — headaches, flu-like symptoms, sore throat, swollen and tender lymph nodes, chronic cough, digestive problems, bloating, intestinal pain, chest pain, and sensitivity to food, alcohol, heat, cold, light, noise, and certain smells.

Because we are all so busy, it can be tempting to return to work and the usual hectic routine when we've not fully recovered from a virus, but this can be counterproductive. If at all possible, when recovering from a virus it's best to take more time than you need to convalesce rather than less. When we're ill, jobs do pile up and there's more on our desk than normal, but somehow we have to avoid the temptation to go back

to a busy lifestyle and ease into things gently. In the long run, this could benefit your health.

Essential oils can be very useful during this stage of recovery. Choose oils that are strengthening and whose aroma you really enjoy. Use at around 2.5% dilution — that's approximately 15 drops to 1 fl. oz. (30 mL) of carrier oil. Choose essential oils depending on the particular symptoms you experience — see the range of blends below. But also use the essential oils you find uplifting, something to cheer yourself up when you feel tender and in need of support. Rose, neroli, or frankincense can be good options, while some people may prefer cedarwood atlas, or clary sage.

Here are two general body oil blends for postviral recovery. They are followed by symptom-specific blends and suggested essential oils.

Postviral Body Blend 1

Cardamom	2 drops
Orange, sweet	9 drops
Geranium	3 drops
Black pepper	1 drop

Dilute in 1 fl. oz. (30 mL) of carrier oil.

Postviral Body Blend 2

Bergamot	5 drops
Immortelle	4 drops
Lavender	4 drops
Chamomile roman	1 drop

Dilute in 1 fl. oz. (30 mL) of carrier oil.

Muscular Fatigue Postviral Oils and Blend

If you're suffering more from muscular fatigue than from headaches and sore throat, use oils such as sweet marjoram, clary sage, vetiver, plai, ginger, black pepper, or immortelle, combined with either sweet orange, lemon, or grapefruit.

Marjoram	5 drops
Immortelle	5 drops
Orange, sweet	5 drops

Headache Postviral Oils and Blend

If headaches are your main symptom, use lavender, spearmint, basil linalol, sandalwood, or rosemary, combined with mandarin.

Spearmint	5 drops
Lavender	5 drops
Basil linalol	1 drop
Mandarin	4 drops

Digestive Problems Postviral Oils and Blend

If you're suffering with digestive problems, try peppermint, ginger, coriander seed, cardamom, or black pepper combined with grapefruit or sweet orange.

Cardamom	3 drops
Ginger	2 drops
Coriander seed	5 drops
Grapefruit	5 drops

Exhaustion Postviral Oils and Blend

If you're tired or even exhausted the whole time, avoid using oils that stimulate the nervous system and instead choose those that work with it, such as chamomile roman, lavender, clary sage, vetiver, frankincense, petitgrain, or bergamot, and combine with grapefruit or lemon.

Petitgrain	8 drops
Lavender	2 drops
Frankincense	2 drops
Lemon	3 drops

Sleep Regulation Postviral Oils and Blend

To assist with the regulation of sleeping patterns, try valerian, spikenard, patchouli, sandalwood, lavender, or chamomile roman, and combine with sweet orange.

Valerian	2 drops
Chamomile roman	2 drops
Lavender	5 drops
Orange, sweet	6 drops

Memory and Concentration Postviral Oils and Blend

To assist with memory and concentration, try myrtle, rosemary, peppermint, bergamot, or basil linalol, combined with lemon.

Rosemary	5 drops
Peppermint	2 drops
Myrtle	5 drops
Lemon	3 drops

Supportive Oils and Blend for Postviral Symptoms

For additional support, try immortelle, lemon tea tree, sweet marjoram, myrtle, bergamot, grapefruit, coriander seed, neroli, rose, or geranium, combined with mandarin, sweet orange, or grapefruit.

Chamomile roman	1 drop
Geranium	5 drops
Lavender	4 drops
Immortelle	1 drop
Mandarin	4 drops

Throughout this book are discussions of conditions and symptoms that may apply to you. Please look at all those sections and pick out those essential oils that seem most helpful to you. There's a profile of each essential oil in chapter 20 (see page 533).

Broad-Spectrum Antimicrobial Room Sprays, Baths, Gel, and Body Oils

The term *broad spectrum* here applies to any microbe, including bacteria and viruses. Sometimes it's impossible to know what the microbial threats are; you just know that "something is going around" and you don't want to catch it.

Colloidal silver is a known antibacterial agent and is a useful addition to general antimicrobial sprays, creams, and gels. Colloidal silver can be used in sprays in conjunction with lavender or tea tree hydrolats, and it can be incorporated into homemade essential oil waters. Blending colloidal silver in antibacterial creams and gels may lessen its effect somewhat, but it's still worth trying.

BROAD-SPECTRUM ROOM SPRAYS

These blends are designed to counter any microbes that may be in the environment. Prevent the water in the spray from falling onto delicate materials and wooden furniture.

Broad-Spectrum Spray 1

Spearmint	10 drops
Lemon	10 drops
Orange, sweet	10 drops
Basil linalol	4 drops
Thyme linalol	4 drops
Lemongrass	6 drops
Bay, West Indian	6 drops
Juniper berry	5 drops
Niaouli	10 drops

Mix the essential oils together, then add to 4 fl. oz. (120 mL) of warm water. Shake well, and leave to cool. Shake well before each use. If you prefer to use a diffuser, use up to 8 drops of the essential oil mix.

Broad-Spectrum Spray 2

Thyme linalol	10 drops
Oregano	12 drops
Palmarosa	10 drops
Lemongrass	9 drops
Clove bud	4 drops

Dilute the blend of essential oils into 2 teaspoons (10 mL) of distilled white vinegar, then add the mixture to around 3½ tablespoons (50 mL) of warm water in a spray bottle. Shake well, leave to cool, and shake well before each use. If you prefer to use a diffuser, use up to 8 drops of the essential oil mix.

BROAD-SPECTRUM ANTIMICROBIAL GEL

Because it is sometimes more convenient to use a gel than a carrier oil as the base for the essential oils, here's a preventative blend that would suit that medium:

Broad-Spectrum Gel Blend

Manuka	4 drops
Lavender	5 drops
Tea tree	2 drops
Thyme linalol	5 drops
Lemon	8 drops
Geranium	5 drops
Eucalyptus radiata	5 drops
Ravensara	5 drops

First blend the essential oils together. Then add to 2 fl. oz. (60 mL) of pure aloe vera or silica gel. Apply a small amount around the neck area — under the ears to the clavicle on both sides, across the top of the chest, and the solar plexus or abdominal area.

BROAD-SPECTRUM ANTIMICROBIAL BATHS

The following blends of essential oils should be diluted in ½ teaspoon (2½ mL) of a carrier oil before being added to the bath.

Broad-Spectrum Bath Blend 1

Fragonia	1 drop
Niaouli	1 drop
Frankincense	1 drop
Palmarosa	1 drop

BROAD-SPECTRUM BATH BLEND 2

Lavender	1 drop
Lemongrass	2 drops
Coriander seed	2 drops

BROAD-SPECTRUM BATH BLEND 3

Eucalyptus radiata	1 drop
Geranium	2 drops
Ho wood	1 drop

BROAD-SPECTRUM ANTIMICROBIAL BODY OILS

If you are not sure whether the bug you're trying to protect yourself against is a bacteria or a virus, try the broad-spectrum blends below, added to a light carrier oil such as sweet almond. For each application use a maximum of 6–10 drops in 2 teaspoons (10 mL) of carrier oil.

BROAD-SPECTRUM BODY BLEND 1

Fragonia	5 drops
Frankincense	2 drops
Palmarosa	5 drops
Geranium	3 drops

BROAD-SPECTRUM BODY BLEND 2

Clove bud	1 drop
Ravensara	5 drops
Lavender	5 drops
Frankincense	2 drops
Lemongrass	5 drops

Note: Any essential oil with a citrus aroma has the potential to cause photosensitivity, so avoid exposure to the sun after applying those oils in a body oil.

Fungal Infections

The following list of essential oils could be used for fungal conditions. Use them moderately in the first instance, either diluted in a carrier oil or aloe vera gel, using methods that are appropriate to the condition and can be found throughout the book.

ESSENTIAL OILS FOR FUNGAL INFECTIONS

Bay laurel (*Laurus nobilis*)
Caraway seed (*Carum carvi*)
Cardamom (*Elettaria cardamomum*)
Cinnamon leaf (*Cinnamomum zeylanicum*)
Clove bud (*Syzygium aromaticum*)
Coriander seed (*Coriandrum sativum*)
Eucalyptus lemon (*Eucalyptus citriodora*)
Fennel, sweet (*Foeniculum vulgare var. dulce*)
Fragonia (*Agonis fragrans*)
Ho wood (*Cinnamomum camphora ct. linalool*)
Kanuka (*Kunzea ericoides*)
Lavender, spike (*Lavandula latifolia*)
Lemongrass (*Cymbopogon citratus/flexuosus*)
Manuka (*Leptospermum scoparium*)
Marjoram, sweet (*Origanum majorana*)
May chang (*Litsea cubeba*)
Melissa (*Melissa officinalis*)
Niaouli (*Melaleuca quinquenervia*)
Oregano (*Origanum vulgare*)
Palmarosa (*Cymbopogon martinii*)
Patchouli (*Pogostemon cablin*)
Peppermint (*Mentha piperita*)
Rosalina (*Melaleuca ericifolia*)
Rosewood (*Aniba rosaeodora*)
Savory, winter (*Satureja montana*)
Tea tree (*Melaleuca alternifolia*)
Thyme (*Thymus vulgaris*)
Thyme linalol (*Thymus vulgaris ct. linalool*)

Hospitals and Nursing Homes

People who are staying in establishments for health reasons, or simply because they're elderly, can be at risk of infection not only because of possible immunodeficiency but also because of cross-infection. This is a major concern both for management and for those of us who are living in or visiting the establishment, or know a loved one who is. Aside from whatever cross-infection avoidance procedures are in place, there are methods we can use to cut down the risk.

By definition, hospitals and nursing homes are places of multiple occupancy, and using essential oils within them requires a degree of sensitivity because aromas can sometimes evoke an emotional response triggered by factors we know nothing about. For this reason, before using them in a shared environment, ask other patients nearby if they would mind that particular aroma being released. Staff too should be consulted. Obviously, the person most directly involved — the patient — should also be consulted.

ENVIRONMENTAL CLEANSING

The first thing to consider is the cleanliness of the environment. However clean things may look, it is always worth taking a few precautions. Cleansing wipes can be used on any hard surface the patient comes into contact with, including the chair, the rails around the bed, the head of the bed, and the bedside cabinet. Try to clean at least those areas the patient can reach. Think too about places the patient may touch when in the room — for example, when they put their slippers on they may touch the soles. These can be wiped. If possible, wipe the chart that hangs on the end of the bed. All this can be done quickly and discreetly so as not to disturb other patients or staff.

THE BED

One drop of lavender essential oil can be put on bedclothes and around the bed. This is a clear oil and should not cause any damage to the material. If possible, and if the patient requests it, a tissue on which a drop or two of anti-infectious or refreshing oils have been placed can be tucked under the pillow, or put by the side of the bed to purify the air.

CUTS AND SCRATCHES

Open wounds are an open door for micro-organisms and should be covered up as soon as possible. Use a Band-Aid or an adhesive dressing on which a drop of lavender has been placed onto the fabric portion of the dressing before applying.

BATHING

Ordinary fine-grain table salt is a disinfectant in its own right, and essential oils can be mixed with it and used in bathing. For a bath, just drop the essential oil/salt mix into the bath and disperse with the hand. For a shower, wash first and then rub the essential oil/salt mixture gently over the body before rinsing off.

Essential oils can be added to a bottle of natural, organic, unscented shower gel. For a bottle size of around 10 fl. oz. (300 mL), use 10 drops of essential oil. Using this method offers some protection in places that can harbor germs — such as the armpits and groin.

THE NOSE

Micro-organisms often enter the body through the nose, and this is one place where preventative steps can be well worthwhile. Many people simply dab a drop of essential oil around the nostrils before visiting a hospital, and patients can benefit from this method as well. Alternatively, dilute essential oil into a natural ointment, like gel, using no more than 2 drops per each tablespoon, and rub a small amount just around the nostrils. Plain gel is used in this method by hay fever sufferers as they find it traps the pollen, and it may trap micro-organisms in the same way. An easy way to protect the airways is simply to inhale through the nose from a tissue on which 1 or 2 drops of essential oil have been placed. If planning to visit a hospital, prepare your tissue at home, place it in a small, sealable plastic bag, and carry it with you.

URINARY TRACT INFECTIONS

A surprising number of people acquire urinary tract infections when staying in hospitals or nursing homes for the elderly. When I see patients wearing gowns that open at the back being pushed around in wheelchairs, I wonder whether the seat has been cleaned between patients. Wheelchair seats are areas that establishment managers might consider as a potential site of cross-contamination. Catheter use can also lead to infection if proper care is not taken.

The area where the catheter has been inserted can get infected and sore. An appropriate method to use in these cases is to add 3 drops of lavender essential oil to 1 fl. oz. of aloe vera gel and 1 teaspoon (5 mL) of colloidal silver. Mix well together and apply a tiny amount to the affected area.

INFECTIONS OF THE DIGESTIVE SYSTEM

Various bacteria and viruses can cause digestion-related infection, the symptoms of which are usually diarrhea, gas, pain, and abdominal swelling. The following blend can be used whether the problem is bacterial or viral-induced, and would also be helpful in cases of food poisoning.

DIGESTION-RELATED INFECTION BLEND 1

Cardamom	10 drops
Ginger	10 drops
Bay, West Indian	4 drops
Black pepper	5 drops
Thyme linalol	8 drops
Cinnamon leaf	1 drop
Lemongrass	5 drops
Geranium	10 drops
Nutmeg	2 drops

Blend the essential oils together and shake well. This blend can then be used in several ways. First, as a body oil for the abdomen: depending upon the severity dilute 15–20 drops in 1 fl. oz. (30 mL) of carrier oil, or a gel such as aloe vera, or a balm type of base. Apply a small amount over the whole abdominal area in a clockwise direction, then apply over the lower back, at least twice a day. Another method involves rubbing 1 drop of the essential oil blend above on the middle of the sole of each foot, and covering with socks prior to sleep. This method should not be used on the very elderly or on children.

The blend above is effective, but it involves quite a number of essential oils that may not be easily available. So I'm also outlining here a simpler alternative:

Ginger	2 drops
Cardamom	4 drops

Dilute the oil in 1 teaspoon (5 mL) of carrier oil. Apply over the whole abdominal area as well as over the lower back, buttocks, and the backs of the thighs.

In cases of digestive system infection it is often helpful to take the following infusion:

DIGESTION-RELATED INFECTION — INFUSION

Cardamom	1 drop
Peppermint	1 drop
Manuka honey	4 teaspoons (20 mL)

Mix the ingredients together well, then dissolve ½ teaspoon in 1 pint (475 mL) of warm water. Sip as needed to help ease the symptoms. Avoid this method if the digestive system has been damaged.

RESPIRATORY SYSTEM INFECTIONS

Various bacteria and viruses can cause respiratory tract infections, which are often called chest infections. The following blend can be used in several ways. First prepare the synergistic blend:

RESPIRATORY TRACT INFECTION BLEND
Eucalyptus radiata	5 drops
Rosemary	5 drops
Niaouli	10 drops
Cajuput	10 drops
Elemi	5 drops
Fragonia	10 drops
Frankincense	10 drops
Thyme linalol	8 drops
Peppermint	2 drops
Myrtle	5 drops

Blend the essential oils together in a bottle and shake well. This blend can be used in several ways. To make a chest and upper back body oil, use 30 drops to each fluid ounce (30 mL) of carrier oil or gel. Also apply it to the glands in the neck — from under the ears to the shoulder on both sides.

To make a room spray, use 20 drops to each 3.5 fl. oz. (100 mL) of water. One drop of the undiluted blend can also be applied onto the balls of the feet, adjacent to the toes, before putting on socks and going to sleep.

The Respiratory Tract Infection Blend is very effective, but it involves quite a number of essential oils that may not be easily available. So here is a simpler alternative:

Niaouli	2 drops
Myrtle	1 drop
Thyme linalol	2 drops

Add the essential oils to 1 teaspoon (5 mL) of carrier oil and apply over the chest and upper back, and over the glands in the neck — from under the ears to the shoulder on both sides.

If working in a hospital, please see the section on hospitals in chapter 4 (page 70).

4

Occupational Oils for the Working Man and Woman

Most of us have absolutely no control over our working environment. We may be at the mercy of building managers who insist that windows can't be opened, install banks of fluorescent lighting above our heads, and don't maintain air-conditioning systems well. Wireless devices are probably all around us, in the form of interactive whiteboards, cell phones, broadband routers, and wireless PC networks. We could be sitting in a sea of invisible waves, courtesy of the wireless local area network. And I haven't even mentioned the electrosmog.

But no complaining. Think of the traffic officer and city taxi drivers who have no choice but to breathe in untold pollutants day in and day out, or the farm workers who are obliged to inhale quantities of pesticides, or the factory workers breathing in all manner of ultrafine industrial particles, or the hospital workers who maneuver among a plethora of antibacterial-resistant microbes each and every day.

Later on in this chapter we'll be looking at remedies for many of the common illnesses that derive directly from the working environment, finding ways of dealing with preinterview or pretest nerves, and reviewing methods for dealing with stress and burnout. But let's first cheer ourselves up by looking at some of the essential oils that can transform the working environment and make it fit for purpose.

ESSENTIAL OILS TO HELP CLEAR BACTERIA AND VIRUSES
Lemon (*Citrus limon*)
Eucalyptus radiata (*Eucalyptus radiata*)
Ho wood (*Cinnamomum camphora ct. linalool*)
Tea tree (*Melaleuca alternifolia*)
Bay laurel (*Laurus nobilis*)
Niaouli (*Melaleuca quinquenervia*)
Oregano (*Origanum vulgare*)
Bergamot (*Citrus bergamia*)
Cinnamon leaf (*Cinnamomum zeylanicum*)
Ravensara (*Ravensara aromatica*)
Thyme linalol (*Thymus vulgaris ct. linalool*)
Clove bud (*Syzygium aromaticum*)
Geranium (*Pelargonium graveolens*)

ESSENTIAL OILS TO CLEAN UP THE AIR
Lemon (*Citrus limon*)
Grapefruit (*Citrus paradisi*)
Lavender (*Lavandula angustifolia*)
Eucalyptus lemon (*Eucalyptus citriodora*)
Rosemary (*Rosmarinus officinalis*)
Cypress (*Cupressus sempervirens*)

Cedarwood atlas (*Cedrus atlantica*)
Pine (*Pinus sylvestris*)
Lemongrass (*Cymbopogon citratus/flexuosus*)
Petitgrain (*Citrus aurantium*)

ESSENTIAL OILS TO AID FOCUS
AND CONCENTRATION
Basil (*Ocimum basilicum*)
Bergamot (*Citrus bergamia*)
Cardamom (*Elettaria cardamomum*)
Grapefruit (*Citrus paradisi*)
Lemon (*Citrus limon*)
Rosemary (*Rosmarinus officinalis*)
Peppermint (*Mentha piperita*)
Eucalyptus lemon (*Eucalyptus citriodora*)

Essential Oils for the Workplace Environment

Essential oils are not only very helpful in the home environment, they are also invaluable for a variety of reasons in specific working environments, such as the office, the industrial workplace, the hospital, and the land.

THE OFFICE

It's hilarious to think that when computers first arrived in offices people were told to get away from the screen for 10-minute breaks every hour. These days, many of us have several screens on the go at the same time, and nobody's thinking about breaks. Indeed, if the internet connection went down for 10 minutes, we'd be nervous wrecks. We're hooked.

The information age has brought with it a dependency on electrical devices that emit electromagnetic radiation. We're all under electromagnetic stress, and terms like *electrosmog*, *electrohypersensitivity*, and *dirty electricity* are all part of the new vocabulary. The small air ions that benefited human beings in the past are being depleted by electromagnetic fields and replaced by large ions. And there does not seem to be much we can do about it, although there are plenty of products out there purporting to be able to help. Let's hope they can. In the meantime, essential oils are little particles of nature, and by bringing them into the office we may be able to regain some of the natural environment we have surely lost. And we do know they can help in specific ways, including with the symptoms that people report from their offices:

Lethargy: grapefruit, eucalyptus lemon, rosemary, niaouli
Stuffy nose: tea tree, fragonia, eucalyptus radiata, ravensara, thyme linalol
Dry throat: grapefruit, lemon, geranium
Dry and itchy eyes: chamomile roman (in humidifier)
Headaches: lavender, peppermint, basil linalol, spearmint

All these physical problems can affect our sense of well-being and our ability to perform in the workplace. Air-conditioned offices can be too cold for some people, and the equipment is not always well maintained. Faulty humidifiers are literally breeding grounds for bacteria, and we've all heard about the buildings that spread Legionnaires' disease to their unsuspecting occupants. Other contributors to sick building syndrome are dust extractors that give off a discharge, carpet cleaning fluids, the chemicals used in furniture making — like pressed woods, adhesives, foams, and veneers — and poorly maintained photocopiers that emit ozone and nitrogen dioxide. All these things add up until we're working in a soup of hazards that we're most often totally unaware of. Maybe we don't feel too well. Maybe we get sick. But who is going around the office keeping a check on all these things? Seen anybody do that lately?

Looking at an entire street of offices, it's hard to see a single window open. Yet even the manufacturers of flooring and furniture recommend that their products be used in spaces with regular ventilation. We have become reliant on mechanical systems of air cleansing, and our health depends on those systems working correctly. If you work in a small office it might be possible, with everyone's agreement, to have a time of the day when you can open the windows for a short while. In larger offices, this might be difficult to arrange. But there are certain plants that clean up the air — please refer to the "Environmental Issues" section in chapter 1 (page 24) — and few would object to you having a plant on your desk. Plants also offer a natural resting place for eyes usually glued to a flickering screen.

During the winter months, when colds and flu are rife and absenteeism is high, any boss would get his or her money back in a day if they invested in a diffusion system for the office and a few antiviral and antibacterial essential oils. Essential oils can help in other ways to contribute to higher productivity and efficiency while lending a sense of well-being to the office. They can be used singly or in blends — the permutations are almost endless, so experiment. Monday morning might need a different combination than Friday afternoon, for example. Most of the room methods can be used in an office environment; essential oils can be used in small humidifiers, in the room spray method, or in one of the purpose-built office diffusing systems.

In a large, open-plan office, your own personal area can be aromatized, but the fragrance sensitivity of your co-workers will have to be taken into consideration because all aromas have the potential to provoke physical or emotional reactions. You might love the smell of frankincense, but it might remind someone else of an incident they would rather forget. Some people are allergic to synthetic perfumes, while others may be subject to asthma or other breathing problems, and you will have to persuade them that essential oils are different. You do not want to be accused of polluting others' working space. Get feedback on the aromas you would like to use.

The citrus essential oil family, including orange, lemon, grapefruit, lime, mandarin, tangerine, and bergamot, all smell very pleasant, and few people object to them. The citrus oils blend well with most other essential oils; an excellent combination would be grapefruit and lemon with a tiny amount of lavender or a small amount of rosemary. Lavender has natural antibiotic properties and also creates a calm and tranquil atmosphere. Rosemary assists with memory, while grapefruit stops you from falling asleep on your paperwork and lemon helps you focus while cleaning up stale air. Together they smell great, please almost everyone, help concentration, and allow inspiration to take place.

THE INDUSTRIAL WORKPLACE

The industrial environment can be debilitating for a miscellany of reasons. Injury, dust, dirt, and grease are obvious hazards to health, but there are also the hidden effects of low-frequency noise vibration, low-grade radioactivity, and electromagnetic activity. Working with chemicals is dangerous because even if the short-term effects are known and deemed harmless, the long-term effects are seldom quantified. Although health and safety measures usually ensure that adequate ventilation and dust-extraction systems are installed, everyone should be vigilant to ensure they are being properly maintained to work efficiently. This is most especially the case when working in places that deal with heavy metals, such as cobalt and titanium. The history of industry is full of instances in which the hazards of particular processes only became evident many years down the line, when groups of co-workers realized the negative health effects they had been suffering as a consequence.

Most factory floors are too big to utilize the usual room methods when using essential oils. But even if the size of your working space seems daunting, the essential oils can be applied to the corner of a tissue or handkerchief and put in your top pocket or protective clothing, so the corner hangs out and allows the aroma to be released into your own body space.

The essential oils that could be used on the factory floor are those that enhance concentration and focus, such as rosemary, eucalyptus, lemon, and grapefruit. These essential oils can be used singly, with slightly different effects, or in an equal mix. Geranium would be a good addition. If you work in an oily, greasy environment the best oils to use are cedarwood atlas and pine. If noise pollution is the problem, cypress, palmarosa, and lemongrass may help: although essential oils cannot affect the noise, they seem to calm the nervous system so the noise ceases to jar quite so much, and you may come to ignore it.

THE HOSPITAL

The average hospital is like a city — it has many districts and people carrying out a variety of jobs. How much more pleasant this city would be if essential oils were routinely employed to fragrance the environment with their uplifting molecules.

Please refer to chapter 3, "The Self-Defense Kit," which is about the antibacterial, antiviral, and antifungal essential oils, including those for MRSA and other infections. See there the section "Hospitals and Nursing Homes" (page 63).

Essential oils that could be used in a hospital to help avoid bacterial infection — alongside all other preventative methods — are thyme, oregano, fragonia, manuka, tea tree, lavender, geranium, or rosalina. All these are thought to offer some action against bacteria.

As antibiotic and antiviral air fresheners, the essential oils obviously have a positive role to play in any hospital, but they are also used to reduce pain, help patients sleep, and enhance the effect of sedative drugs, thus allowing lower doses to be used. As a side benefit, the aroma of the oils makes the whole environment smell wonderful — surely a great improvement on the usual hospital smell.

Here are some essential oil suggestions that will not only help keep everyone "as well as can be expected," as the saying goes, but also uplift the spirit in their own special, subtle way. Simply use in the room spray method or use in a diffuser.

ANTIVIRAL OILS FOR THE HOSPITAL WARD
Oregano (*Origanum vulgare*)
Manuka (*Leptospermum scoparium*)
Lemon (*Citrus limon*)
Niaouli (*Melaleuca quinquenervia*)
Thyme linalol (*Thymus vulgaris ct. linalool*)
Ho wood (*Cinnamomum camphora ct. linalool*)
Cinnamon leaf (*Cinnamomum zeylanicum*)
Fragonia (*Agonis fragrans*)
Tea tree (*Melaleuca alternifolia*)

If you're on night duty and need something to keep you alert but relaxed, use an essential oil that helps clear the air and has antibiotic qualities too. Geranium helps emotionally, while sweet orange essential oil is calming. Place 1 drop of your chosen oil on boiling water in a mug, and allow the molecules to waft around. Not only will this help you in your office, but it may also soothe the patients in the ward.

A mixture of geranium, lavender, and bergamot will alleviate anxiety and depression, while a mixture of thyme, niaouli, lavender, and grapefruit will keep the staff on their toes, even-tempered, and relaxed, as well as benefiting everyone with its refreshing, uplifting, and stimulating aroma.

THE LAND

Those who work the land have humanity's greatest asset in their hands and under their feet. It's their responsibility to think of the future — for the sake of their children, and ours. Most people now agree that monoculture farming methods that rely on chemicals, rather than the inherent goodness of the land, are bad — not only for the land itself and the workers who have to handle pesticides, herbicides, and fungicides on a regular basis but for the consumers of produce so grown. If you are what you eat, most of us are by now, to some degree or other, part chemical. Intercropping, cultivating so that the natural protective mechanisms of plant life can operate, as well as feeding the land organically so that its nutrient qualities are retained and utilizing the essential oils as guardians against pests, would be the best action for anyone concerned enough about the environment to take personal steps to protect it. For more on the subject, refer to chapter 18, "Gardens for the Future."

Visual Stress and Screen Stress

Our eyes were built for natural light, and for looking at things in a green and pleasant environment some distance away. Watching animals on the horizon and stars in the sky exercised our eyes in a totally different way than the way most of us use our eyes today — surfing the web on our smart phones, close up, trying to read small print for hours on end. Our eyes were not designed for this, so it's no wonder that many of us are today suffering with some form of eyestrain or visual stress.

The most commonly reported symptom of visual stress is the inability to focus, but symptoms can also include blurring; seeing colored lights, black specks, or haze around objects; double vision; burning, soreness, dryness, or aching in the eyes; headaches; tiredness or a feeling of sleepiness; red or watering eyes; bags under the eyes; and the feeling of having something in the eye that never goes away. One of the ways to determine if you have eyestrain or visual stress is to quickly look away from what you're focusing on — a book or screen, for example. If it takes a few seconds to refocus, you could have visual stress.

Even though our eyes are one of our most valuable assets, taking care of them is often put to one side simply because we don't know what we can do to protect them aside from what we do already, including regular checkups with the optician to test our vision and check for structural anomalies inside the eyes and ensuring that our lighting at home and work is as natural as possible.

Lighting is incredibly important. Some forms of industrial or commercial lighting give off a gas that can cause blurring, eye ache, and, for some, disorientation. I know this because it's happened to me in places like department stores and shopping malls. I don't consider myself particularly hypersensitive, but in most stores there just seems to be too much lighting — there will be 200 fluorescent tubes where probably 100 would do. This is certainly a waste of energy, but aside from that, building managers could perhaps think more about how to optimize natural light and use forms of lighting that are gentler on the human eye.

We have little control over the lighting in public and work spaces, but at home you can make sure your lighting arrangements are as good as possible. When reading, for example, the light should be behind you, over your shoulder, and move furniture around to utilize as much natural light as you can.

One way to strengthen the eyes and also relieve eyestrain is to splash them with cold water several times a day. This is also generally refreshing. Bathing the eyes in cold mineral water often helps to relieve soreness: fill a small bowl with water — no tap water — put your face into it, and open and close your eyes several times.

Certain foods and vitamins are said to help alleviate visual strain, including lutein, which is a carotenoid and can be found in dark-green vegetables such as kale, spinach, and broccoli as well as in carrots, beetroot, and some fruits. Also helpful are supplements containing omega 3, evening primrose seed oil, riboflavin (B1), vitamin D, vitamin C, and vitamins E and A, and those containing bilberry (*Vaccinium myrtillus*), which belongs to the same botanical family as blueberry and blackcurrant (*Ribes nigrum*).

Rule number one of using essential oils and aromatherapy is: *never put essential oils in the eye*, even if they are highly diluted in water. When using essential oils around the eyes it is absolutely crucial to follow directions to the letter and ensure that the eyes are very tightly closed. As you cannot be sure that children will keep their eyes closed, the following methods should never be used on children.

If you have visual stress, especially if you are sensitive to commercially available products, the following treatment may help. But again, be very careful to keep the eyes closed throughout. Make an eyelid bath by adding 5 drops of chamomile german (this essential oil should be blue in color) to 2 tablespoons (30 mL) of witch hazel water. Mix well, then add to 8½ fl. oz. (250 mL) of mineral water. Shake very well, then filter through an unbleached paper coffee filter twice. Keep this blend in the fridge for up to seven days. At each use take a tablespoon of the refrigerated mixture and dilute it again in 3½ fl. oz. (100 mL) of water. This is your final dilution. Use about 4 teaspoons (20 mL) of this to soak a small piece of natural material — muslin would be ideal — squeeze out any excess, and place over the eyelids, making sure that you are first comfortably positioned and

ready to rest there for 10 minutes. Your eyes must be kept firmly shut throughout.

If your eyes are really aching and you have a heavy head, soak a piece of natural material in 20 mL of the final dilution and place it over both eyes and the head. Store your pieces of soaked material in the refrigerator or freezer for when they are needed.

Marigold flowers (*Calendula officinalis*) make an excellent addition to the method described above, and although they take a little time to prepare, it's well worth the effort if you're suffering from visual stress. With this method, the order of preparation is somewhat different. Mix the essential oils with the witch hazel water, then add 3 organic marigold heads, if you have them growing in the garden, or 2 teaspoons of organic dried marigold petals. Leave to stand and infuse overnight. In the morning, add the mixture to 8½ fl. oz. (250 mL) of mineral water and leave the bottle to stand in the fridge for at least five hours before pouring through an unbleached paper coffee filter. You will now have a clear liquid that makes an excellent eyelid bath.

Mental or emotional stress also causes eyestrain, and if you can alleviate the stress you may find that the eye problem lessens too. Use the oils listed in the stress section in this chapter to scent the air and relieve tension in your workplace.

The list of complaints from people who use computer screens every day, whether at work or in the home, is long. Some people get a red, flushed, sensitive face after a time, some find that their ears pop, or they get headaches. Just tapping away on a keyboard — especially if the chair is too high or too low — can cause problems to the hands, wrists, arms, shoulders, neck, and back. Some people find working on a screen all day makes their skin sallow or spotty. Some of the problems are understandable — our posture is bad, for example — but some are a mystery. What makes the ears pop? That is just weird, but it happens. Something is going on that we just don't understand. What we do know is that we're now living in an era of ubiquitous electromagnetism, radiation, and microwaves. We can't see, hear, smell, or taste these invisible phenomena, but they weave in and out of us with each breath we take. Another thing is the quality of the ions in the atmosphere, in particular the depletion of negative ions caused by computer screens or air conditioning.

Anyone trying to conceive, or a woman in the early days of pregnancy, may need to think of the screen as a biohazard. Sperm, being the smallest cells in the human body, are vulnerable on all fronts, and research has shown them to be affected by computers (see chapter 9, "The Natural Choice for Men"). In Asia, women are encouraged to wear a special type of apron to protect the fetus from invisible waves from computers. There is not a lot of research in these areas, but it is perhaps something to think about if you and your partner are trying to conceive.

Computer screens are only one contributing factor toward the high positive charge found in many offices. The metal frames of modern office blocks, air conditioning, and fixtures and fittings made of unnatural fibers are other factors. The following essential oils are those recommended for use in the high-tech environment: in any of the room methods, preferably in a diffuser; or for personal spaces try the simple water bowl/mug method.

ESSENTIAL OILS FOR THE HIGH-TECH WORKPLACE
Cypress (*Cupressus sempervirens*)
Cedarwood atlas (*Cedrus atlantica*)
Lemon (*Citrus limon*)
Grapefruit (*Citrus paradisi*)
Orange, sweet (*Citrus sinensis*)
Petitgrain (*Citrus aurantium*)
Niaouli (*Melaleuca quinquenervia*)
Bergamot (*Citrus bergamia*)

Patchouli (*Pogostemon cablin*)
Pine (*Pinus sylvestris*)
Sandalwood (*Santalum album*)
Cajuput (*Melaleuca cajuputi*)

Interviews and Exams

The perfume or aftershave you're wearing when you go for a job interview is a crucial factor in "impression management." The interesting thing is that it makes a great deal of difference whether you're being interviewed by a man or a woman. Generally, men who interview aren't impressed with male candidates who wear fragrances, perhaps because of male rivalry, and, surprisingly perhaps, they can consider women who wear perfume at interviews to be frivolous and unprofessional. Female interviewers are much easier to please and consider light, clean-smelling fragrance an integral part of good grooming. But there are perfumes and there are perfumes, and nobody is going to be impressed if you wear a heavy fragrance that you might also use on a seductive date. If you wear one of those fragrances, you might get asked for a date but you won't get the job.

Clearly, if you want to manage the impression you make, the aroma you wear at an interview is an important component of the overall picture. And because odor alters people's perception of each other on a subconscious level, it might even be more important than the qualifications you have in your hand. "I just didn't like him" or "I just had a bad feeling about her" are pretty wishy-washy reasons to turn a candidate down, but according to research it happens — and with predictable regularity. In view of all this, it might be better not to wear a fragrance at all to interviews — especially if you're a man. But we wear fragrances to please ourselves as well as other people and, most importantly, to give us confidence. Somehow a balance has to be struck, and using essential oils is the perfect way to do it.

Certain essential oils are confidence boosters, and their aromas are subtle, so if they're detected on the subconscious level by the interviewers, they will have their confidence raised too. This is all to the good. In view of what we know about the negative impact of heavy scents, it makes good sense to stick to the light floral or citrus types of aroma, even in shower gels and soaps, so if it's perceived on the conscious level it won't make a negative impression. Rather, you will come across as fresh, clean, and confident. Below is a guideline to the essential oils to use, and not to use. Put a couple of drops on a tissue in your jacket pocket and don't use any other fragrance. And if, sometime later, you ask why you got the job and you're told "We just liked you," don't be surprised!

THE RIGHT OILS FOR THE JOB
Lemon (*Citrus limon*)
Neroli (*Citrus aurantium*)
Bergamot (*Citrus bergamia*)
Geranium (*Pelargonium graveolens*)
Melissa (*Melissa officinalis*)
Petitgrain (*Citrus aurantium*)
Eucalyptus lemon (*Eucalyptus citriodora*)

THE WRONG OILS FOR THE JOB
Rose maroc (*Rosa centifolia*)
Jasmine (*Jasminum grandiflorum/officinale*)
Ylang ylang (*Cananga odorata*)
Vetiver (*Vetiveria zizanoides*)
Lavender (*Lavandula angustifolia*)
Clary sage (*Salvia sclarea*)
Cedarwood atlas (*Cedrus atlantica*)
Cistus (*Cistus ladaniferus*)

Avoid essential oils that are strong relaxants because you want to give a fresh and clean impression that also conveys the idea that you are active and ready to make a positive contribution to the

job. The following blend of oils should help boost confidence, increase your memory, and allow you to concentrate — even if you're a nervous wreck. This is perfect for the morning of an interview or exam.

SAILING THROUGH THE INTERVIEW OR EXAM BLEND
Grapefruit	8 drops
Basil linalol	2 drops
Bergamot	5 drops
Petitgrain	2 drops
Rosemary	3 drops

Mix the essential oils together. Then dilute 2 drops in a teaspoon (5 mL) of carrier oil and drop in your bath before you go to the interview or exam. Or put 2 drops on a wet washcloth and rub all over your body while showering. Inhale the aroma deeply to get the full effect.

The evening before an important interview or exam can be dreadful. The anticipation makes you so nervous you can't sleep. To nip this syndrome in the bud and give yourself the refreshing sleep you need, use the following blend in a bath, followed by a massage:

THE NIGHT BEFORE SWEET DREAMS BLEND
Chamomile roman	2 drops
Geranium	6 drops
Sandalwood	4 drops
Orange, sweet	3 drops

Mix the essential oils together. Then dilute 6 drops in a teaspoon (5 mL) of carrier oil and use in a bath, just before bedtime, and dilute 3–5 drops in each 1 teaspoon (5 mL) of carrier oil to use as a body oil. Have a good rest, and in the morning use the Sailing Through Blend above.

The essential oils of rosemary, lemon, and basil linalol are tremendous for helping you concentrate and think straight, and using one or both essential oils in a room diffuser or by simply inhaling while studying during the week before an exam or presentation will really keep you on the ball. (Note: For children's exams, see the section entitled "The Successful Child" in chapter 7, page 138.)

Self-Hypnosis for Relaxation

Self-hypnosis is a technique of suspending normal consciousness for a limited period of time in order to relax and allow the mind and body to recharge. This state of suspension allows complete relaxation and is extremely revitalizing, even if done for only a few minutes. Some people find it easier than others do, but with practice everyone can achieve it. And once you have mastered the technique, a meditative state can be reached without all the preliminary procedure.

Many jobs are extremely stressful, and many of us need a mental oasis to recoup the mental faculties we lose during the course of the working day. Self-hypnosis for relaxation is as relevant for the commodity broker who would prefer not to be burned out by 30 as it is for the teacher of a rowdy bunch of teenagers or for the busy mother of a toddler.

Certain essential oils can help us master the skill of self-hypnosis for relaxation, when used alone or in blends. Always choose oils you like. The heavier absolute oils tend to give a deeper meditative state than the lighter essential oils.

ESSENTIAL OILS TO FACILITATE SELF-HYPNOSIS
Heavier absolutes
Narcissus (*Narcissus poeticus*)
Osmanthus (*Osmanthus fragrans*)
Hyacinth (*Hyacinthus orientalis*)
Tuberose (*Polianthes tuberosa*)
Lotus (*Nelumbo nucifera*)
Jasmine (*Jasminum grandiflorum/officinale*)

Lighter essential oils
Neroli (*Citrus aurantium*)
Geranium (*Pelargonium graveolens*)
Frankincense (*Boswellia carterii*)
Patchouli (*Pogostemon cablin*)
Clary sage (*Salvia sclarea*)
Vetiver (*Vetiveria zizanoides*)
Sandalwood (*Santalum album*)
Cedarwood atlas (*Cedrus atlantica*)
Spikenard (*Nardostachys jatamansi*)
Benzoin (*Styrax benzoin*)

To practice self-hypnosis, first make sure you're comfortable and still. There should be no noise, at least while you are learning the technique. Place 1 or 2 drops of one of the above essential oils or absolutes onto a tissue and inhale. The absolute oils are expensive, so make sure you actually like the aroma before purchasing.

Focus your attention on an object — something light and bright — and keep concentrating. Slowly count from 1 to 50, while all the time maintaining your focus on that object. Close your eyes now and try recalling the object in your mind, seeing it as clearly as possible. Tell yourself that your eyes are heavy and that you couldn't possibly open them until 5 or 10 minutes have passed. When you open your eyes you should feel at ease and relaxed, able to tackle anything or anyone.

The Whole Brain

Once upon a time, management wanted workers who could carry out routine tasks and just do what they were asked. Today, workers are required to "think outside the box" and "come up with ideas to move the company forward." The question is, are we prepared?

The classic example of someone working with the whole brain is the Italian Renaissance artist Leonardo da Vinci, best known for painting the *Mona Lisa* and the *Last Supper* around 1500 CE. But

Leonardo was not only one of the best artists of all time, he was also, among many other talents, a brilliant mathematician, engineer, and inventor of flying machines, submarines, hydraulics, and weaponry. If he were alive today, Leonardo might enjoy a huge salary as head of the R&D department of a multinational corporation. Actually, he'd probably be the CEO of his own vast corporate empire. Leonardo has been called "the complete man," but we can all to some extent be more complete — capable of doing diverse things and, as a consequence, able to enjoy life and work to the fullest.

What often holds us back are teaching methods that categorize children at an early age as either "arty" or "geeky." Gender assumptions, too, cause children to be ushered down avenues that hinder their potential to flourish. For a variety of reasons, then, the perfect balance between arty and geeky, between athletic and intellectual, can be underdeveloped.

Sport is the one area in which business investors have looked into developing the whole brain. It's very easy to concentrate on rigid training, sports science, and strategy planning. But what makes an athlete exceptional is creativity, verve, and inspiration. In full flight, the well-trained athlete who has been allowed to develop their latent artistry can amaze and delight the crowd. Listen to the sound of the cash register! That's why sport has invested in developing the full person — it pays. But as individuals, we too can invest in ourselves.

The brain has two halves, left and right, known as the *cerebral hemispheres*. There are connections between the two, so they're always communicating. But to some extent, it's thought that the two halves of the brain have different functions. For example, the left side of the brain may be good with appropriate vocabulary, but the right side knows how to deliver that information so it makes sense. The right side delivers the words in

the right tone, with appropriate pauses and an up-and-down pitch. It places the words in a fuller context, cognizant of other information that is pertinent to what is being discussed. The right side is more poetic, yet at the same time it's practical because it sees the fuller picture. On its own, the left side could be bland and boring, but without the left side, the right side could be grammatically incorrect and use inappropriate words. Both sides of the brain are important, and they complement each other. By using the whole brain, we are altogether more impressive and effective.

How do you work on developing your whole brain? Begin by sitting or lying down quietly and imagining a small, glowing colored light in your head. The light can be any color. Place the imaginary light inside your head just over the left eyebrow and slowly allow it to explore all over the left side of your brain. Then imagine it crossing over and exploring the right-hand side of the brain. Allow the light to travel along the midline that separates the left and right brain, and then move the light repeatedly, back and forth, crossing over between left and right. Practice this every day for a few minutes. Also, if you are right-handed try to use your left hand instead, or vice versa.

When you feel harassed at work, picture in your mind's eye a scene of great tranquillity and transfer that scene from one side of the brain to the other, back and forth. This method is also useful for particular ambitions — imagine yourself achieving a job you are trying to get done, whether it is getting through a pile of paperwork, completing a PhD, finishing a quilt, or decorating the house. See yourself with the job finished, complete with satisfied grin, and transfer that image back and forth from one side of your brain to the other. You will find that this simple device can motivate you into getting the job done.

Because schooling does a pretty good job of teaching us correct grammar and vocabulary, we are more likely to fall short in putting what we know in context and turning it into an effective message. This is where the essential oils come in, because some oils, listed below, may assist in developing the right side of the brain. Use 1–4 drops in a room diffuser or in one of the other room methods.

THE RIGHT-SIDE BRAIN TRAIN OILS
Bergamot (*Citrus bergamia*)
Geranium (*Pelargonium graveolens*)
Neroli (*Citrus aurantium*)
Myrtle (*Myrtus communis*)
Petitgrain (*Citrus aurantium*)
Palmarosa (*Cymbopogon martinii*)
Grapefruit (*Citrus paradisi*)
Coriander seed (*Coriandrum sativum*)
Chamomile roman (*Anthemis nobilis*)
Melissa (*Melissa officinalis*)
Rose otto (*Rosa damascena*)

If you want to use one of the brain train blends below, mix the oils together using these proportions and bottle. Then use the drops as required.

RIGHT SIDE BRAIN TRAIN BLENDS

BLEND 1
| Palmarosa | 8 drops |
| Petitgrain | 4 drops |

BLEND 2
| Geranium | 4 drops |
| Grapefruit | 6 drops |

BLEND 3
| Myrtle | 4 drops |
| Coriander seed | 4 drops |

BLEND 4
| Melissa | 6 drops |
| Chamomile roman | 2 drops |

Burns

A hospital burn unit is as likely to see a burn from contact with corrosive materials, electricity, radiation, or boiling liquids as from contact with fire. Many of these cases are the result of accidents at work. The depth and severity of a burn is something that should be assessed by a hospital. The classifications of first-, second-, and third-degree burns depend upon the depth of the burn rather than the area concerned, and sometimes a burn can be more serious than it appears. Electrical burns can be particularly misleading because the damage can extend for some distance beneath the skin. One element of all burns is shock, which can develop some hours after the accident. The degree of shock depends on the size of the burn. Infection is another risk with burns. Diluted essential oils should never be used on a burn, nor should any carrier oils, balms, or other greasy mediums. Using appropriate neat (undiluted) essential oils for burns should only be carried out if the skin is not broken.

ESSENTIAL OILS FOR BURNS
Lavender (*Lavandula angustifolia*)
Chamomile german (*Matricaria recutita*)
Chamomile roman (*Anthemis nobilis*)

Any of the above oils used on their own has a remarkable healing capacity on burns and can be used as a complement to any medical treatment, helping with the pain and in many cases preventing blistering and scarring. Using them in a blend can be even more effective.

ELECTRICAL BURNS

Burns caused by electricity are usually worse than they look, so make sure you get a medical opinion. It is vital to immerse the affected area in cold water as soon as possible. Burns of any description involve a process known as *denaturation*, which is the killing of protein, the material of which living matter is composed. If you can imagine the tissue beneath your skin as egg white subjected to heat, turning from the liquid form to the hard, white form of a cooked egg, you will understand why it is so crucial to stop this process as soon as possible. Keep the burned area in the cold water for a good 10 minutes, even if the pain is subsiding. The point is that you want to get all the heat out of the area as soon as possible to prevent further damage to the living tissue beneath your skin.

On no account put butter or carrier oil on the skin, as this will only keep the heat in and make the burn worse. For mild burns, having cooled the burn in cold water, cover the area with a compress. This can be made from clean gauze, if you have it, or a piece of sterile material. If you can't find something really clean it might be better to use nothing. Soak the material in ice-cold water, add the essential oils to the water, and apply the compress to the burned area. Use 1 drop of essential oil for each square inch of skin affected. Use any of the above essential oils on their own, or the blend given below. If burns are a hazard in your workplace, this blend could be ready and waiting in the first aid box.

Burns Blend

Lavender	10 drops
Chamomile german	10 drops
Chamomile roman	5 drops

Mix together in these proportions, then use as required. As lavender is anti-infectious, this also helps reduce the risk of infection.

Also, take 1,000 mg of vitamin C daily to assist the healing, and homeopathic arnica tablets to alleviate the effects of shock. You'll need to replace the fluids that may have been lost through shock, so have plenty of drinks and if possible include honey, glucose, or sugar in them.

CORROSIVE BURNS

Most workplaces that routinely use hazardous chemicals will have appropriate neutralizing agents available, and in the event of a burn these should be used following the manufacturer's instructions. If these are not available, wash the area thoroughly in cold, running water and follow the advice above for electrical burns.

If no other medical advice or treatment has been advised and if the injury is a light surface burn with no broken skin, use 2 drops of the Burns Blend above to 1 tablespoon (15 mL) of aloe vera and apply to the affected area three times a day. Also see "Burns" in chapter 2, "The Basic Care Kit."

The Back: Aches and Pains

According to the U.S. National Institutes of Health, over 25 million Americans experience frequent back pain. This contributes to the national bill for productivity lost to pain in general, which in 2010 was over $300 billion. American employers also suffer because back pain is the number one reason for compensation claims. Yet nobody has come up with a solution to the problem of chronic back pain. And one of the most exasperating aspects of it is that unless you're actually in spasm, nobody can see that you have a problem, so telling the boss you're in agony and can't come into work can be met with disbelief.

Sometimes back pain is due to specific physical conditions such as a herniated, protruding, or ruptured disk. But more often than not it's localized pain that comes from overstraining the muscles and ligaments — simply the pain of strain. The numerous reasons for back pain include typing for long stretches, a sedentary lifestyle, sleeping on an unsuitable mattress, being overweight, or lifting heavy objects all day long. Problems can result from bad posture, digging in the garden, staggering home with the shopping after a long day's work, or carrying too many heavy school books. Falls and whiplash can reappear as back pain years later, and a number of degenerative diseases cause back pain.

There are many types of back pain: lumbago, which affects the lower back; sciatica, which is caused by inflammation of the sciatic nerve and causes pain in the buttocks radiating out to the thighs and legs — even to the ankles in some cases; fibrositis, tender bundles of fibrous tissues within the muscle; arthritis; spondylosis; curvature of the spine; slipped disks; and pains caused by weak back muscles, weak abdominal muscles, and tension.

One of the best preventative measures for back pain involves strengthening the stomach muscles so that compensatory action doesn't need to be taken by the muscles that support the back. Exercise and stretching is especially important for those with poor posture and muscle tone.

Essential oils can provide wonderful relief from back pain. They penetrate deeply into the tense muscle tissues, encouraging contracted muscles to expand, and they help to increase blood flow to the area, allowing torn fibrous tissues to be repaired by the body.

Essential Oils to Treat Back Pain
Rosemary (*Rosmarinus officinalis*)
Ginger (*Zingiber officinale*)
Camphor (*Cinnamomum camphora*)
Lavender (*Lavandula angustifolia*)
Juniper berry (*Juniperus communis*)
Vetiver (*Vetiveria zizanoides*)
Cypress (*Cupressus sempervirens*)
Peppermint (*Mentha piperita*)
Basil (*Ocimum basilicum*)
Eucalyptus radiata (*Eucalyptus radiata*)
Chamomile roman (*Anthemis nobilis*)
Chamomile german (*Matricaria recutita*)
Plai (*Zingiber cassumunar*)

Cardamom (*Elettaria cardamomum*)
Marjoram, sweet (*Origanum majorana*)
Clary sage (*Salvia sclarea*)
Black pepper (*Piper nigrum*)
Immortelle (*Helichrysum italicum*)
Thyme linalol (*Thymus vulgaris ct. linalool*)

Here are three blends that are very good for alleviating back pain. They can be diluted, or in an acute situation 1 or 2 drops can be applied directly to the affected area.

BACK PAIN BLENDS

Blend 1
Rosemary	10 drops
Marjoram, sweet	10 drops
Immortelle	10 drops

Blend 2
Black pepper	3 drops
Ginger	10 drops
Eucalyptus radiata	5 drops
Juniper berry	3 drops

Mix the essential oils of your chosen blend together, then dilute 4–5 drops to each 1 teaspoon (5 mL) of carrier oil.

Blend 3
Rosemary	8 drops
Peppermint	4 drops
Plai	8 drops
Basil linalol	3 drops
Immortelle	6 drops
Marjoram, sweet	3 drops
Lavender	4 drops

Mix the essential oils together to create this synergetic blend. Then dilute 4–5 drops to each 1 teaspoon (5 mL) of carrier oil.

Massage eases any type of backache and is best accomplished with help. If nobody is available, massaging your lower back yourself is relatively easy, although you will find the upper back more difficult. But the oils can still be applied to the skin, as high as you can reach.

Ice pack application can be an effective method of treating lumbago, sciatica, or fibrositis and is also very helpful on an area that feels inflamed. Everyone is different, however, and some people do find that warm or hot application has a better effect on them. It really depends on each case. Generally speaking, ice packs should be applied to inflamed areas, while warm or hot packs are appropriate for muscular contraction or tension.

Repetitive Strain Syndrome

It seems that the human body was not designed to repeat the same movement over and over again, because when it does so it develops all sorts of problems, from writer's cramp to tennis elbow, and from cell phone fingers to computer game thumbs. *Repetitive strain syndrome* (RSS) is a term used to describe a whole range of conditions that come from continuously using the same joints and muscles, whether typing, packing cases, operating machinery, or picking vegetables in the fields. Overusing particular muscles can result in muscle fatigue, inflammation, and various sorts of damage to the bones, joints, cartilage, tendons, and tissue. Apart from pain and discomfort, stiffness and fatigue can also be part of the experience.

It's essential that the first symptoms of RSS are treated, as neglect may lead in later life to the development of conditions such as arthritis. Lessening your chances of developing RSS can often be achieved very simply by using ergonomic furniture, varying the working posture, and breaking up repetitive actions — although all this is easier said than done. And it's no use getting a new chair if you're still going to slump over the keyboard!

Try to get an accurate diagnosis, as there are other conditions that could be classified as RSS, starting with tenosynovitis — a term often wrongly applied to other conditions in this group.

TENOSYNOVITIS

Inflammation of the fibrous sheaths that enclose the tendons of the hands, wrists, and ankles is known as *tenosynovitis*. When these parts of the body become inflamed there's immediate pain and a dull ache that can travel up the forearms or legs. Other symptoms are cracking and grinding noises, numbness, tingling sensations, stiffness, and increasing weakness. Sometimes the joints swell. Tenosynovitis mainly affects people who use their hands and wrists for long periods of time — dressmakers, carpenters, painters, decorators, and anyone using a keyboard, be that a piano or computer.

Treat this condition as soon as you can. Use an ice pack on the affected area and massage frequently. Make up your own blend from the following oils, or use the suggested blend below.

ESSENTIAL OILS FOR TENOSYNOVITIS
Chamomile roman (*Anthemis nobilis*)
Lavender (*Lavandula angustifolia*)
Eucalyptus lemon (*Eucalyptus citriodora*)
Plai (*Zingiber cassumunar*)
Chamomile german (*Matricaria recutita*)
Juniper berry (*Juniperus communis*)
Eucalyptus radiata (*Eucalyptus radiata*)
Cypress (*Cupressus sempervirens*)
Peppermint (*Mentha piperita*)
Immortelle (*Helichrysum italicum*)
Marjoram, sweet (*Origanum majorana*)

TENOSYNOVITIS BLEND

Peppermint	10 drops
Lavender	10 drops
Eucalyptus radiata	10 drops

Mix the essential oils together to create a blend, then dilute 4–5 drops to each 1 teaspoon (5 mL) of carrier oil.

TENDINITIS

Inflammation of the tendons of the wrists can become a work hazard if the fingers and joints start to lock. As with tenosynovitis, this is a condition that affects people who use the hands a great deal. Symptoms usually start with a tingling numbness in the fingers and hand. Apply an ice pack to the affected area, and massage with one of the essential oils listed below, or use one of the blends that follow.

ESSENTIAL OILS FOR TENDINITIS
Rosemary (*Rosmarinus officinalis*)
Plai (*Zingiber cassumunar*)
Lavender (*Lavandula angustifolia*)
Ginger (*Zingiber officinale*)
Peppermint (*Mentha piperita*)
Eucalyptus radiata (*Eucalyptus radiata*)
Immortelle (*Helichrysum italicum*)
Marjoram, sweet (*Origanum majorana*)
Chamomile roman (*Anthemis nobilis*)
Cypress (*Cupressus sempervirens*)

TENDINITIS BLEND 1

Rosemary	10 drops
Lavender	10 drops
Peppermint	5 drops
Plai	5 drops

TENDINITIS BLEND 2

Cypress	10 drops
Immortelle	10 drops
Ginger	3 drops
Chamomile roman	7 drops

Mix the essential oils of your chosen blend together, then dilute 4–5 drops to each 1 teaspoon (5 mL) of carrier oil.

GANGLION

A ganglion is a benign cyst that attaches to a joint or tendon — usually in the hand, wrist, or feet. People who use their hands for work or who play a lot of sports are particularly prone to develop these harmless but sometimes unsightly swellings that appear on the back of the hand or wrist. Ganglia feel like a round, pliable mass or hard nodule of jelly under the surface of the skin and will move around if pressed. They can be dispersed gradually by gentle massage and essential oils, although it may take a long time. When massaging, concentrate on the nodule only, using firm and slow movements. Do not massage in a rough or hard way. You can make your own blend from the essential oil list below, or use one of the blends that follow.

ESSENTIAL OILS FOR GANGLION
Ginger (*Zingiber officinale*)
Basil linalol (*Ocimum basilicum ct. linalool*)
Juniper berry (*Juniperus communis*)
Patchouli (*Pogostemon cablin*)
Chamomile roman (*Anthemis nobilis*)
Black pepper (*Piper nigrum*)
Cypress (*Cupressus sempervirens*)
Cardamom (*Elettaria cardamomum*)

GANGLION BLEND 1

Ginger	8 drops
Basil linalol	5 drops
Patchouli	10 drops
Juniper berry	7 drops

GANGLION BLEND 2

Juniper berry	10 drops
Cypress	10 drops
Lavender	5 drops
Black pepper	5 drops

GANGLION BLEND 3

Cardamom	4 drops
Black pepper	4 drops
Juniper berry	6 drops
Cypress	10 drops
Ginger	4 drops

Mix the essential oils of your chosen blend together, then dilute 4–5 drops to each 1 teaspoon (5 mL) of carrier oil. Massage a small amount over the ganglion at least three times a day.

WRITER'S CRAMP

You don't have to be a writer to get writer's cramp. Students cramming for exams, dressmakers, composers, engravers, and many others who hold their hand and forearm in one position for a long time are all at risk. The main symptom is a cramp in the hand that makes holding a pen difficult — hence the name — and it can be troublesome enough to bring all work to a halt. Massage is one of the best solutions, and increasing your vitamin D intake and taking a complete vitamin B and calcium supplement may also help.

ESSENTIAL OILS FOR WRITER'S CRAMP
Rosemary (*Rosmarinus officinalis*)
Geranium (*Pelargonium graveolens*)
Hyssop decumbens (*Hyssopus officinalis var. decumbens*)
Cypress (*Cupressus sempervirens*)
Marjoram, sweet (*Origanum majorana*)
Plai (*Zingiber cassumunar*)
Immortelle (*Helichrysum italicum*)
Basil linalol (*Ocimum basilicum ct. linalool*)

WRITER'S CRAMP BLEND

Geranium	10 drops
Hyssop decumbens	5 drops
Cypress	15 drops
Marjoram, sweet	5 drops

Mix the essential oils together to create a blend, then dilute 4–5 drops to each 1 teaspoon (5 mL) of carrier oil. Apply a small amount over the affected area twice a day, or as needed.

TENNIS ELBOW

Repetitive use of a screwdriver can result in so-called tennis elbow as easily as can a few games on the courts. The trouble is caused by straining the muscles, specifically those below and on the outer side of the elbow joint. Pain, stiffness, and swelling are the result. Either heat or cold can bring relief. Place an ice pack, or a heat pack — whichever you personally find more effective — around the elbow. If the pack doesn't have a fastener, attach to the area with a bandage or small towel. Make up your own blend of essential oils from the list below. Massage a small amount of your blend directly into the area, then over the whole arm down to the hand.

ESSENTIAL OILS FOR TENNIS ELBOW
Rosemary (*Rosmarinus officinalis*)
Ginger (*Zingiber officinale*)
Cypress (*Cupressus sempervirens*)
Hyssop decumbens (*Hyssopus officinalis var. decumbens*)
Eucalyptus radiata (*Eucalyptus radiata*)
Black pepper (*Piper nigrum*)
Immortelle (*Helichrysum italicum*)
Basil linalol (*Ocimum basilicum ct. linalool*)

TENNIS ELBOW BLEND

Immortelle	10 drops
Ginger	10 drops
Rosemary	10 drops

Mix the essential oils together, then dilute 4–5 drops to each 1 teaspoon (5 mL) of carrier oil, and massage a small amount directly into the area, then over the whole arm down to the hand.

BURSITIS

This is inflammation of the bursae, small sacks of fluid-filled fibrous tissue encased in membrane whose job it is to reduce friction between the body's moving parts — between bone and ligaments or tendons, for example. There are 160 bursae in the body; problems most often occur in the knee, shoulder, and hip. Bursitis can develop as a result of injury or as a result of repetitive movement often integral to a profession, such as carpet laying or roofing.

An ice pack is very helpful for inflamed bursae. Massage the area using the essential oils listed below — either use one on its own or make up your own blend. Alternatively, use one of the blends that follow.

Essential Oils for Bursitis

Juniper berry (*Juniperus communis*)
Cypress (*Cupressus sempervirens*)
Ginger (*Zingiber officinale*)
Rosemary (*Rosmarinus officinalis*)
Chamomile roman (*Anthemis nobilis*)
Geranium (*Pelargonium graveolens*)
Immortelle (*Helichrysum italicum*)

Bursitis Blend 1

Juniper berry	5 drops
Chamomile roman	10 drops
Cypress	15 drops

Bursitis Blend 2

Marjoram, sweet	10 drops
Immortelle	10 drops
Lavender	10 drops

Dilute the blends by mixing 5 drops to each teaspoon (5 mL) of carrier oil, and use enough to cover the affected area.

TORTICOLLIS (CERVICAL DYSTONIA)

Wry-neck or *twisted neck*, as torticollis is sometimes called, can result from constant awkward neck posture, from an unaccustomed sleeping position, or from carrying heavy objects. Watching the assembly line go by to check for errors is one job that may bring it on, especially if the head is turned to one side. A combination that's bound to cause problems is having the head in a taut position too long while also sitting in a draft of cold air — this can cause the head to get stuck in one very uncomfortable position. Some people develop torticollis after a vehicle accident, while for others it develops for no apparent reason.

Several muscles are involved in torticollis. Generally, it's the two sternomastoids — the large muscles at the side of the neck that extend on either side behind the ear down to the sternum and clavicle and the trapezius muscles. To the area that causes the most discomfort apply an ice pack, followed by a warm towel. The cabbage-leaf treatment also helps a great deal (see page 182). Massage with the essential oil blend below, or make your own from the following list:

Essential Oils for Torticollis

Rosemary (*Rosmarinus officinalis*)
Basil linalol (*Ocimum basilicum ct. linalool*)
Thyme linalol (*Thymus vulgaris ct. linalool*)
Marjoram, sweet (*Origanum majorana*)
Chamomile roman (*Anthemis nobilis*)
Plai (*Zingiber cassumunar*)
Immortelle (*Helichrysum italicum*)
Lavender (*Lavandula angustifolia*)

Torticollis Blend

Marjoram, sweet	10 drops
Basil linalol	5 drops
Rosemary	15 drops
Immortelle	5 drops

Mix the essential oils together, then dilute by mixing 4–5 drops to each teaspoon (5 mL) of carrier oil.

The Workaholic Heart

If you answer "yes" to the following questions, you are a workaholic: Do you think you're the only one who can do the job properly? Do you overanalyze your work when you're supposed to be relaxing? Are you neglecting your family, friends, and hobbies? Are you tired all the time? Do you chew over the day's work when you go to bed and then find it hard to fall asleep?

Workaholics have to learn to say "no." Enough is enough. Practice saying the following: "The world will not come to a grinding halt if I don't work late tonight," "I'm going home now," "I'm turning this PC off right now," and "I'm not going to check my emails until I get back to work in the morning."

Being a workaholic is like any addiction — there's always someone around who will convince you to join them in this obsessive behavior. They will phone you at 11 o'clock at night to have a conversation about work — and it's interesting, and it may seem important. That's what you tell yourself. But resist the trap. There is such a thing as a work-life balance.

There's no denying that the pressure is on to become better and faster than anyone else, to absorb ever more information…just in case it's needed. Competition is fierce, and no matter how young you are, there's always someone younger, with perhaps more drive and ambition than you. It's difficult to be laid back when these determined and talented people have their eyes on your job. So the pressure is on — and it's on your heart.

Essential oils may help you cope and calm you down, but you have to be prepared to help yourself too. You really must carve out some time during the week to give your heart a complete rest and recharge. Having a regular aromatherapy treatment is a good way of doing this, or start regular energy-balancing exercise like qi gong, tai chi, or yoga. At the very least, learn to relax. Ask someone to massage you, or if that's too passive for you, massage your partner instead using gentle, rhythmic movements — none of that hard pressure, controlling type of massage.

The following essential oils suit workaholics because they can be gently stimulating while many of them also have relaxant properties. Perhaps you can think of it in terms of people — some are intellectually stimulating while at the same time you feel completely relaxed in their company. A minister or guru might be the kind of person who falls into this group, or a very dear and bright friend. So these are the workaholic's essential oil friends — use them anytime, anywhere, and anyhow:

The Workaholic's Oils
Geranium (*Pelargonium graveolens*)
Basil linalol (*Ocimum basilicum ct. linalool*)
Lavender (*Lavandula angustifolia*)
Petitgrain (*Citrus aurantium*)
Marjoram, sweet (*Origanum majorana*)
Cypress (*Cupressus sempervirens*)
Sandalwood (*Santalum album*)
Cedarwood atlas (*Cedrus atlantica*)
Myrtle (*Myrtus communis*)
Orange, sweet (*Citrus sinensis*)
Lemon (*Citrus limon*)

And here is a blend for the bath:

The Workaholic's Bath
Petitgrain	5 drops
Lavender	1 drop
Geranium	1 drop

Dilute in an equal amount of carrier oil before adding to the bath, and disperse with your hand. This blend could also be used as a body oil by diluting in 2 teaspoons (10 mL) of carrier oil.

You could use this in the morning bath, of course, but it's better to do the whole treatment after work when there is a better chance you may be thinking of relaxing. Lie back in the bath and enjoy the sensation of the water. Breathe deeply. Once out of the bath, apply a body oil using essential oils diluted in a carrier oil or added to a pure, unscented body lotion.

THE WORKAHOLIC'S BODY OIL BLEND

Petitgrain	5 drops
Lavender	10 drops
Geranium	5 drops
Lemon	5 drops
Orange, sweet	5 drops
Niaouli	2 drops

Mix the essential oils together, then dilute by adding 4–5 drops to each teaspoon (5 mL) of carrier oil or unscented lotion, and use as a body oil.

Although workaholics generally have a neat and tidy appearance, their internal physiology isn't always in such terrific shape. Skin care is often neglected, and workaholics often develop dry skin and greasy hair because of the stress (see chapter 13, "The Fragrant Way to Beauty"). A good, nutritionally balanced diet is a must; too many people eat junk food at their desk. Cut out sugary foods and reduce red meats. Try to eat as many fresh green vegetables and raw salads as possible. Take a good all-round multivitamin and mineral supplement, not forgetting essential fatty acids such as omega 3, 6, and 9. Drink plenty of water, and ease back on the sugar, coffee, and alcohol. Just try to remember that you'll need your body longer than you'll need that job!

Stress at Work

There's a world of difference between positive stress, normal stress, and distress. Positive stress can be described as a "high," the excited tension you get when performing your job quickly and efficiently. It is this kind of high that makes people enjoy working in the first place: the sheer joy of accomplishing something, whether that's whizzing through the emails or closing the contract that'll save the company from bankruptcy. Positive stress helps us to aim a little bit higher, to leap over the hurdles life presents to each and every one of us, and it gives us the force to take on life's challenges. This is the kind of energy that increases stimulation, helps our energy level, and makes creativity flow. So not all stress is bad.

Normal stress is a state during which the body performs its functions for survival in response to circumstances. For example, when you have a car accident the body is flooded with adrenaline, which causes all kinds of physical phenomenon — everything can go into slow motion, for example, or pain is not felt. This out-of-the-ordinary stress increases your capacities and efficiency. Your heart may be pounding, you're shaking all over, but somehow you manage to walk away from the vehicle and phone for help. "I don't know how I did it," you say later, looking at the gash in your leg. But your instinctive survival mechanisms took over and enabled you to do what had to be done at the time. These normal stress mechanisms are good — very good. They're there when we need them.

Distress, however, is an altogether different thing. This is when the mechanisms within us to deal with stress become chronically overused, and as a result we have no energy and no will, only frustration at the ever-increasing pressure we're under. Irritability, insomnia, and worry are characteristic of distress.

Everyone suffers from stress at some point in their lives, and it can come about for a variety of reasons. In this section we shall look at environmental stress, chemical stress, physical stress, mental stress, and emotional stress. These come in various degrees, which need different approaches. These different types of stress can exacerbate each other, so, for example, the environmental stress you suffer at work can cause mental stress, which, when taken home, can lead to emotional stress. So stress is not a straightforward subject, yet it is one in which essential oils can help. Use the essential oils listed below in room and inhalation methods.

Environmental stress is caused by, for example, bright lights over your desk, the noise of machinery, the buzzing of PCs, the constant ringing of phones, endless texts and messaging on your cell phone demanding your attention, a cramped office space, or inadequate ventilation.

ESSENTIAL OILS FOR ENVIRONMENTAL STRESS
Cedarwood atlas (*Cedrus atlantica*)
Chamomile roman (*Anthemis nobilis*)
Coriander seed (*Coriandrum sativum*)
Geranium (*Pelargonium graveolens*)
Cypress (*Cupressus sempervirens*)
Lemongrass (*Cymbopogon citratus/flexuosus*)
Marjoram, sweet (*Origanum majorana*)
Frankincense (*Boswellia carterii*)

Chemical stress is caused by, for example, too many cups of coffee, too many lunchtime drinks, too much junk food, too many prescribed drugs, vehicle pollution on the way to work, or chemicals and gases given off by a variety of office equipment and even some types of commercial lighting.

ESSENTIAL OILS FOR CHEMICAL STRESS
Lavender (*Lavandula angustifolia*)
Clary sage (*Salvia sclarea*)
Patchouli (*Pogostemon cablin*)
Grapefruit (*Citrus paradisi*)
Petitgrain (*Citrus aurantium*)
Lemon (*Citrus limon*)
Geranium (*Pelargonium graveolens*)
Rosemary (*Rosmarinus officinalis*)

Physical stress is caused by, for example, constant physical work, pushing your body to the limits, running in the office Fun Run, working out at the gym, or driving long distances.

ESSENTIAL OILS FOR PHYSICAL STRESS
Rosemary (*Rosmarinus officinalis*)
Bergamot (*Citrus bergamia*)
Chamomile roman (*Anthemis nobilis*)
Thyme linalol (*Thymus vulgaris ct. linalool*)
Geranium (*Pelargonium graveolens*)
Marjoram, sweet (*Origanum majorana*)
Fennel, sweet (*Foeniculum vulgare var. dulce*)
Lavender (*Lavandula angustifolia*)

Mental stress is caused by, for example, financial worries, a heavy workload, trying to achieve, anguish over uncompleted jobs, or unemployment.

ESSENTIAL OILS FOR MENTAL STRESS
Geranium (*Pelargonium graveolens*)
Bergamot (*Citrus bergamia*)
Lavender (*Lavandula angustifolia*)
Grapefruit (*Citrus paradisi*)
Sandalwood (*Santalum album*)
Cardamom (*Elettaria cardamomum*)
Basil linalol (*Ocimum basilicum ct. linalool*)
Patchouli (*Pogostemon cablin*)

Emotional stress is caused by, for example, bullying at work, colleagues' jealousy or ambition, fear of losing your job, relationship problems due to working too much, or an inability to express how you feel.

ESSENTIAL OILS FOR EMOTIONAL STRESS
Geranium (*Pelargonium graveolens*)
Vetiver (*Vetiveria zizanoides*)
Sandalwood (*Santalum album*)
Rose otto (*Rosa damascena*)
Palmarosa (*Cymbopogon martinii*)
Cardamom (*Elettaria cardamomum*)
Bergamot (*Citrus bergamia*)
Ylang ylang (*Cananga odorata*)

Also see the section on "Essential Oils for Emotional Problems" in chapter 5, "Emotional Rescue."

STRESS LEVELS

Different types of stress occur in varying degrees, and the oils and blends recommended take these levels of stress into consideration. Identify the degree of your stress from the categories in table 5 below. Then choose from the oils and blends that most closely fit the description of your individual needs. Treat the first level before it develops into the second, the second before it develops into the third, and so forth. Mental health is as precious as physical health; indeed, the sharp distinction so often drawn between the two is misleading. The human being works as an integrated unit of body, mind, and spirit, and to take care of one is to take care of the other.

In the blends that follow in tables 6 (page 88) and 7 (page 89), levels 1 and 3 are grouped together because they both need sedatives and relaxants. At Level 2, however, you need something that will add an element of stimulation to prevent you from slipping into Level 3. This is to get you out of the quagmire and motivated, and to stimulate your immune system to prevent infection.

Only those blends at Level 2 (table 6) and the essential oils listed in the "Stimulants" section on page 90 could be used with permission in an open workspace. All the blends and oils can be used in the atmosphere at work if you have your own office, and in any other method you choose.

At all levels of stress, a bath or shower using essential oils after work every night can help. Use 6–8 drops of your favorite blend or oil in a bath, or take a long, hot shower using 3–4 drops of essential oil on a washcloth. You could also make a

TABLE 5. LEVELS OF STRESS

LEVEL	SYMPTOMS
LEVEL 1	Tiredness, worry over inability to finish tasks, irritability with colleagues, headaches, insomnia
LEVEL 2	All the above plus: feeling tired all the time, depression, chronic aches, feeling uncomfortable at work, being argumentative, paranoid thoughts about co-workers
LEVEL 3	All the above plus: increased depression and insecurity, persecution complex, inability to contribute to tasks, ever-increasing absences from work, starting to resent colleagues who are successful, feeling physically ill, in pain at the very thought of work
LEVEL 4	All the above plus: Now the body-mind connection is really in overdrive and crying for help. Immune function is low and susceptible to airborne infections; you're in meltdown — unable to cope with any kind of work task, unable to accept any criticism without getting angry, in danger of losing employment but not caring, just wanting everyone to go away, increased physical symptoms.

body oil to use before going to work. Any of the room methods can be used at home, and at work a good solution is to have a bottle of oils ready in a tiny spray bottle so you can spray your personal workspace when it's convenient, or use 1 drop of your blend on the soles of your feet. You could also use the tissue or handkerchief method, or just sniff the open bottle. I know company directors who carry a little bottle of their diluted blend and put a little on their upper lip, under their nose, to keep calm when trying to close a deal.

Because the oils for Stress Level 1 are grouped with those for Level 3, we start with the Level 2 blends. Blends of essential oils can be made up using the following proportions, then diluted for the method you're using, as shown in the "Methods of Use" chart (table 2) in chapter 1 (see page 14).

TABLE 6. STRESS LEVEL 2 BLENDS

FOR GENERAL USE					
BLEND 1		BLEND 2		BLEND 3	
Oil	*Amount*	*Oil*	*Amount*	*Oil*	*Amount*
Bergamot	9 drops	Grapefruit	15 drops	Neroli	7 drops
Geranium	11 drops	Rosemary	11 drops	Lavender	3 drops
Ginger	10 drops	Palmarosa	5 drops	Lemon	20 drops
FOR SPECIFIC USES					
APATHY/HELPLESSNESS		DEPRESSION		ANXIETY	
Oil	*Amount*	*Oil*	*Amount*	*Oil*	*Amount*
Grapefruit	15 drops	Geranium	15 drops	Lavender	10 drops
Rosemary	10 drops	Lavender	5 drops	Geranium	10 drops
Lavender	5 drops	Bergamot	10 drops	Palmarosa	10 drops
MUSCULAR PAIN		INFECTIONS, UNEXPLAINED ACHES, AND CHILLS		DIGESTIVE PROBLEMS	
Oil	*Amount*	*Oil*	*Amount*	*Oil*	*Amount*
Lavender	10 drops	Lavender	10 drops	Coriander seed	15 drops
Rosemary	5 drops	Ginger	15 drops	Grapefruit	10 drops
Cypress	15 drops	Cardamom	5 drops	Cypress	5 drops

TABLE 7. STRESS LEVELS 1 AND 3 BLENDS

FOR GENERAL USE					
BLEND 1		BLEND 2		BLEND 3	
Oil	*Amount*	*Oil*	*Amount*	*Oil*	*Amount*
Clary sage	15 drops	Marjoram	15 drops	Petitgrain	17 drops
Lemon	10 drops	Chamomile roman	5 drops	Orange, sweet	5 drops
Lavender	5 drops	Lemon	10 drops	Nutmeg	3 drops
FOR SPECIFIC USES					
TIREDNESS		IRRITABILITY		HEADACHES	
Oil	*Amount*	*Oil*	*Amount*	*Oil*	*Amount*
Lemon	10 drops	Clary sage	10 drops	Lavender	10 drops
Clary sage	5 drops	Orange, sweet	10 drops	Chamomile roman	10 drops
Lavender	15 drops	Petitgrain	12 drops	Geranium	10 drops
INSOMNIA		DEPRESSION		FEARS	
Oil	*Amount*	*Oil*	*Amount*	*Oil*	*Amount*
Marjoram	9 drops	Geranium	15 drops	Rose otto	15 drops
Vetiver	8 drops	Bergamot	5 drops	Chamomile roman	10 drops
Orange, sweet	14 drops	Frankincense	2 drops	Frankincense	5 drops
DESPAIR		GUILT		LOW IMMUNITY	
Oil	*Amount*	*Oil*	*Amount*	*Oil*	*Amount*
Rose maroc	15 drops	Sandalwood	20 drops	Niaouli	10 drops
Petitgrain	10 drops	Chamomile roman	5 drops	Lavender	4 drops
Neroli	5 drops	Clary sage	5 drops	Ravensara	8 drops

MAKING YOUR OWN BLENDS
TO TREAT STRESS

In addition to using the suggested stress blends above you can design your own blends. The essential oils can be used singly or, for the home practitioner, in a blend to a maximum of three oils. You will see that four oils, marked with an asterisk, appear on both of the following lists — for stimulants and sedatives. These are "adaptogens," which vary their action depending on an individual person's physiological and psychological reaction to stress.

Stimulants

Although these are particularly useful in the Level 2 type of stress, to motivate and stimulate, they can be used in the other levels too.

STIMULATING ESSENTIAL OILS
Bergamot (*Citrus bergamia*)
Grapefruit (*Citrus paradisi*)
Lavender (*Lavandula angustifolia*)★
Rosemary (*Rosmarinus officinalis*)
Lemon (*Citrus limon*)★
Geranium (*Pelargonium graveolens*)★
Cypress (*Cupressus sempervirens*)
Neroli (*Citrus aurantium*)★
Coriander seed (*Coriandrum sativum*)
Palmarosa (*Cymbopogon martinii*)
Ginger (*Zingiber officinale*)
Cardamom (*Elettaria cardamomum*)

Sedatives/Relaxants

Although these oils are particularly useful in treating Levels 1 and 3, they can be incorporated into a blend using the oils for Level 2, stimulants, listed above.

Vary the dosages according to the level of stress. If blending for Level 4, for example, use an increased dosage. So whereas you might use a maximum of 30 drops of essential oil diluted in 1 fl. oz. (30 mL) of carrier oil to prepare a bottle of body oil for a Level 2 degree of stress, use a maximum of 40 drops if blending for Level 4. Use only a small amount, 1 teaspoon (5 mL), for each application.

Also use the oils more often if suffering at higher levels of stress, and reduce the frequency when the condition improves.

SEDATING/RELAXING ESSENTIAL OILS
Nutmeg (*Myristica fragrans*)
Geranium (*Pelargonium graveolens*)★
Marjoram, sweet (*Origanum majorana*)
Lemon (*Citrus limon*)★
Lavender (*Lavandula angustifolia*)★
Sandalwood (*Santalum album*)
Neroli (*Citrus aurantium*)★
Clary sage (*Salvia sclarea*)
Rose (*Rosa damascena/centifolia*)
Petitgrain (*Citrus aurantium*)
Vetiver (*Vetiveria zizanoides*)
Chamomile roman (*Anthemis nobilis*)
Chamomile german (*Matricaria recutita*)

STRESS MANAGEMENT AT WORK

Many CEOs of large corporations have realized that stress is eating into their profits. Not only does it cause a huge loss in terms of days taken off for sickness — for stress itself and for conditions exacerbated by stress — but a workforce worn down by stress cannot be as creative and innovative as businesses operating in the global marketplace now need to be. Some managers have introduced flex-time scheduling, a "no work emails after hours" policy, and meditation rooms for staff.

Unfortunately, however, most managers are pretty hopeless at creating a company where all staff can be happy and stress-free. Management is key, not only for how a company runs and how much profit it makes but also for the well-being of its staff, and if your workplace is not up to scratch, maybe you could think about moving to another company. Of course it's difficult to relocate, but searching for a new job is something that can be done in a low-key kind of way, and the process will give you the hope that one day you'll be working in a company that isn't intent on driving you into the ground.

Think laterally about the career you're currently in. Do you enjoy your job, and are you good at it? If you are, that's great. But if you have doubts, maybe there is something else you would prefer to be doing. Perhaps you could enter a new occupation — one that gives you pleasure and fulfillment. People can have all the wealth in the world and still be miserable. You may earn less in your new career, but you may smile more. That's worth a lot.

Studies have shown that most workplace stress is caused by jobs in which high demands are made of the workers, but over which they have little or no control. Firefighters fall into this group, as do police officers, cooks, and waiters. People who work and also have children additionally have the stress of never having guaranteed control over their childcare: What happens if Grandma can't look after the baby today? What happens if the school bus doesn't arrive? What if I get called out of work because little Billy has taken sick? There's stress in contemplating what *might* go wrong, as well as stress when things *do* go wrong. The work situation for many people is characterized by a lack of choice, not the least of which is having no choice about where and when we work; we have to arrive at a particular location by a particular time. Every morning millions of us subject ourselves to tremendous stress just waiting for transport, or sitting in the car in traffic jams. Before the clock strikes nine, people all over the country are already a bundle of nerves!

Suffering from work-related stress is in no way an indication of incompetence. Far from it. Indeed, it's very often those who volunteer for the front line in the "battle of the bucks" who incur the greatest injury through stress because that's where the pressure is greatest. As all our mothers told us, it takes hard work to succeed — and that takes its toll. But who can say whether it's more stressful to be a failure, or to clamber up the ladder of success.

Although using essential oils can help to alleviate the inevitable stress we suffer, there are also many effective relaxation techniques to try, and counseling services to help you sort out your problems. A monthly massage or aromatherapy treatment helps many people to keep on an even keel. Sport and exercise can help tremendously, and those people working out at the gym may be effectively working off the tension they took on at work. Find some time too for your real friends. Maintain the vital links of friendship and you overhaul life's safety net.

Take care of your body. Check your diet and cut down on tea and coffee, which often lead to nervousness and headaches. Take a good multivitamin and mineral supplement. Get some fresh air whenever you can, because the effect of stress can deplete you of oxygen and make you feel sluggish and getting out and about can be a great tonic. Enjoy the world. It's not all about struggle and work. Laugh as much as possible — laughing boosts endorphin levels and makes you feel good. It's true that laughter is the best medicine. Also, refer to chapter 5, "Emotional Rescue," and use essential oils to treat your individual physical symptoms — see the index.

PERFORMANCE STRESS

Performance stress can be caused by onetime events or by the nature of the job. The idea of giving a presentation at a workshop, presenting the company's annual report to the shareholders, giving a presentation to a prospective client, or speaking at a conference induces tremendous stress in some individuals and at least a little stress in most of the rest of us. People who perform in front of others as part of their job often suffer from performance stress every day. When they walk on the stage, performers know there are hundreds if not thousands of people watching their every move and aware of their every mistake. For most performers, exactness is expected of them, whether it's in the notes they play, the dance steps they take, or the words they say. Almost all performers have the added stress of not knowing whether they will still be working in six months' time and able to pay the bills.

Yet giving a performance requires a certain amount of stress. Many maintain that having stage fright before a performance is necessary to provide the sort of energy that enables them to do a good job. The essential oils listed below can help dissipate the sort of stress that undermines the confidence needed to perform, while allowing the positive stress to fuel a good performance.

Essential Oils for Performance Stress
Bergamot (*Citrus bergamia*)
Rosemary (*Rosmarinus officinalis*)
Coriander seed (*Coriandrum sativum*)
Ginger (*Zingiber officinale*)
Neroli (*Citrus aurantium*)
Grapefruit (*Citrus paradisi*)
Palmarosa (*Cymbopogon martinii*)
Rose otto (*Rosa damascena*)
Benzoin (*Styrax benzoin*)
Clary sage (*Salvia sclarea*)
Lemon (*Citrus limon*)

Performance Blend 1
Bergamot	10 drops
Palmarosa	15 drops
Clary sage	5 drops

Performance Blend 2
Patchouli	3 drops
Petitgrain	10 drops
Orange, sweet	10 drops

Performance Blend 3
Cedarwood atlas	10 drops
Bergamot	5 drops
Orange, sweet	3 drops

Combine the essential oils in your chosen blend, then use 3–4 drops in a bath, diluted in a little carrier oil, or 1 or 2 drops in the shower on a washcloth before a performance, inhaling deeply while you do so. If making a body oil, use 5 drops of essential oil to 1 teaspoon (5 mL) of carrier oil.

Often it's more helpful to make up your own blend from essential oils you love to smell, choosing from the list above. Some actors just love the aroma of cedarwood atlas, while others like ylang ylang — it's all a matter of how an aroma makes you feel.

Add a drop to a tissue to take with you and inhale when needed. The essential oils can also be used diluted in water and put into a small spray bottle and sprayed around the dressing room. Ensure that the water droplets don't fall on electrical equipment. Or apply a drop of the blend to the soles of the feet.

BURNOUT

Well, you've done it. You've worn yourself to a frazzle and the cells that haven't seized up have gone on strike. The plant has been shut down. Congratulations! Instead of charging around achieving four things at once, rising at five AM and working until 10 at night, you're now incapacitated by overwhelming fatigue. Relaxation is impossible as your mind goes around in circles, getting nowhere fast. You seem to be a different person and are beginning to think you're cracking up. Your energy is completely and utterly depleted, and you wonder if you'll be able to put a cup under the coffee machine, let alone get through the day.

Burnout is exactly what it sounds like and happens when the body and mind have been under stress for a long time. No one is safe from burnout in this age of increasing pressure, information overload, and being constantly available through text messages and emails. It is vital to build up your energy stores to avoid exhaustion in whatever way you can. Reduce stress and tension, learn to relax more, and let things go. At least breathe in a way that will slow down your pulse rate. Open a window or take a walk in the park, walk barefoot on dewy grass, or stand with your back against a tree. Inhale, and take in large volumes of air, slowly filling the lungs, then exhale slowly. Self-hypnosis is a good way of reaching into what is out of your conscious control and can be used at any time of the day (see "Self-Hypnosis for Relaxation" in this chapter). Lessen your workload wherever possible, and start and finish work at preordained times. Don't let anything interfere with this resolution — work can wait. You have only one body and one mind.

Burnout Relaxation Blend

Sandalwood	8 drops
Palmarosa	5 drops
Lemon	9 drops

Mix together using these proportions. Use this blend in any of the room methods, or add 3–4 drops to the bath. Make a body oil using a maximum of 5 drops of essential oil to each 1 teaspoon (5 mL) of carrier oil and ask a friend to massage you or simply apply it to your body or to the soles of your feet yourself.

To revive yourself at any time, use the following blend in any of the room methods, in the bath (4–6 drops), or in the shower. A foot bath is extremely effective — use 2–3 drops — or make a body rub using 3–5 drops to each 1 teaspoon (5 mL) of carrier oil.

Burnout Reviver Blend

Lavender	5 drops
Eucalyptus radiata	8 drops
Grapefruit	7 drops
Rosemary	4 drops
Peppermint	2 drops

Mix together using these proportions.

After a warm bath, splash yourself all over with an ice-cold reviver. Make up a splash by adding 3 drops of rosemary to 3 teaspoons (15 mL) of witch hazel, then adding this mixture to 5 fl. oz. (150 mL) of water and pouring through an unbleached paper coffee filter. Bottle this blend and keep it refrigerated so it's always cool when you require it. Shake the bottle well and splash all over your body.

Tired eyes respond well to eye pads that have been soaked in an equal mix of cold water and witch hazel, and then squeezed out. See also the section "Visual Stress and Screen Stress" in this chapter, on page 71.

(5)

Emotional Rescue

Emotions are like the winds — we can feel them, but not see them. The wind may be a warm breeze that embraces us, or a hurricane that leaves devastation in its wake. Emotions are not like the physical body, which we can see and explain — the muscles lift the bones, the heart pumps the blood, and so forth. To a large extent, the body is a machine. The mind, to a large extent, drives that machine — it can tell the tired muscles to climb out of bed, for example. The emotions, on the other hand, are something of a mystery. We can't see them, and although we may suspect they're behind a lot that we do with our physical body and know they often inform the decisions we make in our mind, they're more elusive. You can walk into a room and feel the emotions of another person. You may not be able to see their face or read anything in particular from their body language, but emotions seem to emanate into the larger space around a person. When someone says, "You could have cut the atmosphere with a knife," they're not talking about the ideas that were being expressed in that room, but the emotions behind them.

It would be good to think that childhood is a time of carefree joy and that it's only when we're faced with the reality of adult responsibility that stress and anxiety begin. Unfortunately, though, behind many smiling childhood photos lie experiences that bring sadness and pain, not only during those younger years but throughout adulthood too. And it's especially hard to shake off the negative experiences of youth, which can feel embedded in our cellular memory.

Once adulthood begins, life can seem like a race of hurdles, one after the next, a series of challenges unique to each of us. Few people live a charmed life. It seems instead that most human beings have to face challenges, one after the other. This is the human condition, and accepting that may be the first step to good mental health. The next step is to accept that it's the mind that lifts us over the hurdles, which is why taking care of our mental and emotional health should be a priority.

This chapter is divided into two sections. The first looks at ways essential oils can help with some particular emotional problems: stress, anxiety, depression, moodiness and mood swings, trauma, and bereavement. The second section, "Essential Oils for Life Enhancement," is all about enhancing your experience of life, with suggestions for mindfulness, positivity, confidence, concentration, self-esteem, assertiveness, and happiness. These are just a few of the areas in which essential oils can help a person with regard to mind, mood, and emotion that I cover much more extensively in my book *The Fragrant Mind*.

Essential Oils for Emotional Problems

EMOTIONAL STRESS

There are different degrees of emotional stress, and in this chapter I'm breaking it down into three: Stress Level 1 — tiredness, irritability, aches and pains, occasional depression; Stress Level 2 — anxiety/depression, food allergies, persistent infection, subacute disease, hidden weaknesses, such as otherwise dormant viral infections; and Stress Level 3 — a complex pattern of symptoms: anything from suicidal tendencies to stomach pain, fear, withdrawal from society, and despair. So, within the general term *emotional stress*, there's actually a very broad spectrum of symptoms, from irritability to suicidal thoughts. For this reason, choose your essential oils for stress from the applicable categories throughout this section.

Stress is often presented as being the outcome of a person's inability to deal with the normal pressures of life. In my experience, however, stress is the outcome of a person having to deal with more pressure than should reasonably be expected of anyone. To relieve stress, two things need to happen: the circumstances leading to stress have to change, and a person needs to do something to alleviate their symptoms.

For example, a man came to see me at my practice because he felt that the blood flowing through his body was no longer blood, but some other kind of liquid. He felt very uncomfortable in his own skin, as if he was about to physically explode. He was under stress because he was being bullied at work, had taken a lot of time off, and was about to lose his job. His stress was never

going to go away until the work situation could be changed. Luckily, he had a paper trail of the bullying and worked in an organization with a bullying policy. He lodged a complaint against the bully, which he won. When he returned to work, the bully backed off and the stress evaporated. This is an example of how dealing with the source of the stress is sometimes difficult, being itself stressful, but ultimately worth it. Don't just treat stress as your inability to handle a normal life, which requires you to take something to cope — medication, alcohol, recreational drugs, or even essential oils. If you possibly can, deal with the source of the problem.

Human beings are designed to experience a certain amount of stress, which is largely regulated by the adrenal glands and the natural hormones and neurotransmitters epinephrine, norepinephrine, and cortisol. These are released directly into the bloodstream, like a shot in the arm, when we're confronted with an emergency — in ancient times that might have been a herd of buffalo coming toward us, and today it might be a truck out of control. Either way, we need to quickly spring into action and jump out of the way. That is the normal stress mechanism at work, and it's a good thing because it helps us survive.

But stress isn't meant to be an everyday occurrence. What happens is that we get overloaded with the natural stress chemicals because we're stimulated by too many stressful situations. Psychologists call this chronic situation *distress*, and it's dangerous because it can contribute to physiological changes such as hardening of the arteries, heart attacks and strokes, cancer, diabetes, and lesser problems.

Stress can arise from mental causes, such as financial pressure, exams, or work demands; from emotional problems, such as a relationship breakup; from physical pressures, such as too much driving or striving at the gym for physical perfection; from chemical sources, such as too much caffeine or drugs; and from environmental pressures, such as persistent noise on the factory floor. You know you've got distress if everyday annoyances make you blow a fuse — you get angry at the slightest thing. There may be persistent doubts about being able to cope, or feelings of helplessness and being out of control. On the other hand, there are people who are under a tremendous amount of stress but who become emotionally numb to it. It may seem as if they're coping, but physiologically they may be in turmoil.

Symptoms of stress include irritability; loss of sense of humor or memory; difficulty in making decisions, concentrating, or doing jobs in a logical order; feeling defensive and angry inside; and disinterest in large areas of life. Physical symptoms include insomnia, sweating, breathlessness, faints, loss of appetite or bingeing, indigestion, constipation or diarrhea, headaches, cramps, muscle spasms, eczema, psoriasis, and sexual disinterest, but of course the biggest symptom is heart attack or stroke. Stress management is very important, and I have some advice on this at the end of this section.

The Emotional Stress Kit

The following oils could be considered the Emotional Stress Kit oils because various combinations of them would be suitable in most situations. All will be helpful to some extent, either on their own or in combinations, and have long been the basis for aromatherapy relaxation and emotional-stress-relief treatments:

Bergamot (*Citrus bergamia*)
Lavender (*Lavandula angustifolia*)
Geranium (*Pelargonium graveolens*)
Clary sage (*Salvia sclarea*)
Chamomile maroc (*Ormenis multicaulis*)
Chamomile roman (*Anthemis nobilis*)
Ylang ylang (*Cananga odorata*)

Sandalwood (*Santalum album*)
Petitgrain (*Citrus aurantium*)
Mandarin (*Citrus reticulata*)
Orange, sweet (*Citrus sinensis*)
Frankincense (*Boswellia carterii*)
Cedarwood atlas (*Cedrus atlantica*)
Vetiver (*Vetiveria zizanoides*)

As well as those above, there are certain essential oils and absolute oils that are expensive and a luxury for most but that have proven their worth in the treatment of stressful disorders time and time again, and these can be added to your personal stress kit as and when funds allow:

Rose otto (*Rosa damascena*)
Rose maroc (*Rosa centifolia*)
Hyacinth (*Hyacinthus orientalis*)
Carnation (*Dianthus caryophyllus*)
Linden blossom (*Tilia vulgaris/cordata*)
Neroli (*Citrus aurantium*)
Jasmine (*Jasminum grandiflorum/officinale*)

By choosing your additions to the Essential Stress Kit carefully, you can build up a set of oils that will suit all types of stress and the problems incurred because of it. However, using only the emotional stress kit oils, you can make many formulations that will suit most stressful situations.

The following blends have been designed for general use with stress. Dilute 15–30 drops, as indicated, in 1 fl. oz. (30 mL) of carrier oil to make a body or massage oil.

EMOTIONAL STRESS LEVEL 1
Symptoms: tiredness, irritability, aches and pains, occasional depression

STRESS LEVEL 1 — BLEND 1
Orange, sweet	10 drops
Geranium	15 drops
Lavender	5 drops

STRESS LEVEL 1 — BLEND 2

Bergamot	15 drops
Ylang ylang	5 drops
Petitgrain	10 drops

EMOTIONAL STRESS LEVEL 2
Symptoms: anxiety/depression, food allergies, persistent infection, subacute disease, hidden weaknesses (such as otherwise dormant viral infections)

STRESS LEVEL 2 — BLEND 1

Clary sage	10 drops
Chamomile roman	5 drops
Lavender	5 drops
Geranium	10 drops

STRESS LEVEL 2 — BLEND 2

Chamomile maroc	10 drops
Ylang ylang	5 drops
Petitgrain	5 drops
Sandalwood	10 drops

EMOTIONAL STRESS LEVEL 3
Symptoms: complex pattern of symptoms (anything from suicidal tendencies to stomach pain, fear, withdrawal from society, or despair)

STRESS LEVEL 3 — BLEND 1

Chamomile roman	5 drops
Clary sage	15 drops
Chamomile maroc	5 drops
Geranium	5 drops

STRESS LEVEL 3 — BLEND 2

Geranium	6 drops
Bergamot	14 drops
Orange, sweet	5 drops
Frankincense	6 drops
Vetiver	1 drop

As well as the essential oils previously recommended as the Emotional Stress Kit, there's a wider selection of oils that would also be appropriate. A full list is below; they are all in common use and easily available. They blend well with one another and can be successfully interchanged, each having properties that are useful in treating emotional stress. It's additionally helpful to use them in methods that are themselves therapeutic — a massage, for example, or a relaxing bath. Many essential oils also seem to strengthen the immune system, which becomes increasingly weak during stressful periods.

ESSENTIAL OILS TO HELP ALLEVIATE
EMOTIONAL STRESS
Bay laurel (*Laurus nobilis*)
Benzoin (*Styrax benzoin*)
Bergamot (*Citrus bergamia*)
Chamomile maroc (*Ormenis multicaulis*)
Chamomile roman (*Anthemis nobilis*)
Clary sage (*Salvia sclarea*)
Eucalyptus lemon (*Eucalyptus citriodora*)
Frankincense (*Boswellia carterii*)
Geranium (*Pelargonium graveolens*)
Jasmine (*Jasminum grandiflorum/officinale*)
Lavender (*Lavandula angustifolia*)
Mandarin (*Citrus reticulata*)
May chang (*Litsea cubeba*)
Melissa (*Melissa officinalis*)
Neroli (*Citrus aurantium*)
Nutmeg (*Myristica fragrans*)
Orange, sweet (*Citrus sinensis*)
Rose otto (*Rosa damascena*)
Sandalwood (*Santalum album*)
Spikenard (*Nardostachys jatamansi*)
Valerian (*Valeriana officinalis*)
Vetiver (*Vetiveria zizanoides*)
Ylang ylang (*Cananga odorata*)

The much-neglected eucalyptus lemon (*Eucalyptus citriodora*) not only has antibiotic, antifungal, and slightly antiviral properties, but it also appears to boost the immune system, has electrical properties akin to our own energetic force, and is adaptogenic — which basically means it's subtle and adapts to our needs. All these properties make it a must for anyone dealing with stress and its harmful effects.

The following absolute oils and the essential oil of hops are terrific in their own ways when having to deal with emotional stress, and I have separated them from the main list only because they're expensive and often diluted, making good-quality, pure oils sometimes difficult to find.

Tuberose (*Polianthes tuberosa*)
Hyacinth (*Hyacinthus orientalis*)
Narcissus (*Narcissus poeticus*)
Linden blossom (*Tilia vulgaris/cordata*)
Osmanthus (*Osmanthus fragrans*)
Hops (*Humulus lupulus*)

Women in Stress

All the other sections on stress in this chapter apply equally to men and women, but I'm outlining here a few essential oils and blends for the woman who is simply overwhelmed with the number of things she has to do in any given day. The days of women staying home and men going to work are long gone (if they ever existed), and most women today go out to work and still do everything a woman without a job is expected to do in terms of shopping, cooking, laundry, home care, child care, and care of the elderly. It can all be too much! And a man "helping" now and again doesn't really alleviate the interminable regularity of chores, summarized by the expression "a woman's work is never done."

Using essential oils for relaxation is not going to help. The kids need feeding, and you lying back in a bath isn't going to get it done. Likewise, if there's an important meeting to attend, being super relaxed may not give the right impression.

But neither will arriving as if your edges have been frayed!

When looking at the essential oils that follow, don't choose those on the list that you've used before — for example when meditating, or praying, or trying to get yourself or the children to sleep. Also, any oil that for you personally has an association with relaxation should be sidelined when trying, instead, to alleviate stress.

ESSENTIAL OILS FOR THE WOMAN IN STRESS
Basil linalol (*Ocimum basilicum ct. linalool*)
Bergamot (*Citrus bergamia*)
Cardamom (*Elettaria cardamomum*)
Cedarwood atlas (*Cedrus atlantica*)
Chamomile roman (*Anthemis nobilis*)
Clary sage (*Salvia sclarea*)
Frankincense (*Boswellia carterii*)
Geranium (*Pelargonium graveolens*)
Grapefruit (*Citrus paradisi*)
Jasmine (*Jasminum grandiflorum/officinale*)
Lavender, spike (*Lavandula latifolia*)
Lemon (*Citrus limon*)
Marjoram, sweet (*Origanum majorana*)
Melissa (*Melissa officinalis*)
Neroli (*Citrus aurantium*)
Nutmeg (*Myristica fragrans*)
Orange, sweet (*Citrus sinensis*)
Palmarosa (*Cymbopogon martinii*)
Petitgrain (*Citrus aurantium*)
Rose maroc (*Rosa centifolia*)
Sandalwood (*Santalum album*)
Valerian (*Valeriana officinalis*)
Vetiver (*Vetiveria zizanoides*)
Ylang ylang (*Cananga odorata*)

The essential oils can be used singly, but making a unique blend can be advantageous as it's unlikely to have any other associations that may interfere with its job as a stress reliever. Sensory memory is always something we have to think about when using essential oils for mind and emotional relief and enhancement. Use the essential oils neat on a tissue, or in a small bottle, and inhale when needed. If you're in a position where you can use one of the room-diffusing methods, follow their instructions for use. Here are two blends to try, one for the morning and one for the evening:

DAYTIME STRESS BLEND

Lemon	15 drops
Grapefruit	5 drops
Geranium	3 drops
Vetiver	1 drop

EVENING STRESS BLEND

Orange, sweet	15 drops
Petitgrain	6 drops
Valerian	1 drop

Stress Management

If you're under stress, it's time to figure out what got you to this position and try to change it. Money, or rather the shortage of it, is a huge cause of stress — so too is doing a job you don't like, working for a company that doesn't appreciate you, lack of control or decision making, working long hours, and job insecurity. At home, there may be too much to do and too many people making demands.

The first thing to do is write on a piece of paper "What do I want?" and put it somewhere you can see it. Leave it there for weeks, maybe months, until you've figured out what the answer is. Let the empty page taunt you, but ignore it until you're ready. What you eventually write down may surprise you, but make sure it's from the heart. Don't discuss this with anyone; it's between you and the piece of paper. Be patient. See what happens.

Meanwhile, write up a list of all the activities in your life and order them in terms of priorities. The things that come at the bottom of your list, the nonessentials, can be delegated to someone else or simply deleted. Then, look at your list again and ask, "Who am I doing this for — me or someone else?" Then re-evaluate the activities. Are they really necessary? Have a long talk about your problems with someone who knows you well, and see what solutions they can come up with.

Find time to do something for yourself — an activity you enjoy but gave up because you were too busy. It could be something as simple as reading a book or listening to your favorite music. It's often said, and it is very true, that taking a bath with essential oils can be relaxing, so if you have a bathtub, try to make that a regular feature of your life. Meditation, yoga, and tai chi are excellent ways to reduce stress. Any exercise helps to burn off stress and keep you healthy. Take up a hobby that isn't related to work or family responsibilities — art, music, climbing, crafts — anything that gives you pleasure and takes your mind away from daily chores. Don't feel guilty about it either — just an hour or two a week taken entirely for yourself may be a lifesaver. You need it.

ANXIETY

The mind-body connection becomes very clear with the symptoms of anxiety. In some cases, anxiety causes the stomach muscles to tighten up in a spasm, causing terrible pain, while other people can feel stabbing pains in the chest and stronger, faster heartbeats. Not all symptoms are as dramatic. You might find yourself sighing a lot, gasping for breath, or needing to take in large chunks of air. It might even be that you're running to the toilet all the time, getting headaches or back pain, or just unable to relax. A sense of fatigue is common, as are restlessness, insomnia, even tremors. Anxiety can make you dizzy, perspire, or blush, and it can raise your blood pressure. Some people feel dry in the mouth, or belch a lot, feel nauseous, get diarrhea, or vomit. Anxiety can make a person feel so unwell they seriously wonder if there isn't something physically wrong — which causes more anxiety, of course. Anxiety encompasses feelings of worry, unease, and fear. It's as if the day is enveloped in impending doom.

Anxiety is a normal component of the human being and serves to keep us aware of potential danger. But for whatever reason, and there may be more than one, our anxiety fills us with unease. Sometimes the anxiety is transient and can be caused by an identifiable event, but often people are anxious about ongoing issues such as their primary relationship or feeling unsupported, misunderstood, or insecure. For some people anxiety is a daily, generalized feeling of worry — mild to intense — about everything.

Because there are so many symptoms of anxiety, I'm breaking this section into four different types, with blends for each. Please read the symptoms for all types and choose the essential oils most relevant to you. But we start with a general list of essential oils that can help deflate the anxiety and reduce it to a more bearable level.

ESSENTIAL OILS TO HELP RELIEVE
GENERAL ANXIETY
Bergamot (*Citrus bergamia*)
Cedarwood atlas (*Cedrus atlantica*)
Chamomile roman (*Anthemis nobilis*)
Frankincense (*Boswellia carterii*)
Geranium (*Pelargonium graveolens*)
Ho wood (*Cinnamomum camphora ct. linalool*)
Juniper berry (*Juniperus communis*)
Lavender (*Lavandula angustifolia*)
Mandarin (*Citrus reticulata*)
Melissa (*Melissa officinalis*)
Neroli (*Citrus aurantium*)
Orange, sweet (*Citrus sinensis*)
Patchouli (*Pogostemon cablin*)
Rose otto (*Rosa damascena*)
Rosewood (*Aniba rosaeodora*)
Sandalwood (*Santalum album*)
Vetiver (*Vetiveria zizanoides*)

The following blends relate to the four anxiety types. Dilute 15–30 drops in 1 fl. oz. (30 mL) of carrier oil to make a body oil. Or make up a blend of oils using the proportions listed below and use the number of drops recommended for the various methods, such as bath or shower, and in all room and inhalation methods.

Tense Anxiety: Type 1
Symptoms: bodily tension, muscle pain, aches, sore body

Essential oils: sandalwood, lavender, clary sage, chamomile roman, patchouli, ho wood

TENSE ANXIETY BLEND

Clary sage	10 drops
Lavender	15 drops
Chamomile roman	5 drops

Restless Anxiety: Type 2
Symptoms: overactivity, sweating, palpitations, dizziness, lump in throat, frequent urination or diarrhea (overactivity of the autonomic nervous system)

Essential oils: vetiver, cedarwood atlas, juniper berry, chamomile roman, frankincense, mandarin

RESTLESS ANXIETY BLEND

Vetiver	5 drops
Juniper berry	10 drops
Cedarwood atlas	15 drops

Apprehensive Anxiety: Type 3
Symptoms: unease, apprehension, worrying, brooding, overanxiousness, paranoia, sense of foreboding

Essential oils: bergamot, lavender, neroli, rose otto, melissa, geranium, cedarwood atlas, patchouli, orange (sweet)

APPREHENSIVE ANXIETY BLEND

Bergamot	15 drops
Lavender	5 drops
Geranium	10 drops

Repressed Anxiety: Type 4

Symptoms: feeling on edge and irritable, difficulty in concentrating, insomnia, feeling exhausted all the time

   Essential oils: bergamot, melissa, neroli, rose otto, sandalwood, vetiver, cedarwood atlas, ho wood, sandalwood

REPRESSED ANXIETY BLEND

Neroli	10 drops
Rose otto	10 drops
Bergamot	10 drops

DEPRESSION

The main symptoms of depression are feelings of sadness, hopelessness, and pessimism. Another classic symptom is no longer having a positive interest in life's pleasures, including sex. Sufferers may additionally experience the slowing down of physical or mental actions, tiredness, loss of concentration, indecision, and impaired memory. Sometimes depressed people find themselves crying for no apparent reason, and they're unable to control the tears. People react to depression in different ways, particularly in their eating and sleep patterns — which can be either to overeat or to not eat, and to either oversleep or be unable to sleep. Feelings of worthlessness and guilt — excessive and/or inappropriate — often accompany depression, making it easy for someone to say to themselves, "Oh, they'd be better off without me." This is the biggest danger of depression, which is why it must be taken seriously, and why professional help should always be sought.

In many cases, the depression started for no apparent reason. This is known as *endogenous depression*, while depression that results from an identifiable event is called *exogenous depression*. Strangely perhaps, depression can stem from both good and bad life changes — from a promotion or a layoff, from a birth as well as a death. However, depression usually has no single identifiable cause and just comes "out of the blue," which is appropriate because that's what it is — a major case of the blues.

Anyone who feels depressed, for whatever reason, should certainly seek medical advice because there is a chance that there's an underlying physical disorder at fault, possibly involving the thyroid gland, making some cases of depression a form of hormonal imbalance (which we are aware of also in postnatal depression).

Depression might be caused by thyroid disorders, genetic factors, problems in life, either specific or cumulative, by changes in life, either good or bad, or for no apparent reason at all. Psychotherapy can help, especially in cases where the depression started with a bad life experience. There are many different approaches, and it is worth researching which type of therapy might suit you. If you don't want to talk about your problems, look into mindfulness-based cognitive therapy, which uses meditation to treat depression. As depressed people often have trouble receiving loving touch, an aromatherapy treatment can be a great help in overcoming that barrier. Time and love are the greatest gifts, and the concern of loved ones can be a vital component in recovery.

What follows is a range of options in terms of essential oils to use and blends to choose from. Please read through this whole section on depression before choosing your essential oils. You will find subsections for different groups of symptoms, which I categorize under these headings:

"Weepy," "Agitated or Anxious," "Lethargic," and "Hysterical." However, there follows here a list of essential oils that could be called "general" oils for depression that have been traditionally shown to be effective in aromatherapy treatment. They will not provide a magic cure, but they will definitely support and complement any other therapy or help in which the person may be engaged.

ESSENTIAL OILS USED TRADITIONALLY
IN AROMATHERAPY FOR DEPRESSION
Benzoin (*Styrax benzoin*)
Black pepper (*Piper nigrum*)
Mandarin (*Citrus reticulata*)
Chamomile roman (*Anthemis nobilis*)
Lemon (*Citrus limon*)
Bergamot (*Citrus bergamia*)
Grapefruit (*Citrus paradisi*)
Orange, sweet (*Citrus sinensis*)
Jasmine (*Jasminum grandiflorum / officinale*)
Ylang ylang (*Cananga odorata*)
Rose otto (*Rosa damascena*)
Rose maroc (*Rosa centifolia*)
Neroli (*Citrus aurantium*)
Geranium (*Pelargonium graveolens*)
Petitgrain (*Citrus aurantium*)
Immortelle (*Helichrysum italicum*)
Sandalwood (*Santalum album*)
Clary sage (*Salvia sclarea*)
Marjoram, sweet (*Origanum majorana*)
Lavender (*Lavandula angustifolia*)
Frankincense (*Boswellia carterii*)
Nutmeg (*Myristica fragrans*)
Coriander seed (*Coriandrum sativum*)
Cardamom (*Elettaria cardamomum*)

Dilute 15–30 drops in 1 fl. oz. (30 mL) of carrier oil to make a body oil. Or make up a blend of oils using these quantities and use the recommended number of drops for the various methods, such as bath or shower, and in all room and inhalation methods.

Classic Blends of Essential Oils to Use in Cases of Depression

BLEND 1

Benzoin	10 drops
Black pepper	5 drops
Geranium	15 drops

BLEND 2

Clary sage	15 drops
Lavender	5 drops
Bergamot	10 drops

BLEND 3

Rose otto	10 drops
Sandalwood	15 drops
Lemon	5 drops

BLEND 4

Ylang ylang	8 drops
Orange, sweet	14 drops
Cardamom	8 drops

BLEND 5

Neroli	20 drops
Petitgrain	10 drops

Weepy Depression

The weepy depressive will appear normal, carry out their work as usual, function at home, tend to everyone's needs, and then burst into tears. While out and about in public, this type of depressive can be set off into a tearful episode by the words in a song being played at a supermarket, or the sight of a couple in loving embrace in the park, or by a child trustfully grasping its mother's hand. Anything, in fact, can spark off the tearful response, even the smallest gesture of concern or thanks. This tearful response in itself might not be classified as depression, but something is clearly wrong, and the person involved often feels desperate — they don't smile as much as they used to, they feel unwanted, and they often wonder why they bother living. Because weepy depressives usually function so well on a superficial level, few people around them realize what agony they're going through until suddenly they snap and end up in the hospital because, for instance, they were found cuddling a lost kitten in the gutter, crying their eyes out.

Although this person feels overemotional all the time, they may not visit a doctor and may shrug off the crying episodes as a "one-off," not telling those around them how often they occur. Because a person with weepy depression may seem to cope with life's stresses and strains so well, it's quite easy to fail to recognize that the person is really very depressed unless one actually witnesses these crying episodes. Obviously some people cry more easily than others, and we all occasionally cry with pain, rage, temper, frustration, or sadness, but the weepy depressive finds that crying is the only way they can react, and that is a different thing altogether. Quite often, the weepy depressive person has been through an emotional trauma, or a series of traumas, and nobody, including themselves, has realized just how deeply it has affected them. Essential oils that may comfort and bring a sense of relief should be used.

ESSENTIAL OILS TO USE IN CASES OF WEEPY DEPRESSION

Rose otto (*Rosa damascena*)
Neroli (*Citrus aurantium*)
Chamomile roman (*Anthemis nobilis*)
Sandalwood (*Santalum album*)
Patchouli (*Pogostemon cablin*)
Geranium (*Pelargonium graveolens*)
Ylang ylang (*Cananga odorata*)

Whatever the degree of weepy depression, start with the Light Blend below. If things don't improve after three days, progress to the Moderate

Blend. Stay on the Moderate Blend until things improve, and then gradually over the next week or so return to the Light Blend. If things do not improve after a week on the Moderate Blend, go on to the Deep Blend. The essential oils listed above can be used in all the usual methods. The following blends are for body oils:

WEEPY DEPRESSION: LIGHT

Sandalwood	15 drops
Geranium	10 drops
Ylang ylang	5 drops

Blend together, then dilute 15–30 drops in 1 fl. oz. (30 mL) of carrier oil.

WEEPY DEPRESSION: MODERATE

Geranium	23 drops
Chamomile roman	2 drops
Benzoin	5 drops

Blend together, then dilute 15–30 drops in 1 fl. oz. (30 mL) of carrier oil. The chamomile roman can be replaced with 2 drops of an essential oil of your choice, relative to your condition.

WEEPY DEPRESSION: DEEP

Rose maroc	10 drops
Neroli	3 drops
Sandalwood	5 drops

Blend together, then dilute 3–5 drops in 1 teaspoon (5 mL) of carrier oil.

Agitated or Anxious Depression

The agitated depressive can never sit still for long. They're constantly moving, fidgeting, or twiddling with something — with their hair, or fingers, pens on the desk…anything. Although they're very busy, they're not really concerned with whether a job has been done properly, so long as it's been done and they can move on to the next job. They'll have long faces, tired and drawn, but their minds will be racing ahead to all the plans and jobs they've got to get through. This type of depression causes symptoms such as pressure headaches, eye problems, twitches, tics, jumping muscles, and feeling as if a tight band is being gripped around the skull. The head may feel like it's about to explode.

Agitated or anxious depression causes deep anguish that expresses itself as anger over the slightest thing. The person will despair if a little mark has been made on the furniture, as if it were the end of the world, and they can be prone to rapid mood swings. The constant fretting will be covering up deep feelings of worthlessness and fear. There may be palpitations, unexplained tears, and irrational negative thoughts. People suffering from this type of depression usually throw themselves into work, as a means of covering up the underlying feeling of inadequacy.

ESSENTIAL OILS TO USE IN CASES OF
AGITATED OR ANXIOUS DEPRESSION

Melissa (*Melissa officinalis*)
Cedarwood atlas (*Cedrus atlantica*)
Lavender (*Lavandula angustifolia*)
Chamomile roman (*Anthemis nobilis*)
Frankincense (*Boswellia carterii*)
Bergamot (*Citrus bergamia*)
Marjoram, sweet (*Origanum majorana*)
Spikenard (*Nardostachys jatamansi*)
Chamomile maroc (*Ormenis multicaulis*)
Valerian (*Valeriana officinalis*)
Lemon (*Citrus limon*)
Orange, sweet (*Citrus sinensis*)

Whatever the degree of agitated depression, start with the Light Blend. If things don't improve after three days, progress to the Moderate Blend. If things improve, stay on the Moderate Blend until the depression begins to lift, and then gradually over the next week or so return to the Light Blend. If things do not improve after a week on the Moderate Blend, go on to the Deep Blend.

AGITATED DEPRESSION: LIGHT

Lavender	15 drops
Chamomile maroc	5 drops
Bergamot	10 drops

AGITATED DEPRESSION: MODERATE

Cedarwood atlas	20 drops
Orange, sweet	10 drops

AGITATED DEPRESSION: DEEP

Cedarwood atlas	5 drops
Lemon	15 drops
Chamomile maroc	5 drops
Spikenard	5 drops

For any blend, use 15–30 drops diluted in 1 fl. oz. (30 mL) of carrier oil to make a body oil. Or make up a blend of oils using these quantities and use the recommended usual number of drops for the various methods, such as bath or shower, and in all room and inhalation methods.

Lethargic Depression

Many people are struck with a form of depression that makes them want to stay in bed all day, with their head under the pillow. The lethargic depressive doesn't want to go anywhere or do anything. Everything is a huge effort. It's difficult to concentrate on books and papers. It can get very difficult to get out of bed in the morning, wash, and get dressed. Sleep beckons like welcoming arms. Important phone calls are ignored; vital correspondence never gets written. Everything is overwhelming. A cycle begins to develop where the inclination to sleep leads to more tiredness, and more sleeping. And yet despite all this rest, someone with lethargic depression will feel incapable of doing anything without help and encouragement.

Lethargic depressives appear unsociable. Aside from the fact that they won't meet you in town for a social engagement, when you go to visit them they're so unpleasant, you'd think they were trying to drive you away — which they are, of course, but it isn't personal. Anyone can get depressed like this. It might be a creative person being too critical of themselves, or a timid person who has been deeply hurt and emotionally wounded, or even a selfish, domineering person, now criticizing everyone else for not being able to do things properly but having no energy for doing them themselves. People with lethargic depression often display hopelessness and overwhelming desolation.

ESSENTIAL OILS TO USE IN CASES OF
LETHARGIC DEPRESSION
Grapefruit (*Citrus paradisi*)
Cypress (*Cupressus sempervirens*)
Rosemary (*Rosmarinus officinalis*)
Cistus (*Cistus ladaniferus*)
Melissa (*Melissa officinalis*)
Immortelle (*Helichrysum italicum*)
Peppermint (*Mentha piperita*)
Clary sage (*Salvia sclarea*)
Eucalyptus lemon (*Eucalyptus citriodora*)
Eucalyptus peppermint (*Eucalyptus dives*)

Whatever the degree of lethargic depression, start with the Light Blend. If things don't improve after three days, progress to the Moderate Blend. If things improve, stay on the Moderate Blend until the depression begins to lift, and then gradually over the next week or so return to the Light Blend. If things do not improve after a week on the Moderate Blend, go on to the Deep Blend.

LETHARGIC DEPRESSION: LIGHT

Grapefruit	10 drops
Rosemary	10 drops
Frankincense	10 drops

LETHARGIC DEPRESSION: MODERATE

Cypress	10 drops
Eucalyptus lemon	15 drops
Geranium	5 drops

In the Moderate Blend you can substitute another essential oil, relevant to the situations and difficulties that led to the depression. If you do substitute, reduce the cypress to 5 drops and the eucalyptus lemon to 10 drops, and then add 10 drops of your chosen essential oil, making the total of 30 drops again. Dilute in 1 fl. oz. (30 mL) carrier oil.

LETHARGIC DEPRESSION: DEEP

Immortelle	15 drops
Clary sage	5 drops
Vetiver	2 drops
Lemon	8 drops

Dilute 15–30 drops in 1 fl. oz. (30 mL) of carrier oil to make a body oil. Or make up a blend of oils using these quantities and use the recommended number of drops for the various methods, such as bath or shower, and in all room and inhalation methods.

Hysterical Depression

It's sometimes difficult to know whether someone is suffering from hysterical depression or having a bout of bad moods and temper. Hysterical depressives will exaggerate everything, want to be noticed, and let everyone know they are suffering. They will heave great sighs, shout, scream, and cry. They might be vivacious one minute and suicidal the next. Nobody will be able to do anything right. If you tread quietly, you'll be "creeping about," and if you carry on normally, you'll be told you don't care, especially if you're cheerful.

Shy, introverted people can become hysterical depressives, just as the naturally exuberant personality can. This type of depression often affects people who have become depressed through circumstances, such as job loss, bereavement, financial problems, relationship failure, misunderstandings, and loneliness. The person may start having nightmares and become paranoid. Their rapid mood changes make others wonder if they aren't two people in one skin. They often become suspicious and jealous, and they are constantly moaning and feeling miserable — to the point of crying or screaming. Shaking and trembling can be signs of hysterical depression — which is a most unpleasant state to be in.

ESSENTIAL OILS TO USE IN CASES OF
HYSTERICAL DEPRESSION
Mandarin (*Citrus reticulata*)
Chamomile roman (*Anthemis nobilis*)
Frankincense (*Boswellia carterii*)
Linden blossom (*Tilia vulgaris/cordata*)
Vetiver (*Vetiveria zizanoides*)
Bergamot (*Citrus bergamia*)
Neroli (*Citrus aurantium*)
Narcissus (*Narcissus poeticus*)
Lavender (*Lavandula angustifolia*)
Marjoram, sweet (*Origanum majorana*)
Valerian (*Valeriana officinalis*)
Spikenard (*Nardostachys jatamansi*)

Whatever the degree of hysterical depression, start with the Light Blend. If things don't improve after three days, progress to the Moderate Blend. If things improve, stay on the Moderate Blend until the depression begins to lift, and then gradually over the next week or so return to the Light Blend. If things do not improve after a week on the Moderate Blend, go on to the Deep Blend.

HYSTERICAL DEPRESSION: LIGHT
Lavender   10 drops
Chamomile roman   10 drops
Mandarin   5 drops
Valerian   5 drops

HYSTERICAL DEPRESSION: MODERATE
Neroli   15 drops
Mandarin   10 drops
Bergamot   5 drops

HYSTERICAL DEPRESSION: DEEP
Vetiver   10 drops
Bergamot   13 drops
Chamomile roman   7 drops
Dilute 15–30 drops of these blends in 1 fl. oz. (30 mL) of carrier oil to make a body oil. Or make up a blend of oils using these quantities and use the recommended usual number of drops for the various methods, such as bath or shower, and in all room and inhalation methods.

MOODINESS AND MOOD SWINGS

We seem to have an innate ability to harmonize our moods with those of other human beings, which is a strong force for social cohesion. Mood synchronization can also be seen as a form of communication. Some people are particularly responsive to emotional contagion — these are the good listeners who have great empathy with other people and pick up on all their moods, often not expressing their own.

Moodiness is not uncommon in teenagers and during the premenstrual days of a woman's cycle, and there may well be a hormonal factor involved. More generally, moodiness is brought on by particular events during the day, or by life in general. Moody people can be fed up, frustrated, bored, isolated, repressed, irritable, or bad tempered.

ESSENTIAL OILS TO USE WHEN FEELING MOODY
Lemon (*Citrus limon*)
Geranium (*Pelargonium graveolens*)
Eucalyptus lemon (*Eucalyptus citriodora*)
Neroli (*Citrus aurantium*)
Lavender (*Lavandula angustifolia*)
Ylang ylang (*Cananga odorata*)
Chamomile maroc (*Ormenis multicaulis*)
Patchouli (*Pogostemon cablin*)
Sandalwood (*Santalum album*)

ESSENTIAL OILS TO HELP BALANCE
MOOD SWINGS
Geranium (*Pelargonium graveolens*)
Cardamom (*Elettaria cardamomum*)
Lavender (*Lavandula angustifolia*)
Coriander seed (*Coriandrum sativum*)
Cypress (*Cupressus sempervirens*)
Cedarwood atlas (*Cedrus atlantica*)
Linden blossom (*Tilia vulgaris/cordata*)
Immortelle (*Helichrysum italicum*)
Frankincense (*Boswellia carterii*)
Ginger (*Zingiber officinale*)
Cistus (*Cistus ladaniferus*)
Bay laurel (*Laurus nobilis*)

Use between 15 and 30 drops in 1 fl. oz. (30 mL) of carrier oil to make a body oil. Or make up a blend of oils using the quantities listed below and use the recommended number of drops for the various methods, such as bath or shower, and in all room and inhalation methods.

MOODINESS BLEND

Eucalyptus lemon	12 drops
Chamomile maroc	8 drops
Geranium	10 drops

MOOD SWINGS BLEND

Cedarwood atlas	15 drops
Immortelle	5 drops
Cypress	10 drops
Juniper berry	5 drops

TRAUMA

Many emotional problems start during or following a traumatic situation, which could be a deeply personal event, or a crisis or a tragedy that changes a whole life. We know that physical and environmental trauma — caused by accidents, illness, or being in a crisis such as an earthquake — affects the body's structure, causing blockages, stresses, and tensions in the way the body functions. Emotional trauma — such as leaving home,

changing a job, being unjustly accused, losing a loved one — can do the same thing.

Clearly, trauma is an intensely personal thing with many sources, and how much it affects us depends on how we view them. But traumas do affect us all in some way, whether we like it or not. Human beings are mind/body/spirit complexes; we are walking, talking electrical energy, and these integrated aspects of a human being can easily become fragmented in the case of trauma.

ESSENTIAL OILS TO USE IN CASES OF TRAUMA
Thyme linalol (*Thymus vulgaris ct. linalool*)
Lavender (*Lavandula angustifolia*)
Geranium (*Pelargonium graveolens*)
Lemon (*Citrus limon*)
Frankincense (*Boswellia carterii*)
Marjoram, sweet (*Origanum majorana*)
Petitgrain (*Citrus aurantium*)
Clary sage (*Salvia sclarea*)
Chamomile roman (*Anthemis nobilis*)
Vetiver (*Vetiveria zizanoides*)
Spikenard (*Nardostachys jatamansi*)
Valerian (*Valeriana officinalis*)

If you've suffered from trauma, first look at the lists and charts throughout this book for descriptions of any physical symptoms you may have. Choose oils you find there, as well as in the list above. Persons who have suffered trauma need to release the tension and stress to avoid further complications.

BEREAVEMENT

Death is a part of life, the unfortunate part. Whatever the circumstances, bereavement is a most profound loss, a wrenching away of a part of us, and of course it hurts terribly. We will all lose our parents one day, and if they were our anchor in life, we may feel quite alone and adrift in the vast ocean of life. In a long life friends will also be lost, and, though we pray it never happens, some parents will even have to deal with the most heartbreaking loss of all — the loss of a child.

As each death is such an individual experience, no person can be expected to react in a predictable way. I've known people who throw themselves into work to try to blank out the pain, and others who sit in a chair for months, not saying a word. Everyone has to work through it in their own way. Sometimes bereavement counseling can help. Perhaps the worst experience is for those who have unfinished emotional business with the deceased and who never had the chance to say "Good-bye" and "I love you." Around the experience of death there are certainly many emotions aside from the sheer, awful, empty grief — there could be guilt and remorse too.

Clearly, essential oils can only soften the sharp blow of bereavement. But many people have found them a tremendous support and comfort during these deeply sad times, and through any lonely times ahead. They are particularly effective in baths or massage oils. Gently diffused in a room, they can also help provide a calm and comforting atmosphere in which the mourning process can take place.

Essential Oils to Use in Bereavement
Benzoin (*Styrax benzoin*)
Rose otto (*Rosa damascena*)
Neroli (*Citrus aurantium*)
Cistus (*Cistus ladaniferus*)
Linden blossom (*Tilia vulgaris/cordata*)
Lavender (*Lavandula angustifolia*)
Melissa (*Melissa officinalis*)
Chamomile roman (*Anthemis nobilis*)
Vetiver (*Vetiveria zizanoides*)
Patchouli (*Pogostemon cablin*)
Cypress (*Cupressus sempervirens*)
Mandarin (*Citrus reticulata*)
Rose maroc (*Rosa centifolia*)
Frankincense (*Boswellia carterii*)
Spikenard (*Nardostachys jatamansi*)

The essential oils for bereavement reach into the depth of personal emotions, feelings, and aroma connections. Whatever single aroma or combination of oils you choose should make you feel secure and safe. It doesn't matter if no one else likes it. Use what comforts and consoles you. The following paired combinations of oils demonstrate how very different comforting oils can be, but all have been found significantly beneficial by a variety of people coping with loss. These combinations were sometimes chosen to reflect the personality of the grieving person, while others were chosen because the aroma seemed to reflect the personality of the one being grieved for. I hope they will inspire you to look for your perfect combination and find some kind of relief from the grief you're feeling right now.

Lemon	9 drops
Frankincense	4 drops
*	
Rose maroc	5 drops
Bergamot	4 drops
*	
Clary sage	3 drops
Orange, sweet	6 drops
*	
Geranium	6 drops
Lavender	3 drops
*	
Rose maroc	3 drops
Mandarin	6 drops
*	
Neroli	6 drops
Petitgrain	2 drops
*	
Patchouli	1 drop
Orange, sweet	4 drops
*	
Sandalwood	5 drops
Benzoin	2 drops

The essential oils listed at the start of this section can be used singly or made into blends. Aromas have strong associations with the past, and so a particular fragrance can be experienced completely differently by two people — depending on the memories the aroma brings back. Think carefully about each component of the blend you make.

Dilute 15–30 drops in 1 fl. oz. (30 mL) of carrier oil to make a body oil. Or use the recommended number of drops suitable for the various methods, such as bath or shower, and in all room and inhalation methods. The following blends, more complex than the paired combinations, are another option you might like to try:

COMFORTING BLEND 1

Benzoin	5 drops
Rose maroc	10 drops
Chamomile roman	3 drops
Mandarin	5 drops

COMFORTING BLEND 2

Mandarin	15 drops
Geranium	8 drops
Patchouli	7 drops

COMFORTING BLEND 3

Neroli	12 drops
Linden blossom	5 drops
Melissa	8 drops

COMFORTING BLEND 4

Vetiver	5 drops
Geranium	10 drops
Lemon	10 drops
Patchouli	5 drops

Essential Oils for Life Enhancement

Whenever using essential oils, and especially when making a blend, it's important to do so with a certain intent. In fact, three things are needed so that the vibration of positivity enters into the blend. These are (1) focus — focusing the mind on the essential oils, the blend, and the purpose for which they are being prepared, (2) intent — how the oils are going to be used, and (3) concentration — the bringing together of all that is required to make this blend work well, such as knowledge, correct procedure, and love. These things are important when using essential oils for life enhancement.

MINDFULNESS

The idea of mindfulness is not to try and disperse your current problems but to allow yourself to fully focus on them, become fully aware of them and accepting of them, to better deal with them. Mindfulness meditation can help with psychological stresses as well as physical stresses and disorders. There are many ways of practicing mindfulness, and each has its place. Learning to relax the mind in turn relaxes the body, and the practice creates a nonjudgmental awareness and understanding of how the body reacts to stressful situations. This often releases long-held tension that has caused disorder in the physical body.

In mindfulness, it's possible to learn self-compassion through the recognition that situations outside of ourselves, or out of our control, need not disturb our inner quiet moments. Each mind, no matter how full of clutter, is just waiting for a quiet moment to come into focus. And learning to change our response to challenges often also improves our emotional relationships with other people around us.

I've long taught practitioners and therapists a system of aroma exploration called Aroma-Genera, which enables people to recognize long-held emotional patterns of thought that have impeded health and life relationships, as well as the relationship they have with themselves. Aroma-Genera uses aroma to allow the senses to overcome the problems of the day and of the mind so that the subconscious can be heard.

The many benefits of practicing mindfulness or meditation include reduced depression or emotional distress and the ability to cope better with stressful situations, as well as with anticipated stresses and anxieties such as upcoming events. They lead to better health and the ability to better cope with existing health problems.

Aroma is a powerful silent messenger that can prepare the environment for meditation, whether that is to be 2 or 20 minutes. Choose from the oils that appear to connect with your current situation, whatever that may be — oils that promote in you a feeling of calm and tranquillity and, as far as you are aware, have no connections to unpleasant or distressful situations.

Once you have made and used a blend that you enjoy, it can be used for the mindfulness session to prepare your mind and body for the upcoming meditation. Choose from the following, which have been helpful to those practicing mindfulness:

MINDFULNESS ESSENTIAL OILS
Bergamot (*Citrus bergamia*)
Cedarwood atlas (*Cedrus atlantica*)
Chamomile roman (*Anthemis nobilis*)
Clary sage (*Salvia sclarea*)
Cypress (*Cupressus sempervirens*)
Frankincense (*Boswellia carterii*)
Geranium (*Pelargonium graveolens*)
Juniper berry (*Juniperus communis*)
Lemongrass (*Cymbopogon citratus/flexuosus*)

Marjoram, sweet (*Origanum majorana*)
Melissa (*Melissa officinalis*)
Myrtle (*Myrtus communis*)
Patchouli (*Pogostemon cablin*)
Sandalwood (*Santalum album*)
Spikenard (*Nardostachys jatamansi*)
Vetiver (*Vetiveria zizanoides*)
Ylang ylang (*Cananga odorata*)

When devising your special mindfulness blend, try not to use any essential oils that have food connections, such as orange or lemon, or those that you have used on a regular basis for other purposes. For example, if you use lavender to aid sleeping, leave it for bedtime. The idea with the mindfulness blend is to create something unique. Place a few drops of your blend onto a tissue and inhale from it before you start your session, or use it in a room diffuser. These are simple methods, but highly effective.

POSITIVITY

Some thoughts are positive, and some are negative, and some are just a gray porridge of reaction somewhere in the middle — "I'll do nothing and wait for things to happen to me." Positivity is not about gray. It's about being optimistic and proactive — the kind of attitude that creates its own luck.

Positive people construct strategies to improve their chances of success. Rather than leaving things to chance, they put the odds in their favor by planning carefully and learning to deal with different situations. Positive people don't daydream that one day it's all going to get better; they set themselves realistic goals and go for them, step by small step, and they don't blame themselves for every little mishap. Mishaps are to be expected; they are part of the drama, but don't allow them to rule your life.

Life is about good and bad, and the trick is to find a balance in which there is more good than bad. That's all we can do. Optimism is key, and it is the attitude that good will ultimately prevail in the universe.

Pessimists tend to see the worst aspects of everything. But how can we think good must prevail when experience shows us that mean and devious people often succeed in their negative pursuits and the world can be such a rotten place? We can read, hear, and see *that* on the news. But forget the news for five minutes, phone those long-lost friends, and make good contacts again. There is positivity out there, but you have to reach out for it.

Because it's easier to deal with small problems, cut a large problem into several smaller ones. Think of your successes, not your failures. Know what you want and why you want it, then write it all down and draw up a plan of how you're going to get it. Don't wait until tomorrow — if you do just one small thing toward your goals every day, you will get there. Just don't let anyone distract you from your goals or let the psychic vampires get you.

Essential oils are like little packages of positivity, a helping aid in the move toward optimism. They gently nudge you forward until you find yourself saying, "Oh, maybe things aren't so bad!" I don't know of an essential oil that *doesn't* add positivity in some way, but the following have been chosen specifically for their traditional use in this area. In the diffuser method they bring balance and harmony and create a positive atmosphere, at work or at home, and they can also be used in massage oils, baths or showers, or simply inhaled from a tissue.

ESSENTIAL OILS FOR POSITIVITY
Basil (*Ocimum basilicum*)
Grapefruit (*Citrus paradisi*)
Pine (*Pinus sylvestris*)
Patchouli (*Pogostemon cablin*)
Cypress (*Cupressus sempervirens*)
Petitgrain (*Citrus aurantium*)
Frankincense (*Boswellia carterii*)
Lemon (*Citrus limon*)
Cedarwood atlas (*Cedrus atlantica*)
Vetiver (*Vetiveria zizanoides*)
Juniper berry (*Juniperus communis*)
Cardamom (*Elettaria cardamomum*)
Geranium (*Pelargonium graveolens*)
Rosemary (*Rosmarinus officinalis*)

Avoid using basil in baths or showers.

Each blend below includes 30 drops of essential oil. Dilute 15–30 drops in 1 fl. oz. (30 mL) of carrier oil to make a body oil. Or make up a blend of oils using these quantities and use the recommended number of drops for the various methods.

POSITIVITY BLEND 1

Geranium	10 drops
Grapefruit	8 drops
Petitgrain	8 drops
Frankincense	4 drops

POSITIVITY BLEND 2

Cedarwood atlas	10 drops
Pine	5 drops
Cypress	5 drops
Petitgrain	10 drops

CONFIDENCE

Confidence is attractive, and we all recognize it when we see a confident person walk into the room. They may not even say a word, yet they exude confidence. It's not arrogant or loud, it's not aggressive or judgmental. Confidence is subtle, a kind of calm inside the person, bright and light, that says, "This is me. Take me or leave me as I am." Being confident makes it much easier to find a lifetime partner, make friends, or get a job.

We can talk to strangers and feel free in the world at large. Confidence is good because it is liberating. It allows us to live life to the fullest.

Essential oils help build confidence by relieving the fear, stress, and nervous tension that often prevent us from being who we want to be. From the list below, choose an essential oil or oils that you sense a harmony with when you inhale the aroma deeply through the nose. When inhaling the aroma molecules of an essential oil, you might experience an emotional sensation, and if that feeling is negative, avoid that particular oil. The oils you choose should make you feel good, and you should like them.

ESSENTIAL OILS FOR CONFIDENCE
Cedarwood atlas (*Cedrus atlantica*)
Cypress (*Cupressus sempervirens*)
Linden blossom (*Tilia vulgaris/cordata*)
Cardamom (*Elettaria cardamomum*)
Fennel, sweet (*Foeniculum vulgare var. dulce*)
Ginger (*Zingiber officinale*)
Bergamot (*Citrus bergamia*)
Rosewood (*Aniba rosaeodora*)
Grapefruit (*Citrus paradisi*)
Jasmine (*Jasminum grandiflorum/officinale*)
Pine (*Pinus sylvestris*)
Sandalwood (*Santalum album*)
Geranium (*Pelargonium graveolens*)
Rosemary (*Rosmarinus officinalis*)
Orange, sweet (*Citrus sinensis*)
Coriander seed (*Coriandrum sativum*)

The blends below, aside from Blends 2 and 6, comprise 30 drops of essential oil. Dilute 15–30 drops in 1 fl. oz. (30 mL) of carrier oil to make a body oil. Or if making a blend of essential oils, use the recommended number of drops for the various methods.

CONFIDENCE BLEND 1
Orange, sweet	10 drops
Cedarwood atlas	5 drops
Ginger	5 drops
Jasmine	10 drops

CONFIDENCE BLEND 2
Grapefruit	10 drops
Orange, sweet	10 drops
Bergamot	5 drops

CONFIDENCE BLEND 3
Cedarwood atlas	10 drops
Cypress	12 drops
Pine	8 drops

CONFIDENCE BLEND 4
Rosemary	10 drops
Lemon	10 drops
Orange, sweet	10 drops

CONFIDENCE BLEND 5
Cardamom	5 drops
Ginger	15 drops
Coriander seed	10 drops

CONFIDENCE BLEND 6
In 30 mL of carrier oil use 10 drops of *either* jasmine or linden blossom.

CONCENTRATION

There are so many distractions in life today, it's hard to concentrate. If it's not a Tweet, an update, or an email breaking our line of thought, it's the phone ringing. Out of necessity, many of us have learned to concentrate on several things at once. We're becoming used to fragmentation as a way of life. This might not seem important, but if you're trying to write a book, a report for work, or a term paper, lack of concentration might just get you a C instead of an A. But it's not just writing that requires concentration. Practically any job you can think of is going to be carried out better if clarity of thought is brought to it. Dancers need to concentrate, or they might fall. If high-rise window cleaners don't concentrate, they might fall a lot farther. Drivers need to concentrate. Surgeons need to concentrate. The list goes on. Concentration has always been important to human activity, and today is no different.

Used to aid concentration, the essential oils listed here can simply be inhaled from a tissue or gently diffused throughout a room. Used in baths, they can help one concentrate on oneself. Regular use in massage oils will help overall, long-term ability to concentrate.

The following essential oils can be used in all the usual ways except that basil and peppermint should be avoided in baths or showers. For concentrating on efficiency, good choices would be lemon, basil, may chang, or frankincense.

Essential Oils for Concentration

Lemon (*Citrus limon*)
Basil linalol (*Ocimum basilicum ct. linalool*)
Lemongrass (*Cymbopogon citratus/flexuosus*)
May chang (*Litsea cubeba*)
Cardamom (*Elettaria cardamomum*)
Bergamot (*Citrus bergamia*)
Orange, sweet (*Citrus sinensis*)
Cedarwood atlas (*Cedrus atlantica*)
Rosemary (*Rosmarinus officinalis*)
Eucalyptus globulus (*Eucalyptus globulus*)
Peppermint (*Mentha piperita*)
Lavandin (*Lavandula x intermedia*)

Dilute 15–30 drops in 1 fl. oz. (30 mL) of carrier oil to make a body oil. Or make up a blend of oils using these quantities and use the recommended number of drops for the various methods, such as bath or shower, and in all room and inhalation methods.

Concentration Blend 1

Lemon	20 drops
Basil linalol	6 drops
Rosemary	2 drops

Concentration Blend 2

May chang	10 drops
Cardamom	10 drops
Lemon	10 drops

SELF-ESTEEM

Self-esteem is like an eggshell — it's easily broken. It's fragile, and many things can wear it away — bullies at school or at work, a tyrannical boss, a controlling partner, or someone who complains all day long. It's often other people who degrade this delicate shell of ours.

I never cease to be amazed at the low self-esteem so many people have. Perfectly clever, beautiful, and talented people say to me, "I could never do that" or "I'm not smart enough for that." It's utter rubbish. Of course they could do these things. But someone, somewhere in their past or present life, has led them to believe they can't.

Having self-esteem is recognizing your potential and worth, taking pride in what you do, and trusting your own judgment. When you have self-esteem you are secure in yourself, despite your weak points, because you recognize the strong points and appreciate them. Okay, you're not perfect, but nobody is, and you're as good as the next person.

Essential oils won't miraculously turn you overnight from someone with low self-esteem into someone brimming over with confidence, but they will subtly and gently help you cope with any corner of your life with which you are unhappy and so build up your self-esteem and your estimate of what you can do in this world. It's important to use an oil or oils with no previous memory connection that might have negative associations.

ESSENTIAL OILS FOR SELF-ESTEEM
Hyacinth (*Hyacinthus orientalis*)
Sandalwood (*Santalum album*)
Vetiver (*Vetiveria zizanoides*)
Ylang ylang (*Cananga odorata*)
Rose maroc (*Rosa centifolia*)
Jasmine (*Jasminum grandiflorum/officinale*)
Carnation (*Dianthus caryophyllus*)
Bergamot (*Citrus bergamia*)
Geranium (*Pelargonium graveolens*)
Chamomile maroc (*Ormenis multicaulis*)
Cedarwood atlas (*Cedrus atlantica*)
Frankincense (*Boswellia carterii*)
Neroli (*Citrus aurantium*)
Grapefruit (*Citrus paradisi*)
Pine (*Pinus sylvestris*)
Rosewood (*Aniba rosaeodora*)
Orange, sweet (*Citrus sinensis*)
Coriander seed (*Coriandrum sativum*)

Dilute 15–30 drops of the blends below in 1 fl. oz. (30 mL) of carrier oil to make a body oil. Or make up a blend of oils using these quantities and use the recommended number of drops for the various methods such as bath or shower, and in all room and inhalation methods.

SELF-ESTEEM BLEND 1

Ylang ylang	10 drops
Bergamot	4 drops
Vetiver	2 drops
Sandalwood	12 drops

SELF-ESTEEM BLEND 2

Hyacinth	4 drops
Bergamot	5 drops
Rose maroc	5 drops

Blend 2 uses a particularly powerful combination of oils, and only 14 drops or fewer are needed in 1 fl. oz. (30 mL) of carrier oil to make a body oil.

ASSERTIVENESS

Assertive people get what they want. They stand their ground when they've been given shoddy service, and they're not afraid to ask their dream man or woman out on a date. Assertiveness is not just about our relationship with the outside world — it's also about defending our personal integrity and, as a result, maintaining our sense of who we actually are. It's about defending your right to be you, not who someone else wants you to be. Assertive people don't become doormats other people walk over.

Over the years I've seen countless people coming to their first aromatherapy treatment all meek and mild, but blossoming into frank, open, and assertive people after several sessions. Choose individual oils or combinations from the list to suit your choice, or try one of the blends below. They can be used in a bath or shower, in body oil, in diffusers or other room methods, or simply inhaled from a tissue. The change will not happen overnight; it will take about two weeks of regular use. You may not recognize the change in yourself until someone says to you, "Oh, I liked the way you handled that. What's come over you?"

ESSENTIAL OILS FOR ASSERTIVENESS
Fennel, sweet (*Foeniculum vulgare var. dulce*)
Basil linalol (*Ocimum basilicum ct. linalool*)
Jasmine (*Jasminum grandiflorum/officinale*)
Cedarwood atlas (*Cedrus atlantica*)

Cypress (*Cupressus sempervirens*)
Frankincense (*Boswellia carterii*)
Ginger (*Zingiber officinale*)
Patchouli (*Pogostemon cablin*)
Ylang ylang (*Cananga odorata*)
Black pepper (*Piper nigrum*)
Chamomile maroc (*Ormenis multicaulis*)
Bergamot (*Citrus bergamia*)
Coriander seed (*Coriandrum sativum*)
Carnation (*Dianthus caryophyllus*)
Tuberose (*Polianthes tuberosa*)
Lime (*Citrus aurantifolia*)
Cardamom (*Elettaria cardamomum*)
Cistus (*Cistus ladaniferus*)
May chang (*Litsea cubeba*)

Basil should be avoided in baths and showers. With the blends below, first blend the essential oils in the proportions indicated. For a body oil, use no more than 2 drops per teaspoon (5 mL) of carrier oil. Use no more than 3 drops in baths, diluted in a little carrier oil first. For room and inhalation methods, use as directed in "Methods of Use" chart (table 2) in chapter 1 (see page 14).

Assertiveness Blend 1

Cistus	2 drops
May chang	10 drops
Jasmine	6 drops

Assertiveness Blend 2

Patchouli	10 drops
Frankincense	10 drops
Bergamot	10 drops

Assertiveness Blend 3

Cedarwood atlas	15 drops
Cypress	5 drops
Lime	10 drops

HAPPINESS

People often say, "All I want is for my children to be happy." Happiness is top of the list. But what about the grown-ups? For so many people, happiness is a distant magical island they swim toward their whole lives but never quite reach. For others, happiness is like a mist in the dawn, hard to grasp hold of. Happiness can be elusive or fleeting.

The happy person exudes radiance and seems to have found a philosophical position that has banished misery from the soul. Their aura is a delight. But happiness is a very personal thing — what makes one person happy would not necessarily make another one happy. However it comes, though, happiness is glorious. In a sense, it's nothing more than the ability to accept who we are and how we're living — accepting our personal limitations and living in the present instead of always striving for more.

Essential oils will not put a person in a happy state if they've been miserable all their lives, but they will certainly help in a subtle way to amplify the happiness within and bring it into the light. When it comes to choosing a single oil or oils to blend, pick aromas that appeal to you, that feel right.

Some Essential Oils for Happiness

Orange, sweet (*Citrus sinensis*)
Rose otto (*Rosa damascena*)
Rose maroc (*Rosa centifolia*)
Jasmine (*Jasminum grandiflorum/officinale*)
Coriander seed (*Coriandrum sativum*)
Ginger (*Zingiber officinale*)
Clove bud (*Syzygium aromaticum*)
Cinnamon leaf (*Cinnamomum zeylanicum*)
Benzoin (*Styrax benzoin*)
Carnation (*Dianthus caryophyllus*)
Geranium (*Pelargonium graveolens*)
Vanilla (*Vanilla plantifolia*)

Dilute 15–30 drops in 1 fl. oz. (30 mL) of carrier oil to make a body oil. Or make up a blend of essential oils using the proportions below and use the number of recommended drops for each method of use, such as bath or shower, and in all room and inhalation methods.

HAPPINESS BLEND 1

Orange, sweet	19 drops
Rose maroc	5 drops
Jasmine	5 drops
Clove bud	1 drop

HAPPINESS BLEND 2

Bergamot	5 drops
Geranium	13 drops
Cinnamon leaf	2 drops
Ginger	10 drops

6

The Basic Travel Kit

Lavender (*Lavandula angustifolia*) • Peppermint (*Mentha piperita*) • Geranium (*Pelargonium graveolens*)

Chamomile roman (*Anthemis nobilis*) • Ginger (*Zingiber officinalis*)

Eucalyptus radiata (*Eucalyptus radiata*) • Thyme linalol (*Thymus vulgaris ct. linalool*)

Lemongrass (*Cymbopogon citratus/flexuosus*) or Citronella (*Cymbopogon nardus*)

Tea tree (*Melaleuca alternifolia*) • Rosemary (*Rosmarinus officinalis*)

The whole point of traveling is to get away from the same old, same old, and have some fun. By definition we're leaving behind everything we're used to, including our usual safety nets — the local drugstore, our helpful physician, and the medicine cabinet. Everything that happens to us in terms of health issues is going to be unexpected — an accident, an unforeseen circumstance. Vacations are when things happen that we hadn't anticipated, things that just might spoil our fun. This is what the Basic Travel Kit is for.

Travel is an adventure, and that's why we like it. If we didn't think different was good, we'd stay at home. But adventure brings surprises, and some of them aren't so good. This could be in the form of the local flora and fauna — some of which sting and bite — food that doesn't agree with us, accommodation that looks none too clean, and

weather we weren't expecting. Accidents can happen any time, and it's good to be prepared.

For a multitude of reasons, the Basic Travel Kit is useful. Even if you only take one or two bottles of essential oil away with you, this may be all you need to deal with known, recurring problems — sensitivity to the sun, perhaps, or mosquitoes that are insensitive to you. There's also a Mini Travel Kit of four essential oils expressly designed for young people taking a gap year. Even over a long weekend, the unexpected can happen. But first we have to get there, so we start with the journey.

The Journey

Traveling is supposed to be one of life's great pleasures, but you may doubt that if you feel sick in a car or plane. Peppermint oil has a marvelously calming effect on the stomach and is clearly essential for an uneasy traveler. One drop of peppermint oil put on a tissue and placed under the car seat often helps stop the feeling of nausea that comes with travel sickness.

Another excellent general travel oil is ginger, which is well known for alleviating seasickness but is equally effective for other types of travel sickness too. Two drops of ginger oil placed on a handkerchief and inhaled works well, and a drop diluted in a little carrier oil and rubbed over the upper abdomen also helps.

Midsummer traffic jams often make driving to the beach a hot and frustrating time, but passengers and driver alike are kept cool and calm by 1 drop of rosemary, eucalyptus radiata, or lemongrass oil on a cotton ball placed in the car on the floor, away from any sunlight or heat. These oils not only are antibiotic and antiseptic but also soothe the nerves and keep them from fraying. They won't make the driver sleepy, but they will keep him or her on an even keel, relaxed but aware. For more lengthy or tiring journeys the driver can put 2 drops of diluted rosemary, eucalyptus radiata, or lemon oil in the morning bath, or onto the washcloth after washing in the shower, and rub it over the body. This will help to sharpen concentration and keep the driver alert.

Exhaust fumes can cause nausea, so roll up the windows if you're caught in a jam and put a drop of eucalyptus radiata or rosemary on a couple of tissues and place them around the car floor to counteract the smell.

Travel sickness is to a large extent caused by conflicting messages reaching the brain from the eyes, the balancing mechanism of the ears, and the stomach. It helps to look at an unmoving object on the horizon or, if you're in a plane or on a ship, to close your eyes.

FLYING

Flying is a mode of transport that brings its own particular problems. The pressurized compartment causes dehydration and swollen feet and ankles, cramping, dry skin, headaches, and, especially in coach class, painful knees from having them pushed up against the seat in front! Avoid alcohol, tea, and coffee when traveling by air. Do drink plenty of water and fruit juices to keep your sugar level up. During long-haul flights, gases in your intestinal tract can expand, causing bloating and discomfort. To help alleviate this, have a cup of peppermint herb tea before you leave the house, and rub 1 drop of peppermint and 1 drop of lavender essential oil, diluted in 1 teaspoon (5 mL) of carrier oil, over the upper and lower abdomen.

If flying makes you anxious, have ready a tissue with 1 drop of lavender and 1 drop of geranium in a small resealable bag in your pocket. When you're beginning to feel uneasy about the situation, pull the tissue out and hold it to your nose for a moment. Inhale deeply, lie back, close your eyes, and relax. This also works well for people who get irritable on plane journeys.

There are two methods of dealing with swollen feet and ankles, which can become particularly troublesome on long flights. Both work equally well and need preparing in advance. For the first, you will need a piece of cotton — a small handkerchief is perfect — for making a compress. First, put 2–3 drops of lavender on the material, then wet it so it's just damp. Fold it and put it in a small resealable bag to carry with you on the journey. When your ankles swell during the flight, apply the compress to your feet and ankles and gently massage them in an upward direction to the bottom of the calf, both back and front, for a few minutes. For the second method, massage your feet and ankles in an upward direction, as above, with an oil made from adding 5 drops of lavender or eucalyptus radiata to aloe vera gel.

If you're prone to getting cramps while traveling, make a compress as above but using geranium oil and hold the compress over the affected area — usually the calf of the leg or the foot. Also try the old trick of holding your big toe tightly between the thumb and forefinger.

Airlines do give advice during the flight regarding well-being in the air, and it's sensible to follow the instructions being given. Walk around as much as you can; when seated exercise your feet and ankles by moving them in a clockwise and counterclockwise direction.

A particular worry these days, especially with long-haul flights, is the risk of acquiring an infection from fellow travelers in the same confined space. Personally, I travel with a simple paper face mask in case I feel uncomfortable with the health of my seated neighbors. If there's a lot of coughing and spluttering around me, I put into the mask a folded tissue with 1 drop of thyme linalol. More often, I just sniff the tissue occasionally so if anything happens to be in the atmosphere, it's likely to pass me by.

I travel a lot, all around the world, and so far I have never picked up an infection. This may also be because after sitting down, I wipe with essential oil wipes anything I'm likely to touch — the arm rests, table, remote control, and so on. That might sound extreme, but I'm not the only one who does it, and the cabin crew don't bat an eyelid. They've seen it before, obviously! With your travel kit you can easily prepare protective wipes. Use 2–3 drops of the blend below on around 10 dampened tissues, and seal them in a resealable bag. You may not need all the tissues for a single journey, but they're useful to have ready for buses, taxis, and trains too. The wipes smell good and clean up the air as well as being antimicrobial.

TRAVEL WIPES BLEND

Lavender	2 drops
Ginger	2 drops
Thyme linalol	4 drops
Lemongrass	4 drops
Tea tree	2 drops

Children on long flights can get fidgety and irritable — which can make your journey as uncomfortable as theirs. Prepare a bottle containing 5 drops of chamomile roman in 1 tablespoon (15 mL) of a light carrier oil. If things start to get out of control, massage the child's feet and legs with a little of the oil, tuck a blanket around the child, and they'll soon settle down. Only use a tiny portion of the oil — which will also come in handy for other vacation problems.

Jet lag is a set of physical symptoms caused by the body reacting to quick changes in time zones, the most noticeable of which is being unable to sleep at the local time. As we take longer flights, jet lag becomes an increasing problem. Even two or three days of unhappy recovery time are too many for an already short holiday or important business trip — and then there's the journey home to look forward to as well!

Several homeopathic preparations seem to work well for jet lag, such as *Arnica montana, Chamomilla, Lycopodium, Ipecacuanha,* and *Bellis perennis.* Everyone seems to have their own remedy for jet lag, including vitamins, supplements, and dietary advice — and they may all work, for some people. And that's the key: everyone is different. When I travel long haul it's not because I'm going on holiday (unfortunately!) and can relax for the first day or so, but because I'm giving a series of lectures and have to be up and focused bright and early local time. Jet lag is not an option for me! I find that essential oils soften the edges of the time zones, bringing them together and making it possible to avoid fatigue and jarred nerves.

There are several combinations of oils that could be used, but good options would be rosemary and lemongrass for the morning, and lavender and geranium for the evening. Before you set out on your journey, have a bath using 2 drops each of rosemary and lemongrass or, if you prefer to shower, put 1 drop of each onto a wet washcloth and wipe it over your body, once you've washed.

When you arrive at your destination, force yourself to stay awake and go to bed at the local bedtime. Before you sleep, have a bath to which you've added 1 drop each of lavender and geranium oil (or try chamomile, clary sage, or neroli), or use the oils on a washcloth in the shower. If these options aren't available, put a small amount of carrier oil in the palm of your hand, add 1 drop each of lavender and geranium, and rub the oil around your shoulders and neck. Also rub the oil over your lower back and hips to relieve the travel ache and tension that come from sitting for long periods.

This may help alleviate the symptoms, but for the best results continue using the oil over a couple of days. In the mornings, follow the same routine but use rosemary and eucalyptus radiata instead. If your work involves routine intercontinental travel you'd do well to add the fabulous oil of grapefruit to your travel kit. Use it in all the methods described above in the mornings and throughout the day.

Another combination for travelers is peppermint and geranium. This works well for people returning home who, after having spent time unwinding at their vacation destination and getting totally relaxed, find that their vacation has come to an abrupt end and that they're back at their desks with that Monday morning feeling.

Getting back into the routine is very tough, but a couple of drops each of peppermint and geranium in a room diffuser will help you get over the shock of reality.

The Arrival

When we travel to foreign lands we may come into contact with bacteria and viruses against which we have no immunological defense. Not only that, but we sleep and wash where strangers slept and washed the night before. When some of the bacteria and viruses people carry with them are so unpredictable, why take any chances of picking them up? It's not being paranoid to take steps to ensure we don't come home with something longer lasting than a tan.

Even if your toilet facilities look clean, that doesn't mean they've been disinfected. It takes but a minute to wipe the door handle, toilet flush button, and toilet seat with a tissue that has a neat drop of thyme and tea tree essential oil on it. This is a habit I got into before antibacterial wipes became readily available. If you're traveling in particularly suspect areas, you might use a few tissues impregnated with thyme, tea tree, and lemongrass. These three together provide a very powerful bactericide, and few micro-organisms can escape their powerful effect.

As a precautionary measure pull the bedclothes back and wipe the mattress with a tissue on which you have put a few drops of lavender, and depending on where you are in the world, you could add thyme, lemongrass, and tea tree.

The Gap Year…or Weekend!

It's not only young adults who take a gap year traveling, but also adults who never had the opportunity when they were younger. Not everyone will want to pack 10 essential oils, so for them here is a Mini Travel Kit that will be a big help on gap years, and even on mini-breaks!

MINI TRAVEL KIT

Lavender	Thyme linalol
Tea tree	Geranium

Depending on where you're going, you can add to this basic kit other oils that will be particularly useful. For example, if going to a location known as a potential risk for ticks carrying Lyme disease, add eucalyptus lemon. Oregano is a useful antiviral and a good addition as well.

A Home Away from Home

Making a home away from home is easy with essential oils if you take along several that you have already been using at home; the aroma will provide a comforting aura of familiarity and security when used in new surroundings.

Children often feel insecure in unfamiliar places, and familiar essential oils can help calm them because of their association with home. To comfort a child through the sense of smell, pick an oil that you intend to take away with you and use it around the home for a few days before your departure. For example, if you use geranium as a general room fragrance at home, when you arrive at your destination put a few drops of geranium on tissues and place them around the room. The familiarity of the aroma will help children settle down for the night in the pleasantly fresh room that smells just like home.

The Sun

Despite repeated warnings that skin cancer is caused at least in part by exposure to the sun, people still flock to the beach, where they lie prostrate, soaking in as much sunshine as they can. Hopefully, they're wearing a high-factor sunscreen. But lying on the beach more than half naked with nothing much to do does provide the perfect opportunity to make a detailed note, in writing, of the moles we have. And as we seldom lie on the beach alone, our companion can examine the back of our body too. Making a mole map might turn out to be the most useful souvenir you take home with you, especially if you update it regularly to identify any new moles or any changes in existing ones.

One important thing to remember when using essential oils in the sun is that a few of them are what's known as *photosensitive* oils. This means they could increase our skin's sensitivity to the sun.

Sunburn can vary considerably in degree. If the burn is severe and there is blistering, medical assistance may be required. If there is simply redness or a feeling of skin tightness and soreness, one effective first aid treatment is the miraculous oil of lavender.

As with all burns, it's crucial to first get the heat out of the skin, so fill a sink or bath with cold water, add ice if possible, and immerse the sunburnt area as soon as you can. Then apply 1 or 2 drops of neat (undiluted) lavender essential oil over the sunburned area, bearing in mind that 1 or 2 drops of lavender will go quite a long way. You don't need to overdo it; simply make sure that the lavender has covered the reddened area. If you haven't got any lavender with you, use chamomile instead. Then, if you have it to hand, cover the area with cooling aloe vera gel. Pregnant women should not use lavender in this way, but they can use the aloe vera gel on its own.

If you do this, by morning hopefully you won't notice a thing if you weren't sunburned too badly. But do stay out of the sun for at least three days, even if the area looks perfectly healed.

Taking care of skin that's been exposed to more than the usual amount of sunshine makes sense, and the following after-sun oils will also help repair it:

AFTER-SUN OIL

Lavender	10 drops
Chamomile german	5 drops
Geranium	2 drops
Dilute in:	
Sweet almond oil	4 tablespoons (60 mL)
Sesame oil	3 tablespoons (30 mL)

Apply as a body oil after showering or bathing, paying particular attention to areas of skin that have been overexposed to the sun.

AFTER-SUN BATH OIL

Chamomile roman	4 drops
Geranium	2 drops
Lavender	2 drops

Dilute these after-sun bath essential oils in 1 tablespoon (15 mL) of jojoba oil and add it all to a bath. While in the bath, gently smooth the oil over the areas that have been exposed to the sun.

The following body and face oil is very effective in the drying conditions of wind and sun, such as experienced when skiing, sailing, or hiking.

APRÈS SKI, SUN, SAIL, AND HIKE OIL

Chamomile roman	8 drops
Geranium	8 drops
Lavender	8 drops
Dilute in:	
Jojoba oil	2 teaspoons (10 mL)
Sesame seed oil	1 teaspoon (5 mL)
Evening primrose seed oil	1 teaspoon (5 mL)
Almond oil, sweet	2 tablespoons (30 mL)

Blend the ingredients together well and use the oil every night before sleeping.

Hair can also suffer from overexposure to sun, sea, wind, and the chlorine in swimming pools. You can find good natural conditioning treatments in the "Hair Care" section of chapter 13, "The Fragrant Way to Beauty." Bald patches on the head should be protected just as well as the face. Hair on the head provides some natural protection from the sun, but it's always a good idea to wear a hat.

The Heat

HEAT EXHAUSTION AND HEATSTROKE/SUNSTROKE

The symptoms of heat exhaustion or heatstroke can start slowly and appear innocent, but this is a potentially dangerous situation, especially to the young and elderly. A person might feel dizzy, faint, nauseous, or drowsy. They may be confused or disorientated, have a headache, fever, rapid heartbeat, or hyperventilation. A temperature over 104°F (40°C) is a sure warning sign, unless the person has just momentarily become hot from exercising in the sun. When the body's thermoregulation system is overwhelmed, the person stops sweating, which is a sure sign of trouble, especially if the skin becomes hot and dry and flushed red. Also, the person can be feeling cold and shivering, even though heatstroke is the cause. It's easy to think that heatstroke won't happen in humid conditions, but humidity reduces the evaporation of perspiration and so keeps heat in. Whatever the circumstances of heat exhaustion, heatstroke, or sunstroke, it is important to get medical attention as soon as possible.

Meanwhile, get the person out of the sun and into the cool. Remove any unnecessary clothing. Attempt to cool them down in any way possible, using cool water sponging, cool compresses, a water spray, or regularly replaced cold, wet towels. Key areas to try and cool down are the head, neck, armpits, wrists, and groin. If nothing more than water is available, pour it over the person's head and over the key areas. As soon as possible, get the person in a cool shower or, better still, into a bath of cool water. This option, however, is not advisable if the person is elderly or has cardiovascular disease, because it can raise blood pressure.

If pouring water over the body, apply 1 drop of neat eucalyptus radiata to the back of the neck. When sponging, use ice-cold water with eucalyptus radiata and lavender oils added, and continue for at least 24 hours. One quick dowsing with water will only lower the body temperature by one-hundredth of a degree, which isn't going to be enough. Alternatively, if immersing the person in a cold-water bath, add 4 drops each of eucalyptus radiata and lavender essential oil. Apply neat lavender or eucalyptus radiata to their temples, the back of their neck, and the solar plexus — the upper abdomen — and have them breathe deeply.

Although the person with heatstroke may not feel thirsty, they should drink plenty of liquids. If you can't find rehydration packs in the local stores, make up your own as described in the section on page 126 on diarrhea. Heatstroke can develop over a few days, and it takes a few days to recover from it. Keep an eye on the patient throughout this time.

HEAT CRAMPS

Heat cramps can occur after unaccustomed exercise and perspiration, with loss of body fluid and electrolytes. Drink plenty of water and take rehydration drinks, or make your own (see page 127), and massage the legs with the following oil:

HEAT CRAMPS
Geranium   2 drops
Eucalyptus radiata   3 drops
Blend together and then dilute by adding 3–5 drops to each 1 teaspoon (5 mL) of carrier oil.

PRICKLY HEAT

Prickly heat (miliaria rubra) is a rash of tiny blisters that can look like little pink or red spots. Caused by blocked sweat glands, it is extremely itchy. It can affect any part of the body, and the best line of action is to keep as cool as possible and expose the area to air or only cover with light cotton clothing.

Apply a splash to the area, made by diluting 6 drops each of eucalyptus radiata, lavender, and chamomile roman to a teaspoon of alcohol (vodka is fine) and shaking it all in a large cup of spring water. Warm baths are very soothing if you add to them 4 drops each of eucalyptus radiata and lavender essential oil.

Including baking soda in the bath is a good solution. If you can use this method, you only need lavender oil, but — and this is important — add the lavender to the baking soda and mix them together before putting in the bath; don't just put them in separately. Below are the amounts you will need for various age groups. If wanting to help a baby, try to get hold of calamine lotion. Add 2 drops of chamomile german (or chamomile roman) and 2 drops of lavender to 2 tablespoons (30 mL) of calamine lotion. Alternatively, bathe the baby in a warm bath, ensuring the folds of the skin are thoroughly dried afterward.

BAKING SODA BLEND FOR PRICKLY HEAT: BABIES
Baking soda   ½ cup
Lavender   1 drop
Mix the lavender essential oil with the baking soda thoroughly before adding a small amount to the bath. If the baby is under 12 months, this quantity is enough for four baths; if between 12 and 24 months, this makes enough for three baths.

BAKING SODA BLEND FOR PRICKLY HEAT:
CHILDREN AGE 2 TO 7 YEARS
Baking soda   ½ cup
Lavender   2 drops
Mix the lavender essential oil with the baking soda thoroughly before adding to the bath. This quantity is enough for two baths.

BAKING SODA BLEND FOR PRICKLY HEAT:
CHILDREN AGE 8 TO 10 YEARS
Baking soda   ½ cup
Lavender   3 drops

Mix the lavender essential oil with the baking soda thoroughly before adding to the bath. This quantity is enough for two baths.

BAKING SODA BLEND FOR PRICKLY HEAT:
11 YEARS TO ADULT
Baking soda   1 cup
Lavender   3–4 drops
Mix the lavender essential oil with the baking soda thoroughly before adding to the bath.

Fevers

In an adult, a reading above 99.0–99.5°F (37.2–37.5°C) can be classified as a fever, although this can vary with age, time of day, and the person's activity level. In a child, temperatures indicating a fever vary depending on where the temperature is taken — under the arm (99°F/37.2°C), in the mouth (99.5°F/37.5°C), or rectally (100.4°F/38°C).

Fevers that develop on vacation are usually the result of viral or bacterial infection, which can be acquired from food, water, or swimming facilities, for example. Insects that bite and parasites are also vectors of diseases in which fever is a symptom. With a fever, it's very important to get a correct diagnosis. Malaria in its early stages can be mistaken for flu and quickly escalate into a life-threatening situation. Meningitis can cause a fever, as can deep vein thrombosis or appendicitis. This wide range of possible causes is best considered by a local physician, who will be more aware of the local conditions than you, as a visitor, can be.

A body that's feverish can go through many changes, from shivering and coldness to heat, sweating, and delirium. If possible, help to bring the fever down by keeping the body cool with sponging. Add the essential oil of eucalyptus radiata, peppermint, chamomile, or lavender in the water you use to sponge the body.

Give the person plenty of liquids, including fruit juices. Spray the area or room with thyme linalol and tea tree, and use it yourself if you're nursing someone — 2 drops in a bath.

Traveler's Tummy

I asked an intrepid traveler who never has tummy trouble what the secret is. "Only drink bottled water, even if that means taking a crate of your own, never have ice in drinks, avoid all uncooked food, and take a Swiss Army knife." The knife, apparently, is for cutting the skin off fruits. It might seem a bit much to wash your teeth in bottled spring water, but it's a lot less inconvenient than having diarrhea and spending your holiday sightseeing the bathroom!

An amazing number of people get tummy trouble when staying at deluxe hotels, and this may be due to attractive but unprotected buffets — which can be an interesting landing stage for flies. The simple fact of having new foods can cause diarrhea, as can heat. Lemon essential oil will help to purify the water in which you should wash all fruit and vegetables before peeling them. Take with you on vacation a good probiotic supplement especially formulated for travel, as this will increase the good gut bacteria and help fight any invading bacteria.

DIARRHEA

In its mild form, diarrhea usually only lasts up to 48 hours. The main problem with diarrhea is dehydration. If you're unfortunate enough to have a bout of diarrhea, drink plenty of fluids to replace those lost and take a rehydration formula drink to replace electrolytes. If you can't get one, make your own:

REHYDRATION BLEND

Bottled water	1 pint (475 mL)
Sugar	3 level teaspoons
Salt	¼ teaspoon
Lemon essential oil	1 drop (or fresh lemon or lime juice)

Mix together well and drink one small glass at a time.

A warm bath with 4 drops each of geranium and ginger essential oil diluted in a small amount of carrier oil often helps to calm the nerves, and at the very least it will make you feel better.

FOOD POISONING

Food poisoning usually shows up within 24 hours of having eaten the offending meal. It may be caused by bacteria carried by humans or flies or by rotten food. Nausea, vomiting, pain, and diarrhea are the most likely effects, and fever and illness can develop.

Drink plenty of fluids, use rehydration drinks, or use the Rehydration Blend recipe above, and massage the whole body with the following:

Tea tree	2 drops
Geranium	5 drops
Lavender	10 drops

Blend the essential oils together, then dilute by adding 5 drops to each teaspoon (5 mL) of carrier oil.

To help alleviate the physical shock that can result from vomiting and purging, apply 5 drops of ginger essential oil diluted in 1 teaspoon of carrier oil over the whole of the abdomen.

BACILLARY DYSENTERY

Bacillary dysentery, or shigellosis, is carried in contaminated water and food and spread by flies and other carriers, and also by human contacts. It can be distinguished from diarrhea by the fact that the initial watery stools are followed by stools containing mucus and blood. *Bacillary dysentery is infectious* and must be treated by a physician, as saline injections may need to be given. The sufferer could have abdominal pain, fever, vomiting, nausea, chills, and loss of appetite. Rehydration with electrolytes is a must. Keep the person away from others, and spray their room with thyme, lemongrass, and lavender.

Add the following oils to baths (the dose is necessarily high in this case):

Thyme linalol	5 drops
Lavender	5 drops
Ginger	4 drops
Tea tree	1 drop

Dilute first in an equal amount of carrier oil.

If muscle pains occur, use the four essential oils above in a massage oil, in equal parts. Lavender may ease any headache and high temperature, but if it doesn't, use peppermint oil instead — put 1 drop between the index fingers of both hands and rub along the base of the skull and around the temples.

Little Things That Bite

Most travelers are acutely aware of the discomfort and dangers that can be brought about by the smaller creatures living on this earth — and many small creatures seem to make up for their small size by being particularly aggressive. As you'll see from reading this section, dangers are as likely to come from hiking in the mountains, or taking forest walks, or swimming in the sea, or sunning yourself on a beach infested with sand flies, or having a drink on the veranda when the mosquitoes are out. So wherever you go, take your travel kit with you, or at least the oil(s) that are most applicable to the environment you're going to be in. They take up very little room, and if you need them, you'll be glad you didn't leave them behind in the hotel room.

Snakes are just one of the hidden dangers lurking in the undergrowth. A number of harmless-looking plants cause nasty rashes, and many more cause allergic reactions in some people. We share the seas with sea urchins and jellyfish, whose stings come as a nasty shock. The list of insects that bite or sting is almost endless and includes bees, wasps, fleas, bedbugs, gnats, midges, ticks, sand flies, water-ticks, hornets, and that pernicious spreader of disease — the mosquito.

All the oils in the Basic Travel Kit have antiseptic properties and can be applied directly to the skin if you get bitten by an insect — and the sooner, the better. But try to acquaint yourself with the more specific actions and remedies recommended in this section so you're prepared to deal with those little creatures that bite and sting.

PREVENTION

Prevention is better than cure and, as far as insect bites are concerned, a fairly easy option. As a general rule use lemongrass or citronella to keep insects at bay, using the airborne methods of dispersing the oils. Use hot-water bowls, heat sources, paper strings at the windows or ribbons hung from trees, or any other atmospheric method outlined in this book. If you're making a fire outside, put 1 drop of insect-deterrent essential oil on a few pieces of wood about half an hour before putting them on the fire. As they burn, the aroma will be released. To deter insects from landing on your skin, as a general rule lavender is one of the best options.

One of the most helpful things to travel with is a small plastic spray bottle. It will be useful in many ways, including spraying lemongrass or citronella diluted in water around a room. If you have your own en-suite bathroom, let the water run steaming hot into the bath and put a couple

of drops of essential oil on the water before going out for the evening, leaving the steam to waft through the open bathroom door and into your bedroom. Also, put a couple of drops onto the hot tap so its heat releases the aroma molecules into the atmosphere. Alternatively, fill any convenient containers such as cups or glasses with hot water from the bathroom or, preferably, boiling water from a kettle, put a couple of drops of essential oil on the surface of the water, and place the containers strategically by windows or other places where unwelcome visitors may enter your room. If you have a mosquito net, don't forget to use it; as these often have small holes in them, put essential oils on the net itself. In all these methods you can use lavender, lemongrass, thyme, peppermint, or tea tree, or make up the very effective blend below:

INSECT DETERRENT BLEND

Thyme linalol	4 drops
Lemongrass	8 drops
Lavender	4 drops
Peppermint	4 drops
Tea tree	2 drops

It's worth making up quite a bit of this synergistic blend and taking it with you because it can be used in several different ways. Overnight, or during your afternoon siesta, put 2 drops on a cotton ball or tissue and leave it somewhere near your bed. To try and discourage insects from disturbing your meal on the balcony, cut up lengths of ribbon or paper — disposable tissues will do. Put 1 drop of essential oil on each piece and hang them around the balcony. Hanging these aromatic strips above a window may make an insect think twice about entering your room. A good alternative to the essential oil blend above, either to use on its own or in a blend, is eucalyptus lemon (*Eucalyptus citriodora*).

Some people seem to attract little biting insects while others do not, and some people seem to be a magnet for particular insects while others look on, untouched. Clearly there can be no fixed rules here because there are so many species of biting insects — for example, there are over 3,000 different types of mosquito, and to some extent each could be attracted by different bodily chemicals. With insect deterrents, it's very much a matter of personal experimentation. However, people have been using essential oils as insect repellents for a very long time, and certain general observations have been made.

According to one study, the number of mosquitoes observed multiplied 500% when the full moon was out. That's worth remembering when you're wondering whether to apply an essential oil on a moonlit evening to deter them. Also, they apparently prefer people who wear dark clothing, so wearing light-colored clothing in areas where they are rife seems sensible, as does wearing long sleeves and pants. Apparently, mosquitoes are attracted by the smell of beer, and if you're sitting around a table with a group of people and only those drinking beer are getting bitten, that might explain it. Perfumes are said to attract mosquitoes, but as most of the commercial products produced today are more chemical than natural, that's not to say sweet-smelling essential oils will have the same effect.

When diluting an essential oil to make a preventative body rub during a vacation, use 2 drops of the Insect Deterrent Blend, above, diluted in 2 teaspoons (10 mL) of a carrier oil. Or simply add the neat essential oil blend to any body lotion, balm, or cream you may have.

You can make a water-based splash by adding 5 drops of the Insect Deterrent Blend to 1 tablespoon (15 mL) of witch hazel and then diluting it in 3 tablespoons (45 mL) of water. Shake the mixture before each application. Instead of witch hazel you could substitute an alcohol such as vodka, but use 2 teaspoons instead of 1 tablespoon. Splash

the liquid onto your body and smooth it over any exposed areas of skin.

For an evening deterrent, prepare in advance a gel that consists of 2 tablespoons (30 mL) of carrier oil or aloe vera gel, to which you've added 15 drops of lavender or geranium oil. Rub a little of that on the parts of the skin that are exposed, such as arms, legs, and ankles. You can do the same before going to bed to protect you during the night.

BITES AND STINGS: GENERAL ACTION

We usually say insects "bite," and we mostly say that fish "sting," as do certain plants. Either way, the effects are commonly confined to a localized area of reaction — with swelling, redness, soreness, or a rash — but if there's an allergic reaction the effects can be felt throughout the whole body. In all cases of bites or stings, whether from animals, insects, fish, other sea creatures, snakes, or plants, some kind of antidote needs to be applied.

Infection is a risk with many bites and stings. Without a doubt, prevention is the best line of defense, and a few moments spent in applying an oil, cream, balm, or lotion might just save a great deal of time and inconvenience, not to mention danger, later on. Essential oils are well known for their ability to keep a person sting-free and are the active ingredient in many brand-name products. When you use the real thing — the natural product unhampered by chemical solvents and the like — you have tremendous flexibility in their use. The same little bottle can give protection in a room, on the balcony, in a car, on the body, and even on your clothes. And then, if you're unfortunate enough to encounter trouble, the essential oils can help you to deal with the bite or sting while you're on your way to get medical advice. Before looking at particular situations, let's have a look at the general action that can be taken.

In many cases you'll need a disinfectant wash, especially if you are accident-prone. The following blends are extremely effective and can be made up either before you travel or on the spot, if required. To cleanse the area add 8 drops of either blend to a bowl of water. If you don't have a blend pre-prepared, add the number of drops shown in parentheses to a single bowl or cup of water:

DISINFECTANT CLEANSING BLEND

Lavender	10 drops (or 2)
Thyme linalol	20 drops (or 4)
Eucalyptus radiata	10 drops (or 2)

TROPICAL DISINFECTANT CLEANSING BLEND

Lavender	10 drops (or 2)
Thyme linalol	20 drops (or 4)
Eucalyptus radiata	5 drops (or 1)
*Palmarosa or oregano	5 drops (or 1)

These are not in the travel kit but are very useful oils to have.

If you've been stung or bitten, have no idea what caused it, and swelling occurs, first apply a small amount of neat lavender oil to the area, followed by a small amount of neat chamomile roman. One drop can cover quite a large area — apply as needed. If the swelling is excessive as a result of an allergic reaction, seek medical attention.

The following guidelines are first aid measures only:

Animals

General advice for animal bites and scratches: If the skin is broken, medical evaluation and a tetanus injection might be required. In any event, wash the area with a mild soap and warm water to which you've added thyme linalol or lavender essential oils or, if you have it ready, one of the disinfectant blends above. Then add 4 drops of lavender and 3 drops of thyme to a bandage, piece of gauze, or fabric part of an adhesive bandage, and

let it dry. Once the affected area is washed, apply this bandage over this wound.

Rabies is also a concern with animals. Government agencies around the world spend a great deal of money trying to prevent the rabies virus from being brought into the country via animals. But many countries do not. When traveling, be aware of this situation and tell your children not to approach animals in the same way as they might at home.

Rabies is a viral infection that's transmitted by the saliva of an infected animal — usually stray dogs and bats, but it could be any animal, including cattle, foxes, wolves, skunks, and raccoons. Even cute little kittens may carry the virus, so just admire them from a distance. Licks on a small cut or open wound and licks to the mouth, lips, eyes, or nose can also transmit the virus. Hospital attention must be sought immediately if rabies is suspected. If you have been bitten, wash the area as thoroughly as possible and apply neat thyme linalol or oregano essential oil and the strongest alcohol you can lay your hands on while waiting for transport to a hospital.

Insects

General advice for insect bites and stings: If there's a visible sting, remove it but try to avoid squeezing and breaking the venom bag that may be attached. Apply 1 drop of neat lavender oil directly to the site of the sting. Continue to apply neat lavender, a drop at a time, every five minutes or as soon as the drop can be seen to be absorbed, until you reach a total of 5 drops.

Mosquitoes: I don't know anyone who likes mosquitoes. They aren't cuddly, and they don't sing. They just buzz around, threatening to strike. Only female mosquitoes bite, and they do so because they need the blood to help their eggs mature before laying them. But they can be vectors for disease and can ruin a holiday, not to mention a life.

Each year, worldwide, mosquitoes cause one million deaths. The diseases carried by mosquitoes include malaria, West Nile virus, Zika fever, dengue, yellow fever, and chikungunya.

As you can never know who that mosquito diving around your room bit before she started taking a swipe at you, it's only sensible to take all precautions possible to avoid getting bitten yourself. And when you put on your protective oil don't forget your face — it might be life saving as well as face saving! Taking vitamin B1 (thiamin) and garlic oil supplements every day for at least two weeks before going on your travels may discourage bites, as both are disliked by mosquitoes. See "Prevention" on page 128, for other ways to deter mosquitoes. Another thing to keep in mind is that carbon monoxide (CO) and lactic acid are known to attract mosquitoes. CO levels, which are present in a person's breath, are higher in smokers. Lactic acid is present in humans and is also used in soft drinks, candy, processed foods, water, plastic packaging, leather processing, and a whole range of industrial processes.

If you've already been bitten, use neat lavender oil on the bite. If you've been bitten over a large area, take 1 cup of cider vinegar or the juice of two lemons and add to it 10 drops of lavender and 5 of thyme linalol. Put this mixture in a bath, swishing the water around before you get in. Afterward, apply neat lavender oil to all the bites. Each night rub your body with the oil blend given for sand flies, on page 133, adding 5 drops of lemongrass to the mix.

Bees: Bee stings are painful, and if you have an allergy to bees and bee products there's a risk of anaphylaxis and medical attention must be sought. If you experience sudden weakness, your blood pressure may have dropped, which could be an indication of an allergic reaction, so take an antihistamine immediately. Other signs include difficulty in swallowing or breathing due to swelling in the mouth and throat, flushed skin, hives, or nausea. If you feel any of these or other symptoms are developing, seek medical advice.

Most people have no reaction to a bee sting other than pain and swelling at the site. Try to scrape the sting away, rather than pulling, which may cause more venom to enter the skin. Apply a cold compress of chamomile roman or chamomile german to the area. Leave it there for several hours, but if the sting is in an awkward place just hold the compress to it for as long as possible. In both cases, apply 1 drop of neat chamomile twice a day for two days. Bees sting only once, then die.

Wasps and hornets: Wasps and hornets can sting a person several times and they don't die afterward. Plus, if you're bitten by either a wasp or hornet, watch out for more because they both release a pheromone that attracts others of their clan to join in the attack. If you have a can of hair spray handy, spray them! Remove the stings by scraping them sideways.

As wasp stings are alkaline, bathe the area with cider or wine vinegar: into 1 teaspoon put 2 drops each of lavender and chamomile roman essential oil, mix well, and dab onto the stung area three times a day. With hornet stings, follow the treatment recommended for bee stings above, or use undiluted lavender, three times a day.

Spiders: Even the bite of the tiniest of spiders can be fatal. In schools in the United States and Australia children are taught to distinguish safe from unsafe spiders, and many disagreeable bites have been prevented. The first line of defense is to educate yourself about the appearance of venomous spiders. But that only helps, of course, if you saw the one that bit you!

For lethal spider bites, apply 10 neat drops of lavender to the area every 5 to 10 minutes until you get to a hospital and medical care.

For nonlethal spider bites, dilute 3 drops of lavender and 2 drops of chamomile roman essential oil in a teaspoon of alcohol, blend together well, and apply to the area three times over the course of one day. One day of treatment should suffice.

Ticks: Ticks are vectors of many serious conditions, including Lyme disease, Rocky Mountain spotted fever, and Colorado tick fever. They usually feed off the blood of animals but can also attach to humans. Ticks try to attach themselves to new hosts by jumping from tall grass, for example, which is why most bites are on the lower portion of the body. Preventative measures should be undertaken whenever possible.

If hiking or camping in an area known as being tick habitat, try to protect yourself and children in particular by wearing long-sleeved tops and pants, tucking the bottoms of the pant legs into long socks. As a deterrent essential oils can be put onto clothing: use lavender, eucalyptus radiata, peppermint, lemongrass, citronella, palmarosa, or tea tree. Eucalyptus lemon (*Eucalyptus citriodora*) is effective; take it with you if planning a visit into an area known for Lyme disease–carrying ticks. Essential oils that are colorless should not leave a mark on clothing; those that are colored may.

You'll notice the blood-sucking tick by its swollen body attached to the skin. If bitten, remove the tick with a tick-removing implement or pointed tweezers, sliding them along the skin and under the body of the tick and removing it in one swift movement. Keep the tick to show to the physician. Then put 1 drop of thyme linalol essential oil directly on the bite, and apply 1 drop of neat lavender every five minutes, to a total of 10 drops, to try and avoid infection and reduce pain and swelling. If no tick-removing implement or tweezers are available, don't try to pull the tick out of the skin. Carry out the same procedure, dropping the essential oil directly onto the tick until it falls off.

Before leaving the area, check that ticks have not attached themselves to you or your pets and

children — look at small children's heads in particular.

Gnats and midges: There are some parts of the world where gnats and midges are so numerous that they create a cloud of kinetic annoyance. If bitten, dilute 3 drops of thyme linalol, citronella, or lemongrass essential oil in 1 teaspoon of cider vinegar or lemon juice and apply to the bites. This will stop the irritation. As an alternative, you can combine a little neat lavender or tea tree oil with aloe vera gel. Use ribbons or paper strips with essential oils on them to try to deter gnats and midges from entering the area you're in.

Bedbugs and fleas: To deter bedbugs and fleas, when you arrive at your destination pull back the bedclothes and add lavender oil to a tissue and wipe it over the mattress. You might also want to drop lavender oil onto the bedding. If bitten, the important factor is to avoid infection. Bathe the bitten areas and apply neat lavender. Alternatively, dilute 3 drops of thyme linalol in cider vinegar and apply over the bitten area. Eucalyptus radiata is another option — use as you would lavender.

Chiggers and jiggers: *Chiggers* is the name given to the minuscule orange mite of the Trombiculidae family, whose larvae crawl inside human skin, where they inject digestive enzymes so they can more easily eat the skin cells. The tiny female jigger, or chigoe flea, burrows its head into the human host and stays there for a couple of weeks while its eggs develop, the female swelling in size. The flea then dies, which might sound like good news, except it stays in the human host and rots. That's what can cause the infection. These charming little creatures usually enter humans through their feet, as they stroll barefoot in the delightful garden around the hotel or along the beautiful beach.

If you feel a chigger, or see a jigger, dilute 10 drops of thyme linalol in a teaspoon of any alcohol and apply some to the area every three hours.

The next day, and thereafter, apply neat lavender three times a day. If red lines appear up the leg or there's swelling in the lymph glands, consult a physician.

Sand flies: It's hard to avoid knowing that you've been bitten by sand flies because it hurts. With some species, it can feel as if they've crawled right into you and out the other side. As sand flies can cause leishmaniasis and other serious conditions, it's best to deal with the bites straight away. This is why you carry that little bottle of lavender in your beach bag! Apply neat lavender as soon as possible. Then massage the whole of the body twice a day for a week with the following oil:

BLEND FOR SAND FLY BITES

Lavender	10 drops
Eucalyptus radiata	10 drops
Thyme linalol	10 drops
Tea tree	5 drops

Blend the essential oils together, then dilute by using 3–5 drops to each teaspoon (5 mL) of carrier oil.

If you cannot get a container for this quantity quickly, use 3 drops of each oil in 2 teaspoons (10 mL) of carrier oil. If fever develops, see a physician and tell them you were bitten.

Snakes

Snake bites have the potential to be deadly, and the best advice is to get to a hospital quickly. Most of us can't distinguish between a snake that's dangerous and one that's not, so just try to recall what the snake looked like so you can tell the paramedic or specialist. While waiting for help or on the way there, remove any jewelry in case swelling develops and keep the person calm and immobile, especially in the area bitten — for example, make an arm sling if that will help restrict movement. *Do not move* the area of the bite, as this might disperse the venom. Do nothing to the area of the bite itself other than pouring liquid over it to wash away the venom — water is best, but any liquid is better than none — and then dropping neat undiluted lavender essential oil directly on the bite. Use as much as you like, and often… this is an emergency. Lavender has long been used effectively against the venomous adders in mountainous regions of Europe, and it is about the best essential oil from the Basic Travel Kit to use until you can get help.

Fish and Marine Animals

General advice for fish bites: Dry the area and apply 1 drop of neat lavender oil. Continue to apply neat lavender a drop at a time, every five minutes or as soon as the previous drop is absorbed, until a total of 5 drops has been reached.

Poisonous fish and marine animals carry their venom mainly in their tentacles and spines. If spines become lodged within the skin they can be extremely painful to extract, and the risk of infection is always a problem, especially in polluted waters. Any visible spines should be removed and the area washed in clean saltwater; then apply neat thyme linalol and tea tree essential oil.

For stings, wash the area in cold water and immediately apply neat chamomile roman or chamomile german. In many parts of the world, in the absence of other options, fresh urine is used to quash the pain of sea urchin stings.

Portuguese man-of-war: The stings of this long-tentacled creature are extremely painful and cause shock, cramps, vomiting, and difficulty breathing. Medical attention must be sought as soon as possible. Remove any of the remaining tentacles and wash the area with saltwater, not fresh water. Then apply neat lavender all over the area, and as the skin absorbs it, apply some more. If medical treatment has not been possible, wash the area with soap and water and apply chamomile;

continue applying lavender and chamomile every three hours for 24 hours. Keep the person warm and in bed or rested. Give plenty of warm liquids and arnica (a widely available homeopathic preparation) for shock. Apply 2 teaspoons (10 mL) of the following oil to the whole body once a day:

Eucalyptus radiata	10 drops
Peppermint	2 drops
Geranium	10 drops

Blend together, then dilute by adding 3–5 drops to each teaspoon (5 mL) of carrier oil.

Jellyfish: The small common jellyfish can give a slight sting with a reddening effect. Wash the area thoroughly as soon as you can with soap and water, apply 1 drop of chamomile roman, chamomile german, or lavender oil, and then ice.

Sea urchins: If you happen to be unlucky enough to tread on the spines of a sea urchin, the most important thing is to get all the spines out. As these are extremely brittle and break easily, do be careful about it — and make sure that whatever you use to remove them is sterilized first (you can sterilize most any metal with fire, wiping the blackened carbon from the tool before using). After removing all of the spines and washing the area thoroughly, apply 1 drop of neat thyme linalol or lemongrass essential oil over the area every three hours, for 12 hours.

If the spines prove difficult to get out, buy a papaya and use the inside of the skin as a poultice. The enzymes in the fruit help to dissolve the traces of spine left in the skin and also soothe the area. If you are in any doubt that all traces of the spines are gone, seek medical help because if they're left in the skin, usually the foot, this will cause infection.

The pain can be lessened by using the following blend of three essential oils in equal parts:

Chamomile roman or chamomile german	10 drops
Lavender	10 drops
Eucalyptus radiata	10 drops

Blend together, then dilute by adding 5 drops to each teaspoon (5 mL) of carrier oil. Alternatively, use 2 drops of each essential oil listed — for a total of 6 drops — to each teaspoon of carrier oil.

Plants

Some plant species (stinging nettles, poison ivy, and so forth) contain irritants, and these can cause an allergic reaction, such as urticaria, or hives. Intense itching may be a problem, along with areas of raised, often flaky, red or white skin. Wash with soap and cold water as soon as you can, then apply eucalyptus radiata, lavender, or chamomile roman, either undiluted, diluted in aloe vera gel, or on a compress. A cold compress with 2 drops of one of these essential oils often stops the irritation within a few hours.

Pollution

Many vacations feature water as their main attraction — the sea, the lake, or the river. What the glossy images don't tell us, however, is how clean that water is. The lovely color we see on the website has probably been adjusted to make it seem sparkling clean. The problem is that the world's waterways are running with pollutants, dumped there by under-resourced municipalities, irresponsible industries, and ships at sea. If you develop any unusual condition as a result of swimming, treat it as a viral infection — better safe than sorry!

The A–Z Basic Travel Kit Emergency Reference Chart

If you cannot get hold of the botanical species of the essential oils recommended for the Basic Travel Kit, use any close variant that's available to you. For example, *Eucalyptus globulus* may be easier to purchase than *Eucalyptus radiata*. Try to take a small bottle of cider vinegar with you when you travel, or use any vinegar available to you at your destination — even asking for it from a hotel kitchen if needed. Vinegar has antibiotic and antifungal properties and can be used to dilute essential oils.

Animal bites: thyme linalol, lavender, eucalyptus radiata, chamomile roman, tea tree, peppermint

Blisters: geranium, tea tree, lemongrass

Bruises: chamomile roman, geranium, lavender, rosemary

Bumps: lavender, chamomile roman, rosemary, ginger

Burns: lavender

Chills: ginger, geranium, thyme linalol

Colds: eucalyptus radiata, ginger, thyme linalol

Constipation: peppermint, thyme linalol, ginger, lemongrass, geranium

Cramping: geranium, ginger, rosemary, peppermint

Dry, flaky skin: geranium, lavender, chamomile roman

Exhaustion, physical: lavender, chamomile roman, peppermint, geranium, rosemary, lemongrass

Exposure, cold: ginger, thyme linalol, geranium

Exposure, heat: eucalyptus radiata, peppermint, lavender, rosemary

Fevers: eucalyptus radiata, peppermint, lavender, lemongrass, ginger, rosemary

Fractures: ginger, thyme linalol, lavender, geranium, rosemary

Grazes, cuts: lavender, thyme linalol, lemongrass, eucalyptus radiata, tea tree

Hay fever: chamomile roman, eucalyptus radiata, rosemary

Headaches: peppermint, lavender, rosemary, chamomile roman

Heat exhaustion: lavender, eucalyptus radiata, chamomile roman, peppermint

Heatstroke: lavender, eucalyptus radiata, peppermint, chamomile roman

Indigestion: peppermint, ginger, rosemary

Infections: thyme linalol, lavender, chamomile roman, eucalyptus radiata, tea tree

Insect bites: lavender, chamomile roman, eucalyptus radiata, thyme linalol, tea tree

Insect repellent: lemongrass, thyme linalol, lavender, peppermint, tea tree

Itching, summer: eucalyptus radiata, peppermint, lavender, tea tree

Jet lag: lavender, eucalyptus radiata, geranium, peppermint, lemongrass, grapefruit, rosemary

Muscles, overexercised: thyme linalol, lavender, eucalyptus radiata, ginger, lemongrass, rosemary, chamomile roman

Prickly heat: geranium, chamomile roman, eucalyptus radiata, lavender

Rashes: lavender, chamomile roman, eucalyptus radiata, tea tree

Sleeplessness: chamomile roman, lavender

Sprains, strains: ginger, thyme linalol, lavender, chamomile roman, rosemary

Stomach upset: ginger, lavender, chamomile roman, lemongrass, peppermint, geranium

Sunburn: lavender, peppermint, eucalyptus radiata, chamomile roman

Sunstroke: eucalyptus radiata, lavender, peppermint

Swellings: eucalyptus radiata, lavender, chamomile roman, peppermint

Toothache: peppermint, chamomile roman

Travel sickness: ginger, peppermint

Vomiting: peppermint, lavender, ginger, rosemary

Windburn: lavender, chamomile roman, eucalyptus radiata

Wounds: lavender, chamomile roman, tea tree, thyme linalol

7

The Gentle Touch for Babies, Children, and Teenagers

Nothing in the world is more precious to us than our children, and it's a daunting responsibility to care for them. We all rely heavily on the medical professions to keep our children healthy, and we should continue to take advantage of all the benefits modern medicine can offer us. But there are times when help is not available, when we have to fall back on our own resources, and take the care of our children into our own hands.

This quote from the foreword of my book *Aromatherapy for the Healthy Child* sums up the relationship between us, our children, medicine, and essential oils. Our children look to us for help; we are their world. They are our delight and our utmost concern. We all thank goodness for physicians and medicine that can help our children, but there are times when help is simply not available. Maybe the physician can't be reached. If we're traveling, the usual facilities are not at hand. Perhaps the snow has fallen and made a barrier between us and the outside world. For a multitude of reasons, then, having a collection of essential oils nearby can be a blessing, and one that comes straight from nature's hands.

The first section in this chapter is "The Successful Child," where we look at a much-overlooked subject — the stresses faced by children and how to overcome them. Next, there is a chart showing the

essential oils appropriate for each age group. We then come to the problems that can arise in babyhood, followed by a wide range of conditions experienced by children of all ages. This is followed by advice on teenage issues, and then we look at how help can be given to children with 12 very different special challenges, including autism, attention deficit hyperactivity disorder (ADHD) and attention deficit disorder (ADD).

When using essential oils with children we employ a sliding scale of dosage to mirror their growth. It's important to recognize that some essential oils are not suitable for children, depending on their age. This might be because the essential oil has hormonal properties or because it may be unsuitable for the weaker constitutions of children. The most important thing to remember when using essential oils on children is to reserve their use for emergencies only, and not to use them every day. Ideally, all products used on children should be organic.

The Successful Child

Children have to deal with pressure from their peers to conform to group expectations, possible bullying, uncertainty when changing schools and losing lifelong friends, and, of course, years of exams. On top of these things that we recognize from our own childhoods, there are ongoing developments in social media about which we may be unaware. There is a whole digital universe that our children are living in and trying to keep up with, and we may not be in a position to recognize its stresses and possible dangers. At home too there may be issues that children find hard to deal with, including emotional turmoil among the adults in their lives and sibling rivalry. Children today live in the age of information overload, and it can be easy to ignore this fact and accept it as the new normal. But what we can do is stop to consider all these issues, and try to make our children's lives a little easier. If you have a child who is a teenager, please also look at "The Teenage Years" section in this chapter.

ENHANCED MEMORY FOR EXAM SUCCESS

We've all had the experience: a particular aroma instantly reminds us of a special person or place — perhaps from a long time ago. This happens because aroma goes to the limbic portion of the brain, which is the oldest part of the brain and connects aroma with both memory and emotion. This is a powerful connection that can be harnessed to help with studying for exams. Research into learning and memory recall has shown that memory is improved if an aroma is diffused in the room while studying, and then that same aroma is smelled while trying to remember the information studied.

Each essential oil has a unique aroma, of course, but some actually enhance memory recall itself, while others are additionally useful as aids to focus and concentration. These include lemon, peppermint, and rosemary. Bergamot is another useful aroma, as it helps build confidence. It's essential though that your child actually likes the aroma, and they should be consulted about which essential oils you use.

The other key point to remember is that each subject the child studies — for example, math or history — should be allocated its own aroma. When studying for a math exam, use one particular essential oil, and then use that same aroma for the math exam itself. Use a different aroma both while studying history and taking the history exam. The same applies for any other subject.

While studying, the essential oils can be used in one of the room methods; for example use 3–4 drops in a diffuser. When your child has stopped studying, take the aroma away, then open a window or let some fresh air into the room. When the time comes for the exam, the aroma needs to be introduced again. Obviously, you can't have the aroma diffused in the exam room! So you have to find a way for your child to be able to smell the aroma just before the exam. The easiest way is to give them a tissue with a drop of the essential oil on it, which they can inhale before the exam. The aroma should be subtle, so dilute the drop of essential oil in a little carrier oil before putting it on the handkerchief. Some people put the drop of essential oil on the cuff of the shirt or jacket, but that can sometimes be too strong and also damage the clothing.

SCHOOL STRESS

Whatever the age of your child, school can be stressful. Unlike adults who have to compete in only one area — the one for which they have already shown an aptitude and which is their profession — the young person at school is under pressure to succeed in many different subject areas, only some of which they may like. Also, there are peer pressures — which may very well have a social media element — and being liked is important to children. As a parent it's often difficult to know how your child is developing at school or college, as children can find it difficult to talk about what's happening to them.

One of the best ways for anyone to relax is to take a long bath. Younger children should not be left alone while bathing. During the bath or, if your child is old enough to bathe on their own, before or after the bath, invite your child to tell you what's bothering them. Really give them some time to fully express what's on their mind; one of the most precious things we can give a child is our time.

BATH OILS FOR SCHOOL STRESS
Chamomile roman (*Anthemis nobilis*)
Bergamot (*Citrus bergamia*)
Marjoram, sweet (*Origanum majorana*)
Geranium (*Pelargonium graveolens*)
Lemon (*Citrus limon*)
Lavender (*Lavandula angustifolia*)
Clary sage (*Salvia sclarea*)
Mandarin (*Citrus reticulata*)
Sandalwood (*Santalum album*)
Petitgrain (*Citrus aurantium*)

Use 2 drops of one of the essential oils above, or follow one of the blends below, which are designed to help a child cope with school stress. First, though, dilute the essential oil in ½ teaspoon of carrier oil before adding to the bathwater. Make sure the oil droplets are well dispersed by swishing the water about with a hand. Any excessive oil droplets that float on the surface can be removed with a paper towel before the child gets into the bath. The amount of essential oil in Blends 1 and 2 below are enough for four baths each.

BATH BLEND FOR SCHOOL STRESS 1

Bergamot	2 drops
Lavender	2 drops
Marjoram, sweet	2 drops
Lemon	2 drops

Diluted in 2 teaspoons of carrier oil, this makes enough for four baths.

BATH BLEND FOR SCHOOL STRESS 2

Geranium	2 drops
Mandarin	4 drops
Petitgrain	2 drops

Diluted in 2 teaspoons of carrier oil, this makes enough for four baths.

A simple remedy is to add 2 drops of lavender or petitgrain essential oil to ½ teaspoon of carrier oil and drop into the bathtub before the child gets into the bath. Afterward, wrap your child up in something cozy and give them a big warm drink and a gentle foot rub. No child can remain uptight after that!

EXAM STRESS

If your child is under 16 years old, use the following blend in a nightly bath for at least a week before the exams. Don't tell them "it's for nerves" — that puts the idea into their head that they're nervous — but instead say it's to relax and make them feel good. Which it is.

PRE-EXAM BATH BLEND FOR CHILDREN UNDER 16

Lavender	5 drops
Chamomile roman	3 drops
Geranium	3 drops
Mandarin	5 drops

Blend the essential oils together and use 2 drops diluted in ½ teaspoon of sweet almond oil in each bath.

On the morning of the exam, put 1 drop of grapefruit and 1 drop of lavender, diluted in 2 teaspoons of carrier oil (10 mL), in a bath or on a washcloth to be used after washing.

TO HELP SLEEP

Children should be able to sleep soundly without any worries, but life is not always so ideal. Essential oil body oils are very good at reducing stress and helping children to sleep, which will allow them to wake up feeling stronger and ready to face another day. Use a little of the following blend, rubbed onto your child's back before they go to bed.

SLEEP BLEND
Lavender   2 drops
Chamomile roman   1 drop
Dilute in 2 teaspoons (10 mL) of carrier oil.

A GOOD FOUNDATION

Children spend most of their time at home, and parents can provide a relaxing and secure environment for them, where the young person can feel valued and supported. Teenagers in particular need to touch home base, perhaps precisely because they're now extending their sights outward. Touch is extremely important for everyone, but parents tend to hug their children less as they grow older. Cuddles may seem childish to a teenager, and so massage, which is very grown up, is a good way to get in touch with your child, literally and figuratively. You can simply massage their hands or feet, or the shoulders, back, and legs, or, indeed, the whole body. The following essential oils are particularly good for this purpose. The botanical names can be found in the section that follows, which is organized by age.

Boys	*Girls*
Cedarwood atlas	Petitgrain
Marjoram, sweet	Geranium
Bergamot	Lavender
Cypress	Orange, sweet
Lavender	Rosewood
Orange, sweet	Bergamot
Frankincense	Frankincense
Geranium	Ylang ylang

Essential Oils for Babies and Children

What follows are lists of essential oils that can be used on children of particular ages. With each age range, you'll find the dilution ratio — how much carrier oil to use for diluting the specified number of drops of essential oil. Because with children the dilution ratio is so low, it is often necessary to dilute the essential oils into a large volume of carrier oil.

The lists that follow are intended as a general guideline for the home practitioner. Elsewhere in this chapter you'll find blends for specific conditions that use a higher dilution than that recommended for general use in the age-related sections below. This is because those blends address particular problems and are to be used over a short period of time. Generally, refer to the age-related list if using the essential oils for a purpose not covered specifically in this chapter.

Undiluted essential oils are not recommended for use on newborn babies. For the home practitioner, particular carrier oils are recommended instead. When preparing for the birth, gather together good-quality carrier oils, by which I mean non–genetically modified organic oils.

The carrier oils to avoid when caring for babies and children are soy, rapeseed, corn, olive, sunflower, and peanut (groundnut or arachis). Sweet almond is an ideal oil for children of all ages; however, if your child has a sensitivity to nuts it is best to avoid any carrier oil extracted from nuts. In chapter 19 there are detailed profiles for alternative carrier oils to use.

TABLE 8. OILS FOR CHILDREN BY AGE

AGE	DILUTION RATIO AND CARRIER OIL	APPROPRIATE ESSENTIAL OILS
2 WEEKS TO 2 MONTHS	1 drop diluted in 2 tablespoons (30 mL) of sweet almond oil or camellia seed oil	Chamomile german (*Matricaria recutita*) Chamomile roman (*Anthemis nobilis*) Lavender (*Lavandula angustifolia*) Mandarin (*Citrus reticulata*)
3 TO 6 MONTHS	2 drops diluted in 2 tablespoons (30 mL) of sweet almond oil or camellia seed oil	Chamomile german (*Matricaria recutita*) Chamomile roman (*Anthemis nobilis*) Coriander seed (*Coriandrum sativum*) Geranium (*Pelargonium graveolens*) Lavender (*Lavandula angustifolia*) Mandarin (*Citrus reticulata*) Tea tree (*Melaleuca alternifolia*)
7 MONTHS TO 2 YEARS	3–4 drops diluted in 2 tablespoons (30 mL) of sweet almond oil or camellia seed oil	Chamomile german (*Matricaria recutita*) Chamomile roman (*Anthemis nobilis*) Coriander seed (*Coriandrum sativum*) Frankincense (*Boswellia carterii*) Geranium (*Pelargonium graveolens*) Lavender (*Lavandula angustifolia*) Mandarin (*Citrus reticulata*) Manuka (*Leptospermum scoparium*) Orange, sweet (*Citrus sinensis*) Palmarosa (*Cymbopogon martinii*) Ravensara (*Ravensara aromatica*) Thyme linalol (*Thymus vulgaris ct. linalool*)
3 TO 5 YEARS *(continues on next page)*	4–6 drops diluted in 2 tablespoons (30 mL) of sweet almond oil	Cajuput (*Melaleuca cajuputi*) Chamomile german (*Matricaria recutita*) Chamomile roman (*Anthemis nobilis*) Coriander seed (*Coriandrum sativum*) Fragonia (*Agonis fragrans*) Frankincense (*Boswellia carterii*) Geranium (*Pelargonium graveolens*)

AGE	DILUTION RATIO AND CARRIER OIL	APPROPRIATE ESSENTIAL OILS
3 TO 5 YEARS (continued)	4–6 drops diluted in 2 table-spoons (30 mL) of sweet al-mond oil	Ginger (*Zingiber officinale*) Ho wood (*Cinnamomum camphora ct. linalool*) Lavender (*Lavandula angustifolia*) Mandarin (*Citrus reticulata*) Manuka (*Leptospermum scoparium*) Orange, sweet (*Citrus sinensis*) Palmarosa (*Cymbopogon martinii*) Ravensara (*Ravensara aromatica*) Ravintsara (*Cinnamomum camphora ct. cineole*) Rosewood (*Aniba rosaeodora*) Spearmint (*Mentha spicata*) Tea tree (*Melaleuca alternifolia*) Thyme linalol (*Thymus vulgaris ct. linalool*)
6 TO 8 YEARS	5–7 drops diluted in 2 table-spoons (30 mL) of sweet al-mond oil	Chamomile german (*Matricaria recutita*) Chamomile roman (*Anthemis nobilis*) Clary sage (*Salvia sclarea*) Coriander seed (*Coriandrum sativum*) Cypress (*Cupressus sempervirens*) Eucalyptus lemon (*Eucalyptus citriodora*) Fragonia (*Agonis fragrans*) Frankincense (*Boswellia carterii*) Geranium (*Pelargonium graveolens*) Ginger (*Zingiber officinale*) Ho wood (*Cinnamomum camphora ct. linalool*) Lavender (*Lavandula angustifolia*) Mandarin (*Citrus reticulata*) Manuka (*Leptospermum scoparium*) Niaouli (*Melaleuca quinquenervia*) Orange, sweet (*Citrus sinensis*) Palmarosa (*Cymbopogon martinii*) Petitgrain (*Citrus aurantium*) Ravensara (*Ravensara aromatica*) Ravintsara (*Cinnamomum camphora ct. cineole*) Rosemary (*Rosmarinus officinalis*) Rosewood (*Aniba rosaeodora*) Spearmint (*Mentha spicata*) Tangerine (*Citrus reticulata*) Tea tree (*Melaleuca alternifolia*) Thyme linalol (*Thymus vulgaris ct. linalool*) Ylang ylang (*Cananga odorata*)

AGE	DILUTION RATIO AND CARRIER OIL	APPROPRIATE ESSENTIAL OILS
9 TO 12 YEARS	6–8 drops diluted in a carrier oil of choice	Bergamot FCF (*Citrus bergamia*) Cajuput (*Melaleuca cajuputi*) Cedarwood atlas (*Cedrus atlantica*) Chamomile german (*Matricaria recutita*) Chamomile roman (*Anthemis nobilis*) Clary sage (*Salvia sclarea*) Coriander seed (*Coriandrum sativum*) Cypress (*Cupressus sempervirens*) Eucalyptus lemon (*Eucalyptus citriodora*) Eucalyptus radiata (*Eucalyptus radiata*) Fragonia (*Agonis fragrans*) Frankincense (*Boswellia carterii*) Geranium (*Pelargonium graveolens*) Ginger (*Zingiber officinale*) Grapefruit (*Citrus paradisi*) Ho wood (*Cinnamomum camphora ct. linalool*) Jasmine (*Jasminum grandiflorum/officinale*) Lavender (*Lavandula angustifolia*) Lemon (*Citrus limon*) Lemongrass (*Cymbopogon citratus/flexuosus*) Mandarin (*Citrus reticulata*) Manuka (*Leptospermum scoparium*) Marjoram, sweet (*Origanum majorana*) Niaouli (*Melaleuca quinquenervia*) Orange, sweet (*Citrus sinensis*) Palmarosa (*Cymbopogon martinii*) Pepper, black (*Piper nigrum*) Peppermint (*Mentha piperita*) Petitgrain (*Citrus aurantium*) Ravensara (*Ravensara aromatica*) Ravintsara (*Cinnamomum camphora ct. cineole*) Rosemary (*Rosmarinus officinalis*) Rosewood (*Aniba rosaeodora*) Spearmint (*Mentha spicata*) Tangerine (*Citrus reticulata*) Tea tree (*Melaleuca alternifolia*) Thyme linalol (*Thymus vulgaris ct. linalool*) Ylang ylang (*Cananga odorata*)

Newborn Babies

As soon as pregnancy is confirmed, start looking around for suitable pots and bottles to store baby's various creams and potions in. Pharmacies usually sell brown glass bottles, and you can also look for small pots or pillboxes, which should all be washed and then sterilized. When the time comes to make a remedy, nobody wants to be running around looking for a suitable container for the tiny quantities that will be used. Baby's new skin is much more delicate than an older child's, so anything used should always be organic and free from synthetic ingredients and preservatives. Essential oils should be used very sparingly for babies, and not on a regular basis. Save them for emergencies.

These are the essential oils that could be used on babies up to three months old unless specifically directed in this section:

BABIES' FIRST ESSENTIAL OILS
Chamomile roman (*Anthemis nobilis*)
Chamomile german (*Matricaria recutita*)
Lavender (*Lavandula angustifolia*)
Mandarin (*Citrus reticulata*)

One of the gentlest and yet most effective ways to treat various common ailments involves allowing the molecules of essential oil to evaporate and circulate throughout the baby's room. But because the amount of essential oil required for newborns is so tiny, all types of diffuser should be avoided. The only method that gives you complete control over how much essential oil is being evaporated into baby's room is the simple bowl of steaming water. First, add 1 drop of essential oil to 2 teaspoons of water and mix well. From this mix, take a ½ teaspoon and drop it into a bowl of steaming water, placed on the floor in a corner of the room, away from baby's head. This is a tiny amount of essential oil — a quarter of a drop — and not all of it will be evaporated into the room

because the water will go cold before that happens. Clearly, keep other children and pets away from the bowl, to avoid any accidents.

If the baby is suffering from any kind of digestive problem — colic, indigestion, constipation, diarrhea, or regurgitation — coriander seed essential oil is very helpful. Use in the room method just outlined.

If your baby isn't sleeping well, use lavender or chamomile roman. To freshen the air and make it smell delightful, while baby is not in the room use lavender, sweet orange, or mandarin essential oil for their antibiotic, antiseptic, disinfectant, and slightly antiviral properties. Even with the tiny quantity of essential oil recommended, the aroma will be lovely and infinitely better for your baby than any chemical air fresheners — which should definitely be avoided in a baby's room.

THE UMBILICAL CORD

After the birth, the umbilical cord will be cut and tied, leaving a little stump that shrivels up and falls off on its own accord around the sixth or seventh day. Generally, you want to do as little as possible to this area and leave it all to Mother Nature; simply keep the area clean and dry to help avoid infection. If any redness occurs, lavender can help in several ways. The area can be washed in lavender hydrolat or in water that has been boiled with lavender essential oil — use these sparingly on the area and make sure it is absolutely dry before putting clothing on the baby. Also, lavender can be added to pure white kaolin clay, pharmaceutical grade — 5 drops of lavender to 50 mg of clay, mixed in a blender to disperse the lavender thoroughly. Allow to dry, then use a cotton ball to dab up a little of the clay and apply on the umbilical area.

If your baby develops any discharge in the area, or a hernia or swelling, simply leave it alone and point it out to your pediatrician or midwife.

Indeed, you should report any inflammation or redness that occurs.

BABY'S SKIN

What follows is a blend of carrier oils that can be used on a newborn's skin, for various purposes. Opinions vary on what to do with the vernix caseosa, a greasy substance that protects baby's skin as it floats in the amniotic fluid. The vernix, as it's often called, can't be washed off with water because it's oily, and it's either left on, wiped off with a cloth, or taken off with oil. A mother in the hospital often has no control over what oil — processed or mineral — is put on her baby's skin, but if a blend of carrier oils is prepared before the delivery, this could be used. All the following carrier oils are nourishing, and organic versions are available:

BABY'S FIRST BODY OIL

Camellia seed oil	2 tablespoons (30 mL)
Almond oil, sweet	2 teaspoons (10 mL)
Jojoba oil	1 teaspoon (5 mL)

This same oil can be used for dry and wrinkled skin, which is quite usual in babies. And it can also be used as a gentle massage oil for baby (or mom). Babies love being touched and held, and it all helps the baby's development and the bonding process.

CRADLE CAP

Cradle cap, also called neonatal or infantile seborrheic dermatitis, is characterized by yellowish scaly patches, usually found on baby's head but also around the ears and elsewhere. The scales fall off over time on their own and light brushing might help, but never try to remove the scales with your fingers — let them come off in their own time. Cradle cap is not itchy or uncomfortable for the baby, so if baby starts scratching his or her head, it could indicate another condition.

Olive oil is sometimes recommended for cradle cap, but I find it too heavy for a baby's delicate scalp. Jojoba or avocado oil are much better; add 5 drops of borage seed oil (*Borago officinalis*) to every 2 tablespoons (30 mL) of whichever oil is used. Alternatively, use Baby's First Body Oil, outlined above. Other remedies that have been shown to help are baking soda and water mixed into a paste, and a blend of cider vinegar and water — making sure the water is distilled in both cases. Whatever you apply, remember the fontanel. This term applies to several membranous gaps in a young baby's cranial bones, but the one we're most concerned with is the one right at the top of the head. Any touching in this area should be most gentle.

OTHER EARLY PROBLEMS

All young babies sweat slightly, and they occasionally throw up their food and have runny stools. However, excessive sweating, diarrhea, and vomiting can lead to dehydration and affect a baby's health very quickly. If a baby is under three weeks old and has a persistent cough, that's another matter that should be taken seriously. Of course, deciding what's normal or excessive is the tricky part of parenting, but do be demanding of physicians, secure in the knowledge that they have great tolerance for overcautious parents, even if they're impatient or dismissive when you're the patient. Also, have confidence in — and develop — your own intuition. That will be your greatest asset in child care.

Babies from 3 to 12 Months

Babies can't tell us what's making them cry, so the only thing we have to work with is the unspoken communication between child and parent.

Establishing the link between baby and adult is done in a variety of ways, of course, and one of these is massage. The attention given during a massage shows your baby that it's cared for and loved, and that's a priceless message. But massage also relaxes the baby, which makes all the other physiological systems work better. And when that happens, baby stops crying, and everyone else can relax.

BABY MASSAGE

In the blend below we use a carrier oil that's good for skin and essential oils that are good for a great deal more besides. The amount of essential oil used here is about one-tenth that of an adult's massage oil. Even so, this blend can lessen the symptoms of eczema, cradle cap, inflammation, and redness due to teething problems, while boosting the immune system and acting as a general strengthener. It also has a marvelously calming effect on the nervous system, and babies become more content — no doubt appreciating the loving touch they receive.

Massage over the whole of your baby's body, but avoid the face, head, neck, and genitals.

Baby's Massage Oil Blend

Chamomile roman	1 drop
Lavender	1 drop
Geranium	1 drop

Dilute in 2 tablespoons (30 mL) of carrier oil, and use no more than a ¼ of a teaspoon for each massage, depending on the baby's size.

With babies, there's no need to use essential oils on a daily basis, and any remedy should be used on alternate days, or as directed, or when immediately needed. In the case of massage oil, use plain sweet almond oil on the other days.

DIAPER RASH

Diaper rash is the most common of baby problems, and although thought of as a minor inconvenience it's actually very sore and uncomfortable for the baby and worrying for the parent. Pure organic vegetable oils and waxes, plus a little essential oil, provide an easy solution to the problem.

For diaper rash: chamomile german, lavender

When washing baby's bottom, use cotton wool dipped in a bowl of warm water to which you've added either chamomile german or lavender essential oil — 1 drop to each pint (475 mL) of water. Before using, swish the water around well with your hand and then pour through an unbleached paper coffee filter. This is to remove any globules of essential oil that might be remaining. Alternatively, use organic chamomile or lavender hydrolat. Use clean cotton wool each time you make a wipe. Then dry the baby thoroughly.

Diaper Rash Ointment

Tamanu oil	2 teaspoons (10 mL)
Jojoba oil	1 teaspoon (5 mL)
Aloe vera gel	1 fl. oz. (30 mL)

Blend the tamanu oil and jojoba oil into the aloe vera gel and apply a small amount over the sore areas, but avoiding the genital area. As with all baby ingredients, these oils should be organic.

Another method uses zinc and castor oil cream. To each 10 teaspoons (50 mL) of cream add 1 drop of chamomile german or lavender essential oil. (This is when the tiny pots collected earlier will come in handy.) If you make up a blend using equal proportions of the two essential oils, again just mix 1 drop in with the 50 mL of cream. You really won't need much more than this. Use a small amount each time you change the diaper only for as long as required. Do make sure that you blend the essential oil well with the cream before applying it to your baby's bottom.

COLIC

Crying is a baby's way of letting us know that something is wrong. All mothers know that a hungry baby will cry relentlessly until the breast or bottle is presented, when the red-faced, bawling baby is transformed into a preoccupied angel. But if your baby is crying and hunger isn't the reason, don't ignore it. Most probably the reason is colic, and this can usually be helped by rubbing the baby's tummy gently with a baby massage oil. Then turn the baby over and rub the middle portion of the back in gentle circular movements. It's also helpful to massage the soles of the baby's feet, using gentle circular movements.

If the colic is more severe, use the following blend in the same way:

SEVERE COLIC REMEDY
Coriander seed   1 drop
Dilute in 1 tablespoon (15 mL) carrier oil.

Cartoonists have had a field day with the classic image of mother or father walking up and down with baby up against a shoulder, their hand patting and rubbing in an attempt to elicit wind from the usually half-asleep baby. And it's certainly a time-consuming business. Wind can be caused by a baby taking in air during feeding or by crying. Whatever the cause, the treatment is the same.

FRETFULNESS

Fretfulness as a frequent occurrence in a baby is an upsetting business for all concerned, but it also makes it difficult to know when your baby has wind, teething troubles, or a condition that the pediatrician needs to be aware of. Occasional fretfulness affects us all. Babies have frustration to

deal with, and aggravation too — imagine what a baby makes of a blaring TV, complete with gunshots and car chases. Touch works wonders for any anxiety condition, and baby massage is soothing for mother and baby alike. The following massage oils may be applied a couple of times a week or when your baby seems fretful. Choose one of the following blends:

FRETFUL BABY MASSAGE BLEND 1
Chamomile roman   2 drops
Lavender   2 drops
Dilute in 2 tablespoons (30 mL) of carrier oil.

MASSAGE BLEND 2
Chamomile roman   3 drops
Geranium   3 drops
Dilute in 3½ tablespoons (50 mL) of carrier oil.

MASSAGE BLEND 3
Tangerine   5 drops
Chamomile roman   2 drops
Dilute in 3½ tablespoons (50 mL) of carrier oil.

MASSAGE BLEND 4
Mandarin   5 drops
Chamomile roman   2 drops
Dilute in 3½ tablespoons (50 mL) of carrier oil.

One very effective way to bring comfort to a fretful baby is to massage their feet in the following way: holding both feet at the same time, rub your thumbs from the center of the sole of the foot toward the bottom of the toes, over the ball of the foot, in gentle rhythmic movements. You can use this method on bare feet, with or without the massage oil, or by simply using your fingers over the baby's cloth footwear. At first the infant may wiggle around, but you can gently hold both feet between thumb and fingers and the baby will soon settle down. This method is now much in use by nannies all over the world, and you'll be amazed by the calming response this foot massage elicits from an apparently inconsolable baby.

SICKNESS AND VOMITING

If the baby is on formula and constantly being sick it could be that he or she has an intolerance of or sensitivity to cow's milk. Try changing the brand of formula or changing to goat's milk formula, but if the condition continues consult your pediatrician, who might suggest another alternative. Babies who consistently throw up a large portion of their feed can be helped effectively with spearmint or coriander seed essential oils, which calm the stomach and make digestion easier. Put 1 drop on a cotton ball and place this under the baby's crib mattress at the end opposite the baby's head.

Projectile vomiting is when a baby forcefully projects vomit some distance away from the mouth. This could be pyloric stenosis, which is caused by a narrowing of the passage from the stomach to the bowel, and it usually manifests a few weeks after birth. However, if this happens at any time, or if the vomiting is accompanied by other symptoms, seek medical advice.

SLEEPING

When people talk about a "good baby" they most often mean the baby is "good" because he or she sleeps through most of the night. On the other hand, a baby who won't settle or who wakes frequently through the night eventually brings exhaustion to the parents. Plus it can make both baby and parents irritable during the day, which isn't much fun.

Babies wake up during the night because they're hungry or thirsty, they have a dirty diaper, or they've just gotten into the habit of waking up. It's this last reason that essential oils can try to address. The oil is used on alternate days — one day on, one day off — for eight days. Then take a week off, and try again if necessary. When you put baby to bed, place a bowl of hot water on the floor in a corner of the room, not near or under the baby's head. To the water, add 1 drop of chamomile roman and 1 drop of lavender oil. Over a short period of time, hopefully, baby's sleeping pattern will change and baby will wake up only if they have a practical need for the parents' attention. Just take it slowly, and stop using the essential oil when the sleeping pattern has settled down.

TEETHING

By the time a child is two or three years old it will have grown 20 baby teeth. Teething usually begins at around six months, but there's a wide variation in this, as in all aspects of child development: some may not have started by the time they are one year old, others begin very early indeed, and some babies are even born with teeth. Teething may cause inflammation and soreness of the gums, discomfort, and fever. A baby can become very hot, very suddenly, prior to the teeth appearing. Rashes are often associated with teething, but they're more likely to be caused by saliva; if left wet, the skin becomes sore. Some babies seem to suffer more than others, and many sleepless nights are caused by teething, starting a cycle of discomfort and tiredness that makes the baby more irritable.

Giving your baby something to chew on is important at this time — teeth and gums need to be used. Teething can also cause runny stools or a runny nose. Some babies get constipated, and the best thing for them is fruit juice.

Teething can get wrongly blamed for causing just about every problem a small baby might present, so a greater awareness of your baby's condition is important at this stage. Homeopathic teething granules, which are sometimes called *chamomile teething granules*, are of enormous help during this time. Here are the essential oils to use for teething problems:

TEETHING ESSENTIAL OILS
Chamomile roman (*Anthemis nobilis*)
Chamomile german (*Matricaria recutita*)
Lavender (*Lavandula angustifolia*)

There are several remedies that help the teeth and gums and also calm the baby. You can use one of the three essential oils above for this first remedy, singly or in an equal mix (if using one oil, 6 drops; or if combining two oils, 3 drops each). Their effect is equally good:

Chamomile roman   6 drops
or
Chamomile german   6 drops

Dilute in 5 teaspoons (25 mL) of carrier oil (or aloe vera gel), mix well, and leave to stand for 24 hours. Then take 1 teaspoon (5 mL) of the oil blend, put in a glass tumbler, and fill with approximately 1 fl. oz. (30 mL) of ice-cold water (or cold aloe vera gel). *Stir very well.*

You now have two mixtures for this two-part treatment. First, dip a small piece of cotton wool into the cold mixture and gently wipe around baby's exterior jawline (outside, not inside the mouth) to cool any inflammation. Then, using just the oil mix, take a tiny amount and rub between your fingers until dispersed, and then apply to the outside of baby's face along the line of the jaw. You only need 1 drop each time.

Lavender may also be used for teething problems. Put 3 drops of lavender into 1 tablespoon (15 mL) of carrier oil. Mix well. Using only 2 drops of this dilution, apply around the baby's exterior jaw.

COLDS AND COUGHS

We all know how miserable it is to have a cold, and it must be twice as bad for a baby who doesn't know what's happening and can't blow his or her little nose. We might wish to protect baby from this eventuality, and that's understandable, but essential oils shouldn't be applied on your baby just as a precautionary, preventative measure. If everyone else in the household has a cold, just make sure they use a tissue over their noses when they sneeze, then wash their hands. Also, the essential oils can be helpful in freshening up the home environment. The plant spray method is perfect for this because you can spray directly where the essential oils are needed — in the corridor outside your baby's room, but not inside the room. The following essential oils are all useful when used in this way:

Ravensara (*Ravensara aromatica*)
Ravintsara (*Cinnamomum camphora ct. cineole*)
Cajuput (*Melaleuca cajuputi*)
Fragonia (*Agonis fragrans*)
Cypress (*Cupressus sempervirens*)
Niaouli (*Melaleuca quinquenervia*)

If baby already has a cold, feeding can become difficult as baby gasps for breath between sucks. Even the process of breathing can become a struggle. Although it can be distressing, a cold is not actually a serious problem. But colds can be forerunners of other conditions, so if the cold is accompanied by a temperature or fever or your baby is crying a lot or refusing to eat, seek medical advice.

A simple solution to ease the discomfort of a baby's cold involves placing on the floor, in a corner of the room away from the baby's crib, a small bowl of hot water to which you've added 1 drop of ravensara oil. The steam will rise, releasing the molecules of aroma into the room. Or here's a blend you might like to try if your baby is over six weeks old:

SNIFFS AND SNUFFLES BLEND
Ravensara   10 drops
Lavender   10 drops
Thyme linalol   3 drops
Fragonia   3 drops

First, mix the essential oils together using these proportions, then use the number of drops from this mixture as directed in the following method.

If breathing is very difficult, place 1 drop of the blend on a piece of cotton material and place it somewhere away from the baby's bed, where it can't be reached. To prevent the baby from catching a cold or flu from an adult in the household, place 3 drops of the Sniffs and Snuffles Blend on a diffuser in the adult's bedroom overnight.

A massage oil can be made by mixing 1 drop of the blend to 2 teaspoons (10 mL) of carrier oil; massage a small amount of this over your baby's back. Use for three days, then take a break for two days, and resume for another three days if needed.

If your baby has a bad cough, whooping cough, bronchitis, or other chest infection, along with any medication given, you could try the following blend in a room diffusion method — using either a water vapor or steam diffuser, or a simple bowl of hot water left in the baby's room overnight. Use the blend for three consecutive nights, take a break for two nights, and, if necessary, continue once more on this three-on/two-off basis.

RESPIRATORY PROBLEMS BABY BLEND

Ravintsara	3 drops
Niaouli	1 drop
Ho wood	1 drop
Thyme linalol	1 drop

Blend the essential oils together, then use 1 or 2 drops in your chosen diffusion method.

Children's Health

Food provides the nutrients that build our children's cells and bodies, and nutrition has been linked in children to physical health, intellectual development, and behavior. In some cases, specific dietary changes can lead to the elimination of problems — for example, in eczema and attention deficient hyperactivity disorder (ADHD). So when looking for help, the first place to turn to is the refrigerator. What's in it, and what can that tell you? In general, the food in there should be fresh — actual food in the form of meat or fish, vegetables, and fruit, rather than processed foods laden with salt, sugar, fructose, and any number of other things that make food tasty but don't make children healthy.

CUTS, GRAZES, BRUISES, AND BURNS

Children have to learn about their environment through experience. I wouldn't want to climb a tree because I know I'd probably fall out of it. Children, on the other hand, aren't aware of the dangers life presents and, because of that, are constantly getting into scrapes of one sort or another. In learning what "hot" is, they burn themselves. Running around, they fall over. They get so excited playing tag, they simply forget you've told them not to run on the gravel, until they do fall over and end up with blood all over their knees. All we can do is be prepared for the inevitable knocks they're going to take in this action-packed period of their lives.

SCRAPES AND CUTS ESSENTIAL OILS
Lavender (*Lavandula angustifolia*)
Tea tree (*Melaleuca alternifolia*)
Manuka (*Leptospermum scoparium*)
Niaouli (*Melaleuca quinquenervia*)
Lemon (*Citrus limon*)
Chamomile roman (*Anthemis nobilis*)
Palmarosa (*Cymbopogon martinii*)

These essential oils fight infection and promote healing, providing parents with a group of excellent helpmates. First, make absolutely sure that splinters are taken out and that all the dirt is thoroughly bathed away from any cut, graze, or scratch. Then if no other disinfectant is available, bathe the area using 10 drops of lavender, or manuka, in a pint (475 mL) of warm water in a bowl. This doesn't sting as much as disinfectant, and while the aroma gives strength to the fainthearted — you — it also has a calming effect on your child. Allow the damaged skin to heal in the fresh air if at all possible, as it will heal quicker. (Obviously, cover the area if there's danger of infection — if, for example, playtime has just begun.) Repeat the bathing with essential oil a few hours later, whether the cut has been covered or not. If you apply an adhesive bandage, put a drop of neat lavender oil on the gauze pad and let it dry before applying. This will help the skin heal more quickly.

With all scrapes and cuts, avoiding infection is the main concern. When a cut or graze is healing, a scab will often form and — for some unknown reason — children seem to love picking at them. So the wound is revealed and vulnerable again. If this happens, bring out the essential oils, and bathe the area as before.

BRUISES ESSENTIAL OILS
Immortelle (*Helichrysum italicum*)
Geranium (*Pelargonium graveolens*)
Lavender (*Lavandula angustifolia*)
Marjoram, sweet (*Origanum majorana*)

Bruises need another sort of care. First, wrap some ice cubes in a towel and hold this against the area that's received the blow. Then apply a small amount of oil — using just enough to cover the bruised area only — which you've made by diluting 10 drops of immortelle in 2 tablespoons (30 mL) of carrier oil. The homeopathic tincture of arnica is also extremely good blended in aloe vera gel, as are arnica homeopathic tablets. Treat the bruise twice a day.

Burns

The essential oils should be used only in cases of first-degree burns; anything more serious than this requires medical assistance. Burns need the heat taken out of them immediately. Invisible to the eye, a process known as *denaturation* is taking place in the tissues; this is essentially the hardening of proteins. Imagine what an egg looks like when it boils and think how important it is to prevent that happening beneath the surface of the skin. To reach and reduce that heat, run cold water over the burned area for a full 10 minutes.

If that part of the body can't be reached by tap water, apply a cold compress. Prepare a bowl of cold water and add ice cubes. Put 2 neat drops of lavender on a clean washcloth, wring it out in the water, and use it to gently cover the reddened area. If there is no blistering or broken skin, apply 1 drop of neat lavender oil onto the area.

BURNS ESSENTIAL OILS
Lavender (*Lavandula angustifolia*)
Chamomile german (*Matricaria recutita*)
Chamomile roman (*Anthemis nobilis*)
Geranium (*Pelargonium graveolens*)

INSOMNIA

Trying to get children to turn off their phones, tablets, or laptops can sometimes seem like trying to pry a bone from a dog. They growl and complain and won't give it up! Children's obsession with their devices is almost like an addiction, and getting them to give it up at bedtime isn't easy. A child may have a strong desire to stay awake just so they can reach the next level on their game or keep chatting to their friends, but the trouble with this is they go past the stage of natural tiredness and into a kind of zombie-zone of insomnia. Yet we know children need their sleep. So this pattern needs to be broken.

Children develop insomnia for many other reasons, including overanxiety at school, tummy aches, fears, and phobias. Apart from the usual reassurance that a parent can give, help can come in many ways with the essential oils. They've been used by countless families over the centuries, and although children today live in different circumstances, the calming qualities of essential oils are timeless.

One of the best ways to overcome sleeplessness in children, if you have a bathtub, is to give them a warm bath at night and make this a daily winding-down routine just before bedtime. Alternatively, a back massage is very effective. This will relax them before their head hits the pillow. There's also a lot to be said for a warm drink, a cuddle, and a story. The aim is to calm and soothe the growing nerves and brain cells. Choose the essential oils according to the age of the child, as outlined below.

Children's Insomnia Essential Oils

FROM 12 MONTHS TO 5 YEARS
Mandarin
Lavender
Chamomile roman
For baths:
Using 1 drop per year of age, to a maximum of 3 drops, dilute the essential oils in 1 teaspoon (5 mL) of carrier oil before adding to the bathwater.

FROM 5 TO 12 YEARS
Geranium
Clary sage
Mandarin
Chamomile roman
Lavender
Frankincense
For baths:
1 or 2 drops until 7 years old
1–3 drops between 7 and 10
1–4 drops between 11 and 12
Dilute the essential oils in 1 teaspoon (5 mL) of carrier oil before adding to the bathwater.

Insomnia Blends

The essential oils listed above for insomnia could all be used on their own or made into blends of your choice. Alternatively, prepare the appropriate blend for the child's age range, as directed below. First, mix the essential oils together. Then, for baths, use the number of drops required following the age guide above.

For back massage the following amounts are diluted in 1 teaspoon (5 mL) of carrier oil:
1 or 2 drops up to 7 years old
2–3 drops between 8 and 12 years old

FROM 1 TO 7 YEARS
Lavender	10 drops
Chamomile roman	7 drops
Mandarin	7 drops

Blend the essential oils in these proportions and then use 1 drop diluted in 1 teaspoon (5 mL) of carrier oil for a child of 1 to 5 years of age, either for use in the bath or for a back massage. For a child aged between 6 and 7 years old, use 2 drops diluted in 1 teaspoon (5 mL) of sweet almond oil.

FROM 8 TO 12 YEARS
Chamomile roman	5 drops
Lavender	5 drops
Geranium	8 drops
Frankincense	4 drops

Blend the essential oils in these proportions and then use 2 drops diluted in 1 teaspoon (5 mL) of carrier oil for a child of 8–10 years of age, either for use in the bath or for a back massage. For a child between 11 and 12 years old, use 2–3 drops diluted in 1 teaspoon (5 mL) of sweet almond oil.

One thing that's extremely relaxing is a foot massage; carried out after the bath and before bed, it is a real soporific. Using an essential oil from the lists or one of the blends, mix 5 drops into 1 tablespoon (15 mL) of carrier oil for the foot massage oil, using just a small amount of this for each foot. If it's too greasy, you've used too much. And do bear in mind that some oils, if used in high dosage, can become stimulants rather than relaxants, so always underdose, rather than overdose.

COLDS AND FLU

Children often come home from school or from activities with other children carrying cold and flu bugs they've picked up. The following blend can be used in a room diffuser or in a back massage oil:

COLDS OR FLU BLEND
Ravintsara	10 drops
Ho wood	5 drops
Palmarosa	5 drops
Thyme linalol	5 drops

First, blend the essential oils together. Use 6 drops in a room diffuser, and 1–3 drops in 1 teaspoon (5 mL) of carrier oil for a back massage, depending on the age of the child. Use a small amount each time. If you don't have ho wood essential oil, just leave it out.

ACHES AND PAINS

The cause of childhood aches and pains is sometimes easy to identify — perhaps the child has been running around on a playing field or swimming. But children have had unexplained muscle pain for as long as anyone can remember, so the term *growing pains* is something our grandparents would be familiar with. This notion, that the aches and pains children experience are related to growth spurts, is unproven, and these days the term *recurrent limb pain in childhood* is preferred. The aches and pains come and go without apparent reason, usually in the legs and arms, especially in the evening or during the night.

Whatever the cause of muscular aches and pains, massage helps. The blend below is for overexercised muscles, but use single oils or make a blend that is suitable for your particular child, as each ache will be different to some degree. If the legs ache, for example, try a little lavender. Or if your child is over five years old, chamomile roman or sweet marjoram may help. Experiment to find the solution, using the information in this section and the general list of oils for children of your child's age.

OVEREXERCISED CHILD MASSAGE OIL
Cypress	3 drops
Rosemary	2 drops
Lavender	5 drops

Dilute in 10 teaspoons (50 mL) of carrier oil, and use a small amount each time.

Tummy aches can have many causes, from overexercise or overeating to anxiety. But it's worth remembering that appendicitis can start as a mild ache, and that any pain needs to be monitored, and the mind kept open as to its possible cause.

TUMMY ACHE ESSENTIAL OILS
Coriander seed (*Coriandrum sativum*)
Geranium (*Pelargonium graveolens*)
Bergamot FCF (*Citrus bergamia*)
Spearmint (*Mentha spicata*)
Caraway seed (*Carum carvi*)
Lavender (*Lavandula angustifolia*)
Orange, sweet (*Citrus sinensis*)

Make up a massage oil using 5 drops of one of these essential oils to 1 tablespoon (15 mL) of carrier oil. Use a small amount to massage your child's abdomen working around the belly button in a clockwise direction, starting on the child's right side, up and over, down the left side, and repeat. It often helps to massage the back as well — again, in a clockwise direction.

GENERAL TUMMY ACHE BLEND

Coriander seed	4 drops
Geranium	2 drops
Orange, sweet	2 drops

Dilute in 2 tablespoons (30 mL) of carrier oil, and use a small amount each time.

FEVERS

When your child gets sick it can be a frightening experience, perhaps no more so than when they develop a fever. Thankfully, most fevers pass relatively quickly, but we always need to be aware that fever can indicate something serious such as meningitis or septicemia, and finding the right balance between nonchalant cool and sheer panic is difficult. In the decision-making process, as well as when taking a temperature, two things are important: what your child has to say and what you can ascertain about your child's condition. Ask your child if anywhere hurts and make a note of it. Are they unresponsive or confused? Do they have a rash or cold hands or feet? Are their lips or skin bluish in color? Do they have a stiff neck? Are they vomiting? If the fever is occurring without any other symptoms, the chances are that the child's body is fighting an infection, which could be viral or bacterial and in the lungs, ears, or elsewhere. Think back to anything that might have happened recently. If prone to ear infections, has the child been swimming recently? Have they had a cut or wound? Answers to all these questions can help a physician determine how serious the fever is, and what should be done. Information, as they say, is power.

When a child has a fever, try to cool them down. Remove all extra clothing and bedding and cover the child with a sheet. Keep the temperature of the room neither too hot nor too cold. Wipe your child's head, neck, and body continuously with a cool cloth — but not a cold one, as this could be a shock to their body. If cold water is applied to the skin it'll keep the heat in because the blood vessels on the surface contract in response to cold temperature — which we don't want. Also sponge down occasionally using lukewarm water to which you've added cooling essential oil — 2 drops of essential oil to 1 quart of water.

COOLING ESSENTIAL OILS
Spearmint (*Mentha spicata*)
Coriander seed (*Coriandrum sativum*)
Tea tree (*Melaleuca alternifolia*)
Chamomile roman (*Anthemis nobilis*)
Manuka (*Leptospermum scoparium*)
Lavender (*Lavandula angustifolia*)
Lemon (*Citrus limon*)
Grapefruit (*Citrus paradisi*)
Peppermint (*Mentha piperita*) (only for use in a room diffusion method)

Use whichever of the above oils you have in the cupboard. Spearmint and lavender in equal proportions make a useful cooling oil blend.

If the fever has become acute, make up a large bowl of lukewarm water to which you have added 10 drops of essential oil. Swish it around. Make a compress with any clean cotton material you have, soak it in the solution, and wring it out. Put a rubber sheet or piece of plastic underneath your child and apply the oiled water to the armpits, groin (but not the genitals), forehead, and lower back. As soon as the compresses are warm, change them for cool ones. Repeat until the fever subsides.

If the lymphatic glands are swollen, apply the following blend:

SWOLLEN GLANDS / FEVER BLEND

Ravintsara	5 drops
Lavender	5 drops
Palmarosa	5 drops

Make up a blend using these proportions. Put 5 drops in 2 teaspoons (10 mL) of carrier oil and mix well. From this, apply just 1 drop gently onto the glands, neck, and groin (avoid the genitals), once every hour. And continue with the other methods outlined above.

Don't mistake shivering as a sign that your child is cold — the body will use all the methods at its disposal to try to get rid of the fever. A child who has a fever and is shivering should not be made extra warm; nor should you use anything too cold. That will only make things worse. What you can do is cool the body down, and as it cools, the shaking will go.

IMPETIGO

Impetigo is an infection of the outer layers of the skin that can be caused by an infected scratch or insect bite. It starts as tiny red spots, turns into blisters, and can change into a sore, pus-filled area that gets bigger and spreads. Not only is impetigo contagious from person to person but infection can be spread from one area of skin to another on the same person. It is quite a common complaint, and if one child in the school has it you can be pretty sure that others will too.

Impetigo sores do not just go away, and they must be treated as soon as they are noticed. To clean the infected area, prepare a small bowl of around 3½ fl. oz. (100 mL) of boiled water that has been cooled, add 10 drops of lavender, and wash the affected area thoroughly with the solution using clean cotton wool. Now apply a compress.

First, prepare your essential oils — equal amounts of tea tree and palmarosa in a blend. You'll also need a piece of cotton material cut in a rectangle large enough to cover the infected area twice over. Soak the material in water and then put 2 drops of the blend in the center. Fold over the two ends of the material so that the essential oil will not be in direct contact with the impetigo. Use a bandage to tie the material to the body, or if the impetigo is on an awkward part of the body attach it as best you can. Leave the material there for an hour and then remove it so that the area can be exposed to the air. Repeat as necessary.

CONSTIPATION

Constipation in children can be caused by several factors, from a change in food habits to stress, and even by toilet training in the toddler. The stools become dehydrated and difficult to pass. The problem can usually be relieved with a combination of essential oil massage and plenty of fiber, fruit juice, water, and a children's probiotic nutritional supplement.

ESSENTIAL OILS TO EASE CONSTIPATION
Geranium (*Pelargonium graveolens*)
Patchouli (*Pogostemon cablin*)
Rosemary (*Rosmarinus officinalis*)
Mandarin (*Citrus reticulata*)
Chamomile roman (*Anthemis nobilis*)
Orange, sweet (*Citrus sinensis*)

Use any of the oils singly or in combination, or use the following blend:

CHILDREN'S CONSTIPATION MASSAGE OIL BLEND
Geranium	4 drops
Patchouli	6 drops
Mandarin	15 drops

Blend together and use 2 drops for each teaspoon (5 mL) of carrier oil. At bedtime give the child a large glass of natural fruit juice and water to drink. Using a small amount of oil, massage the whole of their abdomen with gentle movements, working around the belly button in a clockwise direction, starting on the child's right side, up and over, down the left side, and repeat.

DIARRHEA

Diarrhea in a child has many causes. It could be a physical problem, such as bacteria, viruses, ear infections, or flu. It could be that the child has a food sensitivity. Nervous tension and stress could also be the culprits: has your child been upset by bullying at school, are they worried about exams, or even made anxious by parental arguments?

With a case of diarrhea it's important that the lost fluid and electrolytes are replaced so dehydration does not occur. If it continues for more than 24 hours you should seek medical advice. Give your child plenty of liquid and offer slightly salty soups and drinks with honey dissolved in them. Avoid dairy products, as they could make matters worse.

The following oils can be included in a body oil to rub gently on the abdomen:

ESSENTIAL OILS TO EASE DIARRHEA
Chamomile roman (*Anthemis nobilis*)
Sandalwood (*Santalum album*)
Ginger (*Zingiber officinale*)
Geranium (*Pelargonium graveolens*)

Or use the following blend:

CHILDREN'S DIARRHEA BODY OIL BLEND
Ginger   5 drops
Sandalwood   8 drops
Chamomile roman   8 drops
Blend together and use 2 drops for each teaspoon (5 mL) of carrier oil.

If your child has a sore bottom, make a chamomile ointment by mixing 3 drops of lavender and 2 drops of chamomile german or chamomile roman essential oil into 1 fl. oz. (30 mL) of aloe vera gel. Apply around the anal area but not directly on the anus to reduce soreness and redness. Keep your child off cow dairy products for at least a week following a bout of diarrhea, and serve gentle foods such as banana, scrambled egg, stewed apple, rice, and oats.

TONSILLITIS

In tonsillitis, the tonsils become enlarged and infected. The swelling may be painful, and the throat is red and sore. Small yellow spots are often seen on the tonsils. The child feels unwell and could be running a temperature or have an earache, headache, neck ache, or tummy ache.

Give your child plenty of drinks, and add manuka honey to soothe and help heal the throat. Honey added to freshly squeezed lemon juice will be helpful. Put the lemon and honey in a glass, then add hot water, stir, and wait until cool enough to drink. Herbal syrups are all extremely useful. (See page 470, in chapter 16, "Cooking with Essential Oils.") They can be used in two ways. If the child likes the taste, simply slide a teaspoon of syrup down the throat. If not, or in addition, dilute a teaspoon of syrup in a small glass of warm water and have your child gargle with it. Do this three times a day to promote healing.

The essential oils can be used in several ways. Use the following oils singly or in a blend, or follow the Tonsillitis Blend:

TONSILLITIS OILS
Lavender (*Lavandula angustifolia*)
Ginger (*Zingiber officinale*)
Tea tree (*Melaleuca alternifolia*)
Chamomile roman (*Anthemis nobilis*)
Lemon (*Citrus limon*)
Niaouli (*Melaleuca quinquenervia*)

TONSILLITIS BLEND
Lavender   10 drops
Tea tree   15 drops
Niaouli   1 drop
Lemon   3 drops
Mix the oils together to make a blend. Use 4 drops of the blend on a warm compress twice a day over the throat area. Also, make up a body oil using 5 drops of the blend in 2 teaspoons (10 mL) of carrier oil and apply a small amount over the upper abdomen and back. The blend could also be used in a diffuser.

An excellent remedy for tonsillitis follows. It can be used as a gargle or as a mouthwash if the child cannot gargle.

Tonsillitis Remedy

Water	3½ fl. oz. (100 mL)
Cider vinegar	3½ tablespoons (50 mL)
Honey	1 tablespoon (15 g)
Ginger	1 drop
Lemon	4 drops

Blend the ingredients together until well amalgamated and put 1 teaspoon in a large tumbler of warm water. Have your child gargle with this mixture twice a day — making sure they don't swallow it, and follow with a teaspoon of organic manuka honey.

SORE THROATS

Sore throats range from the mild, tickly type to the unable-to-swallow type — all irritating and unpleasant. They are usually caused by a virus or by bacteria. Follow the tonsillitis treatments above.

EARS

Earache can make a child very miserable, whether caused by an infection or poking a pencil in the ear! The following remedy may help, whatever the cause. First, make an oil by mixing 2 drops of lavender and 1 drop of chamomile roman in 1 teaspoon (5 mL) of carrier oil, and blend well together. If the child is over nine years old, add 1 drop of geranium oil to the mix. This oil is applied in a very particular place on both sides, even if just one ear is affected: start *behind* the ear and move in a straight line down to the collar bone, or clavicle. Apply a little of the oil twice a day.

Earache that doesn't clear up with antibiotics and has everyone baffled can sometimes be helped by the old-fashioned remedy of putting a piece of cotton wool soaked in warm olive oil in the ear. This is intended to soften the earwax. The cotton wool must be large enough to prevent it being pushed down into the ear. To improve this old remedy, add 1 drop of lavender essential oil to 2 teaspoons (10 mL) of olive oil, mix well and soak a piece of cotton wool in it. After wringing the excess olive oil out of the cotton wool, place it loosely in the ear, changing it twice a day. Do make sure you use pure, virgin, organic olive oil, and squeeze the excess oil out before putting the cotton wool in the ear.

BRONCHITIS

Bronchitis is inflammation of the airways of the lungs. It is usually caused by a virus, but bacteria can sometimes be the trigger. Symptoms are shortness of breath, wheezing, and coughing — often bringing up phlegm. Bronchitis can develop after a cough or cold.

Essential oils help in most cases of bronchial congestion, and children respond well to essential oil treatments of the respiratory tract. Inform your physician if you intend to use essential oils alongside prescribed medication.

Bronchitis Essential Oils for Children under 5 Years

Tea tree (*Melaleuca alternifolia*)
Ravensara (*Ravensara aromatica*)
Chamomile roman (*Anthemis nobilis*)
Lavender (*Lavandula angustifolia*)

Bronchitis Essential Oils for Children over 5 Years

Rosemary (*Rosmarinus officinalis*)
Thyme linalol (*Thymus vulgaris ct. linalool*)
Ravensara (*Ravensara aromatica*)
Niaouli (*Melaleuca quinquenervia*)
Cajuput (*Melaleuca cajuputi*)
Cedarwood atlas (*Cedrus atlantica*)
Pine (*Pinus sylvestris*)
Eucalyptus radiata (*Eucalyptus radiata*)
Eucalyptus lemon (*Eucalyptus citriodora*)
Marjoram, sweet (*Origanum majorana*)

BRONCHITIS ROOM DIFFUSING BLEND
FOR CHILDREN UNDER 5 YEARS

Tea tree	8 drops
Chamomile roman	7 drops
Ravensara	10 drops

First, prepare the blend of essential oils. Use 3 drops in a diffuser or in the steaming water bowl method, three times a day.

BRONCHITIS ROOM DIFFUSING BLEND
FOR CHILDREN OVER 5 YEARS

Niaouli	8 drops
Thyme linalol	10 drops
Cedarwood atlas	7 drops

First, prepare the blend of essential oils. Use 3 drops in a diffuser or in the steaming water bowl method, three times a day.

BRONCHITIS BODY APPLICATION BLEND
FOR CHILDREN UNDER 5 YEARS

Chamomile roman	2 drops
Ravensara	5 drops
Lavender	3 drops

Add the amounts in the blend above to 2 tablespoons (30 mL) of carrier oil. Massage a small amount over the back, up to three times a day.

BRONCHITIS BODY APPLICATION BLEND
FOR CHILDREN OVER 5 YEARS

Thyme linalol	7 drops
Ravensara	8 drops
Chamomile roman	2 drops

Add the amounts in the blend above to 2 tablespoons (30 mL) of sweet almond carrier oil. Massage a small amount over the chest and back, concentrating on the back and lung area, up to three times a day.

CHILDHOOD ASTHMA

The helplessness that parents so often feel in relation to a sick child is very pronounced in the case of the asthmatic child. To have to watch your child wheezing and fighting for breath must be heartbreaking and frightening at the same time. These parents are sometimes asthmatic themselves and so can identify closely with what the child is experiencing. It's encouraging to know that asthma often stops at puberty.

But parents can help in many ways. Keep a diary and note down everything that affects your child — what he or she eats, what exercise is taken, what illnesses and complaints have occurred, events that have preceded the attack, and the pollen count. How far you go with this depends on how much time you have to spare, because asthmatic children have been found to be sensitive to hair spray, deodorant, perfume, polish, dust, grass, animal fur, feathers — not to mention heat, cold, and damp. Look for a pattern and adapt diet and lifestyle accordingly.

Many children respond well to the naturopathic approach: No dairy products. No wheat. No sodas. No additives or preservatives, and nothing out of a can or package. Hard? Yes. But worth it? Most definitely yes, yes, yes. Breathing exercises may help strengthen the lungs and diaphragm, and yoga breathing methods might also be helpful.

Many of the flower essential oils appear to help some children when used in diluted form. They're best used in massage, which in itself is enormously beneficial. Used as a preventative measure, a combination of essential oils and massage can calm the child and reduce tension, which may prevent attacks from occurring so frequently. If the child is known to be sensitive to commercial perfumes, this sensitivity may not occur with essential oils because they're entirely botanical, while commercial perfumes invariably contain synthetic substitutes.

Massage the back in long, sweeping movements. Start at the base of the spine, your hands on either side of the vertebrae, and use upward strokes to the shoulder, over the shoulder, and down the sides of the body. The massage will also be very reassuring to the child. Use the following blends:

Asthma Massage Blend for 2 to 7 Years

Lavender	2 drops
Geranium	2 drops
Frankincense	2 drops

Dilute the blend in 2 tablespoons (30 mL) of carrier oil and use a small amount each time.

Asthma Massage Blend for 7 to 12 Years

Geranium	3 drops
Cypress	2 drops
Frankincense	3 drops

Dilute the blend in 2 tablespoons (30 mL) of carrier oil and use a small amount each time.

ALLERGIES

Why people develop sensitivities and allergies remains a medical mystery. Sensitivities are a very complicated subject, and finding a solution often proves difficult. The best line of defense, until we know more about it, is to remove the offending agent. But finding the cause of the trouble often takes time because almost any substance in the world can trigger a reaction — from the air we breathe to the water we drink, from the people we love to the clothes we wear — and finding the source of the sensitivity, or sensitivities, could be quite a mission! So along with the distressing physical results of an allergy there's the inconvenience of having to change lifestyle, sometimes drastically.

For children, it's often the common, everyday things that produce a reaction: grass, pollen, ragweed, house dust, pets, dairy products, eggs, soybean products, shellfish, nuts, wheat, food colorants, additives, and preservatives are among the culprits. Allergic reactions can manifest as asthma, eczema, hyperactivity, fatigue, itching, runny nose, sneezing, headaches, and lumps and bumps.

Allergic reactions to essential oils are rare if used correctly. A child with hay fever or eczema may be slightly more at risk. In the case of an allergic reaction to one essential oil, don't group similar-seeming oils together and assume there will be a reaction to them too. Sensitivity to orange, for example, does not necessarily mean there will be a reaction to mandarin or lemon. If following the oil recommendations below, only cover a small portion of the skin to begin with, to check there's no reaction.

Eczema

Eczema is very itchy, and this blend can be applied to the affected area once a day:

Chamomile german	8 drops
Manuka	1 drop
Diluted in:	
Camellia seed oil	4 teaspoons (20 mL)
Jojoba oil	2 teaspoons (10 mL)
Evening primrose seed oil	10 drops

Urticaria (Hives)

Urticaria, or hives, are raised patches on the skin that develop from an allergic reaction. They're very itchy and can affect any part of the body. There are three potential options to use. First, follow the same instructions as for eczema. Second, put 2 drops of chamomile german essential oil into a ¼ cup of baking soda, then add to the bath. The third option is to make the oil that follows. Try it first on a small section of skin. If there is no reaction, use a small amount each time.

Tamanu (*Calophyllum inophyllum*)   10 mL
Fragonia (or ravensara)   2 drops

Hay Fever

Hay fever requires a personal approach and a personal blend. Contact a local registered aromatherapist or homeopath.

Bee Stings

Bee stings produce an allergic reaction in a small percentage of children: the body can swell up, and breathing becomes labored. Try to remove the stinger and treat with 1 drop of lavender or chamomile german or, better still, 1 drop of them both combined. Then apply an ice-cold compress. Do be vigilant after a bee sting as the reaction can be unpredictable. See chapter 6, "The Basic Travel Kit."

MIGRAINE

Migraine in children is often caused by a sensitivity to certain foods, and it is certainly worth considering your child's diet if they have migraine. Try changing to a whole-food diet including plenty of fish, chicken, fresh vegetables, fruit, mineral waters, and natural fruit juices diluted with mineral water. Breakfast can consist of real oats or puffed rice with non-GM soy milk, or follow the recipe for real muesli on page 472. Frozen fruit juice popsicles on a stick can be made with natural fruit juices. Give herb teas at bedtime — chamomile sweetened with a little honey, for example. If your child has had sick migraines, give peppermint herb tea during the day; lots of water sometimes helps.

Try to remove from the diet all foods that are not fresh. As well as all the obvious items packed with artificial colorants, flavorings, additives, and preservatives, cut out all canned and packaged goods no matter what promises of purity are made on the label. The child can have grains, but

reduce wheat. Cut out soda and sugary drinks. Also cut out processed meats, and reduce red meat consumption. This new regime could provoke withdrawal symptoms, such as headache or stomachache, in the first few days; this used to be called a *healing crisis*. These symptoms soon pass, hopefully with the migraines.

Common causes of migraine in children are stress, insufficient breakfast and lunch, food intolerances, and a lack of hydration. Many drinks that children consume include sugars or sweeteners, so try to encourage the child to drink filtered water by adding a slice of lemon or strawberry, and dilute fruit juices with water. If a child experiences migraines it might be wise to try to restrict the time they spend on their phones and tablets, and see if that helps. Sleep is one of the best remedies.

Essential oil massages over a period of time can help reduce the number of migraine episodes. Set a time when you can both be relaxed. Ask the child to lie facedown on the bed and massage their back in long, sweeping movements: start at the base of the spine, your hands on either side of the vertebrae, and use upward strokes to the shoulder, over the shoulder, and down the sides of the body. Use the following oils, either singly or in combination:

CHILDREN'S MIGRAINE ESSENTIAL OILS
Grapefruit (*Citrus paradisi*)
Bergamot FCF (*Citrus bergamia*)
Lavender (*Lavandula angustifolia*)
Spearmint (*Mentha spicata*)
Chamomile roman (*Anthemis nobilis*)
Rosemary (*Rosmarinus officinalis*)
Marjoram, sweet (*Origanum majorana*)

CHILDREN'S MIGRAINE BLEND
Chamomile roman   4 drops
Rosemary   4 drops
Marjoram, sweet   6 drops

Spearmint	6 drops
Bergamot FCF	6 drops
Lavender	6 drops

First blend the essential oils together, and then use in the following way depending on the age of the child:

Children between three and seven years of age: dilute in 5 fl. oz. (150 mL) of carrier oil — and use a small amount each time.

Children over seven years of age: dilute in 4 fl. oz. (120 mL) of carrier oil — and use as small amount each time.

Grapefruit essential oil compresses often help in the treatment of this debilitating condition. Add 2 drops of grapefruit oil to 1 pint (475 mL) of cold water and swish the water around well to disperse any essential oil globules on the surface. Soak the compress in this, then squeeze out the excess water, before applying the compress to the back of the neck.

MUMPS

Mumps is a common airborne viral disease whose target is the parotid salivary glands. Two or three weeks after infection the symptoms appear, the most characteristic of these being large, egg-like swellings on one or both sides of the neck just below the ears. Other symptoms are headache, mild fever, muscle ache, earache, pain when eating, and fatigue. Usually mumps is a fairly harmless condition, and the symptoms fade after a couple of days. Sometimes, however, the infection can spread to other glands, and in bad cases, the testes, ovaries, and pancreas become involved. Post-puberty males who haven't had mumps should avoid contact with an infected child, as complications can be more serious in adults. Give the child plenty of fluids and use the following oils in one of the room methods:

ROOM METHOD ESSENTIAL OILS FOR MUMPS
Tea tree (*Melaleuca alternifolia*)
Niaouli (*Melaleuca quinquenervia*)
Ravensara (*Ravensara aromatica*)
Lavender (*Lavandula angustifolia*)
Geranium (*Pelargonium graveolens*)
Ravintsara (*Cinnamomum camphora ct. cineole*)
Eucalyptus radiata (*Eucalyptus radiata*)
Palmarosa (*Cymbopogon martinii*)
Cinnamon leaf (*Cinnamomum zeylanicum*)
Manuka (*Leptospermum scoparium*)

Use a total of 4 drops of any of the above, singly or in combination, in 4 fl. oz. (120 mL) of water.

MUMPS BODY OIL BLEND

Manuka	10 drops
Lavender	10 drops
Coriander seed	5 drops
Lemon	10 drops
Chamomile roman	5 drops

Blend the essential oils together, then dilute 20 drops in 2 tablespoons (30 mL) of carrier oil. Apply a small amount gently around the sore area, the back of the neck, and the abdomen. Use twice a day for seven days. There will be some of the essential oil blend left over — use this in one of the room methods.

MEASLES

Measles is an airborne viral disease that can start as nothing more than a runny nose and a sore throat, and you think your irritable child has just got a cold. Other early symptoms are sore and runny eyes, fever, and enlarged glands in the neck, but symptoms are numerous and vary from child to child. The most telling symptom is spots — small red spots with white centers on the lining of the mouth, followed by spots on the cheeks that turn into a rash around the fourth day, spreading down the body.

Keep the child in bed, in a warm room, and away from other children. The virus is spread by airborne droplets and saliva, so to help protect other family members, use a blend of antiviral oils in any of the room methods, including in the child's room.

MEASLES ESSENTIAL OILS
Thyme linalol (*Thymus vulgaris ct. linalool*)
Fragonia (*Agonis fragrans*)
Ravensara (*Ravensara aromatica*)
Niaouli (*Melaleuca quinquenervia*)
Cypress (*Cupressus sempervirens*)
Palmarosa (*Cymbopogon martinii*)
Ravintsara (*Cinnamomum camphora ct. cineole*)
Geranium (*Pelargonium graveolens*)
Chamomile german (*Matricaria recutita*)
Chamomile roman (*Anthemis nobilis*)
Lemon (*Citrus limon*)
Lavender (*Lavandula angustifolia*)
Eucalyptus radiata (*Eucalyptus radiata*)
Bergamot FCF (*Citrus bergamia*)

It's very soothing for the child and will aid recovery if they're dabbed down with an essential oil water. First, make a blend of essential oils using equal amounts of chamomile german and lavender. Add 5 drops of this combination to a bowl containing 8 fl. oz. (240 mL) of warm, but not hot, water and 1 tablespoon (15 mL) of colloidal silver. Swish the water around with your hand to disperse any floating globules of essential oil. Get a clean sponge or cloth and soak it in the water, wring it out, and gently dab the child. Don't rub, just dab. Do the whole body once or twice a day.

If you want to cover the spots in calamine lotion — a chalky lotion that contains zinc oxide — or aloe vera gel, add 5 drops each of chamomile german and lavender and 4 drops of bergamot

FCF essential oil to 2 fl. oz. (60 mL) of calamine or aloe vera, and blend well.

If the child is over 11 years of age, for one or two days when the rash has first appeared apply 1 drop of eucalyptus radiata essential oil to the sole of each foot.

RUBELLA (GERMAN MEASLES)

Rubella is an airborne viral infection that in many cases is symptom-free. This can be problematic for women in the first four months of pregnancy as rubella can cause miscarriage, or complications for the unborn child. If you know or even suspect your child has rubella, it's most important they are kept away from women who may be pregnant. Rubella usually starts as an itchy rash around the face, then spreads to the rest of the body. The child might be feverish or tired, and the lymph nodes may be swollen.

Treat in the same way as all viral infections by using antiviral oils in one of the room methods to help clear the atmosphere. Also, add 5 drops of chamomile german essential oil or 5 drops of the blend below to a bowl containing 8 fl. oz. (240 mL) of warm, but not hot, water and 1 tablespoon (15 mL) colloidal silver. Swish the water around with your hand to disperse any floating globules of essential oil. Get a clean sponge or cloth and soak it in the water, wring it out, and gently dab the child. Don't rub, just dab. Apply to the whole body once or twice a day.

RUBELLA BLEND
Lavender	15 drops
Chamomile german	15 drops
Tea tree	5 drops

Blend together and use 5 drops in 8 fl. oz. (240 mL) warm water for a body wash dab. Alternatively, make your own blend from the essential oils listed below.

RUBELLA DAB-DOWN ESSENTIAL OILS
Lavender (*Lavandula angustifolia*)
Chamomile roman (*Anthemis nobilis*)
Chamomile german (*Matricaria recutita*)
Tea tree (*Melaleuca alternifolia*)
Frankincense (*Boswellia carterii*)
Bergamot FCF (*Citrus bergamia*)
Manuka (*Leptospermum scoparium*)

If you want to cover the spots/rash in calamine lotion — a chalky lotion that contains zinc oxide — or aloe vera gel, add 4 drops each of chamomile german and lavender and 2 drops of bergamot essential oil to 2 fl. oz. (60 mL) of calamine or aloe vera, and blend well.

CHICKEN POX (VARICELLA)

Chicken pox, or varicella, is yet another contagious viral infection. It's spread by contact with the saliva, mucus, or blisters of a person already infected. Children who've been vaccinated can also develop varicella, but it's usually a milder version. The virus can lie dormant and return as shingles later in life.

After an incubation period of two weeks, the child's temperature may rise and almost immediately a rash will appear. This is made up of small spots that usually turn into blisters, which burst and scab. Trying to stop your child from scratching and picking off the scabs is a full-time occupation. The spots start on the face, back, and chest, and they can then spread all over the body. The child should be isolated until the last scab has fallen off.

Bed rest may prevent fever, and the child should be encouraged to sleep as this is one of the best things for chicken pox. Treatment involves trying to stop the very irritating itching. Add 10 drops of lavender and 10 of chamomile german to a 100 mL bottle of calamine lotion and shake the bottle. Apply all over the body twice a day. Baths

can also relieve the itching: add 2 drops of lavender (or 2 drops of chamomile german), 1 drop of frankincense, and 1 drop of bergamot into 1 cup of baking soda, and put that in the bath. Another itch-relieving bath is an oat bath: add the same essential oils to 1 cup of oat flakes or oatmeal, wrap up well in a piece of natural material such as muslin or undyed cotton, tie very tight, and put in the bath. Squeeze this oat-ball several times to release the oat water and essential oil. Also use antiviral essential oils in any of the room methods. See "Measles" on page 161.

WHOOPING COUGH (PERTUSSIS)

Whooping cough is caused by the bacteria *Bordetella pertussis*, which is why it's often referred to as *pertussis*. It's called *whooping cough* because of the distinctive high-pitched sound, like a "whoop," that can occur when the child tries to breathe in. The coughing is violent and uncontrolled and can last for up to eight weeks. Whooping cough ceases to be contagious after around three weeks of coughing. Try to keep an infected child away from babies and toddlers, as the infection affects them more so than older children.

Whooping cough can start with flu-like symptoms, lasting up to two weeks before the cough — which may not have the "whoop" sound. It affects the respiratory system, causing mucus to accumulate in the airways. For this reason, have a bowl handy so the child can easily cough up the mucus. Disinfect the bowl often. Also, the bowl may be handy if the child vomits as a result of a coughing fit. All this can make the child tired and irritable, and sleeping can be difficult.

Change the diet to one that's light and nutritious. Reduce milk products because they might cause excess mucus in the body. Serve chicken, fish, eggs, whole-meal bread, vegetables, fruit juices, mineral water, and herb teas. Sorbets and frozen treats made at home with diluted natural fruit juices will be soothing. Make soups and broths, and liquidize vegetables to make them easier to swallow. Appropriate children's nutritional supplements at this time would be omega 3, vitamin C, and a multivitamin and mineral tablet that includes zinc.

Let the child have plenty of fresh air, as staying inside in hot stuffy rooms will only dehydrate the body. Open the windows during the day, but ensure the child is well wrapped up. Steam helps a lot. Put bowls of hot steaming water in the child's room at night to keep the atmosphere as humid as possible and to avoid dehydration of the bronchial tract. The essential oils that follow can be used in all the usual room methods, preferably those using water vapor or steam, just 1 or 2 drops each time.

Whooping Cough Room Method Essential Oils
Cinnamon leaf (*Cinnamomum zeylanicum*)
Niaouli (*Melaleuca quinquenervia*)
Lavender (*Lavandula angustifolia*)
Grapefruit (*Citrus paradisi*)
Hyssop decumbens (*Hyssopus officinalis var. decumbens*)
Cypress (*Cupressus sempervirens*)
Thyme linalol (*Thymus vulgaris ct. linalool*)
Palmarosa (*Cymbopogon martinii*)
Frankincense (*Boswellia carterii*)
Oregano (*Origanum vulgare*)
Fragonia (*Agonis fragrans*)
Ravensara (*Ravensara aromatica*)
Cajuput (*Melaleuca cajuputi*)

Whooping Cough Room Method Blend
Hyssop decumbens	5 drops
Thyme linalol	10 drops
Cinnamon leaf	4 drops
Cypress	5 drops
Palmarosa	5 drops
Ravensara	5 drops
Eucalyptus radiata	3 drops

Make into a blend using these proportions, and use 1 or 2 drops each time in one of the room methods.

The following blend can be used in the bath, adding 1 or 2 drops each time, diluted in a little carrier oil. This blend can also be used in the steaming water bowl method, with 3 drops in the bowl, placed near the bed overnight. Alternatively, simply put 3 drops on a piece of cotton material and leave it near the child but out of reach.

Whooping Cough Bath and Water Bowl Blend
Cypress	5 drops
Niaouli	5 drops
Lavender	2 drops
Thyme linalol	3 drops
Frankincense	3 drops

Make into a blend using these proportions. Then use 1 or 2 drops diluted in a teaspoon of carrier oil if using in the bath, or 1–3 drops in a room method.

Back Massage Oil Blend
Thyme linalol	3 drops
Ravensara	3 drops
Palmarosa	3 drops
Frankincense	1 drop
Lavender	2 drops

Blend the essential oils together, then dilute in 2 tablespoons (30 mL) of carrier oil. Use only as much as needed to massage over your child's back, once a day. If your child is under two years old, halve all the suggested essential oil amounts.

Do not use all the methods at once. Use one or two of the methods in any 24-hour period.

VERRUCAS (PLANTAR WARTS) AND OTHER WARTS

Viruses are responsible for both verrucas and warts. Warts can grow anywhere; they're most common on the fingers, hands, and feet. Verrucas most usually grow on the soles of the feet or the underside of toes, but they can also develop on the hands, and instead of growing outward, they tend to grow inward. Verrucas can be extremely painful, and pain is often the first symptom. When you look at it carefully, a telltale black spot is usually seen in the center of a hard piece of skin, which is the painful area. Both verrucas and warts are contagious.

Warts lead a somewhat mysterious life — disappearing and then appearing again in the same place without any apparent reason. They can be embarrassing more than anything else. But verrucas are a real problem because children run about in bare feet at the swimming pool, gym, or locker room, where both catching a verruca and passing it on is a possibility. There are several essential oils that can be a real help to sufferers of verrucas and warts:

Verruca and Wart Essential Oils
Lemon (*Citrus limon*)
Lavender (*Lavandula angustifolia*)
Oregano (*Origanum vulgare*)
Geranium (*Pelargonium graveolens*)
Cypress (*Cupressus sempervirens*)
Tea tree (*Melaleuca alternifolia*)
Manuka (*Leptospermum scoparium*)
Neem (*Azadirachta indica*)
Cinnamon leaf (*Cinnamomum zeylanicum*)
Niaouli (*Melaleuca quinquenervia*)

Because there are different types of warts or verrucas and because people respond differently to particular essential oils, if one essential oil is ineffective, try another. Start with whatever you already have in the cupboard that's on the list.

When using the essential oils on a child who is under five years of age, first dilute your chosen essential oil as best you can in a few drops of cider vinegar. With older children, the essential oil can be applied neat. First, clean the area with soap and water or, better still, colloidal silver. Use any of the oils listed above on their own or in combination, or try the following blend:

Verruca and Wart Blend
Lemon	10 drops
Cypress	5 drops
Manuka (or tea tree)	5 drops

Mix the essential oil together using these proportions. Depending on the age of the child, apply the essential oil neat, or diluted in a few drops of cider vinegar, directly onto the verruca or wart using a cotton ball. Use a clean cotton ball each time the skin is touched, and avoid the surrounding area. Apply once a day.

ATHLETE'S FOOT (TINEA PEDIS)

There are a variety of fungi that cause athlete's foot, and although the word *foot* characterizes this problem, the fungi can be spread to other parts of the body. Anyone with athlete's foot in the household should be extremely careful to avoid spreading it around the family. They should wear shoes at all times — open-toed whenever possible — and wear flip-flops in the shower; they should also avoid touching their feet and should not share towels. This is the only way to prevent the fungus from going back and forth between household members.

Because athlete's foot is contagious, catching it is as easy as walking along the side of a pool where an infected person has walked before. In other words, every pool, gym, and locker room is a potential site of infection. Athlete's foot usually first appears between the toes, and it can affect the toenails, the soles of the feet, and the upper portion of the foot, usually by the toes. The first sign can be itching, and the skin takes on a whitish and flaky or spongy appearance, becoming quite scaly.

ATHLETE'S FOOT ESSENTIAL OILS
Tea tree (*Melaleuca alternifolia*)
Manuka (*Leptospermum scoparium*)
Lavender (*Lavandula angustifolia*)
Cypress (*Cupressus sempervirens*)
Neem (*Azadirachta indica*)
Palmarosa (*Cymbopogon martinii*)
Geranium (*Pelargonium graveolens*)
Eucalyptus radiata (*Eucalyptus radiata*)
Eucalyptus lemon (*Eucalyptus citriodora*)
Bergamot (*Citrus bergamia*)
Coriander seed (*Coriandrum sativum*)

If you have tamanu oil (*Calophyllum inophyllum*), apply it over the affected area, remembering to wash your hands afterward. Alternatively, and depending on the severity of the condition, dilute 3 drops of tea tree or manuka essential oil in 1 teaspoon (5 mL) of tamanu oil, and apply as much as required over the affected area. If you think the condition warrants it, spread a single drop of neat tea tree or manuka essential oil over the affected area, twice a day if necessary but in any event before bed.

Damp conditions around the feet make the condition worse as the fungi just love dark, damp places. Exposing the feet to air is really helpful, so wearing sandals and flip-flops when inside the home makes a lot of sense. Powders help to keep the area dry, and these can be made using either dry white or green clay, talc, or corn flour. To a cup of your chosen base, add 10 drops of tea tree or manuka. This needs to be mixed really well, and an electric blender is perfect for the job because it usually has a tiny hole in the lid that enables the essential oil to be added at intervals to ensure a thorough mix. Hold the lid down, though — you

don't want fine powder flying all over the place! Make sure you get the powder between the toes. Use daily. Natural cotton or wool makes the best sock material at this time, so avoid those made with nylon or other synthetic materials.

RINGWORM

Despite its name, ringworm has got nothing to do with worms. It's a fungal infection passed from person to person, or pet to person, by contact with the skin. Those involved in contact sports are most at risk, but as children are so often in close contact anyway, any child can become infected. The word *ring* in the name is thoroughly appropriate because the fungus moves outward in a circular motion, causing an ever-increasing red ring to appear on the skin. Ringworm can be very itchy, and if it appears on the scalp it can cause small patches of hair to be lost temporarily. Sometimes an allergic reaction to the fungus causes small, itchy blisters to appear on parts of the body that can be far removed from the ringworm itself.

RINGWORM ESSENTIAL OILS
Tea tree (*Melaleuca alternifolia*)
Thyme linalol (*Thymus vulgaris ct. linalool*)
Lavender (*Lavandula angustifolia*)
Manuka (*Leptospermum scoparium*)
Neem (*Azadirachta indica*)
Rosemary (*Rosmarinus officinalis*)
Eucalyptus lemon (*Eucalyptus citriodora*)
Oregano (*Origanum vulgare*)
Geranium (*Pelargonium graveolens*)
Frankincense (*Boswellia carterii*)
Palmarosa (*Cymbopogon martinii*)

Tea tree, manuka, and palmarosa essential oils provide an extremely effective treatment for ringworm. Apply 1 neat drop over the infected area three times a day until it's clear. This should take no more than 10 days. After that, apply an oil composed of 30 drops of tea tree, manuka, or palmarosa diluted in 2 tablespoons (30 mL) of tamanu (*Calophyllum inophyllum*) oil. Apply a small amount over the area daily. Alternatively, try this blend:

RINGWORM BLEND

Palmarosa	10 drops
Oregano	5 drops
Geranium	6 drops
Tea tree	5 drops
Thyme linalol	3 drops

Blend the essential oils together, then dilute in 2 tablespoons (30 mL) of tamanu oil.

PINWORMS

It's extremely unpleasant to think that intestinal parasites may have taken up residence inside your child's body, but, unfortunately, they've found the human body an attractive home since time began, or at least since people started writing about health problems, which was two millennia ago. It doesn't matter one hoot to an intestinal parasite whether your child is angelic or naughty, goes to an expensive private school or the free local one. Parasites love us all, even though we don't think that kindly of them. There are a variety of potential squatters in a child's intestinal tract, the most common of which is pinworm (*Enterobius*), also known as *threadworm* because it looks like a short piece of white cotton thread.

A child becomes infected with pinworm when the eggs get into their mouth and, from there, into the intestine. The eggs can be airborne and just inhaled, or they can be on toilet seats, furniture, or any other surface, including on other people. The eggs are viable for up to 20 hours after being laid, so cleanliness is of the utmost importance. If a child has pinworms, the eggs can get onto night clothing and bedsheets so these should be handled gently, to prevent the eggs from flying off into the

atmosphere, and washed daily. Once inside a body, the males mate and die and are flushed out with the feces. The females have to lay their eggs outside the body because the eggs need oxygen, and that's why around the anus is where they're seen. The females usually emerge from the anus a couple of hours after the child has fallen asleep, and they can be seen as half-inch-long white threads. This is when they lay their eggs.

This activity is excruciatingly itchy for a child, which is why they scratch their bottom. In doing so, they can get more eggs under their fingernails, and if they suck their fingers or bite their nails, the whole cycle continues. The first line of defense is to keep fingernails short, discourage finger sucking, and make sure hands are washed regularly. Although anal itching — especially at night — is the main symptom, pinworms could also be the cause of teeth-grinding, feeling unwell, or being irritable, lethargic, or unable to concentrate. If you suspect pinworms, check stools to see if any are visible. The following essential oils are effective when used as a tummy rub:

ESSENTIAL OILS FOR PINWORMS
Niaouli (*Melaleuca quinquenervia*)
Lemon (*Citrus limon*)
Chamomile roman (*Anthemis nobilis*)
Lavender (*Lavandula angustifolia*)
Eucalyptus lemon (*Eucalyptus citriodora*)
*Eucalyptus radiata (*Eucalyptus radiata*)

Eucalyptus radiata should only be used in reduced amounts, and not on children under two years of age.

Use 15 drops of one of the essential oils listed above, or make a blend using two or more oils, diluted in 2 tablespoons (30 mL) of sweet almond oil. Apply a small amount of the oil as a body oil, morning and night, over the abdomen, for at least two weeks. Aloe vera gel can be applied around the anus to help prevent the itching.

If pinworms are present in the home, the likelihood is that it's not just one child who is infected. The tummy rub could be used on any household member, but use double the dose for adults, and bottle separately.

In France, the first line of defense against worms has traditionally been garlic, which is consumed as garlic soup and garlic bread. Any which way you can get your child to consume garlic would be good, even if that's just in the form of garlic tablets.

Inhaling the essential oils helps too, so make up this blend and use 3 drops in a diffuser in the child's room, or in the hot-water bowl method. This same blend can be used in baths — add 2 drops, diluted in a little carrier oil, to warm baths.

PINWORMS ROOM AND BATH BLEND

Niaouli	10 drops
Lavender	14 drops
Thyme linalol	5 drops

HEAD LICE

Every parent dreads the moment when their child starts scratching their head, particularly if they've heard that an infestation of head lice is going around the preschool or school. By the time a child enters first grade, the chances are they too have heard about "nits." They might not know that the head louse, *Pediculus humanus capitis*, is feasting on their blood, but they will know it makes them itch.

Lice are tiny, six-legged insects that live in hair. They don't have wings and don't hop. They just take up residence in the hair and lay eggs. The eggs are known as *nits*, and because they're white, they are easier to see on dark hair than the lice because the adult louse scuttles away and hides very effectively. Lice will take up camp in any type of hair, clean or dirty, red, blond, black, or brown.

One of the less pleasant parental duties is to check for nits, which are just about as close to the scalp as it's possible for a louse to get. If the white shell is farther away from the scalp, the chances are that the baby louse, known charmingly as a *nymph*, has completed its eight-day incubation period and hatched. It too will now be crawling around the head of your child. The telltale nits are often found by the nape of the neck and above the ears.

As soon as the rumor reaches your ears that lice are in the school, think about taking preventative measures. One thing that can be done at all times is thorough brushing of the hair, morning and night — lice are not so strong that they can survive a vigorous brushing. Use the following essential oils in a lotion or as an addition to the rinsing water when washing the hair. These are the most suitable oils for children:

LICE DETERRENT ESSENTIAL OILS
Rosemary (*Rosmarinus officinalis*)
Lavender (*Lavandula angustifolia*)
Geranium (*Pelargonium graveolens*)
Lemon (*Citrus limon*)
Tea tree (*Melaleuca alternifolia*)
Neem (*Azadirachta indica*)
Eucalyptus lemon (*Eucalyptus citriodora*)
Manuka (*Leptospermum scoparium*)

An excellent preventative blend would comprise equal parts of rosemary, lavender, and lemon. Add 2 drops of this blend to the final rinse after shampooing. Rosemary is used in many Asian hair preparations as it discourages all manner of small creepy-crawlies from making their home in the hair. Neem oil can discourage lice from settling in anyone's hair; however, the smell is pungent. It's best to combine it with other essential oils to disguise the smell. Lavender, of course, is a well-established insect repellent.

Only use the oils in this way intermittently. If you suspect the presence of lice, here's a remedy that could be gently applied to the scalp in sections and left overnight. The mixture can easily be washed out with shampoo and hot water.

LICE BLEND

Rosemary	10 drops
Lavender	10 drops
Geranium	10 drops

Add the blend to 70 grams of aloe vera gel. Neem oil could be substituted for the lavender in the blend — it is very effective, although the strong aroma is not to everyone's taste. This gel can be easily combed through the hair, and then washed out.

If you want to use something that can be left on overnight, make a thicker solution by adding together just under 1 oz. (20 g) of cocoa butter and 3½ tablespoons (50 mL) of castor oil.

First, melt the cocoa butter in a bain-marie (or a dish over a pot of boiling water). Remove from the heat, and add the castor oil until a creamy consistency is achieved. Cool, then add the 30 drops of the Lice Blend, while stirring well. This will thicken, but when it's applied to the skin, it should melt. Apply a small amount directly to the scalp, parting the hair in layers to do so. Cover the head in a scarf or shower cap and leave it on overnight. Wash the hair in the morning using your usual shampoo.

If your child has scratched their head so much that it's caused an inflammatory reaction by breaking the skin, use one of the following oils, or the blend below, in aloe vera gel. These oils are antiseptic and have cooling and calming properties:

ANTISEPTIC COOLING AND CALMING ESSENTIAL OILS

Geranium (*Pelargonium graveolens*)
Chamomile german (*Matricaria recutita*)
Chamomile roman (*Anthemis nobilis*)
Lavender (*Lavandula angustifolia*)

HEAD LICE COOLING BLEND

Chamomile german	20 drops
Lavender	10 drops
Lemon	5 drops

The essential oils can be used in several ways. First, blend them together. Then use 5 drops in 3½ fl. oz. (100 mL) of water and use as a rinse. Or add 10 drops of the blend to the cocoa butter and castor oil mix made as above, apply to the scalp, and leave it on overnight covered in a scarf or shower cap. Alternatively, add 10 drops to 5 teaspoons (25 mL) of aloe vera gel and leave overnight, covered as above. Comb the hair in the morning to remove any eggs or lice before washing thoroughly using your usual shampoo.

The Teenage Years

Teenagers get pretty bad press and are the butt of many jokes. At the same time, they have little control over their lives and are expected to excel at school. Whereas we adults are expected to succeed only in our chosen professions, they're under pressure to achieve high grades in a dozen very different subjects. And while we can come home and relax, they're expected to do homework that can be both extensive and difficult. While all this pressure is being exerted on them, their bodies are going through profound changes, during which there is often an awkward stage.

Boys sometimes suffer from gynecomastia, when the breasts swell as the male and female sex hormones adjust and find their new balance. Hormonal changes lead to involuntary erections and emission of semen, which can make a boy feel his life is totally out of control. Girls may experience irregular or painful periods or premenstrual syndrome. Certain aspects of a child's life during puberty can be anticipated, but as parents we cannot expect to know everything that's bothering our child, especially at school, and the only way we can find out is to talk to them. With our children now so wrapped up in their parallel lives in cyberspace, there's never been a more important time for getting together over a family meal.

SKIN PROBLEMS

The increase in sex hormones that accompanies puberty can cause an increase in sebum production of the sebaceous glands. Exfoliating the skin to remove dead skin cells can help to avoid skin breakouts. The following facial scrub won't damage skin and is equally good for those with skin problems and those trying to avoid them. Use once a week.

THE ESSENTIAL TEENAGE FACIAL SCRUB
Ground almonds   2 tablespoons (30 g)
Raw egg white   2 teaspoons (10 mL)
Palmarosa essential oil   1 drop

These amounts are enough for several scrubs. Bergamot FCF or manuka can be substituted for the palmarosa essential oil. Mix the ingredients together, put a small amount into the palm of the hand, and apply to a previously wetted face. Rub the mixture all over the face in a rolling movement and rinse off with plenty of water. Now dab the face with a lavender hydrolat, using a clean cotton ball. A chamomile hydrolat can be substituted if the skin is reddened or inflamed, and a thyme hydrolat would be effective if there are pimples. Exfoliate the skin no more than twice a week.

It might be worth trying a zinc supplement, not only because many people with acne are shown to be deficient in zinc but because it has many other health benefits. In chapter 13, "The Fragrant Way to Beauty," you'll find other suggestions for acne and a variety of skin problems.

DRUG ABUSE

Illicit drugs have the ability to strip our children of their personality and good character, to the point that we can hardly recognize them. Meanwhile, the children may not recognize that they're losing themselves, like an onion being peeled layer by layer. Parents watching this become enveloped in a terrible fear.

The negative vortex of drug abuse is something that professional aromatherapists, like practitioners in other fields of complementary medicine, are familiar with, having been asked by many desperate parents for help. Withdrawal from drugs is never easy, and the essential oils cannot offer a magical panacea. There will always be a period of difficult emotional and physical transition back to normality. However, the essential oils can help the process in two ways: as a general strengthener to both the emotional and physical systems and in specific treatments of the many side effects of withdrawal. These include insomnia, acute anxiety, night sweats, palpitations, nausea, cramps, headaches, loss of appetite, and trembling.

The following essential oils can be useful in baths and massage oils. Refer to the essential oil profiles in chapter 20, and throughout this book, to find the oils on this list that will be most helpful, given each individual's physical and emotional state.

ESSENTIAL OILS FOR USE DURING
DRUG WITHDRAWAL
Grapefruit (*Citrus paradisi*)
Orange, sweet (*Citrus sinensis*)
Sandalwood (*Santalum album*)
Marjoram, sweet (*Origanum majorana*)
Fennel, sweet (*Foeniculum vulgare var. dulce*)
Bergamot (*Citrus bergamia*)
Basil (*Ocimum basilicum*)
Lavender (*Lavandula angustifolia*)
Eucalyptus lemon (*Eucalyptus citriodora*)

Chamomile roman (*Anthemis nobilis*)

Spikenard (*Nardostachys jatamansi*)

Valerian (*Valeriana officinalis*)

Jasmine absolute (*Jasminum grandiflorum/officinale*)

Vetiver (*Vetiveria zizanoides*)

Patchouli (*Pogostemon cablin*)

Nutmeg (*Myristica fragrans*)

Davana (*Artemisia pallens*)

Basil linalol (*Ocimum basilicum ct. linalool*)

Rosewood (*Aniba rosaeodora*)

Cedarwood atlas (*Cedrus atlantica*)

Ylang ylang (*Cananga odorata*)

Cistus (*Cistus ladaniferus*)

Sage, Greek (*Salvia fruticosa/triloba*)

Guaiacwood, or Palo Santo (*Bulnesia sarmientoi*)

Rose absolute (*Rosa centifolia*)

Children with Special Challenges

Essential oils and aromatherapy are uniquely placed to help children with special challenges. The huge range of different aromas provide a sensory rainbow for the visually impaired and bring a depth of experience to the child with limited physical ability. Aside from this intrinsic value, essential oils can be used in massage, the very act of which provides physical communication between two people and brings reassurance. And the essential oils themselves possess all manner of healing properties. A little box of essential oils, although small, can bring a huge vista of possibilities into the life of a child with special challenges, and indeed their whole family.

Because there's generally so much emphasis on the healing properties of essential oils it's sometimes easy to forget that they're also just nice, and bring charm into any life. They smell delightful, and they uplift the spirit. Many have been cornerstones of the perfume industry for centuries, even millennia in some cases. This is one reason why people have always used them, and why their tradition lives on in aromatherapy. Of course aromatherapy has long been used to alleviate stress and bring relaxation, and the ability of essential oils to positively affect mind, mood, and emotion is a huge aspect of their beneficial range. This is something all children, including those with special needs, can benefit from. For a variety of reasons, then, incorporating essential oils into the daily routine has the potential to enhance many aspects of life.

As well as introducing your child with special needs to a range of possibilities not available by other means, essential oils can also bring benefits to you — the parents and carers. You too face special challenges, both physical and emotional, so please don't forget to take care of yourself. Use the essential oils in a relaxing bath, or ask a family member to massage your shoulders with an essential oil blend. Perhaps your child could massage your hands and arms, allowing them the opportunity to give back; remembering the old adage "it's better to give than receive," this will make them feel positive about themselves. It will also expand their repertoire of activities, add to their confidence, and make them happy that they can help you.

A healthy diet is especially important for children with special needs. If you have a backyard, it would be good to grow your own vegetables, but if not, purchase organic whenever possible. Fresh vegetables and fruit, lean meat, chicken, and fish are the essential building blocks for any child, so try to avoid processed foods, including those in cans, and foods with preservatives and additives. If you have never been a great "from scratch" cook up to now or never had time to become one, try to develop those cooking skills now. If your child needs any teeth filled, avoid the use of mercury fillings.

Although the dosages and methods outlined in this section relate to children, much of the advice applies equally to adults and could be adapted accordingly.

SPINA BIFIDA

There's a huge range in the degree of damage caused by this congenital defect of the neural tube or backbone, so much so that many people don't realize they have a mild form until they go in for a spinal X-ray, for some other reason, and it's pointed out to them. Some children with this diagnosis feel nothing more than a small area of numbness, while others have full paralysis from the waist down. In more serious cases, a baby can be born with a visible gap on the spine, into which the spinal cord pushes. As the spinal cord is an extension of the brain, pressure can be put on the brain because the flow of cerebrospinal fluid is affected.

Because each case of spina bifida is so very unique in terms of both physical and mental development, the aim of using essential oils is to increase general health and well-being and ease any discomfort. Cross-reference this section with the essential oil profiles in chapter 20 to see which oils on the list below are more appropriate for your child, and refer to the chart earlier in this chapter for dosages appropriate for each age group.

ESSENTIAL OILS FOR SPINA BIFIDA
Lavender (*Lavandula angustifolia*)
Chamomile roman (*Anthemis nobilis*)
Chamomile german (*Matricaria recutita*)
Spearmint (*Mentha spicata*)
Rosemary (*Rosmarinus officinalis*)
Orange, sweet (*Citrus sinensis*)
Lemon (*Citrus limon*)
Immortelle (*Helichrysum italicum*)
Mandarin (*Citrus reticulata*)
Clove bud (*Syzygium aromaticum*)

Bergamot FCF (*Citrus bergamia*)
Ravintsara (*Cinnamomum camphora ct. cineole*)
Marjoram, sweet (*Origanum majorana*)
Black pepper (*Piper nigrum*)
Ginger (*Zingiber officinale*)
Patchouli (*Pogostemon cablin*)
Palmarosa (*Cymbopogon martinii*)
Clary sage (*Salvia sclarea*)
Coriander seed (*Coriandrum sativum*)
Ho wood (*Cinnamomum camphora ct. linalool*)
Juniper berry (*Juniperus communis*)
Ravensara (*Ravensara aromatica*)

If making a massage oil, use no more than a total of 15 drops of essential oil to 2 tablespoons (30 mL) of carrier oil. Use a small amount each time, depending on the age and size of your child. Use the essential oils either singly or in any combination you choose. Massage in gentle, stroking movements and work upward, toward the head. A very simple routine is the three-point FHH massage, involving just the feet, hands, and head: start with the feet, then the hands, and finish at the scalp.

Here are some blends to try if a child particularly needs relaxation and calming, or if they need stimulation:

BALANCING AND RELAXING/CALMING
MASSAGE BLEND 1
Lavender	5 drops
Orange, sweet	5 drops
Marjoram, sweet	2 drops

Dilute in 2 tablespoons (30 mL) of carrier oil, and use a small amount each time.

BALANCING AND RELAXING/CALMING
MASSAGE BLEND 2
Chamomile	2 drops
Lavender	5 drops
Mandarin	5 drops

Dilute in 2 tablespoons (30 mL) of carrier oil, and use a small amount each time.

BALANCING AND STIMULATING MASSAGE BLEND 1

Palmarosa	2 drops
Coriander seed	2 drops
Ginger	3 drops
Black pepper	2 drops
Bergamot FCF	3 drops

Dilute in 2 tablespoons (30 mL) of carrier oil, and use a small amount each time.

BALANCING AND STIMULATING MASSAGE BLEND 2

Rosemary	4 drops
Grapefruit	6 drops
Ginger	2 drops

Dilute in 2 tablespoons (30 mL) of carrier oil, and use a small amount each time.

If appropriate, also see "Paralysis" below and "Pressure Sores" on page 179.

PARALYSIS

The suffix -plegia refers to paralysis and is used in paraplegia — paralysis of the lower half of the body; tetraplegia or quadriplegia — when all four limbs have lost their sensation; monoplegia — when only one limb is affected; and hemiplegia — when the paralysis affects one side of the body. This section is intended for all these types of paralysis, whether from accident or a congenital disorder such as spina bifida, and the instructions can be adjusted to match the needs of the particular child.

Hope for children with paralysis came in 2012 when a team from Poland and the UK carried out revolutionary surgery on a man whose spinal cord had been severed in a knife attack, leaving him paraplegic. The patient's severed nerve fibers were gradually regenerated after he was injected above and below the site of injury with a cell culture made from the part of the brain that processes smell — specifically, olfactory ensheathing cells from his olfactory bulb. Two years after surgery, he could walk with the help of a frame, he could drive, and he had some control over bladder and bowel function. This remarkable development in the treatment of paralysis proves the point that we should never give up hope that our child's life can improve.

Every child has special needs, and all would benefit greatly from daily massages. Some muscle wastage is inevitable with paralysis, but manual exercise and massage can greatly improve the overall tone of muscles. That is the objective in daily massage using essential oils.

Essential oils are divided into two sets of oil groups: warm and balancing, and cool and balancing. Use the warm and balancing massage oils on areas of the body that have little movement or have become immobile, such as with muscle wastage. And use the cool and balancing massage oils on areas that feel hot to the child, or to the touch. In some cases it may be that the two massage oils are used on alternate days to help balance the body.

A part of the body that is immobile or without feeling, or that has a loss of sensation, is classed as cool, and the massage oils used would be those chosen from the warm and balancing list. Make your choice dependent upon essential oil availability and both your and your child's personal aroma preferences. Choosing oils that both the massage giver and the receiver enjoy can make a massage doubly beneficial.

Use a maximum of 15 drops of essential oil diluted in 2 tablespoons (30 mL) of carrier oil. Thyme linalol, clove bud, basil linalol, and ginger should be used only sparingly in a massage oil, at no more than 2 drops per 2 tablespoons (30 mL), unless otherwise suggested in a blend.

Some essential oils fall into one of the two groups and some are adaptogens — which means they adapt to what the intended use is. So, for example, although geranium and frankincense are on the warming list, they could also be considered cool and balancing when combined with, say, spearmint, lemon, or eucalyptus radiata essential oil.

WARM AND BALANCING ESSENTIAL OILS
Benzoin (*Styrax benzoin*)
Black pepper (*Piper nigrum*)
Ginger (*Zingiber officinale*)
Basil linalol (*Ocimum basilicum ct. linalool*)
Cedarwood atlas (*Cedrus atlantica*)
Immortelle (*Helichrysum italicum*)
Clary sage (*Salvia sclarea*)
Cardamom (*Elettaria cardamomum*)
Orange, sweet (*Citrus sinensis*)
Rosemary (*Rosmarinus officinalis*)
Thyme linalol (*Thymus vulgaris ct. linalool*)
Patchouli (*Pogostemon cablin*)
Frankincense (*Boswellia carterii*)
Clove bud (*Syzygium aromaticum*)
Geranium (*Pelargonium graveolens*)
Ylang ylang (*Cananga odorata*)

COOL AND BALANCING ESSENTIAL OILS
Chamomile roman (*Anthemis nobilis*)
Lavender (*Lavandula angustifolia*)
Chamomile german (*Matricaria recutita*)
Coriander seed (*Coriandrum sativum*)
Geranium (*Pelargonium graveolens*)
Spearmint (*Mentha spicata*)
Eucalyptus lemon (*Eucalyptus citriodora*)
Frankincense (*Boswellia carterii*)
Bergamot FCF (*Citrus bergamia*)
Lemon (*Citrus limon*)
Cypress (*Cupressus sempervirens*)
Palmarosa (*Cymbopogon martinii*)
Grapefruit (*Citrus paradisi*)
Eucalyptus radiata (*Eucalyptus radiata*)
Rosemary (*Rosmarinus officinalis*)

For a full-body massage, first decide whether to use a massage blend that is warm or cool. Start

the massage on the back of the body, moving in firm but loving upward strokes on either side of the vertebrae. Gently stimulate in this way several times, for two minutes at least. Move downward onto the feet, changing oils if needed. Gently massage the soles of the feet with slow but firm movements. There are reflex healing points all over the soles of the feet that can help balance the body. Don't concentrate on one area but glide over the foot. Moving upward now, massage the back of the legs — first one leg and then the other, and then both together for a balancing effect. Carry on for as short or long a time as requested.

If massaging the front of the body, start by gently holding both feet. Then massage both under and over each foot. Move upward over the front of the legs, concentrating on any really immobile areas to help the blood circulation. From the legs, move on to the shoulders, and then on to the head. Most children like having their head massaged. The arms are massaged last. Make sure your child is kept warm at all times, and after each section is massaged, cover with a towel, just like a professional. Only uncover the part being massaged. Covering each section after it is massaged gives a sense of privacy but also security, and prevents the essential oils from evaporating into the air.

Finish by holding the feet firmly in both hands and sending your love. Imagine a white, shining, sparkling light enveloping your child, or an angel's wing over the child's whole body. Many parents report that this is a special time of exchange between them and their child.

The following blends help with the physical and emotional aspects of the condition:

WARMING AND BALANCING BLEND 1

Ginger	1 drop
Petitgrain	4 drops
Black pepper	1 drop
Geranium	5 drops
Orange, sweet	3 drops

Blend the essential oils together, then dilute as follows: for a child under 11 years of age, dilute in 3 tablespoons (45 mL) of carrier oil; for a child over 11 years of age, dilute in 2 tablespoons (30 mL) of carrier oil.

WARMING AND BALANCING BLEND 2

Benzoin	4 drops
Mandarin	8 drops
Black pepper	1 drop
Ginger	1 drop
Rosemary	2 drops

Blend the essential oils together, then dilute as follows: for a child under 11 years of age, dilute in 3 tablespoons (45 mL) of carrier oil; for a child over 11 years of age, dilute in 2 tablespoons (30 mL) of carrier oil.

COOLING AND BALANCING BLEND 1

Lemon	5 drops
Lavender	4 drops
Chamomile roman	2 drops
Spearmint	4 drops

Blend the essential oils together, then dilute as follows: for a child under 11 years of age, dilute in 3 tablespoons (45 mL) of carrier oil; for a child over 11 years of age, dilute in 2 tablespoons (30 mL) of carrier oil.

COOLING AND BALANCING BLEND 2

Eucalyptus lemon	5 drops
Chamomile german	6 drops
Eucalyptus radiata	3 drops
Juniper berry	4 drops

Blend the essential oils together, then dilute as follows: for a child under 11 years of age, dilute in 4 tablespoons (60 mL) of carrier oil; for a child over 11 years of age, dilute in 3 tablespoons (45 mL) of carrier oil.

ATROPHY

Atrophy refers to the wasting away of a part of the body. The word is generally used to describe muscles that have shrunk due to lack of exercise or immobility, caused by long periods of inactivity or bed rest or by paralysis, or because a bone has been fractured and kept in an orthopedic cast. Follow the advice in "Paralysis" on page 173.

MUSCULAR DYSTROPHY (MD)

The term *muscular dystrophy* refers to a group of conditions, all different in their own ways but similar in that there's increasing muscle weakness and difficulty in carrying out activity. This is one of those conditions that need to be challenged all the way. Children with this condition need to be discouraged from spending hours sitting down and looking at a screen, and encouraged to find friends they can be active with. See if there's a local group they could join to find friends who share their experience.

Bring as much laughter into your lives as you can, and turn off aggression on TV and put away books with morbid stories — they are way too depressing. Massage and movement are cornerstones of the MD challenge.

ESSENTIAL OILS TO USE WITH MD
Lavender (*Lavandula angustifolia*)
Geranium (*Pelargonium graveolens*)
Immortelle (*Helichrysum italicum*)
Rosemary (*Rosmarinus officinalis*)
Basil linalol (*Ocimum basilicum ct. linalool*)
Black pepper (*Piper nigrum*)
Ginger (*Zingiber officinale*)
Cedarwood atlas (*Cedrus atlantica*)
Lemon (*Citrus limon*)
Clary sage (*Salvia sclarea*)
Orange, sweet (*Citrus sinensis*)
Palmarosa (*Cymbopogon martinii*)

Patchouli (*Pogostemon cablin*)
Spikenard (*Nardostachys jatamansi*)
Mandarin (*Citrus reticulata*)
Cinnamon leaf (*Cinnamomum zeylanicum*)
Marjoram, sweet (*Origanum majorana*)
Thyme linalol (*Thymus vulgaris ct. linalool*)
Rosewood (*Aniba rosaeodora*)
Sandalwood (*Santalum album*)

When looking at the lists below, bear in mind that some essential oils, due to their adaptogenic nature, can be used for both restorative and relaxing purposes, depending on which other essential oils they're blended with and the intended use. For example, marjoram and sandalwood are in the relaxing group but can also be restorative when combined with other stimulating essential oils and can adapt to emotional needs — so they are listed in both groups. Essential oils should be chosen on the basis of the symptoms being experienced. Check with the age-related chart earlier in this chapter and the individual essential oils profiles in chapter 20 to help you make the appropriate choices.

RESTORATIVE ESSENTIAL OILS
Immortelle (*Helichrysum italicum*)
Palmarosa (*Cymbopogon martinii*)
Rosemary (*Rosmarinus officinalis*)
Ginger (*Zingiber officinale*)
Eucalyptus radiata (*Eucalyptus radiata*)
Basil linalol (*Ocimum basilicum ct. linalool*)
Black pepper (*Piper nigrum*)
Marjoram, sweet (*Origanum majorana*)
Sandalwood (*Santalum album*)
Cinnamon leaf (*Cinnamomum zeylanicum*)
Thyme linalol (*Thymus vulgaris ct. linalool*)
Geranium (*Pelargonium graveolens*)
Spikenard (*Nardostachys jatamansi*)
Frankincense (*Boswellia carterii*)
Orange, sweet (*Citrus sinensis*)
Lemon (*Citrus limon*)
Grapefruit (*Citrus paradisi*)

RELAXING ESSENTIAL OILS
Lavender (*Lavandula angustifolia*)
Lemon (*Citrus limon*)
Geranium (*Pelargonium graveolens*)
Orange, sweet (*Citrus sinensis*)
Palmarosa (*Cymbopogon martinii*)
Clary sage (*Salvia sclarea*)
Marjoram, sweet (*Origanum majorana*)
Spikenard (*Nardostachys jatamansi*)
Sandalwood (*Santalum album*)
Mandarin (*Citrus reticulata*)
Frankincense (*Boswellia carterii*)
Bergamot FCF (*Citrus bergamia*)

It's nice to have something that smells pleasant as well as being medicinal, so I suggest the following blends for relaxing baths:

RELAXING BATH BLEND 1
Palmarosa	5 drops
Geranium	6 drops
Orange, sweet	7 drops

Mix together in these proportions and dilute 2–3 drops in a teaspoon (5 mL) of carrier oil before adding to the bath.

RELAXING BATH BLEND 2
Lavender	5 drops
Chamomile roman	5 drops
Ho wood	4 drops
Mandarin	3 drops

Mix together in these proportions and dilute 2–3 drops in a teaspoon (5 mL) of carrier oil before adding to the bath.

It would be good if massage could become part of the daily routine, or at least carried out whenever there is time. See the body massage in "Paralysis" on page 174. If it's not possible to massage any part of the torso, do the FHH massage — feet, hands, and head. Each day, try to alternate the type of massage given, depending on personal symptoms, but always use gentle, reassuring strokes — never too hard or too soft. Alternate between a restorative massage and a gentle, relaxing one. The following blends are useful for general symptoms.

RESTORATIVE MASSAGE BLEND

Immortelle	4 drops
Geranium	5 drops
Bergamot	5 drops
Ginger	1 drop
Frankincense	2 drops

Blend the essential oils together, then dilute as follows: for a child under 11 years of age, dilute in 3 tablespoons (45 mL) of carrier oil; for a child over 11 years of age, dilute in 2 tablespoons (30 mL) of carrier oil. For single massages, depending upon the age and size of your child, dilute between 2 and 3 drops of the essential oil blend in 1 teaspoon (5 mL) of carrier oil.

RELAXING MASSAGE BLEND

Lavender	5 drops
Clary sage	2 drops
Orange, sweet	3 drops
Marjoram, sweet	2 drops
Lemon	5 drops

Blend the essential oils together, then dilute as follows: for a child under 11 years of age, dilute in 3 tablespoons (45 mL) of carrier oil; for a child over 11 years of age, dilute in 2 tablespoons (30 mL) of carrier oil. For single massages, depending upon the age and size of your child, dilute between 2 and 3 drops of the essential oil blend in 1 teaspoon (5 mL) of carrier oil.

SPASTICITY

Several conditions can lead to spasticity, which is caused when there's a problem in the central nervous system or spinal cord that causes a disconnect between directions from the brain and the parts of the body the brain should be instructing.

This is most usually experienced as a tightness in the muscles, or as uncontrolled movement in a part of the body. Cerebral palsy is just one of the conditions that can involve spasticity (see "Cerebral Palsy" on page 178).

When using essential oils, the idea is to help release the muscles from being held in a permanent position through exercise and massage. The massage can ease the pain and tenderness associated with the affected areas, and it also facilitates the natural body flow, thereby helping to release any toxins that may not have been sufficiently eliminated from the muscle. Unless you are a trained therapist, massage should only consist of gentle, repetitive stroking movements that become one continuous flow.

ESSENTIAL OILS FOR SPASTICITY
Benzoin (*Styrax benzoin*)
Lemon (*Citrus limon*)
Ginger (*Zingiber officinale*)
Sandalwood (*Santalum album*)
Rosemary (*Rosmarinus officinalis*)
Juniper berry (*Juniperus communis*)
Cypress (*Cupressus sempervirens*)
Lavender (*Lavandula angustifolia*)
Immortelle (*Helichrysum italicum*)
Rosemary (*Rosmarinus officinalis*)
Eucalyptus radiata (*Eucalyptus radiata*)
Basil linalol (*Ocimum basilicum ct. linalool*)
Palmarosa (*Cymbopogon martinii*)
Thyme linalol (*Thymus vulgaris ct. linalool*)
Marjoram, sweet (*Origanum majorana*)
Sandalwood (*Santalum album*)
Geranium (*Pelargonium graveolens*)
Spikenard (*Nardostachys jatamansi*)
Frankincense (*Boswellia carterii*)
Orange, sweet (*Citrus sinensis*)
Lemon (*Citrus limon*)
Grapefruit (*Citrus paradisi*)

All the above essential oils used singly or in blends are effective in massage oils for limbs.

Dilute 10–15 drops in 2 tablespoons (30 mL) of carrier oil. Cinnamon leaf (*Cinnamomum zeylanicum*) and black pepper (*Piper nigrum*) are also useful oils but should be used only in very small quantities, and on children over five years of age.

General Limb Massage Blend

Geranium	2 drops
Black pepper	2 drops
Immortelle	5 drops
Marjoram, sweet	5 drops
Chamomile roman	5 drops

Blend the essential oils together, then dilute 2–4 drops in each teaspoon (5 mL) of carrier oil.

Soothing Blend

Benzoin	8 drops
Lemon	10 drops
Sandalwood	5 drops

Blend the essential oils together, then dilute 2–5 drops in each teaspoon (5 mL) of carrier oil.

Restorative Blend

Rosemary	4 drops
Lavender	4 drops
Ginger	2 drops
Juniper berry	2 drops
Orange, sweet	6 drops

Blend the essential oils together, then dilute 2–4 drops in each teaspoon (5 mL) of carrier oil.

CEREBRAL PALSY

There's huge variation in the degree to which a particular child may be affected by cerebral palsy. Aside from the classic symptoms of involuntary movement, lack of coordination, contracted muscles or joints, and difficulty with posture or gait, a particular child may have difficulty speaking, epilepsy, problems with vision, and some degree of learning difficulty. Cerebral palsy is present from birth and doesn't get worse. Management is the key issue — and keeping the muscles working.

Muscle weakness is common to all sufferers of cerebral palsy, and massage with the essential oils certainly helps in this respect. Include massage of the limbs and spine in any developmental program your child is involved in, and teach self-massage to your child as she or he gets older. The essential oils have such a lovely aroma and massage is in itself so relaxing that this should be a time of enjoyment for your child, as well as being therapeutic. If you would like to give a full-body massage, follow the directions outlined in the section on muscular dystrophy on page 175, adapting it to your particular child's needs.

Essential Oils for Muscular Spasm

Marjoram, sweet (*Origanum majorana*)
Geranium (*Pelargonium graveolens*)
Cypress (*Cupressus sempervirens*)
Lavender (*Lavandula angustifolia*)
Basil linalol (*Ocimum basilicum ct. linalool*)
Chamomile roman (*Anthemis nobilis*)
Clary sage (*Salvia sclarea*)
Immortelle (*Helichrysum italicum*)
Juniper berry (*Juniperus communis*)
Petitgrain (*Citrus aurantium*)
Vetiver (*Vetiveria zizanoides*)
Spearmint (*Mentha spicata*)
Neroli (*Citrus aurantium*)
Grapefruit (*Citrus paradisi*)
Plai (*Zingiber cassumunar*)

Essential Oils for Muscular Weakness

Immortelle (*Helichrysum italicum*)
Basil linalol (*Ocimum basilicum ct. linalool*)
Eucalyptus radiata (*Eucalyptus radiata*)
Rosemary (*Rosmarinus officinalis*)
Marjoram, sweet (*Origanum majorana*)
Patchouli (*Pogostemon cablin*)
Chamomile roman (*Anthemis nobilis*)
Orange, sweet (*Citrus sinensis*)

Plai (*Zingiber cassumunar*)
Cedarwood atlas (*Cedrus atlantica*)

The adaptogenic quality of some essential oils can be used to advantage when relieving some of the symptoms caused by this condition, such as muscular spasm and muscular weakness. To address both, if making your own blend choose oils that are on both lists, such as marjoram, basil linalol, and chamomile roman, and then add a general purpose oil such as lavender or sweet orange. Or choose one oil that's on both lists.

MUSCULAR SPASM BLEND

Clary sage	4 drops
Marjoram, sweet	6 drops
Lavender	5 drops
Eucalyptus lemon	5 drops

Blend the essential oils together, then dilute 2–3 drops in each teaspoon (5 mL) of carrier oil.

MUSCULAR WEAKNESS BLEND

Basil linalol	2 drops
Immortelle	5 drops
Geranium	4 drops
Lavender	2 drops
Ginger	2 drops
Cedarwood atlas	4 drops

Blend the essential oils together, then dilute by mixing 2–3 drops in each 1 teaspoon (5 mL) of carrier oil.

PRESSURE SORES

Pressure sores develop at places on the body that are constantly resting in one position. Children confined to bed could be particularly liable to develop these sores, as can those who spend long periods of time in a wheelchair, for example. The sores can occur pretty much anywhere, but likely places are on the buttocks, thighs, legs, and heels. When there's lack of mobility, it's important to regularly change the position of the body to relieve the pressure on any particular area, and to check for areas of dry and irritable skin that can crack and become a sore.

If an area of the skin looks as if it's irritated or red because of pressure, put 3 cups (700 mL) of warm water in a bowl, add 10 drops of lavender, and bathe the whole area. Then put 2 drops of neat lavender on a sterile piece of muslin and apply to the area once a day.

As an alternative preventative, calendula macerated oil makes a very useful body oil. Blend together 2 teaspoons (10 mL) of jojoba oil and 2 teaspoons (10 mL) of calendula oil, with 3 drops of either lavender or chamomile roman oil, and apply a small amount all over any areas where pressure sores may develop — but not when any sores are present. As calendula macerated oil is bright orange and may stain, avoid getting the oil on any clothing. Geranium is another very useful oil and can be used in the same way as the lavender or chamomile roman.

DIABETES MELLITUS (DM)

Type 1 diabetes, or juvenile diabetes, is often first diagnosed when a child needs to urinate excessively and has excessive thirst or hunger or weight loss. These symptoms can come about rather rapidly, over a few weeks or months, and every parent needs to be aware of them. Diabetes is a serious condition that requires close management, including insulin injections, to avoid complications.

Although essential oils can't alleviate the condition of diabetes, they're very helpful in managing some of the symptoms that result from it. For example, one problem is that the legs and feet can become cold, and numbness and pain can be experienced when walking. Foot baths can really help if your child experiences numbness and pain in their legs. Make a foot bath by adding 3 drops of geranium and 1 drop of rosemary to a teaspoon of carrier oil, then adding this blend to a bowl of warm water and swishing it around. Soak the feet in the bowl for around 10–15 minutes, adding warm water if necessary. Massaging the feet and legs can often help alleviate this problem when it occurs. The following suggestions can also be used on the arms and hands.

MASSAGE BLEND

Geranium	10 drops
Black pepper	1 drop
Cedarwood atlas	5 drops
Rosemary	2 drops
Orange, sweet	4 drops

Blend the essential oils together using these proportions, and bottle. For a massage, dilute 2–3 drops of the blend in each teaspoon (5 mL) of carrier oil.

A twice-weekly full-body massage does in some cases help to prevent some of the complications caused by diabetes in children. Choose from the list below and make your own blend, or follow mine, below:

DM ESSENTIAL OILS

Eucalyptus radiata (*Eucalyptus radiata*)
Geranium (*Pelargonium graveolens*)
Cypress (*Cupressus sempervirens*)
Lavender (*Lavandula angustifolia*)
Ginger (*Zingiber officinale*)
Black pepper (*Piper nigrum*)
Lemon (*Citrus limon*)
Bergamot FCF (*Citrus bergamia*)
Juniper berry (*Juniperus communis*)
Cardamom (*Elettaria cardamomum*)
Coriander seed (*Coriandrum sativum*)
*Cinnamon leaf (*Cinnamomum zeylanicum*)

Use cinnamon leaf only in small amounts — 1 drop per 5 mL of carrier oil.

DM BLEND FOR BODY MASSAGE

Lavender	5 drops
Geranium	9 drops
Coriander seed	5 drops
Cinnamon leaf	1 drop
Juniper berry	6 drops
Eucalyptus radiata	4 drops

Blend the essential oils together using these proportions, and bottle. For a massage, dilute 2–3 drops in each teaspoon (5 mL) of carrier oil. Start with 2 drops, the lower dose.

See other sections of this book for information on how to treat other symptoms.

DOWN SYNDROME

Children with Down syndrome are just like anyone else. They want to be successful in life, find love, and be productive. Because of the distinctive physical characteristics of children with Down syndrome, it is easy to think they are all the same in terms of physical or mental capability. But their degree of ability varies greatly, and like all children, each child with Down syndrome has his or her own unique personality. Generally speaking, though, these children are a diligent, happy, and joyous group with an infectious sense of humor. As they get older they are willing to help at home, and they can pull their weight in their workplace like anyone else.

Use essential oils with this group of children just as you would with any other, using the essential oils and dosages outlined in the chart earlier in this chapter. Down syndrome children will love to be massaged, and to massage in return, so explore those possibilities with them. Within the parameters of the oils recommended for their age group, let your child choose the oils they want used on them. Experiment with blends. Make this a family experience you can all share.

ARTHRITIS

A diagnosis of juvenile arthritis is quite difficult to achieve because there's no specific test, and it greatly depends on eliminating all the other possible causes of your child's symptoms. And there are a variety of forms of juvenile arthritis, so getting to the point where you have a definitive diagnosis probably involved quite an effort.

Many types of arthritis are characterized by inflammation of the tissue that lines the inside of joints, known as the *synovium*, and common symptoms are swollen and painful joints, joints tender to the touch, or occasionally stiffness — usually in the morning. Other symptoms can seem unrelated to arthritis but are part of the autoimmune issues a child may now face, including fatigue, fever, rashes, and difficulties with vision.

Treatment focuses on reducing any swelling around the joints, relieving pain, and improving joint strength and mobility. Any help that can be given toward these ends will help prevent further damage, which in a young person is well worth trying to achieve. Because each case is so individual, take the information given here and elsewhere in this book and adapt it to the needs of your particular child. This section includes essential oils and suggestions for most types of arthritis experienced by children, and if you keep within the recommended dosages and essential oils, it may be good to experiment to find solutions to your individual needs.

In the treatment of all forms of arthritis, nutritional factors are very important. Try to adjust the diet to one that contains organic products in order to avoid residue pesticides, and use olive oil for cooking and in salad dressings. Include in the diet fresh vegetables, including broccoli, and also include avocado, legumes, seeds, fish, and poultry. Grate raw vegetables such as carrots, zucchini, and cabbage into salads. The leafy dark-green vegetables are particularly helpful, so incorporate them into cooked dishes in any way you can. Avoid giving your child processed foods as much as possible. Some people believe that too much citrus can exacerbate symptoms, so try cutting down on orange juice and substitute carrot juice or berry smoothies and see if that helps. Food intolerances can certainly play a part in arthritis for some children, and this is worth exploring. The omega 3 fatty acids seem to help children with this condition, so if your child does not eat oily fish such as salmon, supplements may be useful.

Essential Oils for Arthritis
Geranium (*Pelargonium graveolens*)
Lavender (*Lavandula angustifolia*)
Chamomile roman (*Anthemis nobilis*)
Eucalyptus lemon (*Eucalyptus citriodora*)
Chamomile german (*Matricaria recutita*)
Copaiba (*Copaifera officinalis*)
Cistus (*Cistus ladaniferus*)
Clary sage (*Salvia sclarea*)
Frankincense (*Boswellia carterii*)
Ho wood (*Cinnamomum camphora ct. linalool*)
Rosewood (*Aniba rosaeodora*)
Immortelle (*Helichrysum italicum*)
Juniper berry (*Juniperus communis*)
Spearmint (*Mentha spicata*)
Cedarwood atlas (*Cedrus atlantica*)

Essential oils can be used in the bathtub and in massage. For arthritis conditions, dilute your chosen essential oil or blend and apply it to the affected area *before* entering the bathtub. This method is especially useful in conditions of chronic pain — the oils become effective by a process known as *osmosis*. A cupful of Epsom salts added to the bathtub can also help relieve symptoms.

During flare-ups, a green clay poultice might ease symptoms, as could using the cabbage-leaf method (see page 182) in combination with essential oils.

CLAY POULTICE FOR ARTHRITIS

Eucalyptus lemon	2 drops
Chamomile german	3 drops
Lavender	2 drops

Make a stiff paste by adding water to 1 tablespoon (15 g) of dry clay. Then add the essential oils and mix well. Smear the mixture over the affected joints and painful areas, cover with a piece of white cotton or bandage, and rest.

The cabbage treatment can be very effective, even though it does sound somewhat strange. The cabbages must be organically grown, washed, and dried before use. Use the outer leaves of a winter cabbage — January King for example (*Brassica oleracea var. capitata*). Iron the leaves to release the active properties, and wrap the warm leaf around the affected joint.

Massage is one of the most helpful treatments and can be given regularly, as general pain management and to prevent flare-ups. Single oils or blends could be used.

Here are two blend suggestions:

MASSAGE OIL BLEND 1

Lavender	8 drops
Chamomile german	4 drops
Chamomile roman	3 drops

First blend the essential oils together, then dilute 3–5 drops in each teaspoon (5 mL) of carrier oil, and use a small amount each time.

MASSAGE OIL BLEND 2

Immortelle	8 drops
Clary sage	4 drops
Eucalyptus lemon	3 drops

First blend the essential oils together, then dilute 3–5 drops in each teaspoon (5 mL) of carrier oil, and use a small amount each time.

VISUAL IMPAIRMENT

There are over 130 essential oils in common use in aromatherapy, and they provide a huge spectrum of olfactory stimuli. Some essential oil suppliers sell samples for a few dollars, and it would not be difficult to acquire a wide range of different aromas for a child to experience. Over the years the collection of aromas can be increased, so that by the time your child is a teenager, they'll be a veritable expert in the aromatic rainbow. Once you get into the potential of blending and the variation that occurs depending on the ratio of drops used, the different aromas that can be created become innumerable.

For a small child, developing the skills of aromatic recognition can be a game. As an adult, those skills can become a profession — the design of natural perfumes or working as a highly paid "nose" in the perfume industry. Having a good sense of smell is a valued craft, not only in the essential oil world but in the wine, coffee, and tea businesses too.

Children with visual impairment often use the sensitivity of their fingers as their eyes and are sensitive to the texture of objects in a way the rest of us probably are not. This natural tendency to reach out can be developed into the skill of massage by allowing the child to massage you, starting with just the hands, arms, or feet. Massage gives a visually impaired child the excuse to truly explore the feel of a human body. And to teach them, you first massage your child. This is something that can be done from babyhood and made a routine part of life. When massaging a child just for the fun of it, choose essential oils that are food-related, like sweet orange or mandarin, or those your child enjoys smelling. Use a small amount — 1 drop of essential oil diluted in 1 teaspoon (5 mL) of carrier oil, using only as much as needed each time. Also explore the possibilities of carrier oils, starting with organic sweet almond oil.

CLUB FOOT

When a child is born with one or both feet turned inward, it's called *club foot*. This is a fairly common condition, occurring in around 1 in every 1,000 births. The good news is that in most instances the foot can be manipulated into the correct position. The key is to start as soon as possible after the birth, when the baby is still very flexible. Consult with the pediatrician or physical therapist for advice about which movements to make. Essentially, the idea is to slowly and gently encourage the foot toward a straight position.

Depending on where you live, your child may be given special footwear, a cast, or a stretching device to be used in between physical manipulation sessions. Your therapist may be able to advise you about how to work alongside their own methods and procedures.

Massage the leg from the knee to the ankle in firm but gentle downward strokes. Hold the foot there for a few minutes and gently ease it toward the straight position. Then massage the whole leg to the foot and once again take a fractional step further toward the straight position by gently moving your child's foot. The more times during the day that you can repeat this gentle easing in the right direction, the better, but make it twice a day at least. Use the essential oils suggested below. Whether using one essential oil or a combination, use no more than 5 drops diluted in 2 tablespoons (30 mL) of carrier oil, and use a small amount each time.

ESSENTIAL OILS FOR CLUB FOOT
Lavender (*Lavandula angustifolia*)
Chamomile roman (*Anthemis nobilis*)
Chamomile german (*Matricaria recutita*)
Mandarin (*Citrus reticulata*)

The following soothing blend is not intended to treat or help correct the foot, or feet, but to create a sense of calm while the feet are being massaged:

SOOTHING BLEND FOR CLUB FOOT
Lavender	3 drops
Chamomile roman	3 drops
Mandarin	5 drops

Dilute these amounts in 2 tablespoons (30 mL) of carrier oil, and use a small amount each time.

AUTISM SPECTRUM DISORDER (ASD)

Rates of autism are on the rise. According to the Centers for Disease Control and Prevention, during the 10 years between 1997 and 2008, the incidence of autism had increased in the United States by 289.5% over the previous 11 years. Even between 2002 and 2008 it had increased by 78%. Some of the increase is no doubt due to improved awareness and diagnostic methods. But everyone can see that autism has become more prevalent just from looking around at the people they know, and the increase is happening elsewhere in the world too.

Autism is a condition that's attracting much attention. Research is looking at genetic factors, particularly epigenetics — the way genes are expressed. Something happens to damage the genes contributed by the mother and father at one of several stages: when the gamete cells — the ovum and sperm — are still in separate parental bodies; when they meet and conception occurs, and there's cell division; later, as the baby develops inside the womb; or as the child grows up. Somewhere along this line a genetic change has taken place.

Certain chromosomes and genes have been identified as problematic areas, and researchers now speak of autism as being related to "spontaneous gene glitches," "epi-mutations," "epigenetic silencing," and "de novo events." This work is in its infancy and may at some point lead to treatments, but it doesn't tell us how the glitch happened in the first place, or how to prevent it happening again.

Environmental factors may involve sperm and the genetic translation process, and some people are suggesting that the prevalence of mobile phones, especially those kept in the father's pocket, close to sperm, are changing the DNA of the male gamete before it even gets to the ovum. This is just one of many controversial ideas linking autism to environmental factors, whether to babies' development in utero or to children as they grow. These are important issues being investigated within the relatively new field of study known as *behavioral epigenetics*, which may lead to practical answers in time.

Meanwhile, it's apparently no longer sufficient for parents to worry about their children once they are born; we now also need to consider what dangers they face before conception and in utero from a variety of risks, including those from the polluted environment our society has created. And that includes air pollution, food pollution, packaging pollution, water pollution, and electromagnetic frequencies in the air pollution. Whew! All this adds to the stress of being a parent, which is stressful enough as it is!

Autistic spectrum disorder is a term that encompasses a wide range of individual behavioral patterns that fall into the general diagnosis of autism. Essential oils can provide a variety of options for managing these behaviors, alongside other approaches including diet, exercise, dance, art, and music. For example, the essential oils can be used in massage, but if a child resists the close bond of a loving touch essential oils can still be used in baths — diluted in a little carrier oil — and showers and in all the usual room diffusion methods. This range of options is further amplified by the sheer number of essential oils that exist, which themselves have a variety of useful purposes. For example, in the lists that follow, you can see that grapefruit can be used when a child is non-responsive, and also when they're angry. The skill in using essential oils is recognizing which particular oils a person — either yourself, your child, or a child you care for — responds to. We're all individuals with aroma preferences, and children with autism are no exception. Many aromatic options exist, and because essential oils stimulate

the sense of smell and open up deep emotional pathways, they open doors that might otherwise remain closed.

Smells drift through air, so however distant two people may be in a room they're emotionally linked by that aroma. As you place essential oils in your child's bathwater, you're linked on a deep emotional level. There is an unspoken communication, a message silently drifting on the aromatic highway that says, "I love you and care for you." Nothing may be said, there may be no eye contact, but the message has been delivered.

This is the delight of essential oils, and it highlights an important point. Essential oils need to be reserved for the positive, so they can reinforce that positivity later. By contrast, if you were to use a particular essential oil when you were angry, your child would associate that aroma with anger and bad times. Clearly, when laying down your child's aromatic memories, you want to ensure that they're good memories.

Some of the essential oil aromas are food-based — extracted from foods human beings have been eating and enjoying for millennia. Think of the spices cardamom and coriander, or the fruits orange and lemon. These are enticing essential oils because they tap into our deepest survival mechanisms of hunger and sustenance. Some of these food-derived essential oils can be incorporated into air-freshening sprays and so provide a homeliness that engenders peace and reassurance. An aromatic communication is being built that is designed, on the most subtle of emotional levels, to bring confidence to your child.

The following essential oils can be used in massage oils, in baths and showers, and in all the usual room diffusion methods, or simply inhaled from a tissue whenever needed. The lists below are arranged for a variety of circumstances or needs a child may be experiencing, so choose from the list that most reflects your child's behavior at any particular time. Choose a single oil, make your own blend from the lists, or refer to my general blends suggested below.

Soothing Essential Oils

Chamomile roman (*Anthemis nobilis*)
Lavender (*Lavandula angustifolia*)
Petitgrain (*Citrus aurantium*)
Ylang ylang (*Cananga odorata*)
Bergamot (*Citrus bergamia*)
Rosewood (*Aniba rosaeodora*)
Sandalwood (*Santalum album*)
Cedarwood atlas (*Cedrus atlantica*)
Marjoram, sweet (*Origanum majorana*)
Neroli (*Citrus aurantium*)

Essential Oils for Insomnia

Lavender (*Lavandula angustifolia*)
Orange, sweet (*Citrus sinensis*)
Neroli (*Citrus aurantium*)
Sandalwood (*Santalum album*)

Essential Oils for Restlessness

Geranium (*Pelargonium graveolens*)
Lavender (*Lavandula angustifolia*)
Chamomile roman (*Anthemis nobilis*)
Petitgrain (*Citrus aurantium*)
Orange, sweet (*Citrus sinensis*)
Sandalwood (*Santalum album*)

Essential Oils for Agitation

Clary sage (*Salvia sclarea*)
Ylang ylang (*Cananga odorata*)
Grapefruit (*Citrus paradisi*)
Lavender (*Lavandula angustifolia*)
Chamomile roman (*Anthemis nobilis*)
Spikenard (*Nardostachys jatamansi*)
Geranium (*Pelargonium graveolens*)
Vetiver (*Vetiveria zizanoides*)
Marjoram, sweet (*Origanum majorana*)
Benzoin (*Styrax benzoin*)
Bergamot FCF (*Citrus bergamia*)
Cistus (*Cistus ladaniferus*)

Essential Oils for Nonresponsiveness

Frankincense (*Boswellia carterii*)
Pine (*Pinus sylvestris*)
Cedarwood atlas (*Cedrus atlantica*)
Rosemary (*Rosmarinus officinalis*)
Spearmint (*Mentha spicata*)
Jasmine (*Jasminum grandiflorum / officinale*)
Lemon (*Citrus limon*)
Grapefruit (*Citrus paradisi*)
Eucalyptus lemon (*Eucalyptus citriodora*)

Essential Oils for Anger

Rose otto (*Rosa damascena*)
Frankincense (*Boswellia carterii*)
Spikenard (*Nardostachys jatamansi*)
Vetiver (*Vetiveria zizanoides*)
Lemon (*Citrus limon*)
Orange, sweet (*Citrus sinensis*)
Marjoram, sweet (*Origanum majorana*)
Cistus (*Cistus ladaniferus*)
Grapefruit (*Citrus paradisi*)

When contemplating using massage on your child, the time spent should depend on how much or how little your child will allow. Introduce the experience of massage slowly by just massaging a hand or an arm for a couple of minutes. Gradually extend the time to three minutes, then four, eventually massaging both hands, or arms, or feet. Aim to eventually, over time, reach the stage when your child will welcome an upper-back massage, even a whole-back massage. Play the long game: be patient, don't push, and allow your child to come themselves to a place of acceptance.

A gentle back massage given before bedtime, after a warm bath, can help a child sleep well. Start by gently placing the flat of each hand on either side of the vertebrae around the lumbar region of the back. Glide your hands upward toward the shoulders, and then down the sides of the body. Repeat this movement several times. Repetitive movements such as this are the most useful for children with autism. Then continue to massage over the back using gentle, slow movements. The massage should last around 5–10 minutes, or until your child becomes sleepy.

SLEEPY TIME MASSAGE OIL

| Lavender | 4 drops |
| Mandarin | 3 drops |

Dilute in 1 tablespoon (15 mL) of carrier oil. This amount will be enough for several massages, depending on the age and size of your child.

Sometimes a child with autism can be hard to rouse into action, and the following blend can be used to stimulate a child, either first thing in the morning or during the day. If your child resists massage, or you just don't have the time, use the blend in one of the room methods.

STIMULATING BLEND

Rosemary	2 drops
Spearmint	2 drops
Grapefruit	4 drops

For a massage, blend the essential oils together and then dilute 2–3 drops in each teaspoon (5 mL) of carrier oil. If using in a room diffusion method, use 4 drops of the undiluted blend.

If your child is anxious or even fearful, the following massage oil may help. If they are familiar with the experience of massage and you can apply some of the blend to their back, all to the good. If not, massage their feet, hands, or arms.

BLEND TO ALLAY ANXIETY AND FEAR

Bergamot FCF	7 drops
Geranium	3 drops
Clary sage	4 drops

Blend the essential oils together and dilute 2–3 drops in each teaspoon (5 mL) of carrier oil. If using in a room diffusion method, use 4 drops of the undiluted blend.

Diet

Food intolerances are known to play a part in a child's disruptive behavior. Changing to fresh and organically produced food will reduce exposure to artificial colorants, preservatives, and artificial sweeteners. Adding a children's combined prebiotic and probiotic supplement assists in regulating the gut and digestion, and an omega 3 fatty acid supplement contributes to good overall health.

Exercise and Dance

Exercise has been shown to be highly beneficial to children with autism, perhaps because it grounds energy, releases endorphins, and may balance the hormones. The benefits are many, and finding a physical activity children enjoy will take some exploring but is worth the effort. Some sports involve a group of people and may not be appropriate, but running suits everyone and would be good for Mom and Dad too!

Music and Art

Playing a musical instrument can be an individual activity, but it also allows the possibility of becoming a valued member of a larger group of players. Music provides a potential door to friendship, so for a child with autism it is particularly valuable. Encourage your child to find an instrument that suits them.

Art facilitates creative expression and can provide an emotional outlet for any child. It is, then, valuable to provide a range of art materials because self-expression is crucial for all children, autistic children included.

ATTENTION DEFICIT HYPERACTIVITY DISORDER (ADHD AND ADD)

Just about every reason under the sun has been put forward for the apparent increase in ADHD and ADD over recent years. It's accepted that there are problems with the dopamine and serotonin pathways in the brain, but the question is, what caused them? All the usual culprits, from genetics to environmental factors, are lined up against the wall looking guilty, but that doesn't really help the child who has been branded "naughty" when in reality their body and brain chemicals are in imbalance.

Essential oils can be used in many ways for children with ADHD and ADD. One effective use of essential oils is to apply them to the soles of the feet. The feet have a vast complex of reflex points that are, in a sense, a mirror of internal function. A reflexologist ascertains a great deal about an individual simply from the reflexes on the feet. When using essential oils on the feet in this way, there is no accompanying massage or manipulation — just the application of undiluted essential oils. The oils can be used either individually or in blends, and only 1 single drop is required. Take 1 drop of essential oil between two fingers and rub the fingers together before applying directly on the sole of the foot.

Alternatively, the essential oil can be put on a small piece of tissue and rubbed over the sole of the foot or placed inside the sock or shoe. This is not an everyday thing, but the method can be used when you're aware of a situation brewing that may cause your child to feel anxious, stressful, or even fearful. Vetiver essential oil can be used in this method and is an oil that's long been used by therapists to alleviate stress and anxiety. On the morning of a potentially stressful event, apply 1 drop of vetiver diluted in 2 drops of carrier oil to the soles of the feet to help manage the anxiety and stress of the event. If you prefer, substitute with a drop of another appropriate essential oil or blend.

At home, essential oils can be used in all the usual room diffuser methods. And when your child is going out, a simple option is to put the essential oil on a tissue and place it in their pocket for them to sniff from when they feel they're getting stressed or nervous.

Another method that's been found useful for children with ADHD or ADD is a warm bath at bedtime. As well as using essential oil, diluted in a little carrier oil first, add to the bath a mixture of ¼ cup of Epsom salts and ¼ cup of baking soda. Also have a look at the "Autism Spectrum Disorder" section on page 183 because there may be essential oil categories or blends appropriate to your child, which can also be used in baths or massages.

When it comes to touch or massage, your child may at first be reluctant, so start with a simple hand or foot massage, then work toward arm and leg massage, eventually progressing to massaging the back. See the advice in "Autism Spectrum Disorder." Although the two conditions are almost diametrically opposed — children with autism are generally withdrawn while children with ADHD or ADD are anything but withdrawn — in both cases it can be difficult to entice a child into receiving touch. Look at the essential oil lists and blends in the "Autism Spectrum Disorder" section above, and adjust them according to your own child's behavior pattern.

Choose individual essential oils from the lists below, make your own blends, or use the blends below that seem most appropriate for your child's behavior at any particular time. All can be incorporated into room diffusion blends.

For baths: First blend the essential oils together. Unless otherwise directed, for baths dilute 2–3 drops in a little carrier oil or other medium before adding to the bathwater, swishing it around to disperse any globules on the surface.

For massage: First blend the essential oils together. Unless otherwise directed, for a massage oil dilute 2–3 drops of essential oil to each teaspoon (5 mL) of carrier oil, using only as much as you need depending on the age and size of your child.

ESSENTIAL OILS FOR SLEEPING DIFFICULTIES

Rosewood (*Aniba rosaeodora*)
Valerian (*Valeriana officinalis*)
Lavender (*Lavandula angustifolia*)
Orange, sweet (*Citrus sinensis*)
Petitgrain (*Citrus aurantium*)
Mandarin (*Citrus reticulata*)
Sandalwood (*Santalum album*)
Clary sage (*Salvia sclarea*)
Chamomile roman (*Anthemis nobilis*)
Neroli (*Citrus aurantium*)

SLEEPING BLEND 1

Lavender	8 drops
Valerian	1 drop
Petitgrain	5 drops

First blend the essential oils together. For baths: dilute 2–3 drops in a little carrier oil before adding to the bathwater. For massage oil: dilute 2–3 drops to each teaspoon (5 mL) of carrier oil, and use a small amount each time.

SLEEPING BLEND 2

Lavender	5 drops
Chamomile roman	3 drops
Orange, sweet	5 drops

First blend the essential oils together. For baths: dilute 2–3 drops in a little carrier oil before adding to the bathwater. For massage oil: dilute 2–3 drops in each teaspoon (5 mL) of carrier oil, and use a small amount each time.

ESSENTIAL OILS FOR FOCUS, CONCENTRATION, AND MEMORY

Cedarwood atlas (*Cedrus atlantica*)
Lemon (*Citrus limon*)
Eucalyptus lemon (*Eucalyptus citriodora*)
Patchouli (*Pogostemon cablin*)
Frankincense (*Boswellia carterii*)
Petitgrain (*Citrus aurantium*)
Rosemary (*Rosmarinus officinalis*)

Basil linalol (*Ocimum basilicum ct. linalool*)
Chamomile maroc (*Ormenis multicaulis*)

CONCENTRATION AND MEMORY BLEND

Rosemary	3 drops
Lemon	8 drops
Cedarwood atlas	6 drops

First blend the essential oils together. For baths: dilute 2–3 drops in a little carrier oil before adding to the bathwater. For massage oil: dilute 2–3 drops to each teaspoon (5 mL) of carrier oil, and use a small amount each time.

STRESS AND FOCUS BLEND

Vetiver	7 drops
Bergamot	8 drops
Ylang ylang	3 drops

First blend the essential oils together. For baths: dilute 2–3 drops in a little carrier oil before adding to the bathwater. For massage oil: dilute 1–2 drops in each teaspoon (5 mL) of carrier oil, and use a small amount each time.

ESSENTIAL OILS FOR ANGER AND FRUSTRATION

Lavender (*Lavandula angustifolia*)
Spikenard (*Nardostachys jatamansi*)
Vetiver (*Vetiveria zizanoides*)
Bergamot FCF (*Citrus bergamia*)
Marjoram, sweet (*Origanum majorana*)
Rose otto (*Rosa damascena*)
Ylang ylang (*Cananga odorata*)
Cistus (*Cistus ladaniferus*)
Chamomile maroc (*Ormenis multicaulis*)
Frankincense (*Boswellia carterii*)

ANGER BLEND

Vetiver	8 drops
Bergamot	6 drops
Cistus	3 drops

First blend the essential oils together. For baths: dilute 1–2 drops in a little carrier oil before adding to the bathwater. For massage oil: dilute 1–2 drops in each teaspoon (5 mL) of carrier oil, and use a small amount each time.

Essential Oils for Moodiness
Bergamot FCF (*Citrus bergamia*)
Clary sage (*Salvia sclarea*)
Geranium (*Pelargonium graveolens*)
Lavender (*Lavandula angustifolia*)
Marjoram, sweet (*Origanum majorana*)
Sandalwood (*Santalum album*)
May chang (*Litsea cubeba*)
Frankincense (*Boswellia carterii*)
Benzoin (*Styrax benzoin*)

Moodiness Blend
Geranium	6 drops
Bergamot	7 drops
Lavender	3 drops

First blend the essential oils together. For baths: dilute 2–3 drops in a little carrier oil before adding to the bathwater. For massage oil: dilute 2–3 drops in each teaspoon (5 mL) of carrier oil, and use a small amount each time.

Essential Oils for Anxiety
Spearmint (*Mentha spicata*)
Coriander seed (*Coriandrum sativum*)
Frankincense (*Boswellia carterii*)
Lavender (*Lavandula angustifolia*)
Lemon (*Citrus limon*)
Mandarin (*Citrus reticulata*)
Jasmine (*Jasminum grandiflorum / officinale*)
Sandalwood (*Santalum album*)
Geranium (*Pelargonium graveolens*)
Orange, sweet (*Citrus sinensis*)
Benzoin (*Styrax benzoin*)

Anxiety Blend
Frankincense	3 drops
Sandalwood	8 drops
Mandarin	5 drops

First blend the essential oils together. For baths: dilute 2–3 drops in a little carrier oil before adding to the bathwater. For massage oil: dilute 2–3 drops in each teaspoon (5 mL) of carrier oil, and use a small amount each time.

8

A Woman's Natural Choice

The pressure is on. Women today have pressure on all sides. We're told we have to look fabulous at every stage of life, make a good living in the mean working environment, and maintain a welcoming home. While doing all this, we may be trying to maintain a primary relationship with someone who wants to follow a path going in quite another direction, or location, than our own. If children come along, well, then there's more pressure. The acrobat juggling balls at the circus has nothing on the modern woman, because aside from jumping through hoops and juggling, she's entreated to "find her true self," "find her true calling in life," "follow her dreams," or "express herself." For many women, that self-expression might well be portrayed by the series of four artworks by Norwegian artist Edvard Munch of a woman on a bridge, known collectively as *The Scream*.

The problem with pressure is that it leads to stress, and the problem with stress is that it causes havoc to the mind and to the body, including hormone disruption and autoimmune dysfunction. Stress is a huge subject, and more is to be found in chapter 4, "Occupational Oils for the Working Man and Woman," and in chapter 5, "Emotional Rescue." Because pressure and stress have such far-reaching ramifications, we begin this chapter with a section called "Pressure to Be Perfect." That is followed by sections on breast care; cystitis; ovarian cysts; polycystic ovary syndrome; uterine prolapse; varicose veins; Raynaud's disease; menstrual problems; menopause; pelvic pain, including pelvic venous congestion syndrome (PVCS) and endometriosis; candida; vaginal infections; infertility; miscarriage and preterm delivery; pregnancy; preparing for the birth; and postnatal care, including postnatal depression.

Pressure to Be Perfect

It's a truism that "a woman's work is never done" because most women not only work outside the home to some extent, but when they get home another round of chores is waiting for them. Every tedious aspect of life faced by men — the commute, workplace-related stress, and the commute home — is also faced by women, who additionally, most often, feel responsible for cooking dinner and making sure the laundry is done. Women are thought by society to be the most appropriate primary caregivers, not only for children but for elderly relatives too. This simple picture of the daily division of labor may not be the experience of all women, but it's certainly the experience of many, and some women are operating on low-level anger and exhaustion much of the time. On top of this, women have an additional issue in their daily lives — fear. As well as the fear of being made redundant and the financial consequences that might bring, the number of women who experience domestic violence or psychological control is astonishing in this day and age. The fear of rape is another stress women live with, and although it may not be expressed, it underlies where we feel we can or cannot physically go to maintain personal safety. There is, then, a great deal going on inside the mind of a woman, and whatever the complex of pressures felt, essential oils can have a very helpful effect in managing these stress levels.

ESSENTIAL OILS TO MANAGE FEMALE STRESS

Basil linalol (*Ocimum basilicum ct. linalool*)
Orange, sweet (*Citrus sinensis*)
Geranium (*Pelargonium graveolens*)
Bergamot (*Citrus bergamia*)
Palmarosa (*Cymbopogon martini*)
Marjoram, sweet (*Origanum majorana*)
Petitgrain (*Citrus aurantium*)
Sandalwood (*Santalum album*)
Cardamom (*Elettaria cardamomum*)
Lemon (*Citrus limon*)
Ylang ylang (*Cananga odorata*)
Nutmeg (*Myristica fragrans*)
Rose otto (*Rosa damascena*)
Rose maroc (*Rosa centifolia*)
Chamomile roman (*Anthemis nobilis*)
Neroli (*Citrus aurantium*)
Jasmine (*Jasminum grandiflorum/officinale*)
Valerian (*Valeriana officinalis*)
Frankincense (*Boswellia carterii*)
Vetiver (*Vetiveria zizanoides*)
Melissa (*Melissa officinalis*)
Lavender (*Lavandula angustifolia*)
Tangerine (*Citrus reticulata*)
Cedarwood atlas (*Cedrus atlantica*)
Clary sage (*Salvia sclarea*)
Grapefruit (*Citrus paradisi*)

During the day, when there is so much to be done, it's best not to choose essential oils that you might routinely use in the evening to relax. Try to make a distinction between those that might be used during meditation, prayer, or relaxation in the evening and those to use during the day while out and about or trying to concentrate at work. Refer to the "Quick Reference Chart" in chapter 20 (see table 22, page 534) to help you decide which might be appropriate at particular times.

Aromas can become associated with a particular action, and so even though an aroma might be liked for one purpose, that same association can interfere if the oil is then used for a quite different purpose. Although the essential oils can be used singly, unique blends have the advantage of having no other associations. Use 1 neat drop on a tissue, as needed, or inhale directly from a small bottle. If it's practical to use a diffusing method, follow the general guidelines in "Methods of Use" in chapter 1 (see page 13).

STRESS DAYTIME BLEND

Lemon	15 drops
Grapefruit	5 drops
Geranium	3 drops
Vetiver	1 drop

STRESS EVENING BLEND

Orange, sweet	15 drops
Petitgrain	6 drops
Valerian	1 drop

Breast Care

It sometimes seems that the world is obsessed with breasts. Men pay to look at them, while women worry theirs are too small, too big, unequal in size, or wrongly shaped. We might forget that breasts were designed to provide nourishment to babies, rather than for the adoration of grown-ups. Nevertheless, we know the value of breasts, and many women spend money and effort in finding pretty lace bras and revealing tops that show them off. Many women of course are not satisfied with their breasts and turn to surgery. The vast industry focused in one way or another on breasts can take our attention away from the simple measure that really is important — routinely feeling the breasts for any lumps, bumps, or changes that indicate something is wrong.

There's been quite a controversy over the use of antiperspirants containing aluminum salts and the potential risk of breast cancer. The correlation between the two is unproven, yet the salts have been shown to accumulate in the breast tissue of some women, especially close to the underarms. There's no advantage in having aluminum in the body, but cleanliness is important. How, then, to get through the day smelling nice and clean, while still allowing the body to sweat and rid itself of toxins? The answer in this is a combination of things. First, switch to natural antiperspirants and deodorants that don't contain aluminum salts or, for that matter, parabens or synthetic fragrances, and also wash under the arms with soap and water as often as you can — certainly at night so the pores in the underarm area have a chance to breathe and function as they were designed to do.

Using exercise to keep breasts pert without resorting to surgery takes persistence. Grip your hands together, or hold both wrists, and exercise the pectoral muscles by pushing the arms together so they come up against the invisible force created by your arm pushing in the opposite direction. You should feel the muscles move.

If you plan to have a surgical procedure carried out on the breasts, for example for the removal of a nonmalignant cyst or for cosmetic reasons, it may help to prepare the skin beforehand so it is supple and responsive and heals well.

RESTORATIVE SKIN OIL

Palmarosa	5 drops
Geranium	5 drops
Carrot seed	3 drops
Clary sage	3 drops
Immortelle	7 drops
Lemon	5 drops

First, blend the essential oils together to create a synergetic blend. Then, dilute this in the following two carrier oils:

Camellia seed	4 teaspoons (20 mL)
Rosehip seed	2 teaspoons (10 mL)

Using a small amount of this diluted blend, once a day gently apply over the whole of the breast area in circular movements, avoiding the nipples.

SORE BREASTS

The following blend can be used after surgery and also by those women who routinely suffer from sore breasts for no apparent medical reason. Some women are just sensitive in this area. Also, some women find that their breasts are sore at a particular time in their menstrual cycle.

SORE BREASTS SOOTHING OIL

Chamomile german	5 drops
Geranium	5 drops
Niaouli	5 drops
Lavender	10 drops

First, blend the essential oils together and then dilute in the following two carrier oils:

Calendula (macerated)	2 teaspoons (10 mL)
Camellia seed	4 teaspoons (20 mL)

Using a small amount of this diluted blend, once a day gently apply over the whole of the breast area in circular movements, avoiding the nipples.

BREAST ABSCESS

Breast abscesses can develop if inflammation has been allowed to progress from a bacterial infection, leading to a collection of pus. Women who are lactating should refer to the "Breast Abscess" and "Mastitis" sections on pages 236 and 237. There are two treatments here that can be used either on their own or together. This is the blend of essential oils for the first:

Breast Abscess Blend 1

Fragonia	5 drops
Ravintsara	10 drops
Lavender	10 drops
Chamomile roman	5 drops

Blend the essential oils together using these proportions. Then make a compress by adding 10 drops of the blend to a bowl of warm water, soaking a small piece of material in the bowl, and applying it to the affected area once a day.

A gel can be prepared and stored in the fridge, ready for when required. Thoroughly mix together 1 fl. oz. (30 mL) of aloe vera gel and 1 teaspoon (5 mL) of calendula macerated oil. To this, add 30 drops of the essential oil blend above. Use a small amount, enough to cover the area of the abscess, once a day.

Breast Abscess Blend 2

Palmarosa	2 drops
Tea tree	8 drops
Lavender	10 drops
Chamomile roman	8 drops
Thyme linalol	2 drops

For the second option, mix together the essential oils above. Then dilute 4–5 drops in a teaspoon (5 mL) of sweet almond carrier oil, and apply as required, avoiding the nipples.

FIBROCYSTIC BREAST CONDITIONS

Cystic breasts usually feel lumpy and cause discomfort in either one or both breasts. This is caused by small noncancerous tissue, benign masses, nodules, or small cysts in the breasts. They are often referred to as "lumpy breasts." If these are aspirated by a medical professional, a drop of neat lavender essential oil applied directly to the area will help with the healing and also help avoid infection.

Compresses applied to the breasts can help reduce the pain. This is very personal to each individual woman, with some responding well to ice-cold compresses while others prefer warm. A good supporting bra is essential. This is one of those conditions that respond well to positive changes in the diet. This should involve limiting the amount of fat in the diet and adopting a vegetarian diet for at least two days each week. Probiotics will assist the working of the gut, while milk thistle will help the liver perform well. Try to avoid all caffeine, including black tea, coffee, and sodas, and opt instead for fruit drinks, bottled water, and herb teas, including dandelion. Supplements that may be helpful include iodine and evening primrose, vitamins B6 and E, and the omega 3 essential fatty acids.

Fibrocystic Breast Blend

Lavender	10 drops
Cypress	5 drops
Chamomile roman	15 drops

Blend the essential oils together, then dilute 5 drops to each teaspoon (5 mL) of carrier oil. Gently apply over the breasts daily, avoiding the nipples. Castor oil is sometimes used as the carrier oil to some effect for this condition.

Cystitis

Cystitis is the inflammation of the bladder and, sometimes, its outlet to the urethra. It is extremely painful and troublesome, and although it is mainly suffered by women, men and children can also get cystitis. The main symptom is feeling the need to pass urine, often necessitating getting up many times during the night, only to find that there is little urine to pass and even passing that small amount can be irritating. Cystitis is usually caused by bacterial infection and sometimes by minor bruising of the urethral tube and bladder during sexual intercourse (often called "honeymoon" cystitis for obvious reasons). In older women this can often be avoided by having adequate lubrication. Try a natural lubricant such as organic coconut oil. Treatment of the bacterial form should be prompt to ensure that infection doesn't spread to the kidneys.

The bacteria that cause cystitis can become resistant to antibiotics, elevating an acute case into a chronic one. It is very important to drink a lot of water; also drink pure cranberry juice (or take a freeze-dried cranberry supplement) or aloe vera juice. Avoid coffee and alcohol. A supplement containing vitamin C and zinc may help. D-mannose, derived from the flowering ash tree, is also said to help; however, side effects can include loose stools, and it's not advised for those with diabetes.

CYSTITIS ESSENTIAL OILS
Rosemary (*Rosmarinus officinalis*)
Juniper berry (*Juniperus communis*)
Thyme linalol (*Thymus vulgaris ct. linalool*)
Cajuput (*Melaleuca cajuputi*)
Lavender (*Lavandula angustifolia*)
Oregano (*Origanum vulgare*)
Niaouli (*Melaleuca quinquenervia*)
Cypress (*Cupressus sempervirens*)
Marjoram, sweet (*Origanum majorana*)

Coriander seed (*Coriandrum sativum*)
Eucalyptus radiata (*Eucalyptus radiata*)
Rosewood (*Aniba rosaeodora*)
Chamomile german (*Matricaria recutita*)
Palmarosa (*Cymbopogon martinii*)

You could make up your own blend for a body oil from the list above or use one of the body oil blends below. The quantities of essential oil should be diluted in 2 tablespoons (30 mL) of carrier oil. Use a small amount each time. Apply daily, rubbing the oil over your lower abdomen, hips, and upper and lower back.

BODY OIL BLENDS FOR CYSTITIS

BLEND 1
Lavender	10 drops
Juniper berry	5 drops
Chamomile german	5 drops
Cypress	5 drops
Thyme linalol	5 drops

BLEND 2
Palmarosa	5 drops
Coriander seed	5 drops
Niaouli	15 drops
Ho wood	5 drops

The following four blends can be used either in compresses or in sitz baths. For compresses, use 5 drops per application and apply two compresses at a time — one above the pubic bone at the front, and one across the lower back. One drop of the essential oil blend of your choice can be placed directly on the skin before applying the compresses.

An essential oil sitz bath is particularly effective in easing cystitis. Run a bath to hip level, add into the water 1 tablespoon of bicarbonate of soda, and sit. You can also use a bidet or a large bowl. Use no more than 5 drops of essential oil per bath, diluted in a little carrier oil; the quantities in the blends are for two sitz baths. One drop of the essential oil blend of your choice could be placed directly on the skin, at the front above the pubic bone, and on the lower back, before getting in the sitz bath. Use these methods for between 7 and 14 days.

SITZ BATH BLENDS FOR CYSTITIS

BLEND 1
Eucalyptus radiata	5 drops
Niaouli	5 drops

BLEND 2
Ho wood	5 drops
Chamomile german	5 drops

BLEND 3
Lavender	5 drops
Marjoram, sweet	5 drops

BLEND 4
Coriander seed	4 drops
Palmarosa	6 drops

You can use any of the methods above on their own, or use the body oil method together with either the compress or sitz bath method, depending on the time available to you and the degree of your complaint.

Ovarian Cysts

There are many conditions that cause cysts to develop on the ovary. For example, endometriosis can cause cysts to grow around the ovary, dermoid cysts develop from cells that produce the ovum, the multiple cysts of polycystic ovarian syndrome can gather on the surface of an ovary, and cystadenoma cysts are a form of tumor, usually benign.

The ovaries are two small organs on either side of the womb that hold within them from the girl baby's birth all the ova she will have during her life. Each month, from one or the other ovary, a follicle is released, inside of which is an ovum. The follicle is like a protective shell for the ovum. Once the ovum breaks out of its follicle, it makes its way to a fallopian tube, where it will meet the sperm, if the sperm is there. This process goes on every month, usually without much difficulty. In a well-functioning ovary, the sex hormones estrogen and progesterone are released in a timely manner throughout the cycle, and in good balance.

Ovarian cysts can develop in two ways. If the follicle does not break and release the ovum, it can continue growing as what is called a *follicular cyst*. When a follicle does release the ovum, it transforms into what is known as the *corpus luteum*. But if the break in the follicle where the ovum came out seals itself closed, fluid can accumulate inside, causing a *corpus luteum cyst*. Some cysts are "functional" and tend to disappear of their own accord over time, and some are "pathological" and develop from abnormal cell growth. Essentially, ovarian cysts are fluid-filled sacs that can vary in size from very small to the size of a grapefruit.

Ovarian cysts most often cause no symptoms and go unnoticed until they grow and cause discomfort and pain. They're discovered during an ultrasound, or through a laparoscopy — procedures often carried out to find out why the woman is having fertility issues.

The problem with cysts is that they can rupture and cause scar tissue or adhesions, causing the ovary to attach to various internal tissues. If cysts grow to a large size they can get in the way of the proper working of the reproductive system, including causing a twist in the fallopian tube. Large cysts are often aspirated with keyhole surgery, in which the fluid contents of the cyst are removed.

Because ovarian cysts do not usually, of themselves, cause pain, it's wise to be aware of symptoms that could indicate the presence of a cyst. These include discomfort during intercourse, swelling of the abdomen, pelvic pain, spotting or unusual bleeding, pain while passing stools, frequent urination, fatigue, pain around menstruation, and sudden pangs of pain that could indicate the cyst has ruptured or that it has damaged the ovary in some way.

As with most other medical problems, food plays a big part in the healing of ovarian cysts. Change to an organic whole-food diet, cutting out all refined and processed foods. Cut from your diet all GM foods, white wheat-flour products, and all dairy products including cheese, butter, milk, and milk proteins. Cut out all sugars including corn syrups, maple syrups, and honey products. Avoid red and processed meats, and instead choose fish and organic chicken. Avoid alcohol, smoking, and foods preserved in plastics. And don't use the microwave.

Eat plenty of organic vegetables, especially dark-green ones — cabbages, brussels sprouts, and broccoli. Also good are organic red-colored fruits and vegetables, pulses, nuts, seeds, and as many raw vegetables as possible. Plants should make up the majority of your daily food intake. You can eat fatty fish such as sardines, herring, and wild salmon.

Give your digestion a rest by having one fast day a week, when you only drink organic vegetable juices and spring or distilled water. If you have a juicer and can face it, have an entire week on juices only — making your own from vegetables and fruit. Stress reduction is imperative, and the release of the stress hormone cortisol might just be one of the things responsible for the formation of cysts in the first place.

Take the herbal remedies tribulus (*Tribulus terrestris*), milk thistle (*Silybum marianum*), wild yam root (*Dioscrea villosa*), yarrow (*Achillea millefolium*), maca root (*Lepidium meyenii*), a probiotic, and a vitamin supplement containing all the trace minerals needed by the body.

ESSENTIAL OILS FOR OVARIAN CYSTS
Geranium (*Pelargonium graveolens*)
Cypress (*Cupressus sempervirens*)
Juniper berry (*Juniperus communis*)
Rosemary (*Rosmarinus officinalis*)
Melissa (*Melissa officinalis*)
Cedarwood atlas (*Cedrus atlantica*)
Petitgrain (*Citrus aurantium*)
Lemon (*Citrus limon*)
Rose otto (*Rosa damascena*)
Sandalwood (*Santalum album*)
Immortelle (*Helichrysum italicum*)
Basil linalol (*Ocimum basilicum ct. linalool*)
Patchouli (*Pogostemon cablin*)
Chamomile roman (*Anthemis nobilis*)
Ho wood (*Cinnamomum camphora ct. linalool*)

Compresses can be used to ease any discomfort. Use a large piece of cloth, such as unbleached muslin. Prepare a bowl of hot water to which you have added 4 drops of geranium, 3 drops of patchouli, 3 drops of cypress, and 4 drops of juniper berry essential oil. Lower the material into the water, absorbing the essential oil and water, and place the wet, warm compress over the lower abdomen for 10–15 minutes. Do this once a day for a week, take a week off, and repeat the cycle.

OVARIAN CYST BLEND

Cypress	10 drops
Geranium	20 drops
Basil linalol	5 drops
Juniper berry	7 drops

Add these amounts to 2 tablespoons (30 mL) of carrier oil. Apply a small amount over the abdominal area, from under the breasts to the lower abdomen, and over the lower back — the lumbar region — into the crease of the buttocks but no further.

In addition, geranium oil has been successfully used undiluted over the affected side prior to using the body oil — use 2 drops of geranium oil twice a day for 10 days. Then just use the body oil for 10 days; then repeat with the geranium and body oil for a further 10 days. Continue during the menstrual cycle.

Polycystic Ovary Syndrome (PCOS)

Polycystic ovary syndrome, the most common hormonal condition affecting women of childbearing age, can affect one or both ovaries, appearing as a collection of small cysts on the surface of the ovary, which is often larger than normal. The follicles, which are supposed to release the ovum within them, remain immature, preventing the ovum from escaping and being fertilized. Some women with polycystic ovary syndrome rarely ovulate or release an ovum. However, many women with polycystic ovaries can and do conceive.

One of the symptoms of PCOS is irregular menstrual cycles, and this in itself can make conception difficult as the woman can't judge when she'll be ovulating. Some women have no symptoms at all, while others might experience acne, excessive body hair, mood disorders, mid-cycle bleeding, absent periods, irregular menstrual cycles, heavy menstrual bleeding, and miscarriage.

Although obesity and excessive weight are often associated with PCOS, many women with the condition are slim and otherwise healthy. Anyone suspected of having PCOS should have a series of hormone tests, including those for LH/FSH ratios, testosterone, and progesterone, as well as checks of glucose and cholesterol levels. The adrenal gland produces the hormone DHEA, as well as cortisol — which can be elevated due to stress.

Insulin resistance is thought to be a crucial factor in the development of PCOS, and genetic factors may also play a part. There are many interlocking factors involved in this condition, and a degree of investigation is helpful because it narrows down the approach that should be taken. In general, the aim is to lower androgens in the body and allow the body to process insulin more effectively. Hormonal homeostasis, or balance, is something that essential oils may help with, while regulating insulin can in some cases be accomplished by changes in diet. This is one of those conditions in which a change of diet can really make all the difference, so much so that everything eaten or drunk needs to be thought of as part of a medical campaign.

The first thing to cut out is all highly processed foods, especially refined white flour products, and bring in an organic, whole-food diet full of nuts, seeds, and pulses. Eat lots of fiber as well as plenty of fresh, nutritious vegetables and organic proteins. Cut out all sugar, sugary foods, corn oil, and soy oil, and eat only organically produced pure oils and fats. Try to avoid GM foods. Drink no alcohol, coffee, sodas, or tap water, and instead drink spring or distilled water.

If fertility appears to be a problem, then regulating the amount and times of your meals can be helpful — have a good breakfast, making it the largest meal of the day, a smaller lunch, and an even smaller evening meal. No snacking. Use herbal supplements such as chaste berry (*Vitex agnus castus*), saw palmetto (*Serenoa serrulata*), dong quai (*Angelica sinensis*), sage (*Salvia officinalis*), and black cohosh root (*Actaea racemosa*). And take supplements of chromium (particularly important), magnesium, vitamin D3, vitamin A, and vitamin C; a trace mineral supplement can also help.

PCOS ESSENTIAL OILS
Clary sage (*Salvia sclarea*)
Rose otto (*Rosa damascena*)

Geranium (*Pelargonium graveolens*)
Lavender, spike (*Lavandula latifolia*)
Sage, Greek (*Salvia fruticosa/triloba*)
Juniper berry (*Juniperus communis*)
Carrot seed (*Daucus carota*)
Chamomile roman (*Anthemis nobilis*)
Lavender (*Lavandula angustifolia*)
Myrtle (*Myrtus communis*)

For PCOS the following blend is recommended, diluted and gently rubbed over the abdomen once a day:

PCOS Blend

Clary sage	10 drops
Myrtle	10 drops
Geranium	7 drops
Rose otto	3 drops

PCOS Blend for Hormone Imbalance

Juniper berry	3 drops
Clary sage	5 drops
Geranium	10 drops
Cistus	4 drops
Lemon	8 drops
Carrot seed	4 drops

To make a body oil with either of the blends above, add the amount to 2 tablespoons (30 mL) of carrier oil. Apply a small amount over the abdominal area, from below the breast to the pelvic line, and around the lower back into the crease of the buttocks.

The blends can also be used in baths. Make up the chosen blend, using the proportions shown, and use 6 drops in baths.

Uterine Prolapse

Some women have no idea that they have uterine prolapse until they experience an odd feeling of something in the vagina and maybe also find they're leaking small amounts of urine when coughing. Age is one factor, as is repeated or difficult childbirth that has stretched the ligaments that hold the uterus in place, causing the uterus to displace and drop. In mild cases, no more than an unpleasant dragging sensation is experienced; in severe cases, the uterus may protrude out of the vagina. There are not usually any side effects except that pressure on the bladder sometimes causes slight incontinence.

Pelvic floor exercises that strengthen the muscles are helpful: stand with your legs about two and a half feet apart (or six inches more than is comfortable) and pull the muscles up from the vagina as if trying to stop yourself while urinating. Do this as many times as you can manage during the day, while washing dishes or cooking, for example. It need not take any time out of your day. You could also purchase a vaginal device that produces an electrical current that strengthens the same muscles for you, but as this is inserted into the vagina, its use requires privacy.

The following body oil may help alleviate the feelings of discomfort. Dilute the blend in 2 tablespoons (30 mL) of carrier oil, and use a small amount each time.

Rub over the lower abdomen and lower back, twice a day.

Prolapse Discomfort Blend

Geranium	5 drops
Immortelle	8 drops
Grapefruit	5 drops
Rosemary	9 drops
Lemon	5 drops

Bathing with rosemary, geranium, and lemon essential oils can also help — use 2 drops of each, every time you bathe. Dilute them into a little carrier oil before putting in the bath, and remember to swish the water around well before getting in the bath.

Varicose Veins

It's not only women who get varicose veins; men are just as liable to suffer, although theirs are not so noticeable until summer when the shorts come out of the closet. There are women who will wear only very long skirts and trousers, not because it's part of their style choice but because they don't want to show the veins on their legs. No one wants to have to wear pants — whatever the fashion — to conceal unsightly protruding veins. Nor do we want the ache and fatigue that go with them, and that can be more difficult to hide. Mineral makeup is helpful but can't hide the vein protrusions. Support stockings and tights are fortunately more glamorous than they used to be, and they do have a part to play in prevention.

Indeed, prevention is what this section is all about. There is another section on varicose veins in chapter 10, "Essential Help in the Maturing Years," and you may want to refer there (see page 266) and also to the section on pregnancy further on in this chapter.

People who stand or sit all day are at greater risk of developing varicose veins because the blood can't circulate. Aim to take a walk at lunchtime if your job is a threat to your good-looking legs. And everyone who is confined to a chair all day at the cash register or in an office should get up and stroll around from time to time. If anyone asks what you're doing, tell him or her you're preventing your legs from becoming the subject of a worker's compensation case! Pregnancy, being overweight, constipation, and coming from a maternal line who all had varicose veins can make you predisposed to the condition.

If you already have varicose veins, support tights may help a little to relieve the tiredness caused by the veins, although they do nothing to alleviate the condition itself. That's because 50 denier support tights can't put enough pressure on a dilated vein to send the blood back around

the body and up to the heart. An awareness of the potential problem should encourage us all to take care of our feet and legs. Along with using the essential oils in foot baths, sitz baths, and body oils, try to put your feet up for a while in the evening after work. Herbal remedies are popular in Europe, such as horse chestnut seed extract (*Aesculus hippocastanum*), which is applied topically in a gel or taken as an herbal supplement. Butcher's broom extract (*Ruscus asculeatus*) and gotu kola extract (*Centella asiatica*) may help reduce swelling in the legs and feet due to poor circulation. Vitamins that are helpful include vitamins E and C; also try rutin, which is a bioflavonoid.

VARICOSE VEINS ESSENTIAL OILS
Geranium (*Pelargonium graveolens*)
Cypress (*Cupressus sempervirens*)
Chamomile roman (*Anthemis nobilis*)
Chamomile german (*Matricaria recutita*)
Niaouli (*Melaleuca quinquenervia*)
Peppermint (*Mentha piperita*)
Spearmint (*Mentha spicata*)
Lemon (*Citrus limon*)
Juniper berry (*Juniperus communis*)

Take plenty of calf muscle exercise, such as walking, and find time to relax — and there's no better time to do that than after a foot and leg massage with the following:

VARICOSE VEIN PREVENTATIVE MASSAGE OIL
Peppermint	5 drops
Cypress	10 drops
Lemon	5 drops
Geranium	10 drops

Blend the essential oils together then dilute 3–5 drops to each teaspoon (5 mL) of carrier oil.

Apply lightly in the direction of the heart, from the foot and up the leg. If your feet and legs feel tired after doing any heavy work, carrying the shopping, or just spending a day out, gently apply the oil onto the legs when you get home and again before bedtime.

Tired legs can benefit from a spray or leg splash using witch hazel water (*Hamamelis virginiana*) and cypress and peppermint hydrolat/water. Blend together equal amounts of the three waters or make your own — see page 456. Then add 2 drops of peppermint essential oil and 2 drops of rosemary oil, diluted in a teaspoon of vodka or vegetable glycerin, shake well, and add to the three waters. Put into a spray bottle and use on tired legs. Always shake the bottle before use.

Foot baths are very good at preventing varicose veins. For the following treatment you need two bowls to put your feet into — one filled with cold water to which you have added a few ice cubes, and the other filled with hot water. Add 2 drops of eucalyptus radiata to the cold water and 2 drops of cypress to the hot water. Now put both feet in the cold water and leave them there for three minutes; then put them in the hot water for three minutes. The cold constricts the blood vessels and the hot dilates, sending the blood back around the body. This treatment is also good for tired and swollen legs.

If you stand all day, make the effort at least three times a week to have a foot bath, followed by a leg oil application. Use 2 drops of geranium in a bowl of warm water for the foot bath, for as long as you like, and use the leg oil blend above. Then put your feet up and relax. A foot bath can be taken while watching TV, catching up on paperwork, or peeling the vegetables for dinner. But a more effective treatment is just to sit back and relax completely.

Raynaud's Disease

There are two types of Raynaud's — primary and secondary. The cause of primary Raynaud's is unknown, but it's quite common, and although essential oils cannot cure the condition, they can help in easing the symptoms.

The main symptom of Raynaud's is feeling very, very, *very* cold — usually in the hands and feet but also in other extremities of the body like the ears and nose. Describing the degree of cold to other people can be impossible, but try to imagine a life in which you couldn't take a pack of frozen peas out of the freezer without wearing ice-workers' gloves. I've known women who suffer so badly with this condition that even if they put five pairs of socks on before they go out, their feet will soon be purple and their legs a veritable paint palette, with patches of red, orange, royal blue, mauve, and white showing through the color of their skin. Arriving at a party looking glamorous is a bit difficult when you peel off three pairs of gloves and put away your portable pocket heater only to reveal blue hands!

Raynaud's disease isn't catching and is not really a disease — more an underlying physiological phenomenon relating to blood vessel spasms, which temporary narrow the vessels and can, over time, lead to a thickening of the small arteries, exacerbating the problem.

Normally, blood heat is conserved in the cold by the muscular walls of the arteries constricting a certain amount. Conversely, when it's warm outside, the arteries relax and allow blood to the surface of the skin, where it can cool down. In Raynaud's sufferers, the arteries go into spasm when it's cold, starving the skin of blood. This then turns the skin numb and white and then, as the tissues lose oxygen, blue. As the spasm ends, oxygenated blood flows again, turning the skin red and sometimes causing throbbing pain. Because stress can cause havoc with the body's temperature-regulating system, having something in place to reduce stress levels may be one of the answers to mild attacks.

An attack can last for minutes, days, or weeks, and the sufferer may not know whether a particular attack will last 10 minutes or 2 weeks. The oddest thing can set off an attack — using a power drill, or smoking a cigarette, or holding a bag too tightly, or emotional stress. Nine out of 10 sufferers are women. Some disorders, such as rheumatoid arthritis, lupus, scleroderma, and atherosclerosis, may predispose someone to secondary Raynaud's symptoms.

For those with primary Raynaud's disease, essential oils may be able to provide a remedy. I'll always remember the young mother who after treatment was able, for the first time she could remember, to go out during the cold winter months to play in the snow with her children. Choose from these oils to make your own blend, or follow the blend given below:

RAYNAUD'S DISEASE ESSENTIAL OILS
Geranium (*Pelargonium graveolens*)
Rose absolute (*Rosa centifolia*)
Palmarosa (*Cymbopogon martinii*)
Cardamom (*Elettaria cardamomum*)
Clove bud (*Syzygium aromaticum*)
Lavender (*Lavandula angustifolia*)
Black pepper (*Piper nigrum*)
Ginger (*Zingiber officinale*)
Rosemary (*Rosmarinus officinalis*)
Nutmeg (*Myristica fragrans*)
Cinnamon leaf (*Cinnamomum zeylanicum*)

The treatment is a two-part regime of hand baths or foot baths, combined with massage, using two blends on alternate weeks. Here is the blend for the first week:

RAYNAUD'S DISEASE WEEK 1 BLEND
Nutmeg   5 drops
Clove bud   2 drops
Lavender   5 drops
Geranium   15 drops
Black pepper   3 drops

Make a blend using these proportions. If diluting to make a massage oil, dilute these quantities in 2 tablespoons (30 mL) of carrier oil. As you will need some of the essential oil blend for the hand or foot baths, make up two bottles — one for massage and another of neat essential oil.

Depending on which part of the body is most affected at any time, try to use the hand or foot bath twice a day — in the morning and before going to bed — using 3–4 drops of the blend diluted in 1 teaspoon (5 mL) of carrier oil. The water should be hot but not uncomfortable.

After the hand or foot bath, apply the massage oil over the affected areas, daily. If your toes and fingers are always extremely painful and your skin is perhaps fragile, add 50 drops of geranium essential oil to 2 tablespoons (30 mL) of the pre-prepared massage oil — as given in the blend above. This may seem rather a lot to add, but you are reading it right. Use a small amount of this blend of massage oil during the first two weeks. I've often used undiluted geranium oil on my client's fingers before using a diluted blend.

Now to the second blend. This is used over a full week, then alternate with Week 1 Blend, until the condition eases off and relief is obtained. Use exactly as directed above — in the hand or foot baths and as a massage oil.

RAYNAUD'S DISEASE WEEK 2 BLEND
Clove bud   2 drops
Ginger   2 drops
Black pepper   5 drops
Geranium   15 drops
Cardamom   8 drops

Make a blend using these proportions. If diluting to make a massage oil, dilute these quantities in 2 tablespoons (30 mL) of carrier oil. As you'll need some of the blend for the hand or foot baths, make up two bottles — one for massage and another of neat essential oil.

Several dietary and other measures have been shown to help people with Raynaud's, including vitamin D and E supplementation. Fish oils or omega 3 supplements may help, as can ginkgo biloba and garlic capsules in some cases. Also eat plenty of fresh onions and garlic, if you can, and cut caffeine wherever possible, substituting herbal teas.

Menstrual Problems

Whether a woman has children or not, she menstruates. Different women are affected by menstruation very differently. For some it's hardly noticeable, while at the other end of the spectrum there are women who have three very distressing weeks per month. (Yes, that did read *weeks*!) During menstruation a woman may experience uterine cramps, water retention, bloating, constipation, backache, fatigue, headaches, migraine, nausea, vomiting, and even sinus problems and a runny nose. Premenstrual syndrome may bring additional emotional problems.

The fact that menstruation occurs each month gives a good incentive to find a solution to any related problem. Fortunately, essential oils are very good at establishing hormonal homeostasis and have proved very successful in treating some of the problems associated with menstruation.

This section includes premenstrual syndrome and premenstrual dysphoric disorder, dysmenorrhea, menorrhagia, and amenorrhea. It is followed by menopause and pelvic pain, which includes endometriosis — a condition very much associated with menstruation.

PREMENSTRUAL SYNDROME (PMS) AND PREMENSTRUAL DYSPHORIC DISORDER (PMDD)

Premenstrual syndrome and premenstrual dysphoric disorder — the more severe form of PMS, are hormonal problems occurring during the luteal phase of the ovarian cycle. There is huge variation in how women's hormonal systems react in the days or weeks before their menstruation begins — some having no symptoms and some becoming overwhelmed with a variety of physical and emotional reactions, with most women being somewhere between the two. Essentially, women are reacting differently to fluctuations in the sex hormones: estrogen, progesterone, and testosterone. Other natural chemicals become influenced by this balancing act, including serotonin, which becomes less available and affects mood.

The seriousness of PMS symptoms in some women has led researchers to look at specific women's genes, and it may be possible in the future to routinely obtain a firm diagnosis of PMDD based on those genes that regulate estrogen receptors and the working of the prefrontal cortex — which is an area of the brain that strongly influences mood. It's very good that a physical reason for PMDD may be found because, at present, those women who have extreme physical and emotional reactions in the lead-up time to their menstruation can be left to believe they have serious psychological problems.

The symptoms of PMS and PMDD can include stress, tension, anxiety, panic attacks, mood swings, irritability, anger, sadness, despair, depression, frustration, hopelessness, difficulty concentrating, irrational thinking, apathy, fatigue, problems with memory, hypersensitivity to criticism, sleeping problems, and feeling out of control. The partner of a woman with these symptoms might have to deal with bouts of inexplicable crying, anger, changes in sex drive, and insensitivity to their needs.

On the physical level, a woman may also be having to deal with severe headaches, joint or muscle pain, breast swelling or tenderness, palpitations, actual or imagined weight gain, fluid retention, bloating, swelling around the face, and changes in appetite. This is a huge number of potential symptoms — both emotional and physical — and we can see why so many women dread the approach of their menstruation.

Because all the body's hormones work in an integrated, balancing way, other hormones that affect the salt and sugar levels are also involved in the way the syndrome expresses itself in any particular woman.

For both PMS and PMDD, help is available in the form of nutritional therapies and vitamin and mineral supplementation — such as a course of vitamin B6, vitamin E, evening primrose seed oil, calcium, and magnesium. Herbal remedies such as chaste berry (*Vitex agnus castus*), black cohosh, St. John's wort for depression, ginkgo biloba, and Siberian ginseng can also be helpful. The first step is to reduce your intake of sugar, red meat, soy and corn products, and alcohol, and to eat fresh foods, including dark-green leafy vegetables such as kale and spinach. This is the time many women crave a chocolate fix; if you must, try one that has no dairy, is low in sugar, and has a high dark raw cocoa content. Exercise is also thought to help some women, particularly those who have a sedentary job, sitting at a computer all day. Yoga and tai chi are forms of exercise that help regulate the body's energies, creating more balance.

Aromatherapy and the use of essential oils have proved highly effective in treating this condition or, more accurately, conditions. As each woman experiences the syndromes in her own unique way, it's impossible to provide one simple solution to everyone's problems. A clinical aromatherapist can design blends specific to an individual woman's symptoms and needs, and a woman treating herself can look at the information provided here while also referring to other sections of this book and the "Quick Reference Chart" in chapter 20 (see table 22, page 534).

First comes a general list of oils that help; this information is then broken down into the oils most appropriate for various symptoms under the headings "angry/aggressive," "weepy/depressed," "irritable/disagreeable," "apathetic/tired/listless," and "bloating/heaviness." If you fall clearly into one of these categories, choose from the appropriate list of oils. If your symptoms cross two categories, mix and match your essential oils until you find a blend that exactly suits you. There is also great variation in the length of time any particular woman suffers from PMS. It can start any time from three days before the period to two weeks before, and can disappear between two hours after bleeding starts to three days after. In any event, start the treatment the day after the last day of a period and continue throughout two complete cycles (including the menstruation), plus 14 days. Then break for 14 days so that you can see how your body is reacting and how you feel prior to the next period. If you find that the symptoms have lessened, have an occasional bath or massage using the successful essential oil or blend around the time of ovulation. If the symptoms haven't lessened after two and a half months, try again with an adjusted blend. The aim is to find a blend that personally suits you so the symptoms can be managed and not be life disrupting.

PMS AND PMDD ESSENTIAL OILS
Rose otto (*Rosa damascena*)
Grapefruit (*Citrus paradisi*)
Basil linalol (*Ocimum basilicum ct. linalool*)
Jasmine (*Jasminum grandiflorum/officinale*)

Rose absolute (*Rosa centifolia*)
Geranium (*Pelargonium graveolens*)
Clary sage (*Salvia sclarea*)
Chamomile roman (*Anthemis nobilis*)
Bergamot (*Citrus bergamia*)
Nutmeg (*Myristica fragrans*)
Peppermint (*Mentha piperita*)
Marjoram, sweet (*Origanum majorana*)
Black pepper (*Piper nigrum*)
Cardamom (*Elettaria cardamomum*)
Juniper berry (*Juniperus communis*)
Vetiver (*Vetiveria zizanoides*)
Lavender (*Lavandula angustifolia*)
Ylang ylang (*Cananga odorata*)
Petitgrain (*Citrus aurantium*)
Niaouli (*Melaleuca quinquenervia*)

It's estimated that 40% of women suffer from PMS, and using combinations of the oils above, it would be possible to make each one of them a unique personal blend. The specific blends below reflect a particular emotional state. Add the essential oil blend to 2 tablespoons (30 mL) of a carrier oil such as sweet almond oil and use a small amount each application. Apply over the solar plexus (upper abdomen), the hips, and the lower back to the coccyx — the lower end of the spine, between the crease of the buttocks but not as far as the anus.

ANGRY/AGGRESSIVE PMS ESSENTIAL OILS
Geranium (*Pelargonium graveolens*)
Clary sage (*Salvia sclarea*)
Vetiver (*Vetiveria zizanoides*)
Nutmeg (*Myristica fragrans*)
Palmarosa (*Cymbopogon martinii*)
Bergamot (*Citrus bergamia*)
Lavender (*Lavandula angustifolia*)
Chamomile roman (*Anthemis nobilis*)
Marjoram, sweet (*Origanum majorana*)

BLEND
Palmarosa	6 drops
Bergamot	10 drops
Geranium	10 drops
Clary sage	4 drops

WEEPY/DEPRESSED PMS ESSENTIAL OILS
Rose otto (*Rosa damascena*)
Bergamot (*Citrus bergamia*)
Rose absolute (*Rosa centifolia*)
Geranium (*Pelargonium graveolens*)
Clary sage (*Salvia sclarea*)
Nutmeg (*Myristica fragrans*)
Jasmine (*Jasminum grandiflorum/officinale*)
Orange, sweet (*Citrus sinensis*)
Black pepper (*Piper nigrum*)
Grapefruit (*Citrus paradisi*)

BLEND
Rose absolute	2 drops
Geranium	5 drops
Clary sage	10 drops
Orange, sweet	4 drops
Grapefruit	5 drops

IRRITABLE/DISAGREEABLE PMS ESSENTIAL OILS
Clary sage (*Salvia sclarea*)
Nutmeg (*Myristica fragrans*)
Chamomile roman (*Anthemis nobilis*)
Bergamot (*Citrus bergamia*)
Geranium (*Pelargonium graveolens*)
Cardamom (*Elettaria cardamomum*)
Cypress (*Cupressus sempervirens*)
Juniper berry (*Juniperus communis*)

BLEND
Nutmeg	2 drops
Juniper berry	5 drops
Geranium	5 drops
Bergamot	14 drops

APATHETIC/TIRED/LISTLESS PMS
ESSENTIAL OILS
Grapefruit (*Citrus paradisi*)
Geranium (*Pelargonium graveolens*)
Clary sage (*Salvia sclarea*)
Cypress (*Cupressus sempervirens*)
Bergamot (*Citrus bergamia*)
Chamomile roman (*Anthemis nobilis*)
Black pepper (*Piper nigrum*)
Juniper berry (*Juniperus communis*)
Basil linalol (*Ocimum basilicum ct. linalool*)
Lemon (*Citrus limon*)
Peppermint (*Mentha piperita*)

BLEND

Clary sage	5 drops
Grapefruit	5 drops
Black pepper	3 drops
Basil linalol	5 drops
Cypress	3 drops
Geranium	2 drops

BLOATING/HEAVINESS PMS ESSENTIAL OILS
Geranium (*Pelargonium graveolens*)
Chamomile roman (*Anthemis nobilis*)
Bergamot (*Citrus bergamia*)
Basil linalol (*Ocimum basilicum ct. linalool*)
Black pepper (*Piper nigrum*)
Cardamom (*Elettaria cardamomum*)
Juniper berry (*Juniperus communis*)
Cypress (*Cupressus sempervirens*)
Rosemary (*Rosmarinus officinalis*)
Peppermint (*Mentha piperita*)
Marjoram, sweet (*Origanum majorana*)
Lemon (*Citrus limon*)
Coriander seed (*Coriandrum sativum*)

BLEND

Juniper berry	8 drops
Black pepper	2 drops
Coriander seed	2 drops
Geranium	5 drops
Peppermint	2 drops
Cypress	3 drops
Lemon	8 drops

A friend of mine knew her period was imminent when she found herself rushing around the house cleaning everything in sight. No floor, wall, or surface would escape her frantic action. Every piece of clothing in the house found itself pristinely clean and ironed, hanging in the closet. It wasn't this that constituted her PMS, but the profound listlessness that followed. Knowing that she was going to spend the next few days totally motionless in a miserable heap in bed flung her into action just beforehand, so that at least the house wasn't in as bad a state as she. To an outsider visiting for those few days, this must have seemed the house of a woman with OCD. It is to this propensity for imbalance and extremes that the essential oils address themselves when treating PMS and PMDD. The exaggerated behavior so characteristic is brought into line, so that the naturally quick-tempered woman won't become a violently aggressive one; and the naturally sensitive woman won't end up in a pool of tears. Those who suffer from the syndrome might consider treating themselves to a couple of months with an aromatherapy practitioner — it would be well worth it to ensure that the essential oils bring you back to normal during the crucial premenstrual days.

DYSMENORRHEA

A painful period can be anything from dull ache to a violent cramp that causes you to double over. Most women will suffer some sort of discomfort at some time or other. When emotional factors are involved and we feel particularly fragile, menstrual cramps are liable to be more severe than normal. Pain from other causes, a urinary infection for example, may be amplified during menstruation.

Painful periods fall into two groups: congestive dysmenorrhea, which starts a few days before the period and can cover the whole abdominal area; and spasmodic dysmenorrhea, which comes in a spasm of pain in the pelvis and/or lower back. In either case, avoiding constipation is a must at these times.

Essential Oils for Dysmenorrhea

Chamomile roman (*Anthemis nobilis*)
Clary sage (*Salvia sclarea*)
Frankincense (*Boswellia carterii*)
Cypress (*Cupressus sempervirens*)
Nutmeg (*Myristica fragrans*)
Geranium (*Pelargonium graveolens*)
Peppermint (*Mentha piperita*)
Lavender (*Lavandula angustifolia*)
Rose otto (*Rosa damascena*)
Plai (*Zingiber cassumunar*)
Immortelle (*Helichrysum italicum*)
Cardamom (*Elettaria cardamomum*)
Marjoram, sweet (*Origanum majorana*)
Thyme linalol (*Thymus vulgaris ct. linalool*)
Ginger (*Zingiber officinale*)
Black pepper (*Piper nigrum*)

Which oils are most effective will depend on what is causing the pain or cramps — and that can be many quite different factors. You will have to experiment with oils and blends until you find what works for you. You might like first to try one of the following:

Blend for Stressful Congestive Pain

Chamomile roman	5 drops
Clary sage	5 drops
Marjoram, sweet	10 drops
Juniper berry	5 drops
Lavender	5 drops

Blend for Spasmodic Pain

Lavender	10 drops
Peppermint	5 drops
Cypress	5 drops
Marjoram, sweet	5 drops
Immortelle	5 drops

Blend for Intense Cramping

Cardamom	5 drops
Marjoram, sweet	5 drops
Immortelle	10 drops
Clary sage	5 drops
Nutmeg	3 drops
Plai	10 drops

Make your chosen blend using these proportions. Then use 3–5 drops diluted in a teaspoon (5 mL) of carrier oil, or dilute a larger amount by mixing the essential oils of your chosen blend in 2 tablespoons (30 mL) of carrier oil. Use as much oil as you need to rub over the whole abdomen and lower back area. Use as required, starting a week before the period is due.

Warm compresses can be very helpful. Mix the essential oils below into a blend. Then to make a compress, add the blend to a bowl of hot water, soak a small piece of material in the bowl, and apply it to the abdomen once a day.

Blend for Warm Compress

Lavender	4 drops
Cardamom	4 drops
Geranium	4 drops

MENORRHAGIA

Heavy menstrual bleeding, clotting in normal flow, or irregular bleeding at any time all come under the heading of *menorrhagia*. These are not symptoms that should be taken as part of "a woman's lot" because they can be indicative of serious conditions. Consult with your physician so the situation can be assessed.

Once a proper diagnosis has been given for menorrhagia, use 2 drops of geranium and 1 drop of lemon essential oil in a daily bath, diluted first in a little carrier oil. Make a body oil using the blend below that can be used daily at any time during the cycle:

Menorrhagia Body Oil Blend 1

Chamomile roman	5 drops
Geranium	10 drops
Clary sage	5 drops
Lemon	3 drops
Cypress	7 drops

Dilute in 2 tablespoons (30 mL) of carrier oil, and use a small amount each time.

Or, if you're suffering a lot of stress and anxiety at this time, substitute with the following blend:

Menorrhagia Body Oil Blend 2

Cypress	10 drops
Geranium	10 drops
Lavender	5 drops
Chamomile roman	5 drops

Dilute in 2 tablespoons (30 mL) of carrier oil, and use a small amount each time.

AMENORRHEA

Amenorrhea is the loss of periods. When the period stops during pregnancy and lactation, it is known as "secondary amenorrhea" and is not a medical condition. It is best to avoid using essential oils until you're quite certain that the absence of periods is not actually an unexpected pregnancy.

Stress — whether emotional or physical — is a factor in most menstrual problems and even more so in amenorrhea. The menstrual cycle can also be stopped by an ovarian or hormonal disorder — including a thyroid or pituitary problem, PCOS, or premature menopause — by intrauterine devices, or by some medications, including oral contraceptives. Overexercising can bring about amenorrhea, as can anorexia or bulimia, physical or emotional shock, stress and emotional upsets, and big events in life such as moving, changing jobs, or travel. Lack of good nutrition can also be a factor, and supplementing your diet with a multivitamin and mineral supplement just might help. Make sure it includes zinc, folic acid, iron, and vitamin B12.

If amenorrhea is caused by an emotional problem, the menstrual cycle will usually return to normal once the emotional problem has been addressed. All the following oils have a stress-combating component, although the chamomiles are particularly good during this time. You might also like to refer to other "Stress" sections in chapter 4, "Occupational Oils for the Working Man and Woman" and in chapter 5, "Emotional Rescue."

Essential Oils for Amenorrhea

Chamomile german (*Matricaria recutita*)
Geranium (*Pelargonium graveolens*)
Cypress (*Cupressus sempervirens*)
Chamomile roman (*Anthemis nobilis*)
Marjoram, sweet (*Origanum majorana*)
Clary sage (*Salvia sclarea*)
Rose maroc (*Rosa centifolia*)
Jasmine (*Jasminum grandiflorum / officinale*)
Vetiver (*Vetiveria zizanoides*)
Juniper berry (*Juniperus communis*)
Rosemary (*Rosmarinus officinalis*)

Amenorrhea Blend

Clary sage	4 drops
Chamomile roman	15 drops
Geranium	11 drops

Dilute in 2 tablespoons (30 mL) of carrier oil, and use a small amount each time. Massage over the abdomen and lower back every day for at least two weeks.

You can, in addition, have sitz bath treatments using oils from the list above or the blend. This is a two-part treatment involving a bath of hot water and a bowl of cold water. Add 6–8 drops of one of the essential oils into both bath and bowl; lower yourself alternately three times into the bath of hot water, where you stay for 10 minutes, then the bowl of cold water, where you stay for 5 minutes.

Menopause

Although some people float through menopause without experiencing any of the classic difficulties, most women experience some degree of discomfort in the form of hot flashes, bloating, water retention, and constipation, and after menopause many go on to develop vaginal dryness, circulatory problems, varicose veins, and osteoporosis. These can seem a poor exchange for the premenopausal life of menstruation and contraception.

What's unhelpful is the negativity that so often surrounds the subject of menopause. Women come to me full of dread about what might happen, rather than focusing on what is actually happening. In fact, many of the most glamorous women in the world have been through menopause and still look fabulous and are admired by old and young alike. After menopause loss of sex drive is unlikely to be a problem if there is a desirable partner around, and natural vaginal lubricants are widely available, if that is a problem.

The combination of physical and emotional difficulties that women experience are highly unique to the individual, so to a large extent, using essential oils is a matter of choosing those most appropriate to each woman.

THE MAIN ESSENTIAL OILS FOR MENOPAUSE
Clary sage (*Salvia sclarea*)
Geranium (*Pelargonium graveolens*)
Rose maroc (*Rosa centifolia*)
Jasmine (*Jasminum grandiflorum/officinale*)
Bergamot (*Citrus bergamia*)
Coriander seed (*Coriandrum sativum*)
Nutmeg (*Myristica fragrans*)
Chamomile roman (*Anthemis nobilis*)
Cypress (*Cupressus sempervirens*)
Chaste berry (*Vitex agnus castus*)
Rosemary (*Rosmarinus officinalis*)
Sage, Greek (*Salvia fruticosa/triloba*)
Valerian (*Valeriana officinalis*)
Spikenard (*Nardostachys jatamansi*)
Sandalwood (*Santalum album*)
Lavender (*Lavandula angustifolia*)
Juniper berry (*Juniperus communis*)
Orange, sweet (*Citrus sinensis*)
Peppermint (*Mentha piperita*)
Sage (*Salvia officinalis*) (to be used on the advice of an aromatherapist)

The following is a list of symptoms with appropriate essential oils. They are equally useful for perimenopausal, menopausal, and postmenopausal women. You can design your own blend, depending on the particular symptoms you are seeking to reduce. Incorporate at least two from the lists into your blend. Alternatively, use one of the blends for specific symptoms, which follow after the lists below:

Hot flashes: cypress, geranium, chamomile roman, clary sage, chaste berry, peppermint, niaouli, rosemary, palmarosa

Fluid retention: juniper berry, cedarwood atlas, cypress, rosemary, lemon, sweet orange, coriander seed

Exhaustion/fatigue: basil linalol, bergamot, cardamom, geranium, grapefruit, rosemary, frankincense, eucalyptus radiata, petitgrain, ylang ylang

Depression: bergamot, chamomile roman, clary sage, rose, frankincense, neroli, lavender, ho wood, ylang ylang

Aches and pains: black pepper, cardamom, cypress, ginger, sweet marjoram, plai, immortelle, ravintsara

Anxiety, loss of concentration: cardamom, cedarwood atlas, lemon, rosemary, peppermint, lavender, vetiver, mandarin, petitgrain, neroli

Digestive problems: chamomile german, cardamom, peppermint, lime, coriander seed, spearmint, basil linalol, bergamot

Sleeplessness: valerian, spikenard, vetiver, sweet marjoram, lavender, chamomile roman, cistus, mandarin, sweet orange, petitgrain

Sweats and flashes are caused by the irregular function of the blood vessels when they constrict and dilate, a response to the action of the hypothalamus, itself responding to the fluctuations of the hormone system. Blood flow, temperature, and heart rate can be increased. Probably the main discomfort is embarrassment when you suddenly turn red or break into a sweat while in the company of other people. Avoiding stimulants like tea, coffee, and alcohol is a good idea. Use the following blends when the symptoms occur, and at other times if you so wish:

HOT FLASHES BLEND

Peppermint	2 drops
Cypress	2 drops
Clary sage	10 drops
Spearmint	4 drops
Geranium	6 drops
Lemon	6 drops

Blend the essential oils together and, when required, dilute 4–5 drops in a teaspoon (5 mL) of carrier oil. Apply over the abdomen and lower back. Also use 5 drops of the blend in a bath, diluted in a little carrier oil, whenever you wish.

DAY AND NIGHT SWEATS BLEND

Grapefruit	10 drops
Lime	10 drops
Peppermint	2 drops
Thyme linalol	5 drops

Blend the essential oils together and dilute 3–5 drops in a teaspoon (5 mL) of carrier oil. Apply over the lower back. For baths, mix 1 drop each of geranium and cypress essential oil into a little carrier oil and add to the water, swishing around well before getting in.

WATER RETENTION AND BLOATING BLEND

Coriander seed	5 drops
Juniper berry	5 drops
Lemon	15 drops
Peppermint	5 drops

Blend the essential oils together and dilute 3–5 drops per teaspoon (5 mL) of carrier oil for a body oil. Apply a small amount over the abdominal area, lower back, and upper thighs.

CIRCULATORY PROBLEMS BLEND

Geranium	10 drops
Peppermint	5 drops
Rose maroc	10 drops
Patchouli	5 drops

Blend the essential oils together and dilute 3–5 drops per teaspoon (5 mL) of carrier oil for a body oil. Always massage in the direction of the heart. If it's the legs that are affected, apply from feet to thigh; if the hands, start at the fingers and move up the arm; and if the whole body is affected, apply to the front and back of the torso.

Nutrition is hugely important if facing difficulties with menopause, and the diet needs to be rich in good vegetable proteins, such as tofu, with lots of fresh vegetables and whole grains. Reduce consumption of white flour and refined sugars, and try to eat fewer rich foods, at least until you feel the symptoms have passed. Take a nutritional supplement, such as essential fatty acids — omega 3. Include a vitamin D supplement, unless you live in a sunny state where the sun will help your body produce what it needs. Any multivitamin supplement should include vitamins C, B, and E, calcium, iron, magnesium, and all the trace minerals.

It may take trial and error to find out which natural helpmates minimize each woman's particular symptoms, but those that are known to be invaluable in some cases are evening primrose seed oil, black cohosh, red clover, agnus castus, ginkgo biloba, wild yam, and dong quai. Sage is said to be helpful because it's thought to be a phytoestrogen that mimics our natural estrogen.

Pelvic Pain

Pelvic pain has many causes, including pelvic venous congestion syndrome (PVCS), endometriosis, salpingitis, fibroids, uterine prolapse, chronic interstitial cystitis, urinary tract infection, pelvic inflammatory disease, ovarian cysts, pelvic abscess, irritable bowel syndrome, and many more conditions, including painful ovulation.

Because the female abdominal area has so much potential to cause pelvic pain, it can be difficult to get a quick and accurate diagnosis when problems occur. Recent imaging techniques certainly help, and more readily available information has allowed women to explore the options themselves. But while uncertainty exists, the discomfort is still there. The following essential oils may help reduce the discomfort of any as yet unexplained pelvic pain.

ESSENTIAL OILS TO HELP REDUCE PELVIC DISCOMFORT

Chamomile german (*Matricaria recutita*)
Chamomile roman (*Anthemis nobilis*)
Frankincense (*Boswellia carterii*)
Ginger (*Zingiber officinale*)
Immortelle (*Helichrysum italicum*)
Plai (*Zingiber cassumunar*)
Lavender (*Lavandula angustifolia*)
Thyme linalol (*Thymus vulgaris ct. linalool*)
Geranium (*Pelargonium graveolens*)
Peppermint (*Mentha piperita*)
Cypress (*Cupressus sempervirens*)
Spearmint (*Mentha spicata*)
Fragonia (*Agonis fragrans*)
Cardamom (*Elettaria cardamomum*)
Basil linalol (*Ocimum basilicum ct. linalool*)
Lavandin (*Lavandula x intermedia*)
Marjoram, sweet (*Origanum majorana*)
Cedarwood atlas (*Cedrus atlantica*)

PELVIC DISCOMFORT BLEND

Ginger	5 drops
Chamomile german	10 drops
Lavender	10 drops
Peppermint	3 drops
Geranium	5 drops
Frankincense	10 drops
Marjoram, sweet	5 drops

Blend the essential oils together to create a synergetic blend. Then dilute 3–5 drops in a teaspoon (5 mL) of carrier oil for a body oil. Apply over the abdomen, the lower back, and the upper thighs, once or twice a day.

PELVIC VENOUS CONGESTION SYNDROME (PVCS)

Pelvic venous congestion syndrome occurs when there's damage to the veins in the pelvic area. It's also known as *ovarian vein reflux*. The veins in the pelvic area become unable to function properly, usually after a pregnancy but sometimes later in life, and become rather like varicose veins in the legs — engorged and possibly twisted. The ovarian veins might be implicated in the condition, but other veins may also be involved, such as the internal iliac vein, internal pudendal vein, obturator vein, and ischial veins.

Blood tends to accumulate in the damaged vein, especially after standing or walking for long periods, and because the valves are damaged, the blood cannot move in the right direction.

Most of the time the damaged vein is not visible, but sometimes it can be seen around the inner thigh, upper legs, buttocks, or vulva. A physician might see them near the cervix. MRI, CT, and ultrasound scanning can confirm a diagnosis.

The main symptoms of PVCS are a dragging sensation or pain in the pelvis, a general ache, IBS, and pain on intercourse or during menstruation. The pain can be on one side of the pelvis, or on both. Symptoms usually ease when the woman lies down, or at least sits.

PVCS Essential Oils
Nutmeg (*Myristica fragrans*)
Black pepper (*Piper nigrum*)
Clove bud (*Syzygium aromaticum*)
Ginger (*Zingiber officinale*)
Bergamot (*Citrus bergamia*)
Geranium (*Pelargonium graveolens*)
Coriander seed (*Coriandrum sativum*)
Thyme linalol (*Thymus vulgaris ct. linalool*)
Rose otto (*Rosa damascena*)
Lavender (*Lavandula angustifolia*)
Lemon (*Citrus limon*)
Chamomile roman (*Anthemis nobilis*)
Cypress (*Cupressus sempervirens*)
Immortelle (*Helichrysum italicum*)
Cardamom (*Elettaria cardamomum*)
Juniper berry (*Juniperus communis*)
Rosemary (*Rosmarinus officinalis*)
Niaouli (*Melaleuca quinquenervia*)

Hyssop decumbens (*Hyssopus officinalis var. decumbens*)
Basil linalol (*Ocimum basilicum ct. linalool*)

Treatment involves twice daily oil application, and three sitz baths per week. Ten days before your period is due, begin using the PVCS Blend 1 twice daily — in the morning and evening, and continue for at least eight weeks. Alternatively, make your own blend using the list above, to a total of 30 drops to 2 tablespoons (30 mL) of carrier oil. Apply gently front and back from waist to knees.

PVCS Body Blend 1
Chamomile roman	4 drops
Lemon	4 drops
Geranium	13 drops
Black pepper	4 drops
Ginger	3 drops
Hyssop decumbens	2 drops

Dilute this blend in 2 tablespoons (30 mL) of carrier oil, and use only a small amount each time, just enough to lightly cover the area.

On days when the pain is particularly bad, substitute PVCS Blend 2, below, following the instructions as above, and using a small amount each time. Revert back to PVCS Blend 1 after a day.

PVCS Body Blend 2
Frankincense	3 drops
Peppermint	3 drops
Cypress	7 drops
Niaouli	6 drops
Geranium	8 drops
Marjoram, sweet	3 drops

The second part of the treatment involves alternate warm and cold sitz baths. Follow the sitz bath treatment three times a week, completing at least two cycles each time. Because of the switch in temperature, this method should not be used if there is high blood pressure, deep vein thrombosis, arteriosclerosis, or any heart condition. If you are affected by any of these, use another method.

PVCS Blend for Warm Sitz Bath

Ginger	2 drops
Cardamom	5 drops
Bergamot	8 drops

Make a blend using these proportions and use 3 drops in the warm bath — sit for 10 minutes with the water at hip level.

Then move to the cold sitz bath and stay there for two minutes:

PVCS Blend for Cold Sitz Bath

Coriander seed	1 drop

An alternative method involves using the essential oils in the PVCS Body Blend 1, above, using the stated proportions but using the blend in a compress. Make the compress by adding 10 drops of the blend to a bowl of warm water, soaking a piece of material in the bowl, and applying it to the pelvic area once a day.

Try to adopt a healthy, whole-food diet, avoiding sugars and soda drinks and prepackaged and processed foods. Have at least two vegetarian days a week, and drink plenty of filtered or spring water. A good multivitamin and mineral supplement taken every day may also help, as will the tinctures of agnus castus, hawthorn berry, and horse chestnut seed. Some women find that gentle exercise relieves their symptoms.

ENDOMETRIOSIS

According to the American Society for Reproductive Medicine, up to 10% of all women may have endometriosis, with 20% of women with chronic pelvic pain being affected, along with 24%–50% of women who find it difficult to become pregnant.

These are huge numbers of women, yet the number may be larger because in many cases endometriosis is symptomless; the woman becomes aware of it only after she realizes she can't get pregnant and medical investigation shows she has endometriosis.

Endometrial tissue can potentially deposit itself in a wide variety of places within the abdominal cavity; in some places it causes excruciating pain, while in others it can be painless. This leads to the irony of endometriosis — some women can be symptom-free yet actually have a great deal of endometrial tissue, while other women can suffer agony and only have a few endometrial deposits. It all depends on where the deposits have attached, and their proximity to nerves.

The only reliable diagnosis is made through laparoscopy, which involves the insertion of a fiber-optic tube through the skin to examine the woman's abdominal cavity. The object of this exercise is to look for clumps of cells that usually line the womb — the endometrium — that have managed to get into the abdominal cavity and attach themselves to tissue and organs within: the fallopian tubes, ovaries, bowel, urethra, intestines, and pretty much anywhere else. These cells cause scar tissue and may cause pain, depending on the sites at which they are found and the nerves that have been affected. How these rogue cells manage to displace themselves and relocate is a medical mystery, with several conflicting theories on offer.

The symptoms of endometriosis include chronic pelvic pain, abdominal cramps, pain with menstruation, pain with intercourse, pain with ovulation, backache, heavy or irregular bleeding, pain in the joints, pain in the shoulders, infertility, miscarriage, hot flashes, PMS, bloating, rectal bleeding, pain when emptying the bowels or when urinating, loss of appetite, breathlessness, giddiness, depression, apathy, irritability — and this is not a full list of symptoms. Each woman's symptoms are entirely unique to her because the rogue endometrial cells could be anywhere, causing — or not causing — pain, which itself varies tremendously.

The thing about endometriosis is that it profoundly affects a woman's experience of her womanhood. Pain on intercourse is not sexy. Having so much pain during menstruation and, potentially, at any time of the month makes living day to day really difficult. Many women have to plan their calendar around their menstruation because they know that at that time they won't be able to do anything — no visits, no traveling, no parties, nothing — because they will be in bed, in pain, with a hot-water bottle over their tummy and the duvet over their head.

If this sounds all too familiar, take heart in the fact that essential oils can certainly help the condition. Based upon my research, the International Federation of Aromatherapists carried out a controlled trial of essential oils using my treatments on women with endometriosis, and the results were impressive. I have written a book just on the subject of endometriosis because I know how widespread it is, and how debilitating it can be. That book is called *The Endometriosis Natural Treatment Program*. The following suggestions have been adapted from that more complete treatment plan, which also explains the physiological reasons that certain essential oils are used for this condition.

A general treatment plan for endometriosis includes taking regular gentle exercise such as swimming, eating good nutritious food and excluding all junk food from your diet, and taking vitamin supplements such as a good multivitamin and multimineral and a daily probiotic. Endometriosis is one of those conditions that is a personal challenge in that you need to adopt a positive outlook toward self-healing and be proactive in carrying out any self-help treatments. You might also consider seeing a qualified therapist who understands the condition, has accurate information, and uses only the finest-quality pure essential oils. But many women cannot visit a therapist and can manage the condition at home using fine-quality pure essential oils. It would be good to have a friend give you massages, which are tremendous for de-stressing.

Endometriosis Essential Oils

Basil linalol (*Ocimum basilicum ct. linalool*)
Clary sage (*Salvia sclarea*)
Marjoram, sweet (*Origanum majorana*)
Geranium (*Pelargonium graveolens*)
Immortelle (*Helichrysum italicum*)
Chamomile roman (*Anthemis nobilis*)
Chamomile german (*Matricaria recutita*)
Rose otto (*Rosa damascena*)
Rose absolute (*Rosa centifolia*)
Juniper berry (*Juniperus communis*)
Lavender (*Lavandula angustifolia*)
Cypress (*Cupressus sempervirens*)
Eucalyptus radiata (*Eucalyptus radiata*)
Neroli (*Citrus aurantium*)
Yarrow (*Achillea millefolium*)
Nutmeg (*Myristica fragrans*)
Bergamot (*Citrus bergamia*)
Caraway seed (*Carum carvi*)
Fennel, sweet (*Foeniculum vulgare var. dulce*)
Clove bud (*Syzygium aromaticum*)
Peppermint (*Mentha piperita*)
Cardamom (*Elettaria cardamomum*)
Dill seed (*Anethum graveolens*)
Vetiver (*Vetiveria zizanoides*)

There are several aspects to the endometriosis program. The bath treatment involves taking sitz baths, which are alternate hot and cold sitz baths. Run hot — but not uncomfortably hot — water into the bath and prepare a bowl of cold water for the sitz. A baby bath or even a dishwashing bowl will do, as you need to lower your rear end into it, and "sitz." Ideally, you'd sit in waist-deep water, and in some European health clinics there's specialist equipment to facilitate this. But with ingenuity you might be able to find a piece of suitable equipment such as a baby bath, or even try a garden center for a large plant pot!

The sitz bath method is used for a variety of lower abdominal conditions. Although it's sometimes inconvenient to switch between the two, it's a proven, highly effective form of hydrotherapy and there's no substitute for it. Because of the rapid change in temperature, this method should not be used if there is high blood pressure, deep vein thrombosis, arteriosclerosis, or any heart condition. If these affect you, use another method.

Endometriosis Hot Sitz Bath Blend

Geranium	12 drops
Rose maroc	6 drops
Cypress	3 drops
Immortelle	6 drops
Nutmeg	3 drops
Clary sage	6 drops

Blend the essential oils together to make the blend used in the hot sitz baths. Add 5 drops of the blend to the hot sitz baths, and swish the water around with your hand to ensure there are no globules floating around on the surface of the hot water. To the cold-water sitz bath, add 2 teaspoons (10 mL) of rose water.

The purpose of hot and cold sitz baths is to get the blood vessels to contract and dilate alternately. One hot immersion plus one cold immersion constitutes one "cycle." Aim to do three to five cycles per session. Remain in each sitz bath for two minutes before switching. Ideally, the water will be waist high, but if that's not achievable, make the water level as close to waist high as you practically can. You may need to add a little hot water to the warm sitz bath to keep the temperature up, but

obviously you don't want the water to burn, so test it each time before getting in.

If you find this procedure impossible for practical reasons, you could compromise by using flexible ice packs and heat packs. If nothing else is available, just use a packet of frozen peas wrapped in a thin towel, alternating with a hot, wet towel. Place whatever you're using on your sacrum area — your lower spine, just above the coccyx. Take the cold pack first and hold it in position for five minutes, and then use the hot pack for a further five minutes. This method provides the advantage of alternate hot and cold treatment, but it can't be used with essential oils. A compromise could be to just substitute an ice pack for the cold sitz bath, and use a hot bath for the heat part — including the essential oils.

The second part of the treatment involves massaging twice a day with the following blend. Dilute these quantities in 2 tablespoons (30 mL) of carrier oil, and use as much as needed for each application, massaging over the whole of your abdomen and over the hips.

Endometriosis Body Oil Blend

Rose absolute	5 drops
Clary sage	10 drops
Chamomile roman	2 drops
Geranium	10 drops
Lavender	8 drops

If the pain is particularly bad during menstruation, make up a separate bottle of body oil using double the quantities. (During the week before each period is due you could also use the blends for severe cramps given in the section on page 206 on dysmenorrhea.) This double-strength oil can be used three times a day over the whole of your abdomen and over the hips. So even if you're at work, take the bottle in with you and apply the oil at lunchtime. No excuses — this is your reproductive cycle you're aiming to balance and, possibly, your fertility you're trying to save.

If abdominal bloating is experienced, especially premenstrually, substitute the bloating blend below in a body oil, applied twice a day, morning and night, over the abdomen and hips. The essential oils in the blend are helpful in reducing fluid retention.

ENDOMETRIOSIS BLOATING BLEND

Cypress	5 drops
Caraway seed	2 drops
Rosemary	3 drops
Juniper berry	3 drops
Peppermint	2 drops

Blend the essential oils in these proportions, then dilute the blend by using 5 drops per 1 teaspoon (5 mL) of carrier oil.

Thrush (*Candida albicans*)

The most common yeast infection is caused by the fungus *Candida albicans*, which is an innocuous member of many people's gut flora until there's an overgrowth, causing the condition *candidiasis*. It becomes out of control for a variety of reasons, including the use of antibiotics and certain other pharmaceutical medications.

Candida albicans can affect all parts of the body and may lead to a whole range of symptoms that at first seem unrelated to candida. These might include headaches, extreme fatigue, loss of concentration and focus, depression, bloating, digestive problems, leaky gut, constipation or diarrhea, nausea, sexual difficulties, and even sore gums. When these conditions are actually symptoms of candida, they might be caused by the 80 or so by-products created by candida when it dies, many of them toxins. Treatment for candida might exacerbate these symptoms, at least

for a while, until the candida has been controlled, but in the process it's important to think of the candida treatment as going hand in hand with a detoxification process. This means that the diet is especially important at this time as it's actually part of the treatment program.

Candida thrives on sugar and refined carbohydrates, so the first thing to do is cut out all sugars, not only the obvious ones in cakes and sodas but anything with fructose, artificial sweeteners, and even honey. Some vegetables contain sugar, such as beet and sweet potato, and even fruits should be kept to a minimum for the time being. Processed foods are packed with sugar, ketchup being a prime example. All soy products should be avoided, as well as foods high in gluten, all fermented foods, and foods containing molds or yeasts. The lactose in dairy products may also exacerbate the growth of candida, and many women are lactose intolerant without knowing it.

Change to an organic whole-food diet, cutting out alcohol, tea, and coffee — yes I did say coffee. Try to use garlic in your cooking and apple cider vinegar in your salads, and season with sea salt. Unrefined coconut oil can be used any which way you can find a use for it because it is itself proven to combat candida. The bulk of your diet should be good proteins and fresh, dark-green leafy vegetables, incorporating healthy plant seeds and oils.

Take a prebiotic and probiotic combination tablet daily, one that contains *Saccharomyces boulardii* — these are freeze-dried bacteria that replenish the good bacteria in the gut and help fight candida. Supplement with vitamins C and D3, kelp, which is high in iodine, olive leaf extract, pau d'arco, and supplements containing turmeric, oregano, and cinnamon.

VAGINAL CANDIDA

When treating the vaginal tract bear in mind that some undiluted essential oils could irritate the delicate mucous membrane tissues, so use them in a diluted form.

Candida affects men as well as women, and so whether the thrush is vaginal or penile it can be passed from partner to partner — which is why the treatment is just as important for both of you. For candida in men, see the section on thrush in chapter 9, "The Natural Choice for Men" (page 250).

Essential Oils for Thrush

Chamomile german (*Matricaria recutita*)
Geranium (*Pelargonium graveolens*)
Niaouli (*Melaleuca quinquenervia*)
Lemongrass (*Cymbopogon citratus/flexuosus*)
Tea tree (*Melaleuca alternifolia*)
Myrrh (*Commiphora myrrha*)
Cajuput (*Melaleuca cajuputi*)
Thyme linalol (*Thymus vulgaris ct. linalool*)
May chang (*Litsea cubeba*)
Patchouli (*Pogostemon cablin*)
Lavender (*Lavandula angustifolia*)
Palmarosa (*Cymbopogon martinii*)
Oregano (*Origanum vulgare*)
Lemon (*Citrus limon*)
Manuka (*Leptospermum scoparium*)

There are several ways to treat thrush, so find the most effective methods for you. First, the yogurt way. The yogurt used here must be a live, organic, natural yogurt made from whole milk, with absolutely no sugar, and containing live bacterial cultures. Obviously, the yogurt should contain no additives or preservatives. If you can't find a live yogurt that fits the bill, forget this method for now.

This method is very effective if you have a lot of vaginal soreness and itching. There are two essential oil blends that have been effective in this integrated treatment. You can prepare a carton of yogurt for this purpose and keep it in the fridge.

Thrush Yogurt Blend 1

Chamomile german	5 drops
Lavender	5 drops
Tea tree	5 drops

Thrush Yogurt Blend 2

Manuka	5 drops
Palmarosa	5 drops
Geranium	5 drops

Add one of the above blends to a 2 oz. carton of yogurt (described above) and mix well.

Now we get to the fun part — trying to get the yogurt mixture into the vagina! The simplest way perhaps is to use a long-handled, small-bowled plastic spoon. Some women use an applicator for inserting pessaries, or a tampon applicator. If using the tampon applicator, remove the tampon and scoop as much yogurt into the applicator as you can (in the end that normally holds the tampon). You'll need to close off the end of the applicator that normally pushes the tampon into the vagina; either use a piece of adhesive tape or plug it tightly with cotton wool. Insert the applicator now as you would with a tampon. This will enable you to get as much yogurt mixture into the vagina as is necessary. Apply once a day until the condition has eased. Use this method while lying down with a pillow under the knees, staying there for 10 minutes. It can be messy, but it's worth it.

The second method uses organic, unrefined, virgin coconut oil. This should come as a semi-solid product that melts almost immediately on contact with warm skin. Because the essential oils have to be well mixed in with the coconut oil, put 5 teaspoons (25 mL) of the coconut oil into a small bowl and mix in the essential oils listed in Thrush

Blend 3 below. By this time the coconut will have melted, so cover with plastic wrap and return to the fridge until hard.

The blend makes enough for 10 applications. When required, take ½ teaspoon of the hardened coconut oil, shape into a suppository, and insert into the vagina. Do this while lying down with a pillow under the knees. The oil will melt and may make a mess of whatever is under you, so protect the bed with a towel beforehand. Stay in place for 10 minutes. The coconut oil is itself something that combats candida and should not be substituted with any other product.

Thrush Coconut Oil Blend

Geranium	3 drops
Tea tree	2 drops
Patchouli	1 drop

The third method involves using organic cider/apple vinegar and water. The vinegar should, of course, be an entirely natural, unrefined product with no additives or preservatives — apple vinegar is excellent.

Vinegar Treatment for Thrush

Lemongrass	2 drops
Lavender	2 drops
Manuka	2 drops
Tea tree	2 drops
Niaouli	2 drops

Add the essential oils above to 3½ tablespoons (50 mL) of organic cider/apple vinegar. Mix together well, then add to about 2½ cups (600 mL) of warm water. Use the solution in a douche, daily, for three days.

If you would prefer to use a bath method, add the solution made up as above — but excluding the lemongrass — to a bath that has been run until it's at hip level. Add 1 tablespoon of rock or sea salt. (The salt addition, however, can *only* be used in the bath method, not in the douche method.)

When the mucous membrane of the vagina is inflamed and very sore it's sometimes better to use yet another method — with bicarbonate of soda. First, dilute ½ tablespoon (approximately 7 g) of bicarbonate of soda in 2½ cups (600 mL) of warm water. Then dilute the following essential oils in 1 teaspoon (5 mL) of organic carrier oil. Then mix all the ingredients together well.

Bicarbonate of Soda Blend for Thrush

Lavender	2 drops
Chamomile german	2 drops

Although water and oil don't mix, do the best you can and don't worry about it as this is an effective way to use the bicarbonate of soda with the essential oils. Use the whole solution in a douche. And repeat for two more days. If you prefer, pour the entire solution into a waist-high bath, and again repeat for the next two days.

Vaginal Infections and Inflammation

There are a great variety of possible infections, and sometimes you may not be given a specific diagnosis simply because the organism responsible has not been identified. Sometimes, too, you may have been given a medication that just hasn't worked for you. For these reasons I'm suggesting here some essential oils and methods that could be used when all else has failed.

Hundreds of thousands of women in the United States have been rendered infertile because of unidentified or untreated infections. Any unusual sign or symptom in the reproductive area should most definitely be investigated by a physician because, unchecked, it may lead to all kinds of other problems later.

When essential oils are used alongside any medication your physician prescribes, it's a form of integrative medicine, attacking from all fronts. But when using essential oils for self-treatment in this or in any other way, it's absolutely crucial that you use the purest of products, unadulterated and organic. In this section we're talking about the vagina, which is a mucous membrane — extremely sensitive and absorbent.

ESSENTIAL OILS THAT MIGHT HELP
WITH VAGINAL INFECTIONS
Juniper berry (*Juniperus communis*)
Lemongrass (*Cymbopogon citratus/flexuosus*)
Tea tree (*Melaleuca alternifolia*)
Frankincense (*Boswellia carterii*)
Lavender (*Lavandula angustifolia*)
Eucalyptus radiata (*Eucalyptus radiata*)
Cypress (*Cupressus sempervirens*)
Myrrh (*Commiphora myrrha*)
Sage (*Salvia officinalis*)
Niaouli (*Melaleuca quinquenervia*)
Clary sage (*Salvia sclarea*)
Manuka (*Leptospermum scoparium*)
Palmarosa (*Cymbopogon martinii*)
Chamomile german (*Matricaria recutita*)
Chamomile roman (*Anthemis nobilis*)
Cajuput (*Melaleuca cajuputi*)
Bergamot (*Citrus bergamia*)
Melissa (*Melissa officinalis*)
Sandalwood (*Santalum album*)
Rosewood (*Aniba rosaeodora*)
Ho wood (*Cinnamomum camphora ct. linalool*)
Lemon (*Citrus limon*)
Thyme linalol (*Thymus vulgaris ct. linalool*)

ESSENTIAL OILS THAT MIGHT HELP
WITH VAGINAL INFLAMMATION
Chamomile german (*Matricaria recutita*)
Tea tree (*Melaleuca alternifolia*)
Eucalyptus radiata (*Eucalyptus radiata*)

Lavender (*Lavandula angustifolia*)
Chamomile roman (*Anthemis nobilis*)
Sandalwood (*Santalum album*)

SUMMARY OF METHODS OF USE

When treating the vaginal tract remember that some undiluted essential oils could irritate the delicate mucous membrane tissues, and so you should use them in a diluted form. There are various methods to treat these conditions — just find the method included here that you are most happy with, using no more than two at any time. Please also refer to the "Methods of Use" section in chapter 1 if in any doubt.

Body oils: Make up a blend of essential oils. Then add between 15 and 30 drops into 2 tablespoons (30 mL) of an organic carrier oil such as sweet almond, apricot kernel, jojoba, borage seed, or evening primrose seed.

Cream and gel: Add the blend of essential oils to 3½ fl. oz. (100 mL) of vitamin E cream or aloe vera gel.

Sitz bath: Dilute the essential oil in a small amount of vegetable oil or glycerin before placing in the water and swishing around as usual. The water should be at hip level. Sit in the water for at least five minutes unless otherwise directed.

Douches: Unless otherwise directed, douche no more than once a week. Always add the oils to spring water that has been warmed, and filter through an unbleached, preferably organic, paper coffee filter before use.

Vegetable glycerin: Organic vegetable glycerin is a soothing addition to use in vaginal treatments as it is gentle on mucous membranes and may lessen irritation. Essential oils can be added to glycerin before adding them to water.

NONSPECIFIC VAGINITIS OR BACTERIAL VAGINOSIS (BV)

It is only really now that the huge number of potential vaginal microbiota are being identified. What used to be called *nonspecific vaginitis* has given way to *bacterial vaginosis*, and, in time, that term will break up into a number of conditions made identifiable by the future discovery and classification of the many tiny organisms that apparently reside within women.

Bacterial vaginosis is characterized by an abnormal vaginal discharge with an unpleasant fishy odor. Also, there can be itching around the vagina, discomfort during intercourse, and a burning sensation while urinating. It's very helpful in these cases to take a daily dose of lactobacilli, which add protection against the offending microbe.

BV BLEND
Chamomile german	2 drops
Lavender	2 drops
Cypress	1 drop

Dilute the blend in 2 teaspoons (10 mL) of vegetable glycerin, then add 2½ cups (600 mL) of water and mix well. Strain through an unbleached paper coffee filter.

Once prepared, use this essential oil water in one of two ways:

Method Options
1. Warm sitz bath: add 3½ fl. oz. (100 mL) of the BV Blend water to the water in a sitz bath, daily.
2. Douche: use 10 fl. oz. (300 mL) of the BV Blend water for two days only within a weeklong period.

VAGINAL GARDNERELLA

In vaginal gardnerella the *Haemophilus* bacteria causes an infection of the vaginal secretion. It's normally present in the healthy vagina but gets troublesome when the vagina becomes too alkaline, making the vagina very itchy and producing a white or gray discharge.

VAGINAL GARDNERELLA BLEND
Lavender	1 drop
Tea tree	1 drop
Palmarosa	1 drop

Dilute in 1 teaspoon (5 mL) of organic apple or cider vinegar, plus ½ teaspoon (2½ mL) of fresh lemon juice. Then mix with 2½ cups (600 mL) of water. Use this to douche on two days only within a weeklong period.

ATROPHIC VAGINITIS

Atrophic vaginitis is an inflammation of the genital walls caused by a decrease in the female hormone estrogen, which can leave the vagina vulnerable.

ATROPHIC VAGINITIS BODY OIL BLEND
Chamomile german	5 drops
Lavender	5 drops
Clary sage	5 drops

To make a body oil, dilute the blend in 1 tablespoon (15 mL) of hazelnut, safflower, or sweet almond oil and apply 1 teaspoon (5 mL) a day, over the whole abdomen and lower back — as far as but not into the crease of the buttocks. If there is soreness and dryness, one of the best sexual lubricants is pure organic coconut oil.

LEUKORRHEA

Leukorrhea is a noninfectious condition that causes inflammation in the vagina or cervix. It is thought to be caused by an imbalance of estrogen. The result is an overproduction of dead cells, which resemble a catarrhal-type of discharge from the vagina, usually thick and white but in some cases yellow and with a very unpleasant odor. It is important to try to eradicate the problem because it can get worse over time.

LEUKORRHEA BLEND

Clary sage	2 drops
Juniper berry	2 drops
Bergamot	2 drops
Thyme linalol	1 drop

Dilute the essential oils in 2 teaspoons (10 mL) of vegetable glycerin, then add to 2½ cups (600 mL) of water and mix well. Strain through an unbleached paper coffee filter.

Once prepared, there are two method options to choose from:

Method Options

1. Warm sitz bath: add 3½ fl. oz. (100 mL) of the completed mix above to the water in a sitz bath or bidet, daily.
2. Douche: use 10 fl. oz. (300 mL) of the completed mix above in a douche — use for only two days a week.

Infertility

Each year women from all cultures and corners of the world try to get pregnant and fail, resorting to drug and often multiple in vitro fertilization (IVF) treatments in an attempt to conceive and have a much longed-for child of their own. Infertility is on the increase, and no one really has an explanation for it. We do know that the reasons for infertility divide more or less equally between men, women, and how their two physiologies work together. Many couples' problems are attributable to subfertility, rather than infertility.

When you add up the possible causes of the problems it seems a miracle that anyone makes a baby at all. First, you have to choose the right days and most fertile times of the month to make love, and there are only about 36 of those days a year. Although it takes just one healthy sperm reaching the ovum for conception to occur, the sperm has a long way to go and many hurdles to overcome. For some men, the problem is that the sperm they produce are deformed or diseased. For others, it's that the sperm don't have the mobility to wiggle to their destination. Another hazard is that the sperm may be coated in their own antibodies. Even if there are enough healthy and energetic sperm, they have to be able to speed along the system of tubes without getting stopped by a blockage. Once delivered into the vagina, the sperm face the major obstacle — the cervix. This is coated in mucus that some sperm cannot penetrate. Some women produce a mucus that repels or even kills off sperm.

Now the sperm race to meet the egg. But has the woman's pituitary gland stimulated production of the hormone that will mature an egg that month — and at the right time? Polycystic ovary syndrome may have interfered with the timely release of eggs. A frequent cause of infertility is a blockage in the fallopian tube that prevents the sperm and egg from meeting. There may be something wrong with the glycoprotein that lines the walls of the fallopian tubes and coats a fertilized egg as it travels down the tube to the uterus, or with the endometrium, the lining of the womb that must be prepared to accept it. These are just *some* of the known reasons for infertility.

Although infertility has been an issue for couples both historically and geographically — literature is full of stories in which people could not have a baby — it is on the rise. The increase in infertility has been attributed to the fact that many couples are delaying starting a family — a delay that gives opportunity for an injury to have occurred or for an infection to have taken hold. Also, the environment is awash with hormone-disrupting chemicals, and some medications and so-called recreational drugs are known to reduce fertility. Please refer to the "Infertility" section in chapter 9, "The Natural Choice for Men," where specific treatments for men are suggested.

Being unable to conceive and fulfill parental urges is profoundly stressful, especially when it involves a couple in endless tests and medical examinations — all of which can cause financial stress. Initial testing and examination can often identify the existence of previously unknown medical conditions, such as infections that could have caused scar tissue and structural damage.

The human body works in a remarkably integrated way, with stress and diet playing a huge part in hormone balance. There are at least eight hormones involved in conception, and some essential oils are thought to have phytohormonal properties — plant hormones that are similar to our own. Research has shown that certain essential oils can significantly reduce stress and anxiety, and their significance in conception is best illustrated by a well-known phenomenon — a couple try for years to conceive, then decide to adopt a child or get a pet, whereupon the woman becomes pregnant. Here then are the essential oils for women:

ESSENTIAL OILS TO HELP FEMALE FERTILITY
Cypress (*Cupressus sempervirens*)
Geranium (*Pelargonium graveolens*)
Clary sage (*Salvia sclarea*)
Melissa (*Melissa officinalis*)
Rose maroc (*Rosa centifolia*)
Rose otto (*Rosa damascena*)
Chamomile roman (*Anthemis nobilis*)
Ylang ylang (*Cananga odorata*)
Coriander seed (*Coriandrum sativum*)
Cardamom (*Elettaria cardamomum*)
Frankincense (*Boswellia carterii*)
Sandalwood (*Santalum album*)

Ginger (*Zingiber officinale*)
Chamomile german (*Matricaria recutita*)
Lemon (*Citrus limon*)

The permutations that are possible by utilizing the oils on the list are endless, and which works for you is really dependent on many factors, including medical history, nutritional profile, age, menstrual history, and metabolism. Below are some blends to try that seem to assist women in conceiving:

BODY BLENDS FOR FEMALE FERTILITY

BLEND 1
Rose otto	5 drops
Geranium	20 drops
Clary sage	1 drop
Sandalwood	1 drop
Lemon	3 drops

Dilute in 2 tablespoons (30 mL) of carrier oil.

BLEND 2
Cardamom	5 drops
Rose maroc	5 drops
Geranium	10 drops
Black pepper	5 drops
Lemon	3 drops

Dilute in 2 tablespoons (30 mL) of carrier oil.

BLEND 3
Cardamom	5 drops
Bergamot	4 drops
Clary sage	3 drops
Geranium	8 drops

Dilute in 2 tablespoons (30 mL) of carrier oil.

BLEND 4
Rose maroc	10 drops
Geranium	8 drops
Lemon	4 drops

Dilute in 2 tablespoons (30 mL) of carrier oil.

Whichever blend you choose, first mix the essential oils together. Then dilute in 2 tablespoons (30 mL) of a carrier oil of your choice. Start on the last day of a period. Depending on your size, between 1 and 2 teaspoons of the body oil should be sufficient each time. It's important to cover the whole of the following area: start by massaging the lower back using both hands, then move over the hips and around the whole abdomen, the upper thighs, and the buttocks. Apply twice daily.

Zinc deficiency has been linked with both male and female infertility, but it's thought that many diets do not provide sufficient amounts. Good sources of zinc are fish, meat, organic green leafy vegetables, pulses, nuts, and wheatgerm; or zinc citrate supplements are available. Various complementary medicine systems provide treatment for fertility, including naturopathy, nutritional therapy, homeopathy, Chinese and Ayurvedic medicine, acupuncture, clinical aromatherapy, and massage therapy.

New solutions to the problem of infertility are being found almost yearly, and many of the causes can be treated. Also, conception involves a fair amount of mystery, and miracles are constantly taking place. So, above all, keep hoping.

Miscarriage and Preterm Delivery

The word *miscarriage* is used to describe a spontaneous loss of the fetus prior to the 20th week of pregnancy, while *preterm delivery* describes a loss after this time but before the baby is viable. In either case, this is a highly emotional experience for a woman and her partner. For the woman it's also a shocking physical experience and a profound hormonal one, with metabolic and physical changes.

As important as it is to allow time for your body to recover, it's also important to come to terms with the emotions you experience after a miscarriage. Exploring and expressing your feelings is not easy because miscarriage is a delicate subject for many people, and your partner, friends, or family may not know what to say and may struggle to understand a woman's physical and emotional feelings of emptiness and grief. The body was preparing for nine months of change and ultimate birth and is now having to adjust to the new physical changes, while the emotions are having to cope with loss on a profound level. People's response to the news can often seem like an attempt to close the door on the subject, with comments like "It's nature's way if something is wrong," "It happens all the time — all women miscarry without knowing it," or "Better now than later." These comments don't really open the door for you to talk about your feelings, and so if you find that you need someone to talk to who understands what you are going through, try to find a professional specialist organization that helps women who have been through the same emotional and physical trauma.

Many women who have had a miscarriage worry they may not be able to carry a subsequent baby to full term, but in most cases they can, and do. But women who have Rh-negative blood — or those women who don't know their blood group and may be Rh-negative — need to get an immediate Rh immunoglobulin (RhIG) injection to prevent damage to any future baby.

The essential oils recommended for use after a miscarriage can help to bring the body back into its prepregnancy state and also heal on the emotional and spiritual levels. Aroma preference is always a very personal thing, so when you make individual blends from the list below, choose those oils that are comforting at this time. Use 3–5 drops of essential oil to 1 teaspoon (5 mL) of carrier oil for a body oil, or 6–8 drops diluted in 1 teaspoon (5 mL) of carrier oil in baths:

ESSENTIAL OILS TO USE AFTER A
MISCARRIAGE OR PRETERM DELIVERY

Geranium (*Pelargonium graveolens*)

Rose otto (*Rosa damascena*)

Chamomile roman (*Anthemis nobilis*)

Rose absolute (*Rosa centifolia*)

Melissa (*Melissa officinalis*)

Geranium (*Pelargonium graveolens*)

Grapefruit (*Citrus paradisi*)

Ho wood (*Cinnamomum camphora ct. linalool*)

Palmarosa (*Cymbopogon martinii*)

Frankincense (*Boswellia carterii*)

Jasmine (*Jasminum grandiflorum/officinale*)

Immortelle (*Helichrysum italicum*)

Petitgrain (*Citrus aurantium*)

Neroli (*Citrus aurantium*)

Lavender (*Lavandula angustifolia*)

Orange, sweet (*Citrus sinensis*)

Or try these blends:

BLENDS TO USE AFTER A MISCARRIAGE OR PRETERM DELIVERY

BLEND 1

Frankincense	9 drops
Geranium	5 drops
Grapefruit	7 drops
Chamomile roman	9 drops

BLEND 2

Petitgrain	11 drops
Bergamot	8 drops
Geranium	7 drops
Chamomile roman	4 drops

From your chosen blend of essential oils, use 5 drops to each teaspoon (5 mL) of carrier oil for a body oil, or use 6 drops in a bath, first diluted in a little carrier oil. Alternatively, use a few drops in any of the room methods.

Pregnancy

Despite the myth that all women look and feel marvelous during pregnancy, this is when the body is going through dramatic hormonal changes and incurring great strains. Not only can there be morning sickness at the beginning of the term and extreme heaviness at the end, sebum production increases, and greasy or flaky areas may appear on the skin. Hair might become lank, and fatty areas may develop over the body, besides the lump at the front. Varicose veins appear with no warning, legs swell in summer. With all this going on, for some women it can be difficult to "bloom."

Essential oils can be really helpful during pregnancy, but it is clearly important to avoid those that are contraindicated. A woman who is pregnant is taking care of two people, so twice as much care needs to be taken: please refer to chapter 21, "Safety Information." When you're pregnant, unless otherwise directed by a professional it's better to use the minimum quantities of essential oils and avoid home use during the first trimester. There are many essential oils that are perfectly delightful to use while at the same time alleviating some of the physical stresses pregnancy inevitably brings. As well as the oils listed below, you will find in this section essential oils for the delivery room, for postnatal use, and for use in cases of the baby blues.

PREGNANCY ESSENTIAL OILS

During pregnancy, the bias is toward the gentler oils. The following is a list of essential oils that could, between them, take care of most problems anyone is likely to have, pregnancy-related or not.

The oils can be used in a bath or shower, in a body oil, or in one of the room methods.

Tangerine (*Citrus reticulata*)

Rose otto (*Rosa damascena*)

Cardamom (*Elettaria cardamomum*)

Manuka (*Leptospermum scoparium*)
Mandarin (*Citrus reticulata*)
Neroli (*Citrus aurantium*)
Rosewood (*Aniba rosaeodora*)
Grapefruit (*Citrus paradisi*)
Spearmint (*Mentha spicata*)
Sandalwood (*Santalum album*)
Marjoram, sweet (*Origanum majorana*)
Patchouli (*Pogostemon cablin*)
Black pepper (*Piper nigrum*)
Geranium (*Pelargonium graveolens*)
Coriander seed (*Coriandrum sativum*)
Orange, sweet (*Citrus sinensis*)
Tea tree (*Melaleuca alternifolia*)
Lavender (*Lavandula angustifolia*)
Lemon (*Citrus limon*)
Bergamot (*Citrus bergamia*)
Chamomile roman (*Anthemis nobilis*)
Ginger (*Zingiber officinale*)
Frankincense (*Boswellia carterii*)
Petitgrain (*Citrus aurantium*)
Chamomile german (*Matricaria recutita*)

PROBLEMS IN PREGNANCY

For many women pregnancy may entail a plethora of minor problems, such as backache, swollen legs, heartburn, indigestion, insomnia, hemorrhoids, tiredness, or general aggravation in not being able to accomplish daily tasks with the usual efficiency. If this is so, you need spoiling! Here are some essential oils that, when diluted, can be massaged into your back by yourself, a partner, or a friend — this may alleviate minor physical problems at the same time as it uplifts your spirit.

PREGNANCY PICKUP BACK RUB OILS
Neroli
Rose
*Chamomile roman
Geranium
Lavender
Petitgrain

Choose a single oil from the list above or make a blend using two or three in equal proportions. Dilute between 6 and 18 drops per 10 teaspoons (50 mL) of carrier oil and use a small amount each time.

In some instances chamomile german is more appropriate than chamomile roman if experiencing digestive problems or nerve pain.

If being pregnant is the ultimate high, it is also the original "heavy" experience. But the uplifting qualities of the essential oils are a great help after a tiring day at work or home, when the legs are swollen and the back aches.

Baths and Showers
Relaxing in a bathtub full of warm water and inhaling the aroma of essential oils is a lovely way to relieve the tension of the day. Different essential oils can be chosen, depending on how you feel. Choose your favorites from the above list or try the very relaxing combination of 1 drop each of chamomile roman and lavender oils. Alternatively, try mandarin with geranium.

Generally, for pregnant women, dilute 1 or 2 drops of essential oil in a little carrier oil before adding into the bathtub. If you prefer showers, to capture the relaxing effects of essential oils drop undiluted essential oils onto a washcloth and place the cloth in the shower tray. As the warm water hits the washcloth, the relaxing aroma will rise.

Morning Sickness
Morning sickness or feelings of continual nausea generally start very early on in pregnancy. Most women find that the feelings have gone by the end of the first trimester; however, for some unlucky women the nausea can last throughout the pregnancy. See also "Nausea," below.

For morning sickness, a bowl of boiling water with 4–6 drops of spearmint oil added, placed on the floor by your bed overnight, will help keep the stomach calm. The aroma molecules will waft up and gently work as you sleep, and after using this method for three consecutive nights the morning sickness may have lessened. Alternatively, a combination of 2 drops of ginger oil and 4 drops of spearmint can also be very helpful; while for other women the combination of cardamom, ginger, and sweet orange really helps — 2 drops each. It really is a case of what suits you. If the thought of cardamom brings up memories of a bad curry, that essential oil might not be such a good idea. Here's one blend many women have found useful:

MORNING SICKNESS BLEND

Spearmint	4 drops
Ginger	2 drops
Cardamom	1 drop
Lavender	2 drops

First, blend the essential oils together using these proportions. Then use 2 drops in the bowl-under-the-bed method, or put 1 drop on a tissue and place under your pillow. For all you working women, it's also helpful to keep a tissue in your purse with the blend you find most useful, for those moments when nausea catches you out.

Nausea

Nausea usually clears up by the fourth month of pregnancy, but some unfortunate women go to full term with that feeling of sickness morning, noon, and night, occasionally accompanied by vomiting. The hormones involved in pregnancy affect the digestive system from the esophageal sphincter to the small bowel, so feeling nausea is for many an inevitable discomfort that will disappear when the baby is born and the hormones return to normal. Symptoms can range from a simple loss of appetite to unbearable nausea

when smelling food. This reaction to food can make pregnancy a difficult time in terms of going out and about. Restaurants with an open kitchen area are probably best avoided — just in case! See also "Morning Sickness," above.

ESSENTIAL OILS TO COMBAT NAUSEA

Orange, sweet (*Citrus sinensis*)
Ginger (*Zingiber officinale*)
Cardamom (*Elettaria cardamomum*)
Grapefruit (*Citrus paradisi*)
Coriander seed (*Coriandrum sativum*)
Spearmint (*Mentha spicata*)
Lemon (*Citrus limon*)
Petitgrain (*Citrus aurantium*)
Frankincense (*Boswellia carterii*)
Bergamot (*Citrus bergamia*)

Overall well-being and comfort are greatly helped during pregnancy if the whole gastrointestinal tract can operate efficiently. As a rule, the dosage for nausea treatment should be low. Use 1 drop each of grapefruit, ginger, and cardamom or 3 drops of any of those. Blend the essential oils together, dilute into 2 teaspoons (10 mL) of carrier oil, and rub a small amount onto the wrists or upper chest. Diffusing essential oils can also help: blend 3 drops of grapefruit, 2 drops of ginger, and 1 drop of spearmint together, then use 1 or 2 drops of this mix in a diffuser. If you don't have a diffuser, use the water bowl method. Working moms often find this method useful at work, as the fragrance is quite pleasant. Acupressure bracelets with pressure beads also work for some women — these are often sold to combat sea and travel sickness and are widely available.

Another method involves essential oils of ginger and spearmint. Simply fill a bowl with boiling water, put in 1 drop each of ginger and spearmint per pint (475 mL) of water used, and let the steam circulate in the room.

Stretch Marks

I have treated many women with essential oils during pregnancy, and not one of them had stretch marks. And they all had wonderful babies. For the tummy-rub treatment the carrier oil is as important as the essential oils themselves, and here are two blends that have proved very successful:

BODY MASSAGE CARRIER OIL BLEND 1

Almond (sweet) oil (*Prunus amygdalus var. dulcis*)	2 tablespoons (30 mL)
Wheatgerm oil (*Triticum sativum*)	1 tablespoon (15 mL)
Borage seed oil (*Borago officinalis*)	1 teaspoon (5 mL)
Carrot macerated oil (*Daucus carota*)	1 teaspoon (5 mL)

RICH BODY MASSAGE CARRIER OIL BLEND 2

Avocado oil (*Persea americana*)	2 teaspoons (10 mL)
Evening primrose seed oil (*Oenothera biennis*)	1 teaspoon (5 mL)
Jojoba oil (*Simmondsia chinensis*)	2 teaspoons (10 mL)
Rosehip seed oil (*Rosa rubiginosa*)	1 teaspoon (5 mL)
Almond (sweet) oil (*Prunus amygdalus var. dulcis*)	2.5 fl. oz. (75 mL)

The carrier oils above contain no essential oils. Blend them together well and use as required. Massage into the skin wherever stretch marks may occur — the lower and upper abdomen, thighs, and buttocks. Use the oils regularly or every day to prevent stretch marks. No matter how well protected the skin is during pregnancy, some women will get stretch marks. But by protecting your skin as best as you can it will lessen any effects. Profiles

for alternative carrier oils can be found in chapter 19, "Carrier Oils and Hydrolats."

Although you can add essential oils to the massage carrier blends above, I would suggest that for everyday use, you apply carrier oils without essential oils. Then put aside 2 tablespoons (30 mL) of one of the carrier oil blends above and use this for adding essential oils to — you could use the following blend once a week:

Geranium	2 drops
Mandarin	4 drops
Sandalwood	2 drops

Dilute into your 2 tablespoons (30 mL) of carrier oil, and use a small amount each time.

Constipation

Every pregnant woman knows the importance of eating correctly during her nine months and while breast-feeding. But doing so is by no means as straightforward as it used to be. Unfortunately, many fruits and vegetables can no longer be guaranteed to be nutritious and full of the vitamins and minerals we expect because of monoculture's soil fertility depletion, chemical fertilizers, pesticides and herbicides, and growth-promoting substances. Try to buy organic or biodynamic vegetables and meats, or visit farmer's markets where you can ask about the growing methods.

The unnaturalness of our food plus the hormonal changes, reduced exercise, and the sheer pressure on our digestive system during pregnancy together conspire to make constipation a common complaint at this time. Constipation is often caused by lack of hydration, so drink lots of filtered or mineral water and eat as many raw fruits and vegetables as you can. Good natural laxatives are dried fruits, such as prunes and figs, and greens, such as broccoli and cabbage. Taking a probiotic supplement can also help. Fiber is important, but avoid breakfast cereals that are full of sugar and salt and are so processed that all the natural goodness has been taken out, and then has to be added back — often with synthetic supplements! Try instead the original muesli recipe devised by the Bircher Benner clinic in Zurich, Switzerland (see chapter 16, "Cooking With Essential Oils," page 472). Or make yourself porridge using real oats and water — it's cheap, takes no longer than five minutes, and you can add fruit, nuts, raisins, seeds, and linseeds, which are known to help constipation. Another method involves psyllium husks, which are pure fiber and can be bought raw or in capsule form.

Patchouli and lemon essential oils can be incorporated into a back massage oil if you are experiencing symptoms of constipation. Use a small amount and gently apply over the lower back, on either side of the vertebrae. Alternatively, massage either side of both ankle bones — doing one leg after the other, several times.

PREGNANCY CONSTIPATION BLEND

| Patchouli | 10 drops |
| Lemon | 5 drops |

Blend together, then dilute 1–2 drops per 1 teaspoon (5 mL) of carrier oil.

Hemorrhoids

One problem with being constipated while pregnant is straining to pass a stool, which along with the increased pressure of the swelling abdomen may result in hemorrhoids, a form of dilated veins. A simple measure to relieve the pain or soreness is to hold a washcloth soaked in cold water over the area. Cold lavender hydrolat, or witch hazel water, could be substituted for the plain water. Alternatively, pure aloe vera gel can be kept in the fridge, and a small amount applied over the anal area as required. During the third trimester of pregnancy, the following hemorrhoid blend could be used:

PREGNANCY HEMORRHOIDS BLEND

| Geranium | 10 drops |
| Lemon | 5 drops |

Blend together, then dilute 1–2 drops per 1 teaspoon (5 mL) of carrier oil, and rub a small amount around the anus once a day, before going to bed.

For use in the third trimester, if the anal area is very sore, a cream could be made by adding 10 drops of geranium and 5 drops of chamomile roman essential oil to 3½ fl. oz. (100 mL) of a natural balm, silica gel, or vegetable glycerin ointment. Simply put your chosen ointment into a small, sealable jar, add the essential oils, mix very well, and store in the fridge. When required, apply a small amount around the anus area.

Varicose Veins

Keeping your legs and feet up as often as possible can help relieve the leg ache caused by varicose veins in the legs, so for at least 10 minutes a day lie with a pillow in the small of your back and another at the nape of your neck — not under the head. You may as well take advantage of this time of enforced inactivity to meditate on the well-being of your baby. Send loving, affirmative thoughts to the baby, because positive thinking makes positive things happen. Such thought projection is the oldest of treatments and one whose value is again being recognized.

The extra pressure on the legs caused by pregnancy makes varicose veins a common problem. As well as keeping your feet and legs up as often as possible, try to exercise a little — even if only on the spot. Circle the ankles first one way, then the other — do this five times — then point the foot and relax it. Repeat for a total of five times each leg. This can easily be carried out under your desk at work or while sitting and watching television and may help prevent leg cramps. If you find your leg muscle is cramping, massage the calf muscle. Stroke your legs gently upward while in a bath that contains 2 drops each of geranium and chamomile roman. You'll obviously find this easier in month five than in month nine, but do the best you can. Lavender oil makes an excellent addition to this remedy, so add 2 drops if you have any handy.

A leg oil can be made by blending 10 drops of geranium and 5 drops of lemon essential oil in 2 tablespoons (30 mL) of carrier oil. Use a small amount to stroke the legs very gently, working upward from ankle to thigh. The geranium will encourage the circulation of blood while lemon has an astringent effect. The oil will also help to balance the mind and alleviate doubts and anxieties.

Foot baths can also help, especially if you place a dozen or so small, round pebbles at the bottom of the bowl of water and rub your feet gently back and forth over them. Add 2 drops each of geranium and spearmint essential oil to a bowl of warm water.

Cramps

Cramps during pregnancy might be caused by the position of the baby, or by how your body is processing calcium, or by a shortage of calcium, magnesium, potassium, or any number of other micronutrients, or for no apparent reason at all. The muscular spasms are often felt in the feet, toes, or calf muscles and are usually more common in the second and third trimesters. Cramps are often worse during the night or during an afternoon nap, and they usually come on suddenly. Stretching the muscles in the foot or leg before bedtime can sometimes help, as can massaging the leg with or without essential oils. Many women find that the relaxing effect of foot baths helps reduce incidents of cramp, and women have been using the following foot baths with success for many years:

LEG CRAMPS FOOT BATH BLEND 1

Marjoram, sweet	2 drops
Geranium	5 drops
Rosemary	2 drops
Plai	3 drops

LEG CRAMPS FOOT BATH BLEND 2

Geranium	5 drops
Lavender	9 drops
Marjoram, sweet	2 drops

Blend the essential oils together, place 4 drops of the blend into a bowl of comfortably warm water, and swish the water around before putting your feet in the bowl.

You could also take a good nutritional supplement designed for use during pregnancy, which should include all the minerals and trace elements needed. Dehydration can be a factor, so increase your fluid intake if you're experiencing muscular leg cramps.

If you've experienced a night cramp, before going to bed the next evening massage half a teaspoon of the following leg cramp oil onto both legs and feet:

LEG CRAMP MASSAGE OIL

Marjoram, sweet	2 drops
Geranium	4 drops
Black pepper	1 drop
Lemon	2 drops

Blend the oils together, then dilute in 2 tablespoons (30 mL) of carrier oil.

Cramps in the abdomen are a completely different subject and should always be checked immediately by your obstetrician.

Edema

One of the things that often happens during pregnancy is swelling — a buildup of fluid within the tissues, mainly of the lower limbs. It's quite normal during pregnancy to experience a certain degree of swelling, usually of the feet and ankles; it can happen, for example, during hot weather or when standing for long periods of time. Edema is extremely common and is usually nothing to worry about, but if it occurs in conjunction with high blood pressure and high levels of protein in the urine it can indicate preeclampsia, which can lead to eclampsia. So if there's any sudden swelling in the hands, face, or other parts of the body, report that to your obstetrician.

If you're experiencing feet or ankle swelling, spend at least 10 minutes a day lying down with a pillow under your feet. The important thing is to have your feet higher than your heart, so just sitting down won't help. Counterintuitive as it may seem, drinking plenty of water will help at this time, as can herbal teas such as dandelion or nettle, twice a day.

A cold foot bath can be extremely helpful. First, blend these essential oils together:

EDEMA FOOT BATH

Lemon	3 drops
Coriander seed	2 drops
Lavender	2 drops
Black pepper	1 drop

From this blend add 4 drops to a bowl of cool water and swish them around. Put some round pebbles in the bottom of the bowl, if you can find them, and roll your feet back and forth over them. The water in the bowl can also be used for a cold compress: just lower a piece of natural material into the water — the colder, the better this time — squeeze out, and apply to the ankles or lower legs, while lying flat on the bed or sofa.

Exhaustion

Exhaustion can occur at any stage of pregnancy, especially if you already have one or two little ones to take care of. Here is a reviving blend that

you can use for a body oil, bath, or foot bath. There's nothing to stop you from using it after the birth too — when you're just as likely to need it! First, blend together the following essential oils:

EXHAUSTION BLEND

Lavender	8 drops
Grapefruit	7 drops
Frankincense	5 drops

For a body rub, dilute 2 drops in 1 teaspoon (5 mL) of sweet almond oil. In a bath, use 3 drops, diluted in a little carrier oil. And for a foot bath, add 4 drops to a bowl of comfortably warm water.

Preparing for the Birth

Massage can help prepare for childbirth the bridge of muscle and tissue that lies between the vagina and anus, known as the *perineum*. Massage softens the skin and makes it more pliable, which may help avoid tearing during childbirth. First, prepare the oil:

PERINEUM OIL

Almond (sweet) oil	10 mL
Sesame oil	5 mL
Jojoba oil	10 mL
Olive oil	5 mL

Always use organic oils. Starting around week 34, apply a small amount of the oil once a day directly on the perineum, and massage gently. There is no need to go anywhere near the urethra. To avoid the risk of infection, only carry out the massage immediately after washing hands. If an infection is already present anywhere in the area, don't carry out this massage. Keep the bottle of oil in a dry, cool place, away from heat.

Gently stretching the vagina can also be helpful in preparing for the birth: place your thumb or two fingers just inside the vagina and gently stretch the vaginal walls by moving the fingers back and forth, particularly toward the back. This, in conjunction with the perineum massage, will help stretch the combined area — ready for the biggest stretch of your life! From about the seventh month the uterus can be prepared for labor by drinking raspberry leaf tea: 1 teaspoon of organic raspberry leaf tea in a cup of boiling water.

THE DELIVERY ROOM

During labor a baby's body produces special stress hormones called *catecholamines* that increase blood flow and immune response and help baby's lungs expand so it can clear amniotic fluid and breathe well.

The mother's uterus has been having trial runs of contractions during the pregnancy — sometimes hardly noticeable — and has been rehearsing for the big performance over and over again. Increased levels of progesterone have been softening up the pelvis, uterus, and cervix, as well as the surrounding muscles and ligaments.

Labor, as it is so aptly known, is work. It is, indeed, probably the hardest work that a woman will do in her life. What's needed is to make the experience as easy as possible — for both the mother and the baby. Obstetric practices change from year to year and also vary from place to place, but these changes are determined to a large degree by the expectations and demands of the mothers themselves. If our suggestions facilitate an easier delivery for both the mother and baby, there's no reason to assume that midwives and doctors will object.

Your choices in using essential oils or indeed any aspect of the delivery will depend to some degree on whether you're having a home or a hospital delivery. Water births are popular, but don't under any circumstances use essential oils in the birthing pool — or have any essential oil left on the body prior to delivery in the pool. Diffuse the essential oils outside of the pool, or have them on a tissue to inhale.

A cesarean can be planned, or it can be an emergency procedure. If planned, it's easier to use essential oil, but even in an emergency, essential oils can still be used before and after.

Along with other methods, warm compresses often help during labor, and these can be used at home quite easily. First, prepare the material to be used, add your chosen essential oils or blend to a bowl of warm water, soak the material in the bowl, and then apply to the back or wherever the pain seems to be worse — excluding the genital area.

Babies are remarkably aware of the environment outside the womb, and it's now thought that as well as being aware of the emotional state of the mother and the sounds she hears, baby is also aware of the smells its mother inhales. If the mother is aware of this, she can prepare the environment so that it will be reassuring for the newborn baby. For a few days before the birth, at least, spend some time quietly relaxed — listening to soft and gentle music, rubbing your tummy, and letting your baby know that everything is all right. The same music can be played in the delivery room, thus reducing the contrast between the womb and the outside world. While you relax at home listening to the music and communicating with your baby, use the essential oils you intend to have in the delivery room so that all the senses become inextricably linked in baby's mind: relaxation, welcome, music, and aroma. When the baby is born it will be into an environment he or she recognizes as being related to the mother, and moreover, to the mother being relaxed.

If you intend to use essential oils as part of your birth plan, inform the hospital where you're planning to have your baby. Discuss with them your music playing options, and ask whether it would be possible to reduce the lighting, at least part of the time. If you were having a home birth none of these plans would be a problem, but hospital rules vary greatly and it's important that the staff know your wishes before the event. Some of the larger hospitals have widely differing requests from their patients, who come from all cultures and backgrounds, and they usually recognize the need to be aware of each mother's birthing wishes.

To ease the mother's task during delivery, massage is widely recommended these days, especially as the partner is often present to do the job. Using a special mix of essential oils, we can incorporate the benefits of massage with those of the oils and at the same time ensure the baby will have a pleasant natural aroma to greet him or her. As you can see from the list below, rose and geranium both have excellent properties for use during delivery, and although a combination works very well, it's really important (and never more so than now) that the aroma of the oil you choose suits your taste. It's always wise to try out any essential oil blend before you go into labor, to make sure you really like it. If you have a favorite essential oil, now may be the time to include it in your delivery room diffusing blend.

I always suggest to my clients that they have ready several essential oils or blends, one to help relax and calm, one to stimulate, and one that seems to have a great spiritual connection or just makes the woman feel peaceful and at ease. Other blends could be prepared to ease intense discomfort, and it's great to have on hand a ready-made refreshing face spray containing a cooling hydrolat or essential oil blend.

ESSENTIAL OILS FOR THE DELIVERY ROOM
Geranium (*Pelargonium graveolens*)
Rose absolute (*Rosa centifolia*)
Jasmine (*Jasminum grandiflorum/officinale*)
Lemon (*Citrus limon*)
Mandarin (*Citrus reticulata*)

Neroli (*Citrus aurantium*)
Orange, sweet (*Citrus sinensis*)
Lavender (*Lavandula angustifolia*)
Frankincense (*Boswellia carterii*)
Grapefruit (*Citrus paradisi*)
Clary sage (*Salvia sclarea*)
Chamomile roman (*Anthemis nobilis*)
Rose otto (*Rosa damascena*)
Petitgrain (*Citrus aurantium*)
Sandalwood (*Santalum album*)
Patchouli (*Pogostemon cablin*)
Spearmint (*Mentha spicata*)

To help choose which oils you might like to incorporate into blends, there are some delivery room profiles below. Some oils have a role in making the blend uplifting and refreshing, such as lemon, sweet orange, and mandarin.

DELIVERY ROOM ESSENTIAL OIL PROFILES

ROSE OTTO (*Rosa damascena*)
Uterine relaxant
Helps ligaments to soften, enabling the pelvic bones to expand
Helps regain elasticity after the birth
Natural antiseptic
Slight analgesic effect
Good cardiac tonic

NEROLI (*Citrus aurantium*)
Assists the nervous system and helps relieve feelings of anxiety
Calming
Confidence boosting
Antidepressant
In low doses (1 or 2 drops per day on a diffuser), has a sedative and calming effect; in higher doses, can be a stimulant
Antiseptic; disinfectant

FRANKINCENSE (*Boswellia carterii*)

Helps respiration

Useful in labor to alleviate stress or anxiety

For some women, gives a sense of comfort as it is used in spiritual practices and, in some cultures, is said to create positive energy

CHAMOMILE ROMAN (*Anthemis nobilis*)

Has a calming effect on the nervous system, helping to relieve stress and anxiety

Can give a feeling of ease from the discomfort of contractions

Helps relieve aches and pains, and headache

LAVENDER (*Lavandula angustifolia*)

Slight analgesic effect

Calming

Antibiotic, antiseptic, disinfectant, slight antiviral properties, anti-inflammatory

Promotes healing of open wounds — can be used instead of antiseptics

Accepted by everyone

Good for headaches, fainting, and bringing around after shock

JASMINE (*Jasminum grandiflorum/officinale*)

Antispasmodic

Slight analgesic effect

Strengthening and calming

Reduces anxiety and fear and elevates mood

Some women love the aroma of jasmine, and it will assist those women through the discomfort of childbirth. Other women do not like the aroma, so ensure the woman feels comfortable with the fragrance before using it.

CLARY SAGE (*Salvia sclarea*)

This essential oil must not be confused with sage.

Mild analgesic

Helps respiratory and muscular systems

Thought to facilitate birth; uterine tonic

GERANIUM (*Pelargonium graveolens*)

Circulation stimulating; one of the best circulatory oils — and if the circulation is good, breathing will be easier.

Good for the uterus and endometrium

Contractive effect — may pull dilated tissues together, so excellent for after the birth

Good for the whole female reproductive system

Antidepressant, known for its uplifting effects

MASSAGE

Being massaged during labor helps relieve the pain and discomfort a woman will experience. Massage over the whole back during the onset of labor, and as the labor pains increase concentrate on the lower back to the crease of the bottom. Some women find massage of the buttocks and back of the legs helps with the more intensely painful contractions. The pressure used will depend on the woman — some women like deep pressure; others, light gentle massage.

DELIVERY ROOM MASSAGE BLEND

Spearmint	1 drop
Marjoram, sweet	2 drops
Plai	2 drops
Immortelle	2 drops
Lavender	2 drops
Chamomile roman	1 drop
Clary sage	2 drops

Blend the essential oils together to create a synergistic blend. Then dilute into 2 tablespoons (30 mL) of carrier oil.

Foot Massage

Many women find that a foot massage is relaxing. Take a small amount of your prepared back massage oil and use that in a foot massage. This is very useful for women who don't want their torso being touched during labor.

INHALATION

Essential oils or blends can be dropped onto a tissue and inhaled as needed. Many facilities allow diffusers in the labor room. They won't allow the candle type and may object to electrical ones, so look for a different type of diffuser — possibly using simple blotting paper. Ask about this at the facility when you make a predelivery visit. The most simple diffusion method involves putting the essential oils on tissues and spreading them around the room. I doubt anyone will object to that — especially as the aromas you'll be using are so delightful. The cold vaporizers designed for clinic use are inappropriate in the delivery room.

HYDROLAT BODY SPRAYS

Body sprays are ideal at this time, as are cooling face sprays. Use the water method to make your own floral water, or use a hydrolat or a blend of hydrolats. A combination of lavender, spearmint, and lemon hydrolat would be refreshing for a body spray. For the face, a combination of lavender, rose, and orange blossom hydrolat would be a good choice, and these could be used on their own as well. Clearly, when using a spray on the face, close your eyes.

Postnatal Care

Now it's time to really enjoy yourself and the baby. The essential oils are ideal to use after the birth, not only because of their excellent antibiotic, antiseptic, and disinfectant properties but because they are emotionally and spiritually uplifting. You can't use every essential oil at this time because you're still very delicate, but among those recommended here there's something for every mother to enjoy pampering herself with — in the knowledge that she's doing herself good at the same time! All those below can be used in a bath (4 drops), incorporated into a body oil (a total of 20 drops per 2 tablespoons, 30 mL, of carrier oil), or used in any of the room methods. If you shower rather than bathe, simply put 1 drop of essential oil on your facecloth after you have finished washing yourself and wipe it over your body.

POSTNATAL ESSENTIAL OILS

Rose maroc (*Rosa centifolia*)
Jasmine (*Jasminum grandiflorum / officinale*)
Neroli (*Citrus aurantium*)
Chamomile roman (*Anthemis nobilis*)
Ylang ylang (*Cananga odorata*)
Mandarin (*Citrus reticulata*)
Lavender (*Lavandula angustifolia*)
Frankincense (*Boswellia carterii*)
Rose otto (*Rosa damascena*)
Myrrh (*Commiphora myrrha*)
Clary sage (*Salvia sclarea*)
Patchouli (*Pogostemon cablin*)
Geranium (*Pelargonium graveolens*)
Sandalwood (*Santalum album*)
Ho wood (*Cinnamomum camphora ct. linalool*)
Grapefruit (*Citrus paradisi*)
Lemon (*Citrus limon*)
Bergamot (*Citrus bergamia*)
Cardamom (*Elettaria cardamomum*)
Cedarwood atlas (*Cedrus atlantica*)
Immortelle (*Helichrysum italicum*)

INFECTION

Infections after birth are fairly common, and, as usual, nature has provided help for that event. This can be seen in action throughout the world, as mothers apply a little colostrum — the food that comes from the breast for the first couple of days — to any infection the baby may have. Colostrum is packed with antibodies that give resistance to infections, which is why it proves to be such a remarkable remedy for all sorts of ailments.

After the birth it's important to keep the whole genital area clean and free from infection. A saline wash (salt and water mix) is excellent for this purpose:

Postnatal Saline Wash

Salt	4 tablespoons
Lavender	4 drops
Chamomile roman (or chamomile german)	2 drops
Tea tree	1 drop

Add the essential oils and salt together, and store in a small clean jar. Add 1 teaspoon of the mix to the water you use to wash the genital area — use a bowl or bidet, swishing the water around to make sure there are no globules of essential oils on the surface before lowering yourself into the water. For some women, this simple procedure ensures a chemical-free genital wash that is effective in both keeping infection away and facilitating healing.

If you do have an infection in the vagina or cervix following delivery, you could use one of the suggestions below, and either blend could be used alongside any medication being given. Put 3 drops in 2 tablespoons of salt and then add the whole mixture to a bowl of warm water, or to a bidet. Swish the water around well to disperse any essential oil globules — if any remain, remove them with a paper towel before lowering your bottom into the water. Repeat three times a day. Ensure that your genital area remains submerged in the warm water for three minutes to allow the essential oils to do their job. First, choose which of the blends you are going to make, and bottle it for future use:

Blend for Infections 1

Lavender	20 drops
Tea tree	5 drops
Chamomile roman (or chamomile german)	10 drops

Blend for Infections 2

Lavender	20 drops
Fragonia	10 drops
Chamomile german	5 drops

Your chosen blend of essential oils is worth making up in some quantity because it'll be very useful to treat all manner of possible minor infections. Blend the essential oils in a clean, brown glass bottle that has a dropper for easy measurement, and store in a dry, cool place. Never use this blend neat in any bodily orifice — mouth, ears, rectum, or vagina.

Minor injuries: For treating cuts, grazes, or open wounds, bathe the area with sterilized gauze that has been soaked in 1 pint (475 mL) of water to which you have added 2 drops of essential oil or blend.

Rashes: Rashes can be treated by mixing 1 drop of essential oil or blend per 2 tablespoons (30 mL) of a natural organic vitamin E cream or aloe vera gel. Mix it well, and use only a small amount.

Recovery: If you've not been healing or recovering from the delivery as quickly as expected, it indicates that your immune system may need nutritional support in the form of a multivitamin or a probiotic supplement. In addition, a body oil can be made by adding 3 drops of your chosen essential oil or blend to 1 teaspoon (5 mL) of carrier oil.

Uterine infection: If you've contracted an infection of the uterus, make a body oil using 5 drops of your chosen infection blend in 1 teaspoon (5 mL) of carrier oil, and massage over your stomach and lower back.

CARE OF THE BREASTS

Breast and nipple care becomes very important after a birth for the comfort and well-being of the mother. Cracked nipples are a fairly common problem and surprisingly painful. This reason alone would warrant taking good care of them, but the possibility of subsequent infection makes it vital. Whatever you put on the nipples to alleviate the pain of cracking or soreness, wash it off before you put your baby to the breast.

Nipple Soreness

This is a problem that can affect all new mothers; the symptoms can vary from soreness, swelling, inflammation, and pain to eventually cracking and splitting of the nipples. This is not confined to the act of breast-feeding; it can be uncomfortable throughout the day and night.

To help avoid nipple problems, massage the blend below over the whole nipple and areola area in the weeks prior to giving birth. Also spend some time stimulating the nipples in preparation by rolling them between well-oiled thumb and forefingers.

SORE NIPPLE OIL

Almond (sweet) oil	40 mL
Avocado	20 mL
Jojoba oil	40 mL

Mix the oils listed above together, then add 4 teaspoons (20 mL) of calendula macerated oil.

You can also add calendula macerated oil to vitamin E cream, aloe vera gel, or a natural plant-derived ointment. Add 10 drops of the calendula oil to each teaspoon of your chosen cream or gel, and mix together well.

Nipple and Breast Soreness

Compresses may relieve the soreness for a while. Organic herbal teas can easily be incorporated into compresses. Chamomile, peppermint, spearmint, and lavender teas can all be prepared in a bowl. If you're using fresh herbs, infuse the herb in boiling hot water and leave it to stew for at least three hours, squeezing out the very last drops of plant goodness before putting the infusion through a sieve, then boil the liquid again and leave to cool. Having prepared the liquid, pour some into a large soup plate, soak in this a piece of unbleached cotton muslin or cotton, and place it over the nipple. Use as and when required. Store in the fridge and use within seven days.

To use essential oils, add to 1 pint (475 mL) of boiling water 7 drops of the essential oils of either chamomile german, chamomile roman, or lavender. Two of these oils could be combined — using 3 drops of each. Pour the liquid through an unbleached paper coffee filter, let it cool, and use for a compress, as above.

Special Compress Fusion

The following special fusion is particularly useful and utilizes essential oils with hydrolats. Mix 4 fl. oz. (120 mL) of lavender hydrolat and 2 fl. oz. (60 mL) of peppermint hydrolat in a stainless steel saucepan, bring to a boil, and then remove from heat. Then add 7 drops of lavender, 7 drops of chamomile roman (or chamomile german), 4 drops of geranium, and 3 drops of lemon. Cover tightly with a lid and leave to cool. When cool, filter the blend through an unbleached paper coffee filter or through a piece of unbleached muslin cloth to remove any essential oil globules. Bottle the mixture and keep it in the refrigerator. Use it for the compress method, in the same way as directed above, before applying a soothing cream or gel.

Breast Abscesses

Breast abscesses can occasionally occur before birth but are more usual afterward. The breast becomes hard and painful and feels very hot to the touch; often there's redness and a feeling of pulsation. You should always seek help from your physician with this condition. Whatever treatment the doctor decides to employ, in addition you could use the following blend to help relieve the redness and soreness. The following suggestion could be used alongside any oral medication if your physician approves, but not alongside any other external/topical medicated solutions because the action of one may interfere with the action of the other.

BREAST ABSCESS BLEND

Chamomile german	15 drops
Lavender	10 drops
Eucalyptus radiata	5 drops

First, make up a blend using these proportions. Put 10 drops of the blend into a saucer of warm chamomile tea, to which has been added 2 teaspoons (10 mL) of colloidal silver. Soak a piece of unbleached muslin or cloth in the mixture and place the compress over the breast. Repeat this treatment twice a day for five days only.

If there's still discomfort after this time, prepare a topically applied soothing oil, using the quantities of essential oil above diluted in 4 tablespoons (60 mL) of carrier oil. Gently apply a small amount on the affected breast(s), twice a day, until the condition eases. It is not recommended to breast-feed if you develop a breast abscess. Stop using the blend once the condition has cleared and particularly if you intend to commence breast-feeding. The cabbage-leaf method is also helpful to this condition — please see page 304.

Mastitis

Mastitis is mostly caused by a bacteria that causes symptoms such as a hot, red swelling or a hard lump in the breast. Sometimes, as with any infection, it's accompanied by a fever. There are treatment options; use the information for breast abscess above. Plus, to help relieve the redness and soreness, try an ironed cabbage leaf (see page 304) or applying the juice of organic raw potatoes. However, as this is a bacterial infection I would suggest adding 4 teaspoons (20 mL) of colloidal silver and 5 drops of fragonia (or tea tree) essential oil to the Special Compress Fusion above.

Breast-Feeding

All agree that the best possible start in life for an infant is being breast-fed, if only for the first few days of life, but sometimes this isn't as easy as the mother would wish. With the best will in the world, problems can still occur — including engorged breasts, lack of milk flow, an inverted nipple, breast abscess, a weak mother, or a baby who cannot suck strongly enough to stimulate the flow of milk or who just doesn't want to suckle.

No woman should be made to feel guilty about not breast-feeding a baby when there are other options available. Some new mothers find the whole process uncomfortable and don't like the sensation; for others breast-feeding is just not an option because of ill health, substance addiction, or even work commitments. If you're in good health, expressing your milk does mean that the father or other members of the family can help to care and share in those first months of life.

Whatever the situation, if you decide that feeding by breast is the only option for you and problems do occur, help should be sought. If milk flow is the problem, massaging the breasts is thought to help, although this method cannot solve all breast-feeding problems. The following method can sometimes help if the supply of milk is insufficient for the baby's needs. Using either an organic almond or jojoba oil, massage the breasts in a circular movement: start under the arms, then gently massage under the breast, then in toward the cleavage, then up between the breasts, and continue around the breast in a circular movement, avoiding the nipple. Do this once a day, remembering to wash off the oil before feeding your baby.

Postnatal Boost

Carrying a baby and giving birth is surely the ultimate example of human beings expending their energies to good purpose. But it does take a lot out of the mother. What follows is something for the woman who has been through a lot, has given a lot, and would like to feel a lot better! This is an all-round oil that helps to bring you, physically and emotionally, back to normal:

POSTNATAL LIFT BLEND

Ho wood	6 drops
Bergamot	5 drops
Frankincense	2 drops
Lemon	5 drops
Jasmine	4 drops

First, blend the essential oils together to create a blend. For a body oil, dilute 3–5 drops of the blend to each teaspoon (5 mL) of carrier oil. Or use 2–4 drops in a diffuser or other room method, or use 1 drop on a tissue and sniff whenever needed.

The following blend differs slightly from the previous one and can be used when the mind has "baby brain fog":

POSTNATAL FOG BLEND

Bergamot	10 drops
Rosemary	2 drops
Eucalyptus radiata	2 drops
Lavender	5 drops

Make a blend using these proportions and use in the same way as the Postnatal Lift Blend, above.

These blends are entirely different from those found in the following section on postnatal depression, and are intended for all mothers who feel they need a boost. So if someone wants to give you a treat and you've already got more bunches of flowers than vases to hold them, suggest they give you a bottle of essential oil instead…and maybe you feel you deserve more than one.

POSTNATAL DEPRESSION

Pity the women who had postnatal depression before it was a recognized medical condition. They and their families could find no justification for the feelings of depression that overcame the new mother, often accompanied by rejection of her baby. It must have seemed the height of ingratitude for her to cry and bemoan what was, as we all logically know, a reason for gratitude and profound joy — the birth of a healthy baby. We now know that when a woman sheds the placenta at birth, a massive hormonal change takes place and her body has to make profound adjustments, and this process sometimes doesn't go according to plan.

There are degrees of postnatal depression, ranging from the baby blues, which affects so many women around three days after the birth that it's come to be seen almost as an integral part of giving birth, to postpartum psychosis. Giving birth is not only the most profound chemical change a human body can go through in the space of a few hours, it's also the most profound social change for the mother and will affect every move she makes for the next decade, at least.

There are many pressures after the birth of a child and many causes for concern. As well as the unrelenting demands of the baby itself, there's the unremitting rounds of washing and cleaning, relatives and friends all offering conflicting advice, another child who may feel resentment that their position as baby in the family has now gone, a partner who may feel left out and jealous, single friends zooming off to exciting activities, and images of the perfect and happy mother in a thousand advertisements. And as if this weren't enough, there may be the background fear that something might happen to the baby in its sleep, or that it has some undiagnosed condition nobody knows is in the family gene pool.

Essential oils can redress the balance on the hormonal and emotional levels so that motivation and feelings of self-esteem aren't allowed to get out of balance. Socially, those around you need to recognize the complete change that's taken place in your timetable and give you some time for yourself. You need as much support as you can get from your partner, friends, and family. However, with a little support most new mothers will find they can not only cope but handle the situation with renewed confidence and energy.

Choose your essential oils from the following list: these will make you feel special, calm you down, strengthen your nervous system, and, in their own unique way, lift depression.

GOODBYE BABY BLUES ESSENTIAL OILS
Bergamot (*Citrus bergamia*)
Immortelle (*Helichrysum italicum*)
Neroli (*Citrus aurantium*)
Mandarin (*Citrus reticulata*)
Rose otto (*Rosa damascena*)
Geranium (*Pelargonium graveolens*)
Clary sage (*Salvia sclarea*)
Rose absolute (*Rosa centifolia*)
Grapefruit (*Citrus paradisi*)
Orange, sweet (*Citrus sinensis*)
Lemon (*Citrus limon*)
Ylang ylang (*Cananga odorata*)

You can use any of the essential oils above on their own or in any combination: between 20 and 30 drops in 2 tablespoons (30 mL) of carrier oil for a body oil — use a small amount each time; up to 2–4 drops in a room diffuser; or 3–6 drops in a bath diluted in 1 teaspoon (5 mL) of carrier oil.

If you feel in need of a real lift, give yourself some time of total indulgence every couple of days. Ask your partner to babysit, remembering that they too need time to form a close bond with the baby. Choose one of the single oils above or one of the following blends. If you have a bath, retire to the bathroom and shut the door. Run the bath and put in up to 6 drops of your chosen oil or blend of oils, diluted in a little skin-nourishing carrier oil. Agitate the water with your hand to disperse any essential oil globules, lower yourself into the water, and breathe deeply to inhale the aroma. If you use a shower, wash as usual and then put 2 drops of essential oil onto a wet washcloth and wipe it over yourself, avoiding the genital area, and then let the water run over you. The combination of water and aroma creates a calming, healing effect.

Retreat to your bedroom and, taking your time, rub the body oil into your body, concentrating on the tummy, from breast to pubic line. Breathe deeply as you apply the oil and do some gentle stretching exercises. Stroll about doing nothing in particular, painting your nails or whatever you want to do — even if it's just lying back on the bed and listening to music. Try to ignore all the sounds coming from the other room, without feeling guilty about leaving your baby in the hands of your partner. You're not asking for too much: you're trying to preserve your sanity for the benefit of the whole family, and it's surprising how just a little time of cushioned indulgence with the essential oils can strengthen and revitalize you.

Banish the Baby Blues Blends

BLEND 1

Geranium	5 drops
Neroli	10 drops
Grapefruit	15 drops

BLEND 2

Bergamot	10 drops
Rose absolute	2 drops
Clary sage	5 drops

BLEND 3

Neroli	6 drops
Petitgrain	4 drops
Orange, sweet	8 drops

BLEND 4

Jasmine	5 drops
Geranium	8 drops
Bergamot	6 drops

BLEND 5

Grapefruit	10 drops
Geranium	10 drops
Mandarin	5 drops

BLEND 6

Geranium	8 drops
Lavender	5 drops
Spearmint	5 drops
Lemon	7 drops

Mix your chosen blend of essential oils beforehand in a clean brown or blue glass bottle using the proportions shown. From this bottle, use 3–5 drops per teaspoon of carrier oil when making a body oil. Use up to 6 drops in a bath. Use up to 8 drops in a room diffuser, or put 1 or 2 drops on a tissue and inhale whenever needed. You can also make a blend yourself by using a combination of oils on the "Goodbye Baby Blues" list on page 239. Some women find help by simply using one essential oil — choose an oil from the list that you really like and that makes you feel relaxed and at ease.

9

The Natural Choice for Men

In this chapter you'll find sections on exhaustion, androgen decline in the aging male (ADAM), sexual vigor, infertility, the reproductive system, certain conditions that seem to affect men more, hair loss, and shaving. There are many other subjects of special interest to men's health, and they can be found throughout this book. In particular refer to chapter 4, "Occupational Oils for the Working Man and Woman"; chapter 5, "Emotional Rescue"; chapter 10, "Essential Help in the Maturing Years"; chapter 11, "Assertive Oils for Sports, Dance, and Exercise"; and chapter 12, "Major Health Concerns."

Exhaustion

The human male is socially conditioned to ignore biological signs that protect him from stress and illness. All too often the fatigue that warns him against going on any further and protects him from exhaustion is pushed aside heroically, or it may be that a sense of duty or the circumstances of his responsibilities prevent him from taking heed of the warnings. Whatever the reason, pushing yourself beyond the limits of healthy fatigue over a period of time leads to the gradual breakdown of bodily systems and mental health.

Having body and mind awareness is being able to chart the difference between extending ourselves and overextending ourselves. The problem with this whole subject is that once we've become exhausted it is difficult to recognize that things have gone too far. We blame the escalated problems, frayed tempers, and fractured relationships on other things.

You can be pretty sure you're heading for trouble when you find you have no reserves for unexpected situations. Even something as simple as the phone ringing — again — can seem like a huge aggravation. Your goodwill seems to be wearing very thin indeed, but you may experience it as a feeling that the world is full of idiots and incompetents. Some men get into the state of being unable to distinguish between what's good for them and what's bad for them, and this sensation of turning in circles and getting giddy brings an unnerving sense of lack of control. A common sign that things are not as they should be comes when your partner asks you to mow the lawn and you think that they've just asked you to climb Mount Everest. Every little molehill has become a mountain. You feel that your partner, by asking you to do these insurmountable tasks, is picking at your self-esteem. Naturally, this causes more friction in the family unit, arguments become commonplace, sleep becomes impossible, sexual relations dwindle, and separation may seem inevitable. "You're impossible to live with," says your partner; "My partner doesn't understand me," you say.

A crucial factor in this scenario is the pressure imposed by society on men always to be able to handle life's problems. Employment brings enormous pressures, but not as great as those that result from being unemployed. Mental ill-health is greatest among the unemployed, and those who drink heavily are far more likely to find themselves on the psychiatrist's couch than those who do not.

Denying that problems exist is a common practice among men, to the extent that men are less likely to seek professional help for mental and emotional problems from a counselor, or for physical problems from a doctor. But what results from all this is a commonly felt sense of profound isolation among men, and that shows up in the high statistics of male suicide.

Maybe the pressure on men to cope with life and present a tough exterior to the world is the very thing that's causing their demise. And for every man that cannot take any more, there are thousands who silently put up with a wide range of problems that are actually exacerbating their stress and potential physical collapse.

This is why it's important to be honest with yourself. Do you sometimes feel anxiety, rage, and despair? Are you tired of trying to succeed, tired of feeling responsible for providing for the family, tired of younger people being promoted over you, tired of watching other people accumulate wealth, tired of feeling like a loser, tired of trying to maintain success, tired of your job, or tired of looking for a job — just tired, tired, tired?

Mental and physical exhaustion manifests itself in a myriad of different ways. Common manifestations are angina pectoris, high blood pressure, low blood pressure, fluid retention, ulcers, bowel disorders, breathing problems, hyperventilation, and inexplicable pains. Medications that are often prescribed in these situations may not provide an answer to the fundamental problem — exhaustion; of far more use is the awareness needed to recognize the symptoms for what they are. Looking at how family and friends react to you is also helpful. If they jump out of the window every time you enter the room, you know that it may be time to slow down. Pushing yourself beyond the limit to get the house painted over the weekends is all very commendable, but is it worth it if it makes you so grumpy that nobody dares talk to you? And think about that pain you have in the leg or back — it may have more to do with sheer exhaustion than rheumatic problems.

Relaxation is the key word, but without help it is easier said than done. For someone in an exhausted state massage provides a particularly good way of relaxing, although it may take three or more sessions for relaxation to be complete. Using essential oils could help the body to cope, which in turn may enable an exhausted person to sleep better so reserves of energy can be put back. A rested person is also better able to deal with emotional situations and can avoid the dramatic emotional swings characteristic of the exhausted state. Recovering from exhaustion takes two distinct steps, and these are the oils for that First Step:

First-Step Essential Oils to Use for Exhaustion

Vetiver (*Vetiveria zizanoides*)
Marjoram, sweet (*Origanum majorana*)
Frankincense (*Boswellia carterii*)
Lavender (*Lavandula angustifolia*)
Bergamot (*Citrus bergamia*)
Melissa (*Melissa officinalis*)
Chamomile roman (*Anthemis nobilis*)
Benzoin (*Styrax benzoin*)
Clary sage (*Salvia sclarea*)

Valerian (*Valeriana officinalis*)
Cedarwood atlas (*Cedrus atlantica*)
Pine (*Pinus sylvestris*)
Neroli (*Citrus aurantium*)

FIRST-STEP EXHAUSTION BODY BLEND

Vetiver	3 drops
Frankincense	5 drops
Bergamot	5 drops
Marjoram, sweet	8 drops
Clary sage	5 drops
Chamomile roman	2 drops
Valerian	2 drops

Blend the essential oils together to create a synergistic blend, then dilute by mixing 3–5 drops to each teaspoon (5 mL) of carrier oil.

Initially, exhaustion is not overcome by stimulating an already overstimulated body, so we start with oils that calm and relax. It's a process of deprogramming, so it will take time — don't expect miracles overnight. Use the blend above, or make your own from the selection of oils above, and apply over your solar plexus and over as much of the back as you can reach, every night. If someone else can do this for you, all the better. When you're sleeping well and find that you can forget about the list of things you have to do, move on to the Second Step.

SECOND-STEP ESSENTIAL OILS TO USE FOR EXHAUSTION

Lavender (*Lavandula angustifolia*)
Black pepper (*Piper nigrum*)
Rosemary (*Rosmarinus officinalis*)
Petitgrain (*Citrus aurantium*)
Basil linalol (*Ocimum basilicum ct. linalool*)
Lemon (*Citrus limon*)
Ginger (*Zingiber officinale*)
Lime (*Citrus aurantifolia*)
Sandalwood (*Santalum album*)
Grapefruit (*Citrus paradisi*)

Immortelle (*Helichrysum italicum*)
Bay laurel (*Laurus nobilis*)
Myrtle (*Myrtus communis*)
Niaouli (*Melaleuca quinquenervia*)

SECOND-STEP EXHAUSTION BODY BLEND

Lemon	6 drops
Black pepper	2 drops
Ginger	2 drops
Rosemary	10 drops
Basil linalol	8 drops
Lavender	2 drops

Blend the essential oils together to create a synergistic blend, then dilute 3–5 drops per each teaspoon (5 mL) of carrier oil. Use the Second-Step Blend, or make up one of your own using the Second-Step list of essential oils. Use this oil in the mornings, applying over your solar plexus area and as over much of the back as you can reach. Continue to use the First-Step body oil in the evenings, leaving it on overnight.

Androgen Decline in the Aging Male (ADAM)

Men in their 30s or 40s can have androgen decline in the aging male, or ADAM, although it's usually associated with men in their 50s or older. This is a relatively recently recognized condition, so much so that it goes by a variety of names, including *male climacteric andropause*, or simply *andropause*. If that sounds a bit like *menopause*, that's because it's likewise related to a decrease in sex hormones. In men, the decline does not come with an obvious physical symptom such as women experience when their menstruation stops, but the decline is slow, occurring over a period of years. The changes may be imperceptible, yet a man reaches a point when he realizes he's no longer the man he was.

Symptoms can be general, such as muscle and joint pain and just feeling unwell for no apparent reason, gaining weight, and feeling tired or even exhausted yet having difficulty sleeping. A man might find his beard growing less, have night sweats, or develop "man boobs." There could be emotional problems such as depression, anxiety, nervousness, or irritability. But the symptoms that make most men sit up and notice something is wrong is when they no longer have as many erections in the morning, have difficulty in achieving an erection during sex, produce less ejaculate, or are just not interested in sex at all.

All these symptoms might be interpreted as a midlife crisis, and a man may take the lack of sexual interest as a problem with his home life, rather than a problem with himself. Many men might have left a loving relationship in the hope that a younger partner could rekindle his sexual fire when, all the time, ADAM was the source of the problem.

The cause of this condition is still very much a topic of debate. The simple idea is that men lose the levels of testosterone being produced. But men with the above symptoms might have normal levels of this male hormone, while, conversely, men with low levels of testosterone have none of the symptoms. This hasn't stopped the market in testosterone replacement therapy products, including patches, gel, gum, injections, and implants.

To some extent, the symptoms of ADAM could be caused by other factors that need addressing, such as being overweight, or drinking too much alcohol, or taking certain medications. Diabetes is linked to ADAM, as is having had infections or inflammation of the testicles, prostate, or urinary tract. In other words, treating ADAM is not always a simple case of being given the "he-hormone." A true deficiency in serum testosterone levels is associated with a condition called *late-onset hypogonadism*, which is a biochemical syndrome quite different than what many are calling "the male menopause."

The following essential oils can be used to help ease specific symptoms, in all the usual methods, following the "Methods of Use" guidelines on page 14:

Anxiety: bergamot, lavender, sweet marjoram, basil linalol, lemon

Anguish: clary sage, lavender, cistus, geranium, grapefruit

Grumpiness and irritability: lavender, chamomile maroc, chamomile roman, davana, clary sage, geranium

Mood swings: geranium, sweet orange, rosemary, sandalwood, rose, ylang ylang

Depression: bergamot, geranium, neroli, cedarwood atlas, patchouli, sandalwood, cistus

Memory and concentration: lemon, rosemary, pine, eucalyptus lemon, peppermint

Fatigue: rosemary, peppermint, spearmint, grapefruit, cypress, pine, cistus

Sleeplessness: sweet orange, lavender, valerian, nutmeg, vetiver, spikenard

Unexplained aches and pain: sweet marjoram, peppermint, ginger, plai, clove bud, immortelle

Sudden sweats: cypress, rosewood, juniper berry, peppermint, lime, fragonia

Sexual Vigor

Since time began, and all over the world, men have been concerned with enhancing their sexual vigor, and probably since time began, men have been utilizing natural plant products to address that problem. The following blend is a massage oil that you apply on the lower back, down just into the crease of the buttocks but not as far as the anus, and also on the upper thigh but avoiding the genital area:

MEN'S VIGOR BLEND

Ginger (*Zingiber officinale*)	2 drops
Black pepper (*Piper nigrum*)	2 drops
Cardamom (*Elettaria cardamomum*)	2 drops
Damiana (*Turnera diffusa*)	2 drops

Blend these quantities into 1 tablespoon (15 mL) of carrier oil, and use as much as required to cover the area described above, once a day. Use for two weeks, break for two weeks, and resume if required.

Potency problems can be associated with medications, so if you're taking any, speak to your physician about this subject. Natural products that are said to aid sexual vigor include ginseng root (*Panax ginseng*), Peruvian ginseng or maca root (*Lepidium meyenii*), catuaba bark (*Erythroxylum catuab*), the shrub-like tree huanarpo macho (*Jatropha macrantha*), the bark of the pine pycnogenol (*Pinus pinaster*), yohimbe bark (*Pausinystalia yohimbe*), and ginkgo. Also being used to enhance male sexual vigor is carnitine — an amino acid — particularly two forms in combination: propionyl-L-carnitine and acetyl-L-carnitine. Another amino acid used for this purpose is L-arginine, but this should be avoided if you have or have had cardiac problems.

It can be hard to hold back during the throes of passion, and the following blend may address that problem. Make up the Holding Back Blend and rub it over your abdomen — avoiding the genital area — before having sex. Do not make the mistake of thinking the blend will be more effective if you use more essential oils. Use these quantities; they are perfectly adequate.

HOLDING BACK BLEND

Clary sage (*Salvia sclarea*)	2 drops
Davana (*Artemisia pallens*)	2 drops
Vetiver (*Vetiveria zizanoides*)	2 drops

Dilute in 2 teaspoons (10 mL) of carrier oil, and use a small amount each time.

Infertility

Sperm are the smallest cells in the human body, and they're vulnerable to the heat generated by a laptop and the radio-frequency electromagnetic radiation (RF-EMR) emitted by mobile phones. There's been a great deal of debate over the years about the dangers of electronic devices to sperm, but the argument now seems to have come down on the side of caution, with an 8% drop in male fertility being attributed to them. It's not so much the concentration of sperm — the number of them — that's at risk, but their viability and motility — their ability to get to their goal. Given what we know, routinely carrying a phone around in the pants pocket seems unwise, as this is as close to sperm as a phone can get.

Another hazard for male fertility comes in the form of xenoestrogens, a group of chemicals used in industry and now widely dispersed in the environment. Xenoestrogens leach from plastic and find their way into the water supply. They're everywhere, and this may explain why male fertility is decreasing all over the world — and that's true for animals, as well as for men. These endocrine-disrupting compounds are causing worldwide concern. For an individual man, this just illustrates that the potential for fertility has to be protected more than ever before. We all love our devices, but when researchers put sperm into pots next to laptops, it took just four hours for them to become damaged. It's worth remembering that when you're sitting with a tablet on your lap searching for solutions to male infertility!

Essential oils can't directly address the problems associated with male sperm viability and motility. However, there may be an underlying condition that's not been diagnosed for which essential oils are effective, and that may be why some people believe they do have a positive effect on male fertility.

MALE INFERTILITY ESSENTIAL OILS
Sandalwood (*Santalum album*)
Rosewood (*Aniba rosaeodora*)
Patchouli (*Pogostemon cablin*)
Chamomile german (*Matricaria recutita*)
Damiana (*Turnera diffusa*)
Cardamom (*Elettaria cardamomum*)
Geranium (*Pelargonium graveolens*)
Cedarwood atlas (*Cedrus atlantica*)
Frankincense (*Boswellia carterii*)
Palmarosa (*Cymbopogon martinii*)
Clary sage (*Salvia sclarea*)
Sage, Greek (*Salvia fruticosa/triloba*)
Angelica seed (*Angelica archangelica*)
Basil linalol (*Ocimum basilicum ct. linalool*)

Choose a single oil from the list above, or make a blend that both you and your partner enjoy. Use 5 drops in each teaspoon (5 mL) of carrier oil to make a body oil, which is applied in a very specific area: the upper and lower abdominal muscles, the pelvis, the lower back area where the nerves to the gonads lie in the vertebrae (lumbar regions 3 and 4) — just into the crease of the buttocks but not as far as the anus. Be careful to avoid the genital area. The oils can also be used diluted in baths, 2–4 drops, or in showers, 1 or 2 drops on a washcloth after washing, rubbed on the body while avoiding the genital region. Carry on using the essential oils in your daily routine for 3–6 months to see if they have been effective.

The Reproductive System

The male genital system is a complex production and delivery network that consists of many parts. As well as the penis and scrotum, there are the testes, prostate gland, seminal vesicles, vas deferens, and urethra, all connected by a system of tubes. The interrelationship between the parts of the whole means that a problem in any one system can cause problems elsewhere, and can even lead to relationship difficulties. Having an awareness of potential trouble spots within the network is important to ensure a smoothly running system. One such spot is the testicles, because testicular cancer is the most common cancer in young men and it's on the increase. The two testicles are often slightly different in size, but when one begins to change in relation to the other, or its consistency changes, or you feel a hard lump or nodule, it is time to visit your physician. Swelling can be painless and quite generalized, and the testicle may feel numb or slightly numb. Other symptoms are back pain, dull aches in the lower abdomen or groin, tenderness, a wart-type growth on the foreskin or glans, a pus discharge, blood passed in urine, pain on urinating, or the need to pass urine frequently. All men should make a point of checking for any changes in their testicles once a month. Do this in the bath while the supporting muscles are relaxed, by rolling each testicle in turn between the thumbs and fingers of both hands.

Many of the symptoms listed above could relate to all sorts of other conditions, and it goes without saying that anything unusual should be checked by your physician.

PAINS AND SORES

Any pain or sores on the penis must be seen by a medical practitioner. Don't ignore them. Pain can mean kidney, bladder, or prostate disorders. Sores can be caused by sexually transmitted diseases, gout, diabetes, and lack of hygiene. Cleaning with salt and essential oil every day will help to relieve soreness and heal sores. Washing around the genitals is important for health and relationship happiness alike. Washing well under the foreskin with soap and water, enhanced by the antibacterial and antiviral properties of the essential oils, can be helpful in combating genital smell and infection.

SOOTHING BATHING SOLUTION

Lavender   5 drops
Natural rock salt   1 teaspoon

Put the essential oil into the salt before adding to 1 pint (475 mL) of warm water, stirring thoroughly to disperse any globules of essential oil. Use the solution to wash the genital area, avoiding the penile gland.

ESSENTIAL OILS FOR THE MALE

When using the essential oils from the lists below, mix 2 drops in a little carrier oil before adding to a bowl containing a pint (475 mL) of warm water. Agitate the water to disperse the oil as much as possible, then wash your penis and scrotum in the water. Use only the essential oils listed below, which are grouped into various therapeutic roles.

Infection

Tea tree (*Melaleuca alternifolia*)
Niaouli (*Melaleuca quinquenervia*)
Lavender (*Lavandula angustifolia*)
Patchouli (*Pogostemon cablin*)
Fragonia (*Agonis fragrans*)
Thyme linalol (*Thymus vulgaris ct. linalool*)
Manuka (*Leptospermum scoparium*)

Inflammation

Chamomile german (*Matricaria recutita*)
Lavender (*Lavandula angustifolia*)
Chamomile roman (*Anthemis nobilis*)
Eucalyptus radiata (*Eucalyptus radiata*)

Swelling

Cypress (*Cupressus sempervirens*)
Lavender (*Lavandula angustifolia*)
Juniper berry (*Juniperus communis*)
Chamomile german (*Matricaria recutita*)
Chamomile roman (*Anthemis nobilis*)

Niaouli (*Melaleuca quinquenervia*)
Immortelle (*Helichrysum italicum*)
Rosemary (*Rosmarinus officinalis*)

ABRASIONS

The delicate mucous membrane of the penis can suffer minor abrasions, or the foreskin can split, either of which may lead to infections. Treatment with essential oils can be effective — the antibacterial properties of lavender help to avoid infection while encouraging healing:

FOR MINOR ABRASIONS OF THE PENIS

Lavender   3 drops

Add to a bowl of warm water, agitate the water to disperse any essential oil globules, and wash twice daily until healed.

INFLAMMATION

Never be tempted to use neat essential oil to speed up the process of reducing swelling — the essential oils must be diluted as directed. Here are two methods of treating an inflamed, swollen testicle:

ANTI-INFLAMMATORY 1 FOR SWOLLEN TESTICLES

Chamomile german   6 drops

Use in a sitz bath. Or add to 1 pint (475 mL) of cold water for sponging.

ANTI-INFLAMMATORY 2 FOR SWOLLEN TESTICLES

Chamomile roman *or*
   chamomile german   10 drops
Lavender   10 drops

Blend together, and dilute 2 drops in 1 teaspoon (5 mL) of jojoba oil or centella oil (*Centella asiatica*). Mix again well and, from this, use just enough to cover the testicle, each time you apply the oil.

COOLING BLEND FOR PENIS AND TESTICLES

Chamomile roman
Chamomile german

Using either oil singly, or both in combination. Add a total of 4 drops to ½ pint (240 mL) of water and mix well. Apply with a washcloth or sponge.

Or

Use 2 drops of either oil, mixed with 1 drop of lavender, in ½ pint (240 mL) of water, and mix well. Apply with a washcloth or sponge.

BALANITIS

This is an inflammation of the penile glans. It can cause a burning sensation when urine is passed. As with any condition with symptoms of this sort, a diagnosis must be sought from your physician to rule out the possibility of sexually transmitted disease. Self-help involves bathing the area twice a day.

BALANITIS BLEND

Lavender	3 drops
Chamomile german	2 drops

Add the essential oils to a pint (475 mL) of warm water to which 2 teaspoons (10 g) of rock salt or sea salt has been added. Agitate the water with your hand to disperse any globules of essential oil.

HYDROCELES

Fluid that gathers in the layers of tissue around a testicle is often harmless and painless, but it can cause swelling and discomfort. Hydroceles are often caused by an inguinal hernia, which may require surgery. When the fluid is simply drawn off, the problem may reoccur. Another cause of hydrocele is injury to the testicle.

Gentle massage may help to reduce the fluid: massage around the lower abdomen and the swollen testicle, once a day, for 15 days. There are two blends to choose from:

HYDROCELE BLEND 1

Juniper berry	10 drops
Niaouli	5 drops
Lemon	10 drops
Immortelle	5 drops

HYDROCELE BLEND 2

Juniper berry	5 drops
Cypress	10 drops
Lavender	10 drops

Blend the essential oils together. Then dilute by mixing 2–3 drops in 1 teaspoon (5 mL) of carrier oil.

ORCHITIS

Orchitis is an inflammation of the testes. It can be a complication of mumps and can occur at any age. Symptoms are painful swelling of the testes, fever, and pain when passing urine. The following treatment is in two parts, body massage and testicle massage, using two different oils, twice a day:

ORCHITIS BODY OIL

Chamomile german	5 drops
Geranium	5 drops
Lemon	10 drops
Ho wood	2 drops
Thyme linalol	3 drops

Blend the essential oils together, then dilute by mixing 3–5 drops in each teaspoon (5 mL) of carrier oil. Apply over the lower back and lower abdomen twice a day.

ORCHITIS TESTICLE OIL

Lavender	10 drops
Chamomile german	10 drops
Cypress	5 drops
Palmarosa	5 drops

Blend the essential oils together, then dilute by mixing 2–3 drops to each teaspoon (5 mL) of carrier oil. Apply a small amount over the affected area.

PROSTATITIS

There are many causes of an inflamed prostate gland, including prostatitis — which can be chronic or acute. Symptoms are pain, burning sensation when passing urine, lower abdominal pain, heaviness, the inability to retain urine, frequent urination, fever, and a general feeling of tiredness and lethargy. It can occur at any time and is most uncomfortable.

Apply around the lower abdominal area, over the lower back, and around the upper buttock area with the following blend. Use a small amount, as needed, to a maximum of three times a day:

PROSTATITIS BODY OIL

Lavender	5 drops
Cypress	5 drops
Eucalyptus radiata	5 drops
Geranium	3 drops
Niaouli	3 drops
Tea tree	3 drops
Chamomile german	2 drops
Thyme linalol	4 drops

Blend the essential oils together to create a synergistic blend, then dilute by mixing 3–5 drops in each teaspoon (5 mL) of carrier oil.

INTERTRIGO

Soreness and inflammation can affect skin that's in contact with another skin surface, especially in a damp, sweaty area such as around the groin. If the skin doesn't have a chance to breathe or dry, intertrigo can be initiated by a bacterial, viral, or fungal infection, although it can also be caused by vitamin B6 deficiency. The skin can take on a disagreeable appearance and odor. Intertrigo can be a consequence of obesity, and of incontinence in the elderly.

Bathe the affected areas with the following wash twice a day for one week:

INTERTRIGO BLEND

Lavender	5 drops
Eucalyptus lemon	10 drops

Add the essential oils to 2½ cups (600 mL) of water, and use about 3½ fl. oz. (100 mL) each time.

Also prepare the following body powder using a natural, finely powdered white clay. Mix the ingredients thoroughly, in a blender if available, being careful not to inhale. Dust a small amount over the area after washing and drying:

INTERTRIGO POWDER

White clay/kaolin (powdered)	4 oz.
Lavender	10 drops
Rosemary	10 drops
Chamomile german	10 drops

VARICOCELE

A varicocele is a varicose swelling of a vein leading from the testicle, usually on the left side for anatomical reasons. The soft swelling is usually harmless and often painless, but it can ache, especially after standing for long periods.

Massage around the lower abdomen and the lower back just above the crease of the buttocks (sacrum area) daily with the following:

VARICOCELE BODY BLEND 1

Geranium	15 drops
Cypress	10 drops
Chamomile roman	5 drops

Blend the essential oils, then dilute by mixing 3–5 drops to each teaspoon (5 mL) of carrier oil.

Also, the ice-cup method could be applied (see page 303) to the swelling once a day, and then gently massage the area with the following:

VARICOCELE BODY BLEND 2
Chamomile roman   2 drops
Cypress   3 drops
Dilute in 1 teaspoon (5 mL) of evening primrose seed oil or jojoba oil. This quantity is enough for two applications.

Other Problems

FOOT ODOR

Having feet that smell less than sweet is by no means an entirely male condition, but men do seem more prone to it. This embarrassing and inhibiting problem can be caused by a number of fungal disorders. And if a fungal infection is your problem, add 2 drops of tea tree essential oil to the foot powder blend below:

FOOT ODOR POWDER
Baking powder   1 tablespoon
Peppermint   1 drop
Pine, Scots (or Greek sage
    or rosemary)   2 drops
Put the baking powder in a plastic bag, add the peppermint and your additional choice of essential oil, and shake the bag well. Allow to dry, and separate the mixture by running a rolling pin over the bag.

Add a zinc supplement to the daily diet, as this can help enormously. Bathing the feet in a bowl of water with 2 drops of either Greek sage, manuka, palmarosa, or tea tree essential oil, every day for a week, will help too. Dust the feet regularly with the foot powder above and also leave half a teaspoon in your shoes overnight — this will provide good bacterial protection. Tap the powder out in the morning. Change your shoes regularly too.

JOCK ITCH

Jock itch is a problem familiar to men, especially athletes, and it is often caused by wearing tight briefs or jeans. The symptoms are a scaly type of itchy rash, which can become sore. The fungus that causes this infection of the skin, *Tinea cruris*, thrives in a moist area, so the groin area should be kept as clean and dry as possible. Boxer shorts help to keep the air circulating. Oiled skin is also better for keeping the fungus at bay, which is why it features in the two-part treatment below:

JOCK ITCH ESSENTIAL OILS
Lavender (*Lavandula angustifolia*)
Fragonia (*Agonis fragrans*)
Patchouli (*Pogostemon cablin*)
Tea tree (*Melaleuca alternifolia*)
Manuka (*Leptospermum scoparium*)
Dilute 2 drops of any one of the essential oils above in a bowl of water. Wash the area, and dry well. Also, use 2 drops of any one of the essential oils listed, diluted in 1 teaspoon (5 mL) of your chosen carrier oil or centella oil (*Centella asiatica*), and apply to the area morning and night.

CANDIDA/THRUSH

Thrush is often thought of as a woman's problem, but it affects men too and can be passed back and forth during sexual activity. Symptoms include a red rash on the penis or a burning or itching sensation on the tip of the penis. A physician should be consulted, and the recommended medication taken. Thrush is caused by the fungal infection *Candida albicans*, which lives in the bowel or stomach and can infect not only the genitals, mouth, throat, and skin but even the fingernails. Essential oils can be used in baths or in the sponging method. This involves first making up the blend of essential oils, then taking from the blend 4 drops and adding them to a bowl of warm water, and using this to sponge down the genital area.

Three Candida Baths

BLEND 1

Patchouli	6 drops
Palmarosa	2 drops
Immortelle	2 drops

BLEND 2

Fragonia	6 drops
Bergamot	2 drops

BLEND 3

Manuka	1 drop
Patchouli	2 drops
Lavender	2 drops

Blend the essential oils together, then use 4 drops diluted in a small amount of carrier oil in the bath. Alternatively, use 2 drops of the blend, diluted in ½ teaspoon (2½ mL) of carrier oil in a sitz bath.

The following blend can be used in a bath or body oil, or both:

CANDIDA BLEND

Niaouli	5 drops
Patchouli	5 drops
Tea tree	5 drops
Lemon	5 drops
May chang	3 drops
Eucalyptus radiata	5 drops

Mix the essential oils together to create a synergistic blend, which can then be used in two methods. For baths — use 4 drops diluted in a little carrier oil. For a body oil — dilute by mixing 3–5 drops in 1 teaspoon (5 mL) of carrier oil and apply over the abdomen and lower back area: use once a day for a week, giving the body a chance to respond to the treatment.

For suggestions on dietary changes and supplementation in cases of *Candida albicans*, please refer to the section on thrush in chapter 8, "A Woman's Natural Choice" (see page 216).

PRURITUS ANI

Pruritus ani is the medical term for an itchy anus. This can be caused by a multitude of reasons, from the use of certain soaps and detergents or the chemicals in toilet tissue to antibiotics and laxatives. Emotional factors are also thought to play a part, and there is always the possibility of threadworms, which although usually associated with childhood, can easily spread to adults within the household — all of whom will need treatment with medication. The anal area is moist and warm and is an ideal breeding ground for fungi and bacteria, and any such infection can lead to inflammation too. The very act of scratching the anus itself evokes the release of inflammatory chemicals that lead to further itching, and a cycle develops in which there is no end to the problem.

The first step, after ruling out parasitic worms, is to use a hypoallergenic soap when washing the area twice a day, preferably after passing stools, and adding 2 drops of the following blend of oils to the water:

PRURITUS ANI WASHING BLEND

Geranium	5 drops
Lavender	4 drops
Bergamot	3 drops

Also, make a gel to apply directly to the area, using the following ingredients:

Pruritus Ani Gel Blend

Aloe vera gel	1 fl. oz. (30 mL)
Jojoba oil	1 teaspoon (5 mL)
Eucalyptus lemon	3 drops
Chamomile roman	3 drops
Palmarosa	2 drops
Geranium	2 drops

To prepare this gel, first add the essential oils into the jojoba oil and mix in well. Then add the jojoba mixture to the aloe vera gel, mix well again, and store in a sealed jar, which can be kept in the fridge. Use a small amount each time, applied directly to the area around the anus, as needed.

HEMORRHOIDS

While we're in the general area, let's discuss hemorrhoids. This is a problem that seems to affect men more so than women, and it is best treated early on. Start to drink plenty of water and take vitamin E supplements. Many people have reported complete relief of the symptoms after following the method below for 7 to 10 days.

Hemorrhoids Essential Oils

Geranium (*Pelargonium graveolens*)
Cypress (*Cupressus sempervirens*)
Lavender (*Lavandula angustifolia*)
Immortelle (*Helichrysum italicum*)
Lavandin (*Lavandula x intermedia*)
Patchouli (*Pogostemon cablin*)
Niaouli (*Melaleuca quinquenervia*)

Hemorrhoids Blend 1

Cypress	2 drops
Geranium	2 drops
Patchouli	2 drops
Immortelle	4 drops

Hemorrhoids Blend 2

Geranium	2 drops
Cypress	3 drops

Hemorrhoids Blend 3

Lavandin	3 drops
Immortelle	2 drops

Dilute your chosen blend in 1 tablespoon (15 mL) of carrier oil or ½ fl. oz. (15 mL) of aloe vera gel. Use a small amount each time, applying directly to the area around the anus, as needed.

The Liver

The largest internal organ in the human body is the liver, which sits quietly under the diaphragm while carrying out around 500 crucial functions. Because the liver has no pain receptors, other than on the membrane, identifying a problem with it can be difficult. The liver has a remarkable capacity for compensatory growth, which means that healthy cells can increase their cell size or improve their rate of cell division to compensate for damage or loss. This tells us that the body knows how important the liver is, even if we don't.

This section has been put in the chapter for men because the most likely cause of damage to the liver is overconsumption of alcohol, and men are twice as likely to have an alcohol use disorder (AUD) as women. But the consumption of fatty foods also causes the liver no end of difficulty, as does infection, which can lead to inflammation of the liver tissues.

Because the liver is involved in so many important functions, symptoms may appear elsewhere in the body, but when they're tracked back to their source, the liver is often identified. The liver sits behind the ribs, mostly on the right side of the body, so any dull ache in that area can indicate a problem, as can right shoulder pain or even back pain. Jaundice — yellowing of the skin — is a classic sign of problems in the liver, and dark-colored urine or light-colored feces can also indicate a liver-related condition. Less obvious symptoms might be itchy skin or general fatigue.

Every single minute, the liver is taking in around 2½ pints (1.2 liters) of blood and reprocessing it. Some waste products in the blood are converted into helpful elements for use elsewhere, while harmful waste is sent off for excretion. But the liver isn't just a recycling plant. It's more like the most complicated chemical factory imaginable, doing a whole number of vital things all at the same time. It's involved in the metabolism of carbohydrates, proteins, and fats, including cholesterol, and in the process of bone and muscle growth. The liver produces the hormone thrombopoietin, which regulates platelet and blood production; it synthesizes amino acids and glucose; and it stores vitamins A, D, and B12. The liver does more than just clean the blood of toxins. That would be like comparing the liver to a butler who just takes out the rubbish when, in fact, that butler is also building the house we live in, keeping our blood flowing, and basically attending to all our needs while being unassuming, quiet, and efficient.

Alcohol is by far the biggest problem a liver has to deal with, so next time you have a large bourbon and ruminate on how the world puts its troubles on your shoulders, just remember that you're leaning on your liver and that it, ultimately, gets the brunt of the world's problems. This is literally true, because the liver may have to process toxins we take in from the environment, including those we inhale at work. Even certain medications make the liver work harder, and, needless to say, all the junk food we throw into our supermarket cart ends up in some form in the liver. Convenience foods might suit us, but pity the poor liver that will have to clear up the mess.

But there is a lot you can do to help yourself. The first thing is to prevent any further damage to liver health by subjecting it to fewer toxins. Nonorganic red meat, fish, chicken, wheat, and dairy products may all contain traces of chemicals and pollutants used in their growth. So eat plenty of organic raw or steamed vegetables — including dark-green leafy ones such as spinach and kale — whole grains, pulses, nuts, apple cider vinegar, and all fruits except citrus. Pineapple is a good fruit for the liver because it contains bromelain. Drink filtered or bottled water, green tea, ginger and dandelion teas, and fresh carrot juice — which also blends well with apple juice. Take herbal extracts of milk thistle and artichoke, as well as at least 1,000 mg of vitamin C a day and a good multivitamin and mineral supplement.

To help with the elimination of toxins, carry out daily skin brushing using a body brush, always moving in the direction of the heart, take daily showers, saunas whenever possible, and ask a qualified therapist to carry out a lymphatic drainage massage for you. Weekly massage is a great help, and you can do this yourself.

ESSENTIAL OILS FOR LIVER SUPPORT

Chamomile roman (*Anthemis nobilis*)
Chamomile german (*Matricaria recutita*)
Lavender (*Lavandula angustifolia*)
Geranium (*Pelargonium graveolens*)
Cypress (*Cupressus sempervirens*)
Immortelle (*Helichrysum italicum*)
Rosemary (*Rosmarinus officinalis*)
Juniper berry (*Juniperus communis*)
Greenland moss (*Ledum groenlandicum*)
Carrot seed (*Daucus carota*)
Peppermint (*Mentha piperita*)
Cardamom (*Elettaria cardamomum*)
Ginger (*Zingiber officinale*)
Grapefruit (*Citrus paradisi*)
Turmeric (*Curcuma longa*)
Patchouli (*Pogostemon cablin*)

Use the essential oils in the usual ways, referring to the "Methods of Use" section on page 14.

LIVER SUPPORT BLEND 1

Rosemary	5 drops
Juniper berry	4 drops
Chamomile german	3 drops
Cypress	4 drops
Ginger	6 drops
Carrot seed	3 drops
Geranium	5 drops

LIVER SUPPORT BLEND 2

Carrot seed	3 drops
Rosemary	5 drops
Juniper berry	7 drops
Ginger	9 drops
Cypress	2 drops

Mix your chosen essential oil blend together, then dilute 3–5 drops in 1 teaspoon (5 mL) of carrier oil. Apply over the midsection of the body including the abdomen, around the ribs, both sides of the body, and the upper/middle back.

HEPATITIS

Hepatitis is inflammation of the liver cells and can take several forms. Symptoms can seem initially to be very similar to those of the flu. They include muscle ache, headache, nausea, poor appetite, digestive upsets, stool changes, drowsiness, rashes, fever, lack of focus, mental confusion, or just generally feeling unwell. A yellowing of the skin, mucous membrane, and parts of the eye can be indicative that hepatitis has developed.

Viruses cause hepatitis A, B, C, D, and E, but liver inflammation can also come about because of alcohol use, certain medications, industrial toxins, and even autoimmune disease. People contract the hepatitis viruses for a multitude of reasons. A pretty salad washed in contaminated water or unknowingly handled by someone with hepatitis can pass on infection. Dentists and other healthcare professionals come into contact with people with hepatitis. Children may pick up something off the ground that's been contaminated with feces. Water is a potential risk in many countries, and travelers need to be particularly aware of the risks. Ice in drinks is often made from nonbottled water, and the virus can be innocently sipped along with a nice cool drink in the sun. Because so many people with hepatitis are symptom-free and the condition is so contagious, we're all vulnerable. The symptoms of hepatitis can be similar to those of chronic fatigue syndrome (CFS), which emphasizes the need for testing in these cases.

If intending to use essential oils in cases of hepatitis, first inform your physician and take their advice. A clinical aromatherapist may be able to provide essential oil formulations tailored to your particular symptoms.

SUPPORT ESSENTIAL OILS IN CASES OF HEPATITIS

Chamomile german (*Matricaria recutita*)
Thyme linalol (*Thymus vulgaris ct. linalool*)
Tea tree (*Melaleuca alternifolia*)
Chamomile german (*Matricaria recutita*)
Eucalyptus lemon (*Eucalyptus citriodora*)
Eucalyptus radiata (*Eucalyptus radiata*)
Cinnamon leaf (*Cinnamomum zeylanicum*)
Oregano (*Origanum vulgare*)
Patchouli (*Pogostemon cablin*)
Carrot seed (*Daucus carota*)
Cypress (*Cupressus sempervirens*)
Immortelle (*Helichrysum italicum*)
Greenland moss (*Ledum groenlandicum*)
Grapefruit (*Citrus paradisi*)
Ginger (*Zingiber officinalis*)
Peppermint (*Mentha piperita*)

Use the essential oils in baths or body oils. Use the following blend for the first two weeks.

HEPATITIS BATH OR BODY OIL BLEND:
FIRST TWO WEEKS

Chamomile german	5 drops
Greenland moss	5 drops
Oregano	5 drops
Cypress	5 drops
Ginger	3 drops
Grapefruit	4 drops
Manuka	3 drops

First mix the essential oils together to create a synergistic blend. Use 2–3 drops in a bath diluted in a little carrier oil. For a body oil, dilute 3–5 drops per each 1 teaspoon (5 mL) of carrier oil.

HEPATITIS BATH OR BODY OIL BLEND:
FOLLOWING WEEKS

Juniper berry	5 drops
Peppermint	3 drops
Greenland moss	5 drops
Chamomile german	4 drops
Carrot seed	4 drops
Oregano	5 drops
Eucalyptus lemon	4 drops

First mix the essential oils together to create a synergistic blend. Use 2–3 drops in a bath diluted in a little carrier oil. For a body oil, dilute 3–5 drops per each 1 teaspoon (5 mL) of carrier oil.

Other suggestions that may help with the symptoms are extract of milk thistle and artichoke, drinking green tea and fresh carrot juice, sticking with a high-fiber diet, and incorporating apple cider vinegar, a daily probiotic, and a good vitamin and mineral supplement.

Hair Loss

A gradual loss of hair leading to baldness is something many men worry about. It's long been said that bald men have too much testosterone so are probably sexier, and women as a rule don't care as much about their man being bald as the man does. And it's probably no consolation to know that baldness is indeed attributed to high levels of dihydrotestosterone (DHT), a derivative of testosterone. This binds onto hair follicle receptors, causing them to reduce in size and making it more difficult for hair to grow. Surprisingly, perhaps, essential oils do help in some cases and are certainly worth a try. For this treatment the choice of carrier oils is also very important, and recommended oils are listed below the essential oils that could be tried.

HAIR LOSS ESSENTIAL OILS
Rosemary (*Rosmarinus officinalis*)
Sage, Greek (*Salvia fruticosa/triloba*)
Hyssop decumbens (*Hyssopus officinalis var. decumbens*)
Cedarwood atlas (*Cedrus atlantica*)
Lavender (*Lavandula angustifolia*)
Thyme linalol (*Thymus vulgaris ct. linalool*)
Geranium (*Pelargonium graveolens*)
Lemon (*Citrus limon*)
Basil linalol (*Ocimum basilicum ct. linalool*)
Grapefruit (*Citrus paradisi*)
Ginger (*Zingiber officinale*)
Cypress (*Cupressus sempervirens*)
Black pepper (*Piper nigrum*)
Bay laurel (*Laurus nobilis*)

HAIR LOSS CARRIER OILS
Coconut oil (*Cocos nucifera*)
Babassu oil (*Attalea speciosa*)
Sesame oil (*Sesamum indicum*)
Andiroba oil (*Carapa guianensis*)
Argan oil (*Argania spinosa*)
Rice bran oil (*Oryza sativa*)
Jojoba oil (*Simmondsia chinensis*)
Hemp seed oil (*Cannabis sativa*)

This following method may prevent hair from falling out, strengthen and thicken the hair you still have, and in some cases if the hair follicle is still productive, grow new hair. Initially, the hair will be vellus, or downy hair. Premature balding can be lessened by the oils, but don't be impatient — treatment must be continuous, and don't expect to see results for at least four months. However, patience is rewarded with a bonus — while you're following the treatment you may find that you have fewer coughs, colds, and outbreaks of flu. First make your blend of oils, choosing from the blends below. If the first one you try isn't effective, try one of the others.

Hair Loss Blend 1

Rosemary	5 drops
Geranium	6 drops
Lavender	7 drops
Cypress	6 drops
Juniper berry	4 drops

Hair Loss Blend 2

Basil linalol	4 drops
Rosemary	8 drops
Peppermint	2 drops
Elemi	6 drops
Palmarosa	5 drops
Geranium	2 drops

Hair Loss Blend 3

Ginger	5 drops
Black pepper	5 drops
Thyme linalol	5 drops
Rosemary	5 drops
Cedarwood atlas	5 drops

First, mix your chosen blend together and bottle it. Then prepare a second, larger bottle of filtered or mineral water to which you have added 1 drop of essential oil for each 2 teaspoons (10 mL) of water. For example, if the bottle holds 100 mL, add 10 drops of your chosen essential oil blend. Shake this bottle well before each use. Each day, pour 1 teaspoon (5 mL) from this larger water-filled bottle into a saucer, from which you pat the water onto your head, taking care that none goes near the eyes. Apply just a little of the water with each pat so none goes to waste.

On alternate days, starting on day 2, before putting the essential oil water on the head, wrap the head in a hot towel, turban style, and leave it in place for two or three minutes. Remove the towel, and rub the head gently using an ice cup (see page 303). When the scalp is icy cold, apply another hot towel. Repeat this alternate hot and cold procedure for at least five hot and cold cycles. Then apply the essential oil water on the head, and leave it on the scalp overnight.

On the 15th day, combine 2 teaspoons (10 mL) of argan oil with 1 teaspoon (5 mL) of jojoba oil to use as your hair carrier oil. Add 4–5 drops of the essential oil blend to 1 teaspoon (5 mL) of your hair carrier. Massage into the scalp, using as much as needed. For most people, this 1 teaspoon should be enough for two days. Leave the oil on overnight.

When shampooing, use a hypoallergenic shampoo — one that doesn't contain detergent. As a simple measure to strengthen hair, add 1 drop of rosemary oil to a cold-water rinse when you've finished washing your hair. There's no need to rinse the rosemary out — it will give your hair a nice sheen — while the cold water stimulates the blood capillaries, causing them to contract and then dilate, stimulating the movement of nutrients from the blood into the hair follicle.

Shaving

The ancient Roman poet Ovid, who wrote *The Art of Love*, said, "Men should not care too much for good looks; neglect is becoming." Well, maybe women two thousand years ago admired a scruffy man, but today it's another story. We're in a very competitive society, and if stress and fatigue show, the boss might decide you're looking a bit rough and give the promotion to someone else — someone with a bright and clean image. This need not be someone younger because the older man can be very attractive and sexy if he takes care of himself, and facial lines add character. Neglect, on the other hand, shows a lack of care and perhaps laziness, which is never a good thing, especially in the workplace.

Some careers that are traditionally more often taken up by men subject the skin to rigors the rest of us can hardly imagine. Fishermen out on the raging seas are beaten by howling salt-bearing winds; while the heat in the steel mill exerts a drying effect on the skin that's impossible to avoid, and miners emerge from the bowels of the earth covered in grime. On a somewhat less dramatic note, I know that one of the most grueling experiences my skin has had to endure was a day of mixing cement — it was weeks before the dryness and soreness disappeared.

In certain respects male and female skin is the same, but men produce more sebum, which, combined with the 20% additional thickness of their skin, ensures that wrinkles don't come so early. However, the thickness of male skin means that when middle age comes, the wrinkles can be deeper.

Facial hair is of course the major feature distinguishing male from female skin, and the average man will spend approximately 4,000 hours of his life standing in front of the mirror with a shaver in his hand. The sheer inevitability of having to shave every morning has driven most men, at some time in their lives, to the decision to grow a beard or at least a mustache.

Shaving can bring about all kinds of problems to the skin, including cuts, razor burn, razor bumps, irritant contact dermatitis, general irritation, inflammation, rashes, exfoliation, itching,

and lipid barrier compromise. Some men have a problem with ingrown hairs, which are sometimes difficult to manage. Certainly, they don't make shaving any easier, and they can cause an inflammatory response. The skin might have to deal with poor water quality, blunt razor blades, and products containing ingredients that cause a reaction. All these things conspire to make shaving a trial many men endure rather than enjoy.

SHAVING OIL

Shaving oils are becoming more popular because they're generally nonirritating and are far better for skin condition and skin protection, and it's easy to make your own personal customized version. Shaving oils can be used either on their own or under the regular shaving foam or gel to improve the slide of the razor. They may take a bit of getting used to if you've used shaving foam all your adult life, because only 2–3 drops of shaving oil are needed and this doesn't seem a lot. But, in this case, a little goes a long way. The benefits are many — fewer rashes and less razor burn, irritation, redness, and soreness. This list is a guide to those carrier oils suitable for use in a shaving oil:

GOOD SHAVING CARRIER OILS
Jojoba oil (*Simmondsia chinensis*)
Hemp seed oil (*Cannabis sativa*)
Argan oil (*Argania spinosa*)
Camellia seed oil (*Camellia japonica*)
Rosehip seed oil (*Rosa rubiginosa*)
Macadamia oil (*Macadamia ternifolia*)
Avocado oil (*Persea americana*)
Coconut oil (*Cocos nucifera*)
Sesame oil (*Sesamum indicum*)
Meadowfoam oil (*Limnanthes alba*)

Either use the oils listed above on their own, or use a combination of two or three, finding a blend that's most appropriate to your skin type. Here are a few suggestions:

Four Shaving Oils

BLEND 1

| Jojoba oil | 2 teaspoons (10 mL) |
| Argan oil | 1 teaspoon (5 mL) |

BLEND 2

| Jojoba oil | 2 teaspoons (10 mL) |
| Coconut oil | 1 teaspoon (5 mL) |

BLEND 3

| Jojoba oil | 2 teaspoons (10 mL) |
| Meadowfoam oil | 1 teaspoon (5 mL) |

BLEND 4

| Jojoba oil | 2 teaspoons (10 mL) |
| Rosehip seed oil | 1 teaspoon (5 mL) |

The following oils can be added in smaller amounts (about 5% dilution) to your chosen basic shaving blend to improve its skin-protective and anti-aging properties.

ADDITIONAL SKIN-CARE OILS

Evening primrose seed oil (*Oenothera biennis*)
Borage seed oil (*Borago officinalis*)
Cranberry seed oil (*Vaccinium macrocarpon*)
Raspberry seed oil (*Rubus idaeus*)
Sea buckthorn oil (*Hippophae rhamnoides*)

Essential oils are today found in a multitude of men's facial products, but they're made on an industrial scale using low percentages of essential oils. It can be difficult when making your own shaving oil at home to apply such low dilutions for everyday use unless making a far larger amount than you personally might need. This is especially so when trying out blends that suit your shaving needs. So dilute 1 drop of a single essential oil, or blend, into a teaspoon (5 mL) of carrier oil, and then add 2 or 3 drops of this diluted oil to your daily shaving oil.

Sandalwood or geranium essential oils would be good additions to a shaving oil if the skin tends to be dry or even flaky. Lavender essential oil is appropriate for any kind of irritation; while tea tree is great if there's an infection. Avoid using citrus oils if leaving the oil on the skin and going into sunlight.

ESSENTIAL OILS TO USE IN SHAVING OILS

Antiseptic: tea tree, manuka, lavender, palmarosa, geranium

Soothing (for sensitivity and redness): lavender, chamomile roman, chamomile german, sandalwood, cedarwood atlas

Cooling: eucalyptus radiata, peppermint, spearmint, coriander seed

No matter how careful you are, shaving can bring the following problems:

Shaving cuts: Make up this shaving cut mixture to keep in the bathroom cabinet for when it's needed. Put all the ingredients in a bottle and shake it well each time before using. Dab a little onto cuts to stem bleeding and as an antiseptic.

Witch hazel	2 teaspoons (10 mL)
Lavender	10 drops
Chamomile roman	10 drops

Shaving rash: Apply a little over the rash after shaving in the morning, and before going to bed.

Evening primrose seed oil	2 teaspoons (10 mL)
Tamanu oil	2 teaspoons (10 mL)
Almond (sweet) oil	4 teaspoons (20 mL)
Lavender	10 drops
Chamomile german	10 drops

Shaving itch: The blend above for shaving rash can also be used for itchy skin that accompanies dry skin resulting from shaving. Make it up as above, but dilute it further by adding the total ingredients shown above to 2 tablespoons (30 mL) of jojoba oil.

Shaving inflammation and sensitivity: This blend should be splashed on the face after shaving if your skin is inflamed or sensitive. First, dilute the essential oils in the tincture of myrrh and then add that to your choice of hydrolat. Shake the bottle well after preparing, and shake again before each use.

Tincture of myrrh	2 teaspoons (10 mL)
Chamomile german	5 drops
Lavender	10 drops
Peppermint	1 drop
Lemon	1 drop
Lavender or chamomile hydrolat	5 fl. oz. (150 mL)

Oily skin: Gentle exfoliation or facial exfoliating masks are ideal for men who have an oily complexion. Refer to chapter 13, "The Fragrant Way to Beauty," where there are instructions for various masks. Some masks have an anti-aging and moisturizing effect and are as good for men as they are for women.

Beards

A beard should be in good condition — shiny, healthy, and well groomed — but a dull-looking, bristly, patchy one looks unkempt. Essential oils diluted in a conditioning medium are extremely useful during the growth period, and make a good conditioning treatment for the beard that's already grown. These can be used at night before going to bed.

ESSENTIAL OILS FOR THE BEARD
Rosemary (*Rosmarinus officinalis*)
Lemon (*Citrus limon*)
Lavender (*Lavandula angustifolia*)
Cypress (*Cupressus sempervirens*)
Sandalwood (*Santalum album*)
Cedarwood atlas (*Cedrus atlantica*)

CONDITIONING MEDIUMS
Argan oil (*Argania spinosa*)
Avocado oil (*Persea americana*)
Jojoba oil (*Simmondsia chinensis*)
Coconut oil (*Cocos nucifera*)
Macadamia oil (*Macadamia ternifolia*)
Safflower oil (*Carthamus tinctorius*)
Pataua/ungurahui oil (*Oenocarpus batauva*)

BEARD CONDITIONING BLEND

Rosemary	3 drops
Lavender	5 drops
Sandalwood	5 drops
Lemon	2 drops

Mix the essential oils together to create a blend, then dilute 2 drops in 1 teaspoon (5 mL) of argan oil.

During the growth period, apply a little of the conditioning oil on the beard once a day, massaging it in well and wiping off the excess. If your beard has already grown, use the oil as a conditioning treatment by adding the whole blend to 2 teaspoons (10 mL) of jojoba oil, and use a small amount each time.

10

Essential Help in the Maturing Years

Most seniors say they *feel* themselves to be the same person they were in their youth. Experience has taught them to think differently about a few things, but essentially, they're the same person as they were then. Reconciling these inner feelings with the mature body can be difficult, especially in a society that venerates accumulation in everything but years. But getting to know the essential oils can help us mature gracefully by bringing the body more into line with the young person we feel inside. Remember, you're never too old for an activity unless you're physically incapable of doing it. And there's no law that says you can't go dancing every night.

Whatever you do, make this time of your life one of enjoyment. Once you are retired there is more time to enjoy the simple pleasures of life, like music, picnicking in the park, traveling, and volunteering — not to mention starting a new blog or business! Of course, we all need a little help sometimes, so if you wake up feeling listless and tired, here is the regime for you: when you get up, take a bath or shower using the essential oils below. If you opt for the bath, dilute the essential oils in 1 teaspoon (5 mL) of carrier oil before adding to the bath, lie back, and breathe deeply, inhaling the delicate, revitalizing aroma molecules.

WAKE-UP ESSENTIAL OILS FOR THE
MATURING YEARS
Bergamot FCF (*Citrus bergamia*)
Rosemary (*Rosmarinus officinalis*)
Niaouli (*Melaleuca quinquenervia*)

WAKE-UP BLEND
Bergamot FCF   2 drops
Rosemary   1 drop
Grapefruit   1 drop
Whether using oils singly or in a blend, use 3–4 drops in the bath or 1 or 2 drops in the shower method.

If you find that as far as exercise is concerned, the mind may be willing but the body is not, things will seem much easier after the wake-up bath or shower. This doesn't extend to an intense, extreme cardiac workout — it's more like a cat stretching in the morning. Just stretch each muscle as best you can, paying attention to each part of the body in turn, or try some tai chi, qi gong, or yoga. You may also find that gently brushing the skin with a stiff body brush — always in the direction of the heart — will help stimulate that wake-up feeling.

By this time you'll be ready for a balanced, nutritional breakfast. So many health problems have been linked to poor diet that the maturing years are the time to stop gambling with health and ensure that the diet is full of fresh fruits and vegetables, whole foods, nuts, seeds, and similar good things.

High Blood Pressure

Arterial hypertension, or high blood pressure, can go unnoticed for many years. For some people with this condition, there's no apparent cause, and you may have high blood pressure without suspecting it, even though it can lead to heart disease, kidney failure, and stroke.

It is a well-established fact that those with high blood pressure tend not to thrive as long as those without it. This is in part due to the complications that can arise from it, including strokes, angina, and thrombosis. High blood pressure can cause hardening of the arteries and the loss of elasticity, which can lead to arteriosclerosis. The causes of hypertension are still unclear, and so treatment is therefore limited to the high blood pressure itself, unless there is a known underlying cause. Since symptoms may be nonexistent, or as vague as headaches, tiredness, and dizziness, the only way to keep track of blood pressure is to have it checked regularly.

Anyone who has high blood pressure needs to look for ways to reduce stress. Keep active and exercise — but don't overdo it. When measuring blood pressure, bear in mind that it rises and falls throughout the day, depending on our activities and emotional state.

Dietary changes are particularly effective. Eat plenty of fruit, vegetables, fish, poultry, pulses, and grains. Use olive oil, spices, onions, garlic, and ginger, and eat raw foods whenever you can. Make your own muesli (see page 472 for the recipe). Avoid animal fats, sugars, refined wheat, red meats, and dairy foods, and reduce salt intake. Also cut down on coffee, tea, and alcohol. One vegetable that has been shown to reduce high blood pressure is beetroot. Fresh raw or ready-cooked beetroot can be eaten hot or cold, made into juices, and incorporated into chocolate cake. If juicing, drink 4 fl. oz. a day. Beetroot has the added advantage of providing the body with measurable extra energy.

Supplements may also help, such as vitamin A in the beta-carotene form, vitamins C, E, and D3, selenium, germanium, and the remarkable coenzyme Q10 (CoQ10). Try to include essential fatty acids in your diet, such as omega 3, and eat three proper meals a day, avoiding salty or sugary snacks. And find things that make you laugh, because laughter lessens blood pressure and releases feel-good hormones in the brain.

Many essential oils have a profound effect on the cardiovascular system. Use them in baths and body oils; with the latter, apply the oil in strokes that move toward the heart, for example, from foot to thigh. Ask a friend or your partner to massage your back — and perhaps you could return the favor (for we all need a little help from our friends). The massage should be gentle and with a rhythmic flow, as that type of massage can help reduce blood pressure even without essential oils.

ESSENTIAL OILS THAT COULD BE USED
IF YOU HAVE HYPERTENSION
Clary sage (*Salvia sclarea*)
Lavender (*Lavandula angustifolia*)
Geranium (*Pelargonium graveolens*)
Neroli (*Citrus aurantium*)
Marjoram, sweet (*Origanum majorana*)
Rose otto (*Rosa damascena*)
Melissa (*Melissa officinalis*)
Ylang ylang (*Cananga odorata*)

Frankincense (*Boswellia carterii*)
Chamomile roman (*Anthemis nobilis*)
Petitgrain (*Citrus aurantium*)
Sandalwood (*Santalum album*)

The following body oil is especially designed for those with high blood pressure:

HIGH BLOOD PRESSURE BODY OIL

Lavender	5 drops
Marjoram, sweet	10 drops
Geranium	15 drops

Blend the oils together, then dilute by mixing 3 drops in 1 teaspoon (5 mL) of carrier oil.

HIGH BLOOD PRESSURE BATH BLEND

Clary sage	2 drops
Marjoram, sweet	5 drops
Lavender	5 drops
Geranium	5 drops
Chamomile roman	3 drops

Blend the oils together, then dilute 4 drops in 1 teaspoon (5 mL) of carrier oil per bath.

Circulation

Poor circulation in the limbs is a problem that can affect a person of any age. The first place any circulatory problem may become apparent is in the feet and legs. Symptoms may include more noticeable vascular veins, cold feet, swelling ankles, and discolored skin. Consequently, taking care of the feet and legs is of the utmost importance as we get older.

Circulatory problems can also be associated with diabetes, tissue breakdown, and leg ulceration. Exercise, good eating habits, and reducing cholesterol levels are all part of keeping our vascular network system in good working order, while taking care of dry and fragile skin on the legs and feet can help avoid ulceration. A major factor that often goes unnoticed is how stress affects circulation. Stress produces a hormone called *cortisol* that is good in small quantities but that can have a destructive impact when stress is continual.

Preventive measures include exercise — walking or jogging depending on how fit you are, cycling if you can manage it, and golf and tennis. Cut out dietary fats, and start eating a mainly plant-based diet — limiting red meats and other acid-forming foods. Good nutritional supplements would be those that contain hawthorn berry (*Crataegus oxyacantha*), ginkgo (*Ginkgo biloba*), bilberry (*Vaccinium myrtillus*), turmeric (*Curcuma longa*), and cayenne pepper (*Capsicum annuum, C. frutescens*). The vitamins E, D, and C, selenium and beta-carotene, and an omega 3 supplement can all help. Plus, if you have digestive concerns take a daily probiotic supplement. Eat oily fish while reducing red and processed meats, and add more fruits and vegetables into the diet, as well as whole grains, pulses, seeds, and nuts. Try cutting out refined white sugar altogether — substituting it with unrefined brown sugar, crystallized coconut, agave sweetener, organic honey, or maple syrup.

Using essential oils and massage helps the circulation, as does hydrotherapy — the use of alternate hot- and cold-water treatments.

ESSENTIAL OILS FOR CIRCULATION

Marjoram, sweet (*Origanum majorana*)
Galbanum (*Ferula galbaniflua*)
Geranium (*Pelargonium graveolens*)
Basil linalol (*Ocimum basilicum ct. linalool*)
Cubeb (*Piper cubeba*)
Ginger (*Zingiber officinale*)
Black pepper (*Piper nigrum*)
Cinnamon leaf (*Cinnamomum zeylanicum*)
Clove bud (*Syzygium aromaticum*)
Immortelle (*Helichrysum italicum*)
Lavender (*Lavandula angustifolia*)
Rosemary (*Rosmarinus officinalis*)
Niaouli (*Melaleuca quinquenervia*)

FOOT AND LEG MASSAGE OIL

This massage oil is specifically for use on the feet and legs for those with poor circulation in these areas:

Black pepper	3 drops
Geranium	10 drops
Clove bud	2 drops
Basil linalol	4 drops

Blend together, then dilute in 2 tablespoons (30 mL) of a light carrier oil such as sweet almond oil. Apply a small amount and massage over the feet first, then gently massage up the back of the leg to behind the knee on one leg, and then do the same with the other leg. Then repeat the whole process, always making sure you massage upward toward the thigh.

Some people have very dry, delicate skin that could split with the slightest bump. This type of skin benefits from being moisturized every day to help the skin remain supple. There are three carrier oil choices below for the foot and leg delicate skin massage oil blend.

FOOT AND LEG MASSAGE BLEND FOR DRY, DELICATE SKIN

Geranium	5 drops
Chamomile german	5 drops
Lavender	5 drops

Dilute these quantities into 3 tablespoons (45 mL) of carrier oil — either jojoba, avocado, meadowsweet, or a combination of all three carrier oils. Apply a small amount every day, massaging the oil into the feet and legs, always upward toward the heart. This blend could also be added to 1½ oz. (45 g) of an unscented vitamin E cream base.

GENERAL BODY OIL

Body massage always helps increase circulation, but the massage should be gentle rather than overly vigorous. Always massage, or simply apply, in the direction of the heart.

Immortelle	8 drops
Marjoram, sweet	4 drops
Ginger	3 drops
Lavender	2 drops
Basil linalol	2 drops

Blend the essential oils together, then add to 2 tablespoons (30 mL) of carrier oil, and use a small amount for each massage. To make enough for an individual massage, add 3 drops to a teaspoon (5 mL) of carrier oil.

FOOT BATH AND HAND BATH

Although this might seem a little odd, hand and foot baths can help increase circulation. Use the General Body Oil essential oil blend above, adding 3 drops to a bowl of comfortably warm water with some small round pebbles placed on the bottom. Put your feet into the bowl and gently roll the soles of your feet over the pebbles.

If you're suffering from bad circulation in the hands, fill two small bowls with warm water and add 1 drop of the essential oil blend above into each bowl, then put a hand in each and leave them there for three minutes. If the water gets too cold, just top off with a little hot water. It's even better if you can use both the foot and hand baths simultaneously.

Swollen Ankles and Feet

Ankles can swell for many reasons, including arthritis, rheumatism, heart problems, varicose veins, high blood pressure, fluid retention, and even constipation. Resting with the feet up is always an effective measure, as is the following two-stage treatment: a pebble bath followed by massage.

Swollen Ankles and Feet Stage One: Water Bowl

Cypress	1 drop
Lavender	1 drop
Peppermint	1 drop
Juniper berry	1 drop

Place a dozen or so smooth, round pebbles in a bowl of comfortably warm water, and then add the blend, diluted in a little carrier oil. Roll the soles of your feet slowly over the pebbles for a few minutes, and leave the feet soaking in the bowl.

After drying the feet, massage with the following oil, starting at the feet — as low as you can manage — then moving to the ankles and then upward toward the knees, including behind the knees.

Swollen Ankles and Feet Stage 2: Massage Oil

Immortelle	5 drops
Cypress	5 drops
Juniper berry	5 drops
Peppermint	1 drop

Dilute in 2 tablespoons (30 mL) of carrier oil and use a small amount each time. Rest a while afterward with your feet up and drink plenty of water.

If the swelling happens in hot weather, before massaging the feet and ankles carry out this ice-pack procedure: fill a plastic bag with ice cubes, wrapping a towel around the bag to prevent ice burn. Wrap it around the back of the knees until they feel quite cold, and then rub the bag in the center of the soles of your feet.

Leg Cramps

Leg cramps can cause a great deal of anguish, not only from the painful muscle contraction but, if they occur during the night, from the interrupted sleep pattern that results. A cramp is a painful, spasmodic contraction of a muscle that can come on day or night. The cause is often unknown (idiopathic), but cramps can be due to circulatory conditions, overexercising, injury, infection, dehydration, neurological disorders, or a lack of potassium, magnesium, calcium, or B vitamins in the diet. Cramps most often occur in the calf, thigh, or foot muscles, and the ache can be felt long after the spasm has passed. If leg cramps occur while carrying out any type of exercise or after exercise, it could be that the body is not efficiently dealing with the lactic acid (lactate) in the muscles.

In Asia and some parts of Europe people use a simple first aid remedy that's often effective: hold the big toe joint very firmly — almost like a pinch — with the thumb on the big toenail and a finger at the back, and press hard until the cramp passes. Stretching the leg or foot may help, as does massaging the affected muscles. Anything that gets the circulation flowing during the day will also help.

Prevention is always the best option. Calcium, zinc, and magnesium supplements are recommended, as are garlic capsules and quinine — which is found in tonic water. Vitamins such as complete B complex — B1, 6, and 5 — vitamins D, E, and C, and folic acid also should be included in a supplement regime. Herbal remedies such as hawthorn berry (*Crataegus oxyacantha*) and horse chestnut (*Aesculus hippocastanum*) could also be helpful if the cramps are due to insufficient circulation. Include in your diet magnesium- and potassium-rich foods. Warmth and massaging with essential oils really help.

Essential Oils to Help Prevent Cramps
Geranium (*Pelargonium graveolens*)
Marjoram, sweet (*Origanum majorana*)
Immortelle (*Helichrysum italicum*)
Ginger (*Zingiber officinale*)

Peppermint (*Mentha piperita*)
Clary sage (*Salvia sclarea*)
Black pepper (*Piper nigrum*)
Cypress (*Cupressus sempervirens*)
Patchouli (*Pogostemon cablin*)
Rosemary (*Rosmarinus officinalis*)
Orange, sweet (*Citrus sinensis*)
Lavender (*Lavandula angustifolia*)
Hyssop decumbens (*Hyssopus officinalis var. decumbens*)

Leg Cramp Massage Oil

Rosemary	10 drops
Geranium	5 drops
Lavender	5 drops
Marjoram, sweet	10 drops

Blend the essential oils together, then dilute by mixing 5 drops in 1 teaspoon (5 mL) of carrier oil, for a single massage. Or mix the whole blend in 2 tablespoons (30 mL) of carrier oil, and use a small amount each time.

Warming Leg Cramp Oil for Night or Day

Immortelle	10 drops
Black pepper	4 drops
Geranium	8 drops
Ginger	4 drops
Marjoram, sweet	4 drops

Blend the essential oils together, then dilute by mixing 4–5 drops in 1 teaspoon (5 mL) of carrier oil, for a single application. Or mix the whole blend in 2 tablespoons (30 mL) of carrier oil, and use a small amount each time.

If you are prone to cramps when exercising or even when the legs and feet are being massaged, use the warming oil in upward movements all over the legs and feet before exercise.

If you suffer from cramps before going to bed, massage the whole leg in an upward direction and lastly, massage the feet. Then put on a pair of warm socks. This should be done every night for at least two weeks. Treating reoccurring cramps is also a deprogramming process — you have to put a stop to the message that says, "There'll be a cramp tonight, as every night."

Incidentally, one of the most effective ways to combat cold feet during the night is to place a soft pillow between the sheets at the end of the bed and use it as a sort of hot-water bottle. The difference is that while a hot-water bottle starts warm and gets progressively colder during the night, the pillow starts cold and gets progressively warmer as it absorbs your body heat. If you can heat the pillow on a radiator before putting it in the bed, you have the best of both worlds.

Varicose Veins

There are two interconnected systems of veins in the legs — the deep veins and the so-called superficial veins, which are near the surface. It is the latter that are prone to the unsightly and painful condition known as varicose veins, in which they become swollen and engorged, bulging and standing out from the surface of the skin. This is a result of the small valves in the veins being weak or damaged and not working properly. The muscular tissue lining the walls of the veins relaxes and weakens — sometimes as a result of a hormonal imbalance.

Although they're not dangerous, varicose veins can cause a great deal of discomfort, swelling in the feet, and general fatigue. Inflammation can occur, and varicose veins can be prone to bruising and, in the more mature person, varicose ulceration. Avoiding all this is why it's important to take care of the circulatory system, any enlarged veins, and also the smaller capillaries.

General massage may cause damage to the fragile capillary wall in those who are weak and frail. Since essential oils can be highly beneficial by lessening the pressure on the defective valves, you can apply them, but only when using a particular massage technique. Please note that deep and strong massage techniques should not be used with this condition. Grip the ankle gently and, using the whole of the hand, sweep upward in one gentle and smooth movement, using one hand only, avoiding the varicose vein area.

Essential Oils to Use with Varicose Veins

Geranium (*Pelargonium graveolens*)
Cypress (*Cupressus sempervirens*)
Peppermint (*Mentha piperita*)
Lemon (*Citrus limon*)
Rosemary (*Rosmarinus officinalis*)
Black pepper (*Piper nigrum*)
Carrot seed (*Daucus carota*)
Chamomile roman (*Anthemis nobilis*)
Chamomile german (*Matricaria recutita*)
Immortelle (*Helichrysum italicum*)
Patchouli (*Pogostemon cablin*)
Niaouli (*Melaleuca quinquenervia*)

Daytime Varicose Vein Leg Oil

Geranium	10 drops
Cypress	15 drops
Lemon	5 drops

Blend the essential oils together, then dilute by mixing 3–5 drops in 1 teaspoon (5 mL) of carrier oil, or add the 30 drops of essential oil to 2 tablespoons (30 mL) of carrier oil, and use a small amount for each massage.

Nighttime Varicose Vein Leg Oil

Cypress	10 drops
Peppermint	1 drop

Blend the essential oils together, then dilute by mixing 4–5 drops in 1 teaspoon (5 mL) of carrier oil or add the total amount to 2 teaspoons (10 mL) of carrier oil.

It's important to avoid constipation, as this increases the pressure on the veins. Increase the fiber in your cooking. Garlic capsules, vitamin E, and rutin (a bioflavonoid) supplements are helpful aids in the treatment of varicose veins. The herbal tinctures of horse chestnut (*Aesculus hippocastanum*), hawthorn berry (*Crataegus oxyacantha*), butcher's broom extract (*Ruscus asculeatus*), and gotu kola (*Centella asiatica*) may all help to reduce swelling in the legs and feet and increase circulation. Walking is the best form of exercise for anyone with this condition, but any gentle exercise is better than none. After long periods of standing, sit with your feet up and, following the advice often given on airlines, circle the feet. Another helpful exercise is to raise the heel of the foot while pushing down with the ball of the foot, then putting the heel down, and repeating.

Leg Ulcers

Venous leg ulcers, also known as *stasis ulcers*, are caused by wounds unable to heal properly due to various blood circulatory problems. They can start with an innocent-looking discoloration on the skin that has a dry, papery feel and look. As well as high blood pressure and age, risk factors include insufficient circulation to the area, diabetes, being overweight, varicose veins, peripheral arterial disease, and deep vein thrombosis (DVT). The ulcers tend to get worse over time, becoming larger and deeper, especially if there's accompanying infection, cellulitis, and water retention.

Certain nutritional supplements are useful as a preventative measure. These include zinc, vitamins E, C, D, and A (beta-carotene), evening primrose seed oil, and essential fatty acids such as omega 3. The following treatment is an example of integrative care — where conventional treatment is complemented with other methods such as essential oils. In this case a physician's advice would be followed concerning dressings, compression, and any prescribed medication; the essential oils would be added to this regimen.

ESSENTIAL OILS FOR USE WITH LEG ULCERATION
Lavender (*Lavandula angustifolia*)
Chamomile german (*Matricaria recutita*)
Myrrh (*Commiphora myrrha*)
Geranium (*Pelargonium graveolens*)
Lemon (*Citrus limon*)
Fragonia (*Agonis fragrans*)
Chamomile roman (*Anthemis nobilis*)
Tea tree (*Melaleuca alternifolia*)
Frankincense (*Boswellia carterii*)
Thyme linalol (*Thymus vulgaris ct. linalool*)
Cypress (*Cupressus sempervirens*)
Immortelle (*Helichrysum italicum*)

Organic aloe vera gel, pure vitamin E, propolis, manuka honey, and colloidal silver are all useful additions to an ulceration treatment plan. Treatment of the area surrounding the ulcer is relatively straightforward and involves two steps — using essential oils in the water to wash the surrounding skin, and applying essential oils to the dressing.

LEG ULCERATION BLEND

Lavender	10 drops
Chamomile german	5 drops
Geranium	5 drops
Thyme linalol	5 drops
Lemon	5 drops

Prepare the blend above. If your doctor has asked you to clean the affected area with water, add 2 drops of the blend, or 2 drops of one of the other essential oils listed above, to a cup of warm water. This may not sound like very much, but it is enough to bathe the whole leg below the knee. Bathe around the affected area, avoiding the ulcer itself, then bathe the unaffected part of the leg. It's crucial to avoid infection, and using colloidal silver

combined with essential oils, to bathe around the area, can be valuable.

If using essential oils on dressings, place 4 neat drops of the blend, or 2 drops of one of the essential oils listed above, onto a sterile piece of gauze and let it dry for a little while before applying to the skin. Change the dressing every day. Moisturize the nonulcerated areas of both legs regularly to avoid further splitting of the skin, using calendula oil, jojoba oil, or avocado oil, which are helpful in keeping the skin supple.

Pressure Sores

Anyone at any age can suffer from pressure sores if they are left immobile or bedridden for any reason, but the elderly are more prone to them simply because at that age they're more likely to spend time in bed recovering from various health conditions. No matter how good the quality of care provided, when a person becomes bedridden or spends a considerable length of time sitting in a chair, there's always the risk of pressure sores developing.

Pressure sores are skin lesions, where the skin has become damaged due to blood flow restriction. They can develop on any part of the body where the weight of the body applies pressure. The danger is that they can become infected — whether at home, in a nursing home, or a hospital — and that infection can become fatal. Preventative measures are important; these simply require that the person's body be turned onto another position every two hours to reduce the pressure on one area of the body, and to avoid friction on fragile skin. Also, the body should be kept dry and clean, and dry fragile skin should be moisturized daily using natural products that help strengthen the skin. Or use a natural baby powder. Keep bedding fresh and dry, and try to use equipment especially designed to help relieve physical pressure — such as air beds. Eating a well-balanced diet and keeping hydrated really helps, as do the vitamins C, D, and E, zinc, and essential fatty acids such as omega 3.

The carrier oils used to dilute the essential oils can be important. These can be either used individually or made into a blend. Use jojoba, avocado, rose hip seed, sesame seed, virgin cold-pressed olive oil, macadamia oil, hemp seed oil, or calendula macerated oil.

ESSENTIAL OILS TO HELP PREVENT PRESSURE SORES
Immortelle (*Helichrysum italicum*)
Frankincense (*Boswellia carterii*)
Myrrh (*Commiphora myrrha*)
Geranium (*Pelargonium graveolens*)
Chamomile roman (*Anthemis nobilis*)
Chamomile german (*Matricaria recutita*)
Tea tree (*Melaleuca alternifolia*)
Carrot seed (*Daucus carota*)
Palmarosa (*Cymbopogon martinii*)
Cardamom (*Elettaria cardamomum*)

PRESSURE SORE PREVENTION BLEND
Lavender   5 drops
Chamomile roman   5 drops
Tea tree   3 drops
Add the essential oils above to 3 tablespoons (45 mL) of your chosen carrier oil. Apply a small amount twice daily on areas of pressure that may be at risk of developing sores, but not directly on any existing pressure sores.

Insomnia

Sleep patterns can become a problem if we hold on to the idea that everyone needs a good eight hours' sleep each night when the fact is that many people function very well throughout their lives on less than eight hours. A vicious cycle may begin after retirement, when catnapping becomes possible during the day, leading to waking during the night because the body just doesn't need all that sleep.

Generally people sleep a lot longer than they think they do, with the loss of sleep being exaggerated. "I haven't slept all night" can, on examination, really mean that someone woke a couple of times for two or three minutes. The time involved becomes amplified by the aggravation it caused.

There's nothing wrong in waking with the dawn chorus, but if you're starting to worry about it, feel tired all day, or are not mentally alert then you possibly have true insomnia. If this is the case, there are several possible causes, including pain, cramps, fatigue, diet, stimulants, stress and anxiety, insufficient food, and even certain medications. Removal of the cause, if possible, is the first and most important step. If the problem is diuretic and you frequently need to pass urine during the night, there may be an underlying health problem that you need to check with your physician. Flatulence can cause pain and discomfort and is often caused by eating too late — so eat earlier. Fatigue can be caused by working late into the night, and even reading a book can cause overstimulation and the tired-but-can't-sleep syndrome. The glare from e-book readers, TVs, laptops, and tablets can contribute to the suppression of melatonin production, and these are probably best avoided in the bedroom if suffering from insomnia.

Look at your habits in the hours prior to going to bed. Stimulants such as caffeine in the form of coffee, tea, or sodas should be avoided after four o'clock in the afternoon if you go to bed at ten. Instead, drink herbal teas such as chamomile, lemon balm, and passion flower seed, and avoid alcohol. Try to remove from your sleeping area all external disturbances such as electronic clocks or any other electrical machine with a humming sound, however slight.

Emotional problems and anxiety are more difficult to control. It's understandable that people think deeply about their problems at night because this is often the only opportunity for the mind to sort through the events of the day with no interruptions. So do take some time to think through everything that may be concerning you, but tell yourself you'll have another think about it tomorrow if you can't figure out a solution right that minute. Or write down the problems, so you can deal with them in the morning. In fact, one of the best pieces of advice for overthinking problems is to "sleep on it." Address concerns in the morning, rather than at night.

At night, anxieties can be eased by using the essential oils and listening to music that relaxes you. A lack of fresh ventilation while sleeping may cause waking in the night. Most importantly, stop worrying about not sleeping!

The essential oils below can be used in a warm, sensuous bath (as opposed to a hot, stimulating one) before bedtime. You may prefer to use them in a foot bath. Also, essential oils can be used in a body oil that can be gently rubbed onto any easy-to-reach parts of the body. An aromatic diffuser in the bedroom often helps when used prior to going to sleep. People have very different responses to individual essential oils, so do experiment with those on the list. Bear in mind that some oils can become stimulating, rather than relaxing, when used in doses that are too high, depending on each individual's response.

Essential Oils for Insomnia

Lavender (*Lavandula angustifolia*)
Benzoin (*Styrax benzoin*)
Marjoram, sweet (*Origanum majorana*)
Clary sage (*Salvia sclarea*)
Chamomile roman (*Anthemis nobilis*)
Vetiver (*Vetiveria zizanoides*)

Ylang ylang (*Cananga odorata*)
Neroli (*Citrus aurantium*)
Valerian (*Valeriana officinalis*)
Petitgrain (*Citrus aurantium*)
Mandarin (*Citrus reticulata*)
Cistus (*Cistus ladaniferus*)

General Blend for Insomnia

Clary sage	3 drops
Vetiver	2 drops
Valerian	1 drop
Lavender	2 drops

Blend the essential oils together, then use 3–4 drops per bath, diluted in a small amount of carrier oil. Or use 3 drops diluted in 1 teaspoon (5 mL) of carrier oil for a body oil, and apply a small amount over the solar plexus area — the upper abdomen.

Warming Blend for Insomnia

Benzoin	4 drops
Mandarin	2 drops
Nutmeg	1 drop
Chamomile roman	2 drops

Blend the essential oils together, then use 3–4 drops per bath, diluted in a small amount of carrier oil. Or use 3 drops diluted in 1 teaspoon (5 mL) of carrier oil for a body oil, and apply a small amount over the solar plexus area — the upper abdomen.

Calming Blend for Insomnia

Lavender	7 drops
Ylang ylang	8 drops
Clary sage	2 drops
Vetiver	1 drop

Blend the essential oils together, then use 3–4 drops per bath, diluted in a small amount of carrier oil. Or use 3 drops diluted in 1 teaspoon (5 mL) of carrier oil for a body oil, and apply a small amount over the solar plexus area — the upper abdomen.

FOOT BATH BLEND FOR INSOMNIA
Lavender	1 drop
Marjoram, sweet	3 drops
Chamomile roman	3 drops
Valerian	1 drop

Blend the essential oils together, then use 4 drops in a warm foot bath.

Another simple method for trying to alleviate sleeplessness is to put a drop of essential oil onto a tissue and place it under the pillow. Ensure it is located somewhere that avoids direct contact with the eyes. Use lavender, chamomile roman, or clary sage. Alternatively, put the essential oil directly on the underside corner of a pillowcase or on nightwear, before going to bed. Choose from the essential oils on the Insomnia list above, but do be aware that some of the more viscous or colored oils, such as vetiver, could stain materials such as bed linen and bedclothes.

Breathing Difficulties

The three most common types of breathing problems in the maturing years are painful breathing, shortness of breath, and noisy, wheezing breathing.

PAINFUL BREATHING

Chest pain when breathing is often an indication of a disorder of the lungs, muscles, or bones. It can be accompanied by a cough, which is also painful, and inflammation. A physician must be consulted for a diagnosis of the symptoms, which may be caused by pneumonia, pleurisy, a pulmonary embolism, or a chest injury. Another cause could be costochondritis — inflammation of the joints and cartilage attaching the ribs to the sternum (breastbone). The following essential oils may help ease the symptoms:

ESSENTIAL OILS FOR PAINFUL BREATHING
Eucalyptus radiata (*Eucalyptus radiata*)
Chamomile roman (*Anthemis nobilis*)
Rosemary (*Rosmarinus officinalis*)
Cajuput (*Melaleuca cajuputi*)
Ginger (*Zingiber officinale*)
Cinnamon leaf (*Cinnamomum zeylanicum*)
Ravensara (*Ravensara aromatica*)
Hyssop decumbens (*Hyssopus officinalis var. decumbens*)
Frankincense (*Boswellia carterii*)
Cypress (*Cupressus sempervirens*)
Niaouli (*Melaleuca quinquenervia*)
Ho wood (*Cinnamomum camphora ct. linalool*)
Oregano, Moroccan (*Origanum compactum*)

Use the essential oils above to make your own body oil, or make up the blend below, and rub a little of the diluted oil all around the chest area, and the back too, if possible.

BLEND FOR PAINFUL BREATHING
Niaouli	5 drops
Chamomile roman	5 drops
Rosemary	5 drops
Frankincense	10 drops
Cajuput	5 drops

Blend the essential oils together, then dilute 4–5 drops in 1 teaspoon (5 mL) of carrier oil. Rub a little over the chest and back, up to three times a day.

SHORTNESS OF BREATH

Shortness of breath can become a problem when age brings lack of mobility. If you find yourself breathless when climbing the stairs, walking to the end of the garden, or going to the store, you may have to adjust your lifestyle no matter how much the rest of you says "go." There are many causes of breathlessness, including chest infection, chronic obstructive pulmonary disease (COPD), asthma, airway obstruction, and heart disease, so these potential conditions need to be ruled out by a physician before attempting to alleviate any symptoms.

Another type of shortness of breath is brought on by emotional anxiety, and almost anything can spark it off. As with all kinds of breathing difficulties, it helps enormously if you learn to control your breathing. Practice taking deep breaths, like sighs, and holding them for a few seconds before releasing. Also, as you breathe in, raise your arms above your head, and lower them as you breathe out, as this will exercise the intercostal muscles — the muscles in between the ribs. It can be helpful to learn the breathing techniques used in yoga, tai chi, and qi gong.

Use the following essential oils to make a body oil, or use the blend. Also use the oils in warm baths or showers.

Essential Oils to Help Breathlessness
Eucalyptus lemon (*Eucalyptus citriodora*)
Geranium (*Pelargonium graveolens*)
Hyssop decumbens (*Hyssopus officinalis var. decumbens*)
Rosemary (*Rosmarinus officinalis*)
Benzoin (*Styrax benzoin*)
Cardamom (*Elettaria cardamomum*)
Marjoram, sweet (*Origanum majorana*)
Juniper berry (*Juniperus communis*)
Thyme linalol (*Thymus vulgaris ct. linalool*)
Lavender (*Lavandula angustifolia*)
Chamomile roman (*Anthemis nobilis*)
Clary sage (*Salvia sclarea*)
Mandarin (*Citrus reticulata*)

Blend for Breathlessness
Benzoin   15 drops
Geranium   5 drops
Mandarin   5 drops

Blend the essential oils together. Then dilute 4–5 drops in 1 teaspoon (5 mL) of carrier oil, for a body oil, or dilute 3 drops in a little carrier oil for a bath, or use 3 drops in the usual shower method.

NOISY BREATHING

Noisy breathing can be wheezy or hoarse, and it can come suddenly (acute) or be a chronic wheeze that increases in intensity. Often the simple common cold is to blame, but the cause may be more serious, such as an obstruction, asthma, bronchitis, or certain viral infections.

For acute conditions, rest and steam inhalations are often all that are needed. Float 4 drops of eucalyptus radiata or ravensara in a bowl of hot water, and breathe over the bowl as deeply as you can for around three minutes. Your head needs to be covered with a towel to keep the steam in, and you will need to come out for a second or two every now and again. Keep your eyes closed when under the towel.

Steam in the bedroom helps at night. Boiling a kettle repeatedly helps to clear the room of dry dust particles, or invest in an ionizer. Sitting in a steamy bathroom may help too. Chronic conditions are eased by massage and steam. Massage with the following blend over the chest first, then the neck and the back if at all possible:

Noisy Breathing Body Oil
Eucalyptus radiata   15 drops
Rosemary   10 drops
Chamomile roman   5 drops
Blend the essential oils together, then dilute 4–5 drops in 1 teaspoon (5 mL) of carrier oil.

Bronchitis

Bronchitis is inflammation of the bronchi, the air passages in the lungs. It can be acute or chronic.

Essential Help in the Maturing Years 273

The condition can be caused by viral or bacterial infection, or by inflammation caused by irritants such as tobacco smoke, air pollution, and chemicals, both domestic and industrial. During the acute stage there is often wheezing, expectoration of phlegm, and a persistent cough, and there may also be a headache or fever.

The first thing to do if you have been diagnosed with bronchitis is to keep warm, stay in bed, and avoid all smoke — whether from cigarettes or fires. When the cough is painful and dry, gentle inhalation of essential oils during the night will help tremendously. These can be used in a diffuser or any of the room methods, or simply put the essential oil in a cup or bowl of steaming hot water placed in the room — the ideal place would be on the floor near where you sleep so the steam and aroma molecules can rise near you. However, if children or pets come into the room, the bowl must be kept well out of their reach to avoid accidents.

A virus is often the root cause of the problem, with secondary infection being caused by bacteria; to deal with these infections refer to the lists of essential oils in chapter 3, "The Self-Defense Kit." The oils can be used in whatever inhalation method you decide to use. A body oil could also be made and rubbed on the chest — all around the rib cage and along the entire length of the front torso, from the throat and neck to the abdomen. If possible, ask someone to rub the oil on your back as well. One or 2 drops of neat ravensara oil rubbed over the back and chest area often helps the body to fight the infection.

All types of eucalyptus essential oil are useful in the treatment of bronchitis; there are three types in the list below. Use the oils listed individually or make your own blend, and massage twice a day:

BRONCHITIS ESSENTIAL OILS
Benzoin (*Styrax benzoin*)
Eucalyptus radiata (*Eucalyptus radiata*)
Frankincense (*Boswellia carterii*)
Eucalyptus peppermint (*Eucalyptus dives*)
Marjoram, sweet (*Origanum majorana*)
Chamomile german (*Matricaria recutita*)
Ho wood (*Cinnamomum camphora ct. linalool*)
Clove bud (*Syzygium aromaticum*)
Eucalyptus globulus (*Eucalyptus globulus*)
Ginger (*Zingiber officinale*)
Niaouli (*Melaleuca quinquenervia*)
Cinnamon leaf (*Cinnamomum zeylanicum*)
Cajuput (*Melaleuca cajuputi*)
Thyme linalol (*Thymus vulgaris ct. linalool*)
Tea tree (*Melaleuca alternifolia*)
Ravensara (*Ravensara aromatica*)
Immortelle (*Helichrysum italicum*)
Cypress (*Cupressus sempervirens*)
Pine (*Pinus sylvestris*)
Ravintsara (*Cinnamomum camphora ct. cineole*)

BRONCHITIS BLEND
Thyme linalol	10 drops
Eucalyptus radiata	5 drops
Ravensara	5 drops
Niaouli	3 drops
Frankincense	5 drops
Ginger	2 drops

Blend the essential oils together, then dilute 4–5 drops in 1 teaspoon (5 mL) of carrier oil.

Although it may sound a bit strange, putting essential oil onto a tissue and into the bottom of the socks is an extremely effective measure. Tear a tissue in half and on each piece put 2 drops of ginger essential oil. Arrange both pieces in the sock so the tissues are against the soles of your feet. Change tissues at night, this time using thyme linalol, and leave the socks on overnight. If the ginger irritates your foot, change the oil used to ravensara or eucalyptus radiata — used in the morning and at night. These two oils could be applied neat — 1 drop each time — to the soles of the feet, the area between the toes and the arch. Another method involves cabbage (see page 304) — putting the ironed cabbage leaves into the socks before wearing them overnight.

Bronchitis becomes chronic when the bronchi become inflamed, swell, and narrow, there's an overproduction of mucus, and the tiny air sacs of which the lungs are composed are distended. This inflammatory response can be from a virus or bacteria, but it's not helped by irritation caused by exposure to various pollutants, including indoor airborne chemicals — such as dust particles, synthetic air fresheners, and cigarette smoke. As your bronchi are disturbed already, before choosing any essential oil, make sure you don't have a sensitivity to it by using just a very small amount of that essential oil to begin with. If you're not sensitive, carry on with the treatment.

Rest is extremely important. Try to avoid getting cold — stay out of cold air and keep yourself warm, especially the hands and feet. Diet should be attended to: cut out all dairy products (except eggs) as these are mucus forming, as well as all white-flour and sugar products. Also avoid toxins as far as possible, including all forms of caffeine. Drink herbal teas instead, or try fresh lemon juice with manuka honey. Other alternatives are licorice (*Glycyrrhiza glabra*) tea or tincture, thyme (*Thymus vulgaris*) herbal tea, or the herbal tincture of common ivy (*Hedera helix*).

If the bronchitis is ongoing, try an old-fashioned remedy, made in the following way: add about 2 tablespoons (60 g) of fresh, grated ginger to 3½ fl. oz. (100 mL) of brandy, and leave it to stand for a week in an airtight container; then strain, and add the liquid to 4 tablespoons of manuka honey; blend them together well; and bottle. From this bottle, take 1 teaspoon in a cup of hot water. This remedy can be part of the treatment or used as a preventative if someone is prone to developing bronchitis through the winter months. An alternative method involves substituting 2 drops of essential oil of ginger for the grated ginger and leaving it to infuse in the honey for a week, before adding 3½ fl. oz. (100 mL) of brandy. Also massage with the blend above or choose from the essential oils recommended, following the instructions at the beginning of this section.

Pneumonia

There are various types of pneumonia, most being caused by bacteria or viruses, but some also by other micro-organisms. It causes inflammation of the lungs and a variety of symptoms that vary from person to person, depending on the type of pneumonia. For example, pneumonia caused by the bacteria *Streptococcus pneumoniae* tends to produce a reddish-colored mucus when coughing, while that caused by the bacteria *Legionella* can bring on abdominal pain and diarrhea. Pneumonia that has been caused by a virus tends to produce more wheezing than the bacterial versions. It's important to be aware of the symptoms, as this can lead to a more accurate diagnosis and targeted treatment. Symptoms can include chest pain, a cough that produces sputum, fever and/ or shaking chills, increased rate of breathing, temperature fluctuation, vomiting, lack of thirst, and in the elderly, confusion.

Pneumonia can appear out of the blue, for no apparent reason, after feeling not too well for a while, and in the maturing years, this may just feel like a common cold. The people at most risk of developing pneumonia are the very young and the elderly. Antibiotics are often prescribed, and the full course should be taken, even if you begin to feel fine or generally don't like taking antibiotics. Having a probiotic every day will help rebalance the intestinal flora while you're taking the antibiotics. This is one of those conditions where a symbiosis of different methods of treatment, or integrative medicine, is brought into play.

Bed rest is essential, as is drinking plenty of

fluid and keeping your feet and hands warm. Use essential oils in bed socks, as outlined on page 272 in "Bronchitis." Essential oil inhalations are an extremely good way to help the body recover from pneumonia and can be used alongside your prescribed medication. These are the essential oils you could use:

PNEUMONIA: OILS FOR INHALATIONS AND ROOM DIFFUSION
Ravensara (*Ravensara aromatica*)
Niaouli (*Melaleuca quinquenervia*)
Tea tree (*Melaleuca alternifolia*)
Ginger (*Zingiber officinale*)
Clove bud (*Syzygium aromaticum*)
Cinnamon leaf (*Cinnamomum zeylanicum*)
Cajuput (*Melaleuca cajuputi*)
Lemongrass (*Cymbopogon citratus/flexuosus*)
Star anise (*Illicium verum*)
Eucalyptus globulus (*Eucalyptus globulus*)
Thyme linalol (*Thymus vulgaris ct. linalool*)
Melissa (*Melissa officinalis*)
Manuka (*Leptospermum scoparium*)
Kanuka (*Kunzea ericoides*)
Oregano (*Origanum vulgare*)
Ho wood (*Cinnamomum camphora ct. linalool*)
Hyssop decumbens (*Hyssopus officinalis var. decumbens*)
Cypress (*Cupressus sempervirens*)

Use in any of the room methods, following the general directions. For inhalation, use 6 drops on a bowl of steaming hot water, covering the head with a towel while inhaling the vapors through the nose. Ensure your eyes are closed while under the towel. Also, make a body oil from the following essential oils, which can be used all over the body, except for the face:

PNEUMONIA: BODY OIL ESSENTIAL OILS
Niaouli (*Melaleuca quinquenervia*)
Eucalyptus radiata (*Eucalyptus radiata*)
Ho wood (*Cinnamomum camphora ct. linalool*)
Ravintsara (*Cinnamomum camphora ct. cineole*)
Tea tree (*Melaleuca alternifolia*)
Eucalyptus lemon (*Eucalyptus citriodora*)
Thyme linalol (*Thymus vulgaris ct. linalool*)
Cinnamon leaf (*Cinnamomum zeylanicum*)
Ravensara (*Ravensara aromatica*)
Cajuput (*Melaleuca cajuputi*)
Ginger (*Zingiber officinale*)
Clove bud (*Syzygium aromaticum*)
Hyssop decumbens (*Hyssopus officinalis var. decumbens*)
Manuka (*Leptospermum scoparium*)
Fragonia (*Agonis fragrans*)
Cypress (*Cupressus sempervirens*)

BLEND 1: GENERAL BODY OIL
Eucalyptus lemon	10 drops
Niaouli	10 drops
Thyme linalol	5 drops
Ravensara	5 drops

Blend the oils together, then dilute 4–5 drops in 1 teaspoon (5 mL) of carrier oil for each application, and apply over the front of the body — from navel to neck, and over the upper back.

BLEND 2: STRONGER BODY OIL
Ginger	3 drops
Clove bud	2 drops
Thyme linalol	7 drops
Cinnamon leaf	2 drops
Hyssop decumbens	3 drops
Fragonia	5 drops
Oregano	2 drops
Ho wood	6 drops

Dilute this synergistic essential oil blend into 1 fl. oz. (30 mL) of carrier oil, and apply as much as required over the front of the body — from navel to neck, and over the upper back.

Try to keep your diet as healthy as possible — eat fresh foods and drink plenty of honey-and-lemon water drinks, plus herbal teas such as thyme, oregano, ginger, nettle, rosehip, and peppermint. Take a good multivitamin supplement. Vitamins D3 and C will help your body fight both bacterial and viral lung infections.

Occasional Loss of Memory

Occasional loss of memory or absentmindedness is entirely different from dementia or Alzheimer's disease, both of which are discussed further below.

Have you ever gone to dial a number but forgotten who you were supposed to be calling by the time you picked up the phone? Or walked into another room to fetch something, and forgotten what it was by the time you got there? Experiences such as these are common to us all, so don't start to panic just yet. Forgetfulness affects children, teenagers, and middle-aged adults, as well as many in their maturing years. Lapses in concentration account for much of this: having too much on your mind or thinking of three things at once.

To describe how the volatile aromatic molecules contained in essential oils can help in enhancing memory, I am going to quote from another of my books, *The Fragrant Mind*:

Using essential oils regularly seems to give access to areas of our memory that might otherwise be overloaded with the plethora of daily events, or ignored by a conscious mind that has its own ideas about what is important. Aromas are the direct route of access into the brain, stimulating brain cells to respond. Aroma probably works well to retrieve memorized information because it stimulates the hippocampus, which seems to be responsible for storing information, both about experiences (*episodic memories*) and facts (*semantic memories*), in the brain.

Aroma evokes memories — it presses a button and flash, the memory is there. How it does this, we do not know.

ESSENTIAL OILS FOR MEMORY ENHANCEMENT AND CONCENTRATION
Ginger (*Zingiber officinale*)
Basil linalol (*Ocimum basilicum ct. linalool*)
Lemon (*Citrus limon*)
Grapefruit (*Citrus paradisi*)
Thyme linalol (*Thymus vulgaris ct. linalool*)
Rosemary (*Rosmarinus officinalis*)
Cardamom (*Elettaria cardamomum*)
Black pepper (*Piper nigrum*)
Coriander seed (*Coriandrum sativum*)

The following three blends can be either simply sniffed from a tissue when needed or used in one of the room methods — a diffuser or water spray would be simple and effective. Mix the essential oils together using these proportions, then store in a small bottle. Use 2 drops for the tissue method and 8 drops in your chosen room method.

MEMORY ENHANCEMENT BLEND 1

Ginger	7 drops
Lemon	8 drops
Cardamom	10 drops
Black pepper	5 drops

MEMORY ENHANCEMENT BLEND 2

Rosemary	10 drops
Basil linalol	5 drops
Thyme linalol	7 drops
Grapefruit	8 drops

MEMORY ENHANCEMENT BLEND 3

Basil linalol	3 drops
Rosemary	3 drops
Black pepper	3 drops
Lemon	3 drops

If you think of your brain as an electrical circuit that can short when switching from one circuit to another, you can get an idea of what happens when the mind goes blank or gets confused. Fortifying the brain with the food it needs is very important. This is a very complex subject, as you can imagine, but certain vitamins, minerals, and micronutrients do seem to have a profound effect on brain function, notably zinc, vitamins C, D, and B12, and, with some people only, lecithin. Having a good level of potassium is important for memory but supplements are not recommended for people with high blood pressure, who should instead eat potassium-rich foods such as dried figs, dates, apricots, raisins, bananas, and baked potatoes.

Dementia and Alzheimer's Disease

Dementia and Alzheimer's disease are quite different conditions, yet both create a distance between people that can be truly upsetting. There are many symptoms that occur in both conditions — for example, finding the right words, the inability to follow a conversation, social withdrawal, and difficulty in reading and writing. Because the essential oils used for both conditions are mostly the same, I've listed them together in this section. Further down, you'll find essential oils suggested for many of the difficulties faced by people with either dementia or Alzheimer's: general memory loss, short-term memory loss, long-term memory loss, decreased alertness and awareness, frustration, mood swings, irritability, restlessness, agitation, stress, anxiety, depression, sleeplessness and disturbed sleep, headaches, indigestion, and loss of appetite.

DEMENTIA

Dementia is a term used to describe neurodegenerative diseases that diminish the ability to think rationally, causing difficulties in daily life. It can lead the affected person to total dependence on others to carry out the simplest of tasks. Dementia is often characterized by repetition — the person asks the same question, or gives the same information, over and over again. Short-term memory is almost nonexistent in some cases, and so we have the relative with dementia phoning to ask, "Why have you not phoned?" when you've just put the phone down after speaking to them. They might say someone has not been to visit them when that person is actually right there, in the room. Circulatory conditions most certainly play a part in age-related dementia, so improving circulation and nutrition may help in delaying the progression of the disease.

Essential oils can't stop the onset of dementia or prevent it, but they can provide a link into parts of the brain connected with focus and concentration, which in turn could be used for memory recall. Use an essential oil that has an aroma experienced in previous happy times as a food or a perfume. Bay or cinnamon can bring back memories of the family around the table at Thanksgiving, or neroli may recall the memory of a favorite perfume used in youth. Although we may not consciously remember the complete aroma, the limbic system of the brain will remember neroli as one of the ingredients. Aromatic memories associated with happy times can be drawn upon when the person with dementia is irritated or upset, or showing signs of anxiety. There are lots of hypotheses around the connection between the mind, smell, and memory recall — no one can honestly say how it works, but it does.

TABLE 9. ESSENTIAL OILS FOR COMPLICATIONS OF DEMENTIA AND ALZHEIMER'S

COMPLICATION	OILS
GENERAL MEMORY LOSS	Rosemary (*Rosmarinus officinalis*) Lemon (*Citrus limon*) Orange, sweet (*Citrus sinensis*) Basil linalol (*Ocimum basilicum ct. linalool*) Black pepper (*Piper nigrum*) Cardamom (*Elettaria cardamomum*)
SHORT-TERM MEMORY LOSS	Rosemary (*Rosmarinus officinalis*) Peppermint (*Mentha piperita*) Frankincense (*Boswellia carterii*) Lemon (*Citrus limon*)
LONG-TERM MEMORY LOSS	Rosemary (*Rosmarinus officinalis*) Geranium (*Pelargonium graveolens*) Lemon (*Citrus limon*) Orange, sweet (*Citrus sinensis*) Melissa (*Melissa officinalis*) Cardamom (*Elettaria cardamomum*) Grapefruit (*Citrus paradisi*)
DECREASED ALERTNESS AND AWARENESS	Peppermint (*Mentha piperita*) Black pepper (*Piper nigrum*) Cinnamon leaf (*Cinnamomum zeylanicum*) Rosemary (*Rosmarinus officinalis*) Basil linalol (*Ocimum basilicum ct. linalool*) Lemon (*Citrus limon*)
FRUSTRATION	Chamomile roman (*Anthemis nobilis*) Lemon (*Citrus limon*) Petitgrain (*Citrus aurantium*) Geranium (*Pelargonium graveolens*) Frankincense (*Boswellia carterii*)

COMPLICATION	OILS
MOOD SWINGS	Neroli (*Citrus aurantium*) Petitgrain (*Citrus aurantium*) Rosewood (*Aniba rosaeodora*) Clary sage (*Salvia sclarea*) Bergamot (*Citrus bergamia*) Lavender (*Lavandula angustifolia*) Orange, sweet (*Citrus sinensis*) Frankincense (*Boswellia carterii*)
IRRITABILITY	Lavender (*Lavandula angustifolia*) Bergamot (*Citrus bergamia*) Geranium (*Pelargonium graveolens*) Petitgrain (*Citrus aurantium*) Mandarin (*Citrus reticulata*) Palmarosa (*Cymbopogon martinii*) Chamomile roman (*Anthemis nobilis*)
RESTLESSNESS	Lavender (*Lavandula angustifolia*) Chamomile roman (*Anthemis nobilis*) Marjoram, sweet (*Origanum majorana*) Ylang ylang (*Cananga odorata*) Mandarin (*Citrus reticulata*) Petitgrain (*Citrus aurantium*)
AGITATION	Bergamot (*Citrus bergamia*) Geranium (*Pelargonium graveolens*) Melissa (*Melissa officinalis*) Mandarin (*Citrus reticulata*) Clary sage (*Salvia sclarea*) Cedarwood atlas (*Cedrus atlantica*)
STRESS	Lavender (*Lavandula angustifolia*) Clary sage (*Salvia sclarea*) Bergamot (*Citrus bergamia*) Ylang ylang (*Cananga odorata*) Mandarin (*Citrus reticulata*) Chamomile roman (*Anthemis nobilis*) Palmarosa (*Cymbopogon martinii*)

COMPLICATION	OILS
ANXIETY	Geranium (*Pelargonium graveolens*) Lavender (*Lavandula angustifolia*) Chamomile roman (*Anthemis nobilis*) Ylang ylang (*Cananga odorata*) Neroli (*Citrus aurantium*) Bergamot (*Citrus bergamia*) Melissa (*Melissa officinalis*) Marjoram, sweet (*Origanum majorana*) Frankincense (*Boswellia carterii*)
DEPRESSION	Clary sage (*Salvia sclarea*) Bergamot (*Citrus bergamia*) Geranium (*Pelargonium graveolens*) Grapefruit (*Citrus paradisi*) Lemon (*Citrus limon*) Orange, sweet (*Citrus sinensis*) Neroli (*Citrus aurantium*) Rose maroc (*Rosa centifolia*) Rosemary (*Rosmarinus officinalis*) Frankincense (*Boswellia carterii*) Mandarin (*Citrus reticulata*) Ho wood (*Cinnamomum camphora ct. linalool*)
HEADACHES	Peppermint (*Mentha piperita*) Marjoram, sweet (*Origanum majorana*) Lavender (*Lavandula angustifolia*) Basil linalol (*Ocimum basilicum ct. linalool*) Rosemary (*Rosmarinus officinalis*) Chamomile roman (*Anthemis nobilis*)
INDIGESTION	Peppermint (*Mentha piperita*) Ginger (*Zingiber officinale*) Cardamom (*Elettaria cardamomum*) Coriander seed (*Coriandrum sativum*) Grapefruit (*Citrus paradisi*)

COMPLICATION	OILS
LOSS OF APPETITE	Lemon (*Citrus limon*) Orange, sweet (*Citrus sinensis*) Black pepper (*Piper nigrum*) Cardamom (*Elettaria cardamomum*) Coriander seed (*Coriandrum sativum*) Ginger (*Zingiber officinale*)
SLEEPLESS-NESS AND DISTURBED SLEEP	Lavender (*Lavandula angustifolia*) Orange, sweet (*Citrus sinensis*) Mandarin (*Citrus reticulata*) Valerian (*Valeriana officinalis*) Melissa (*Melissa officinalis*) Petitgrain (*Citrus aurantium*)

ALZHEIMER'S DISEASE

Alzheimer's disease causes a person to inexorably drift away to a place where they can't remember their family, or even who they are. It is perhaps the most disturbing condition to affect our loved ones, and many people live in fear that Alzheimer's will creep over them too.

Communicating with someone who has become a stranger even to themselves may seem an entirely hopeless task, but one thing that can encourage closeness between people is touch. This is especially the case when the person with Alzheimer's is a member of the family. This is not the time for therapeutic massage; it's just an opportunity to convey love with a gentle body or shoulder massage, or even a simple foot or hand massage. Not only will the essential oils used be pleasing to the Alzheimer's sufferer's senses, and to your own, but if you use aromas the person experienced in the past, memories may be rekindled.

Any essential oils can be used, but it's helpful to cast your mind back to the aromatic likes of the person and try to re-create those aromas now. For example, if the person with Alzheimer's is your mother and she always wore a rose-based perfume, then rose oil may be the perfect choice. Generally good choices are the citrus essential oils of lemon, grapefruit, and sweet orange plus the spices, such as coriander seed, cardamom, and ginger, because these also stimulate the gastric juices and touch upon the primeval senses of feeding and survival. Try to establish a communication pattern based on appetite, smell, memory, love, and trust. It doesn't matter that the person, who may be a parent, doesn't know who you are; the loving energetic exchange between the two of you, even if not apparent at the time, will touch their heart.

In newly diagnosed and less advanced cases of Alzheimer's you can be more adventurous and utilize the gentle fragrances of flowers — lavender, rose, geranium, and neroli would be good examples, perhaps used in conjunction with the spices mentioned above or basil, rosemary, and juniper berry. Make a massage oil using the essential oils and use them in a hand or foot massage, or on the very important neck and shoulder area. You could try the following blend:

ALZHEIMER'S MASSAGE BLEND

Rose	5 drops
Geranium	5 drops
Basil	2 drops
Lavender	10 drops
Rosemary	2 drops

Blend together, then dilute 3–5 drops per 1 teaspoon (5 mL) of carrier oil.

If you use a particular essential oil, or blend, or several different blends when the person developing Alzheimer's can still communicate with you and recognize your warmth, concern, and love, then when you use the same aroma(s) some time later, when the disease has developed further, the aroma may on some level communicate your enduring love and give comfort to them. The sense of smell operates within the limbic system, which is the most ancient part of the human brain, very much connected with both survival and emotion.

It's amazing what deeply hidden emotions can be felt through the power of aroma.

Alzheimer's is thought to be caused by the development of neurofibrillary tangles and senile plaques in the brain. The question is, why do they develop? There could well be a genetic factor in this, and very likely there is an environmental element. Curiously, at the core of some tangles and plaques are found aluminosilicates that form a variety of lattice shapes. These are precipitates — they have formed a solid out of two previously nonsolid elements, aluminum and silicon. This precipitation is a seemingly unique phenomenon in inorganic chemistry.

It was once suspected that too much aluminum floating around the bloodstream was the cause of the problem. Then it was discovered that people who had absorbed large quantities of aluminum for one reason or another — working in the aluminum industry, for example, or being on dialysis — were not more prone to develop Alzheimer's than other people. However, studies have shown that people living in areas with high aluminum in the water or using antiperspirants that contain aluminum were at higher risk. The mystery deepened.

The tangles and plaques that seem to cause Alzheimer's congregate around precipitates made up of both aluminum and silicates — the latter of which may have come from silicic acid, because it's the form that's water soluble, and could have crossed the blood-brain barrier. What appears to happen when molecules of silicic acid and aluminum meet is that they come together and form insoluble lumps. If this happens outside the brain these lumps could be excreted, but when they form inside the brain they may contribute to Alzheimer's. So, it's not about having too much aluminum, or too much silicic acid, but having an imbalance. Any extra aluminum can be carried to the brain by transferrin, and if it connects with extra silicic acid there, precipitation can occur.

To be realistic, none of us is going to be able to absorb a perfectly balanced amount of aluminum and silicon, at the exact same time, so if they precipitate it's *inside* the body and gets excreted before any extra gets into the brain, thereby preventing it from connecting with the other extra and causing problems.

Aluminum is the most widespread metal in the natural environment and can be absorbed into the food we eat. Because of this it has been deemed safe, and so it's added to raising agents — in breads, cakes, cookies, etc. — as well as to most processed foods. It's also used in the production of food coloring, sweets, cocoa, tea, sodas, and infant formula. Aluminum is found in vaccines, aspirin, antacids, antiperspirants, cosmetics, sunscreen, and many other products. Most of the aluminum ingested comes from leavening agents (such as baking soda and baking powder), but you can buy aluminum-free varieties and bake your own cakes and cookies. Fifty to 80% of the silicon we absorb comes through the water supply — and it gets there via minerals in the soil. It's also in antacids and other pharmaceuticals, and in foods — mostly cereals.

Anyone whose symptoms seem similar to those of dementia or Alzheimer's should have a complete evaluation of the medications they're taking — both prescription drugs and over-the-counter preparations. This is recommended by Prof. Shelly Gray of the University of Washington, who carried out a seven-year study and showed that the long-term use of high doses of medications correlates with the development of these conditions. The drugs in question, known as *anticholinergic medications*, include tricyclic antidepressants, antihistamines, and antimuscarinics. It is easy to find alternatives for the first two groups here, but less so for the third group — which are for bladder control. Anticholinergic drugs encompass a wide group, including some used as sleeping aids and antihistamines, and others for the treatment of irritable bowel syndrome, asthma, bronchitis, COPD, and Parkinson's disease. The evaluation should involve the person's physician, who should also be made aware of all products routinely bought over the counter at drugstores.

Parkinson's Disease

Parkinson's disease (PD) is a degenerative disorder of the central nervous system that occurs when dopamine ceases to be generated from the pars compacta region of the substantia nigra portion of the midbrain. This interrupts the transmission of messages to the nerves and muscles, causing tremors, rigidity, slowing down of movement, and instability on the feet. As the disease progresses it can affect cognitive function and emotions. Each case is unique, depending on the location and degree of cell damage and the progression of the disease.

Some help with the symptoms can be offered by medications and other alternative treatments, forming an integrated management plan. As stress, anxiety, trauma, shock, and depression may all play a part in the onset and progression of the disease, the essential oils can be very helpful to a Parkinson's sufferer because they are able to address both the physical and emotional symptoms a person may be showing. Massage can help prevent muscles from stiffening and can help maintain mobility, while warm, fragrant, sensual baths can help alleviate the depression that can accompany this condition.

If you have Parkinson's, massage yourself as often as possible, as best you can. Better still, ask someone to massage you. And if possible visit a qualified registered aromatherapist once a month; that will make all the difference. Use the following essential oils in baths and massage oils.

ESSENTIAL OILS USEFUL FOR PEOPLE WITH PD
Rosemary (*Rosmarinus officinalis*)
Marjoram, sweet (*Origanum majorana*)

Lemon (*Citrus limon*)
Lavender (*Lavandula angustifolia*)
Basil linalol (*Ocimum basilicum ct. linalool*)
Geranium (*Pelargonium graveolens*)
Orange, sweet (*Citrus sinensis*)
Valerian (*Valeriana officinalis*)
Bergamot (*Citrus bergamia*)
Mandarin (*Citrus reticulata*)

PARKINSON'S GENERAL BATH BLEND

Orange, sweet	5 drops
Bergamot	5 drops
Lavender	10 drops

Blend the essential oils together, then dilute 4 drops per 1 teaspoon (5 mL) of carrier oil and put into the bathtub, swishing it around well before getting in.

PARKINSON'S GENERAL BODY OIL

Orange, sweet	5 drops
Valerian	2 drops
Geranium	5 drops
Rosemary	18 drops

Blend the essential oils together, then dilute 2–5 drops per 1 teaspoon (5 mL) of carrier oil.

PARKINSON'S BODY OIL FOR MUSCLE STIFFNESS

Marjoram, sweet	10 drops
Basil linalol	5 drops
Rosemary	10 drops
Lemon	5 drops

Blend the essential oils together, then dilute 5 drops per 1 teaspoon (5 mL) of carrier oil.

Diet is of the utmost importance. Try to eat a well-balanced, nutritious, organic diet, avoiding all dairy, wheat, and corn products. Avoid all processed fats and foods. Use bottled spring or distilled water, drink green tea, and take supplements such as essential fatty acids omega 3, 6, and 9 in the form of cold-pressed hemp seed oil, and omega 6 and gamma linolenic acid (GLA) in evening primrose seed oil. Also helpful are the

coenzyme Q10, vitamin B12, magnesium, and herbal supplements such as ginkgo (*Ginkgo biloba*) and turmeric (*Curcuma longa*).

Trembling

Trembling that is unrelated to a physical disorder such as Parkinson's disease (PD) can sometimes be helped by applying the following body oil. People with PD may also find the blend helpful.

BLEND FOR TREMBLING

Chamomile roman	3 drops
Clary sage	2 drops
Geranium	4 drops
Lemon	2 drops

Blend the essential oils together, then dilute 2–5 drops per 1 teaspoon (5 mL) of carrier oil.

If the trembling is more pronounced in the upper body, apply the body oil over one arm, across the chest, down the other arm, and over both hands. If the trembling tends to be in the lower portion of the body, apply the body oil over the lower back, hips, legs, and feet. It is helpful to get the blend down the length of the spine — about four inches on either side — although this will probably require help. If no one is available, just do what you can.

Arthritis

Arthritis is a term that applies to several diseases of the joints, the most common of which are rheumatoid arthritis and osteoarthritis. Both are discussed much more fully under their own section headings below. Pain is the common characteristic, and millions of people suffer varying degrees of it. Essential oils may help reduce the symptoms of arthritis, not only in helping retain the mobility of the joints, but also in providing some pain relief and helping to reduce inflammation and swelling. In all cases of arthritis, however, the first line of defense must be diet. In some patients, changing to a more healthy diet produces a transformational change. In others, the progression of the disease can be slowed, and prevented from worsening.

Naturally, if you have pain and movement restriction, being overweight doesn't help. If this is the case, reducing weight will lighten the stress load on your knees and feet. The hips will be less stressed because they won't have to try to compensate for lack of mobility in the knees. Following the nutritional suggestions below may be a challenge for some, but your knees will thank you.

NUTRITIONAL CHANGES

In some cases dietary changes can stop the advance of arthritis in its tracks. I remember seeing a man who could hardly walk for the pain but who, after it was identified that he was eating apples sprayed with an insecticide and he eliminated them from his diet, could walk easily and with much less pain. You too may be someone whose arthritis is the result of a chemical sensitivity or food allergy. If so, allergy testing may be helpful, or limit certain suspect foods and then reintroduce them into your diet to see if there's a difference.

The following regime should be carried out for at least six weeks, longer if you can. Even if you do not instantly change your diet to the one below, start noting the date and time when your symptoms seem to worsen, and the foods you ate prior to that. Try to be as thorough as possible. "Tea" should read, for example, "black tea, cow's milk, white sugar" or "herb tea — nettle, wild honey," if those things apply. In some people a reaction can be felt just half an hour after eating the responsible food, while in others it may be weeks afterward. For this latter group of people, identifying the cause might be difficult, but keeping a food diary allows any emerging pattern to be noticeable. In many cases of food sensitivity, it's not the food itself causing the problem but the additives or enzymes that may have been added — which does sometimes make things a little harder to identify. To test if a food is increasing your symptoms, gradually reintroduce each food — if the symptoms worsen, you may have found your culprit.

Start by cutting out or reducing all the following from your diet: processed meat and red meat; alcohol; dairy products; all sugar; refined flour and refined flour products (biscuits, cakes, white bread); fried foods; peanuts; lemons, grapefruit, oranges, and limes; root vegetables, including potatoes; tomatoes; and all preservatives and additives, including natural ones.

You could eat lots of fish, such as salmon, herring, mackerel, sardines, and tuna, including canned; plenty of green vegetables, such as those with calcium, like broccoli and kale; salads; pulses; nuts; seeds, such as sunflower and pumpkin; whole-grain bread; chicken; and figs, grapes, apricots, and peaches. Drink filtered, distilled, or bottled water and herbal teas.

Simple meals can be made quite quickly without dipping into the freezer section at your local store. Try spinach with a poached egg on top with whole-grain toast, or poached white fish with herbs served with steamed broccoli and green beans. A large tuna salad mixed with all your favorite allowed ingredients is a good standby, and chicken stuffed with chestnut and whole-grain stuffing makes a healthier alternative to pot roast and loads of gravy.

Supplements can be very helpful. Take at least 1,000 mg per day of vitamin C, along with a good multivitamin and mineral supplement; glucosamine with chondroitin is known to be beneficial, as is methylsulfonyl methane (MSM). Omega 3 fatty acids should be always included, and the seed oils that contain a balance of omega 3, 6, and 9 are beneficial — such as hemp seed and flax seed oils. Anti-inflammatories that could be incorporated into a healthy lifestyle include supplements of turmeric (curcumin) and Indian frankincense (*Boswellia serrata*). To help with pain and stiffness of joints try pycnogenol from maritime pine bark and bromelain extract. Also try to eat as many antioxidant-loaded fruits as possible, such as berries and cherries. Cod liver oil and organic virgin olive oil are also beneficial: take at least 2 teaspoons with 5 drops of evening primrose seed oil or borage seed oil — this can be added to milk or orange juice and should be sipped slowly. Try to purchase organic foods whenever possible.

For the first two weeks treatment is the same for all types of arthritis. This concentrates on detoxification, and takes the form of baths.

Arthritis Stage 1: Detox Bath Blend

Fennel, sweet	5 drops
Cypress	15 drops
Juniper berry	15 drops
Eucalyptus lemon	10 drops

First, blend the essential oils together. From this mix, take 3 drops and dilute them in ½ teaspoon (2½ mL) of carrier oil for each bath. The quantity of essential oils listed above is enough for 15 baths. After running the bath, add two large handfuls of Epsom salts and one large handful of rock salt or Dead Sea salt, then add the ½ teaspoon of carrier oil in which you've diluted the 3 drops of essential oil. Following the detoxification period, the different forms of arthritis are treated individually.

RHEUMATOID ARTHRITIS (RA)

Rheumatoid arthritis is a type of autoimmune disease where the body turns upon itself, causing an inflammatory response that mainly affects flexible joints but that can progress to the membranes of the lungs and around the heart, and even the whites of the eyes. At this point nobody knows why rheumatoid arthritis develops in some people and not in others — there are many theories, but no certainty.

What we do know is that rheumatoid arthritis can be extremely painful and can lead to deformity and loss of mobility in the joints. It's easy to recognize by the shiny tight skin around and over the affected areas, the swelling around joints, and by stiffness.

The first thing to think about is diet. Follow the advice given on page 283 in "Nutritional Changes." Foods to avoid include all those listed above, but do also cut out pre-prepared processed foods. Instead of using general vegetable oils, switch to virgin olive oil, hemp seed oil, or flax seed oil — in both cooking and on salads. Cut out all red meat. Eat garlic in your food or take a garlic supplement, and add fresh herbs and spices to your food for flavor. And cut all processed bottled or canned condiments if at all possible — try making your own instead; it's not as difficult as it sounds.

Essential oil treatment has three stages, the first of which has already been described above. The next two stages take two weeks each; throughout the total period of time continue with the diet outlined previously, along with the suggested supplements.

Rheumatoid Arthritis Stage 2
Essential Oils

Chamomile roman (*Anthemis nobilis*)
Peppermint (*Mentha piperita*)
Niaouli (*Melaleuca quinquenervia*)
Eucalyptus radiata (*Eucalyptus radiata*)
Chamomile german (*Matricaria recutita*)
Plai (*Zingiber cassumunar*)
Lavender (*Lavandula angustifolia*)
Eucalyptus lemon (*Eucalyptus citriodora*)
Juniper berry (*Juniperus communis*)

Rheumatoid Arthritis Stage 2 Bath Blend

Cypress	5 drops
Juniper berry	5 drops

Lavender	10 drops
Eucalyptus radiata	20 drops
Chamomile roman	16 drops

First, blend the essential oils together. To each bath add 4 drops of the blend diluted in ½ teaspoon (2½ mL) of carrier oil. As with Stage 1, add two handfuls of Epsom salts and one handful of rock or Dead Sea salt to the daily bath.

RHEUMATOID ARTHRITIS STAGE 2 BODY OIL

Chamomile german	8 drops
Lavender	10 drops
Peppermint	2 drops
Ginger	8 drops
Plai	10 drops

Also massage morning and night over the painful areas using a little of the Stage 2 Body Oil. First, blend the essential oils together, then use 3–5 drops diluted in 1 teaspoon (5 mL) of carrier oil for each application.

Carry out the Stage 2 treatment for two weeks, and then progress to Stage 3. These are the essential oils to use:

RHEUMATOID ARTHRITIS STAGE 3 ESSENTIAL OILS
Ginger (*Zingiber officinale*)
Chamomile german (*Matricaria recutita*)
Black pepper (*Piper nigrum*)
Rosemary (*Rosmarinus officinalis*)
Chamomile roman (*Anthemis nobilis*)
Lavender (*Lavandula angustifolia*)
Eucalyptus radiata (*Eucalyptus radiata*)
Frankincense (*Boswellia carterii*)
Plai (*Zingiber cassumunar*)
Eucalyptus lemon (*Eucalyptus citriodora*)

The baths taken during the two weeks of Stage 3 alternate between the blend already given in Stage 2 (omitting the Epsom salts but still using the rock or Dead Sea salt) and the following blend:

RHEUMATOID ARTHRITIS STAGE 3 BATH BLEND

Ginger	4 drops
Lavender	4 drops
Rosemary	15 drops
Frankincense	5 drops

Blend together, then use 3 drops diluted in 1 teaspoon (5 mL) of carrier oil per bath, adding one handful of rock or Dead Sea salt.

During Stage 3, massage the affected joints only. Use the following oil and the Stage 2 Body Oil on alternate days:

RHEUMATOID ARTHRITIS STAGE 3 BODY OIL

Rosemary	8 drops
Lavender	7 drops
Frankincense	10 drops
Ginger	5 drops

Blend the essential oils together, then dilute 3–5 drops in 1 teaspoon (5 mL) of carrier oil for each massage.

After completing Stage 3, move to the Maintenance Program, which follows on page 287.

OSTEOARTHRITIS (OA)

Osteoarthritis is a degenerative condition that may have an inflammatory component — affecting joints such as the hips, knees, and fingers — in which the cartilage wears away, causing damage to the bones. It can be very painful and lead to immobility in the joints, with muscle atrophy and ineffective ligaments. It can start innocently enough with just an ache and stiffness, yet feel progressively worse as time goes on. It's very important to keep the affected area active so as not to allow immobility to set in. Follow the suggestions in the "Nutritional Changes" section on page 283, along with the recommendations for useful supplements. Stage 1 of treatment comprises the Stage 1 Detox Baths, also described above. Stage 2 uses the following essential oils:

OSTEOARTHRITIS STAGE 2 ESSENTIAL OILS
Cedarwood atlas (*Cedrus atlantica*)
Ginger (*Zingiber officinale*)
Sandalwood (*Santalum album*)
Lavender (*Lavandula angustifolia*)
Petitgrain (*Citrus aurantium*)
Rosemary (*Rosmarinus officinalis*)
Cypress (*Cupressus sempervirens*)
Black pepper (*Piper nigrum*)
Pine (*Pinus sylvestris*)
Patchouli (*Pogostemon cablin*)

OSTEOARTHRITIS STAGE 2 BATH BLEND

Petitgrain	5 drops
Cedarwood	15 drops
Marjoram, sweet	8 drops

First, blend the essential oils together. Then put two large handfuls of Epsom salts and one large handful of rock salt or Dead Sea salt in the bath, and add 3 drops of the blend, diluted in 1 teaspoon (5 mL) of carrier oil.

OSTEOARTHRITIS STAGE 2 BODY OIL

Ginger	8 drops
Geranium	5 drops
Black pepper	8 drops
Cedarwood atlas	4 drops
Cypress	5 drops

First, blend the essential oils together, then dilute 3–5 drops in 1 teaspoon (5 mL) of carrier oil. Apply the Stage 2 massage blend to the affected areas once or twice a day.

Stage 3 of the treatment also lasts two weeks, and these are the essential oils:

OSTEOARTHRITIS STAGE 3 ESSENTIAL OILS
Lavender (*Lavandula angustifolia*)
Ginger (*Zingiber officinale*)
Black pepper (*Piper nigrum*)
Nutmeg (*Myristica fragrans*)
Rosemary (*Rosmarinus officinalis*)
Marjoram, sweet (*Origanum majorana*)
Sandalwood (*Santalum album*)
Cypress (*Cupressus sempervirens*)
Petitgrain (*Citrus aurantium*)
Pine (*Pinus sylvestris*)

The baths taken during Stage 3 should alternate daily between the blend already given for Stage 1 and the Stage 3 bath blend.

OSTEOARTHRITIS STAGE 3 BATH BLEND

Black pepper	5 drops
Rosemary	15 drops
Marjoram, sweet	8 drops

First, blend the essential oils together. Put one handful of Epsom salts and one handful of rock or Dead Sea salt in the bath, and add 4 drops of the blend, diluted in 1 teaspoon (5 mL) of carrier oil.

During Stage 3 massage only the affected joints. Alternate between the body oil blend in Stage 2 and the following:

OSTEOARTHRITIS STAGE 3 BODY OIL

Sandalwood	15 drops
Ginger	5 drops
Lavender	10 drops

First, blend the essential oils together, then dilute 3–5 drops in 1 teaspoon (5 mL) of carrier oil for each massage.

After this six-week treatment, move on to the maintenance program below. If your arthritis developed during or after menopause, add geranium or rose otto essential oils to your treatment. If your condition gets worse during periods of stress, add to your blend those oils that are helpful in alleviating stress — you will find relevant lists in several sections of this book.

MAINTENANCE PROGRAM FOR RHEUMATOID ARTHRITIS AND OSTEOARTHRITIS

The six-week treatments above for rheumatoid arthritis and osteoarthritis may be repeated. In between these cycles, massage can be carried out using the essential oils below using 1 drop of essential oil per teaspoon (5 mL) of carrier oil — either used singly or in blends.

ARTHRITIS MAINTENANCE OILS

Mandarin (*Citrus reticulata*)
Chamomile roman (*Anthemis nobilis*)
Chamomile german (*Matricaria recutita*)
Marjoram, sweet (*Origanum majorana*)
Geranium (*Pelargonium graveolens*)
Lavender (*Lavandula angustifolia*)

Other Skeletal Disorders

Every person is different, and the onset of any musculoskeletal condition will have a series of common symptoms, along with other symptoms unique to each individual. Variable factors include genetics, dietary habits, and previous health conditions. Although it's not generally recognized, there can also be an element of emotion involved in the development of musculoskeletal conditions, and emotional factors also have an influence on the range and degree of symptoms.

If you're suffering from ankylosis or spondylosis, follow the treatment for osteoarthritis; if you suffer from lupus erythematosus, follow the rheumatoid arthritis treatment.

Gout

Gout is a form of inflammatory arthritis that can become unbearably painful on occasion. It's caused by an overproduction of uric acid in the body, which forms into crystals that gather, usually around joints and tendons. There can be a burning sensation, as well as swelling. The good news is that gout can be managed and the symptoms reduced; the not-so-good news is that gout is often associated with serious health problems such as diabetes, high blood pressure, raised cholesterol, and heart disease. Back to the good news: steps to reduce the excruciating pain of gout can also reduce the risk of the other health problems mentioned, which may not have such obvious symptoms. In other words, gout provides a flashing, warning red light that tells you something needs to be done. Gout can also be the result of other factors, including genetics and physical trauma.

About half of gout sufferers experience it in their feet, especially in the metatarsal-phalangeal joint at the base of the big toe. Other commonly affected joints are the fingers, heels, knees, and wrists, although it can affect all parts of the body, including the earlobe. High levels of uric acid can also cause kidney stones. If there's swelling and accompanying redness of the skin, gout could be suspected.

The aim of any treatment of gout is to dissolve the monosodium urate crystals that are causing the pain. More than that, the aim is to reduce the production of the crystals in the first place, which involves reducing the level of uric acid concentration in the body, which in turn is a consequence of inefficient purine metabolism. Improving kidney function is a key element in the picture, as this allows uric acid to leave the body efficiently.

Purine is something found in all food groups and is clearly something to consider, but most purine — around 80% — comes from normal physical processes happening within any healthy body. Specifically, the millions of cells that die within us each and every day break down and release purine, most of which is taken up again in the formation of new cells. The excess purines get sent to the liver for processing into uric acid, which then moves via the bloodstream to the kidneys, where it is urinated out. This is where the first problem can occur if the kidneys don't have enough water to flush out the uric acid. Drinking plenty of water is the first step to reducing the degree of gout, but it should be drunk slowly, in small amounts throughout the day rather than in a few large glasses, allowing hydration to take place rather than a quick balancing-out of fluid in the form of immediate urination. Over time, the uric acid in the body can be expelled from the interstitial fluid — the fluid between cells — and from the synovial fluid — the fluid inside joints — and eventually the crystals can be reduced. This takes time, but anyone suffering the pain of gout will know it's worth it.

Good kidney function is essential to anyone, including people with gout, and this is closely related to the function of the adrenal glands, which sit on top of each kidney. The adrenals respond to stress, which is why, disconnected as it may first appear, stress reduction becomes a factor in kidney function and gout. Taking time out to reduce stress is easier said than done, but if it's thought of as a way to alleviate adrenal fatigue and as an important element in a healthy lifestyle, more value may be given to finding the time. Physical activities that reduce stress include tai chi, qi gong, and yoga, but just take time for yourself and do whatever it is that makes you relaxed. If you can relax in the sun, even better, as that provides vitamin D. Try not to think of relaxation as "wasting time" but as "taking nature's meds."

ESSENTIAL OILS THAT COULD BE USED
FOR GOUT
Basil linalol (*Ocimum basilicum ct. linalool*)
Pine (*Pinus sylvestris*)
Grapefruit (*Citrus paradisi*)

Plai (*Zingiber cassumunar*)
Juniper berry (*Juniperus communis*)
Spearmint (*Mentha spicata*)
Peppermint (*Mentha piperita*)
Chamomile german (*Matricaria recutita*)
Chamomile roman (*Anthemis nobilis*)
Cypress (*Cupressus sempervirens*)
Geranium (*Pelargonium graveolens*)
Thyme linalol (*Thymus vulgaris ct. linalool*)
Eucalyptus radiata (*Eucalyptus radiata*)
Bergamot (*Citrus bergamia*)
Immortelle (*Helichrysum italicum*)
Eucalyptus peppermint (*Eucalyptus dives*)
Rosemary (*Rosmarinus officinalis*)
Fennel, sweet (*Foeniculum vulgare var. dulce*)

The intense pain of an inflamed, or hot-to-the-touch, gout episode can be unbearable, and it's good to have something ready-prepared that can alleviate the symptoms. In general, ice-cold compresses can help, applied over the area. Simply soak a piece of material, or a facecloth, in water and keep it in a plastic bag in the ice compartment of the fridge until needed.

A gel can also be stored in the fridge, ready for an inflamed episode. Use enough to cover the affected area. When making this pre-prepared gel, first blend the essential oils together in the order in which they appear on the list, and put to one side. Ensure that the aloe vera gel and arnica oil are well combined before adding the essential oil blend, and mix well.

GEL FOR GOUT

Aloe vera gel	2 fl. oz. (60 mL)
Arnica macerated oil	2 teaspoons (10 mL)
Chamomile german	5 drops
Lavender	10 drops
Peppermint	3 drops
Juniper berry	5 drops
Chamomile roman	5 drops

The following two body oil blends have different properties, so choose the one that is more appropriate at any given time. First, dilute your chosen blend in 2 teaspoons (10 mL) of arnica macerated oil or organic cold-pressed virgin olive oil. Use a small amount to gently massage the affected joint. Drink plenty of water after the massage.

BLEND FOR RED, SWOLLEN, AND INFLAMED JOINTS

Cypress	5 drops
Peppermint	3 drops
Juniper berry	5 drops
Eucalyptus radiata	10 drops
Chamomile german	5 drops

BLEND FOR PAINFUL AND STIFF JOINTS

Immortelle	5 drops
Peppermint	2 drops
Rosemary	10 drops
Chamomile german	10 drops

Purines are a key factor in gout, and although our bodies produce the vast majority of purines in our system, we can control the purines we choose to ingest in food. The purines in plants don't seem to cause any problems, but the purines found in certain other foods, if eaten in excess, may be exacerbating the condition. These include offal from animals, such as liver, kidney, heart, and brain; shellfish, such as mussels and scallops; and fish, such as anchovies, mackerel, herring, and sardines. Historically, gout was associated with the wealthy, hard-drinking man, but although alcohol certainly doesn't help, the drinks that cause the modern man and woman more problems these days are sodas made with fructose corn syrup. Any processed foods are likely to contain purines that won't help anyone with gout, and, being really straight about this, a vegan or plant-based diet is the best way forward.

Change to an organic diet using fresh products, cooking from scratch. Olive oil is the better oil to use in cooking; try to avoid corn oil. Cheese and yogurt are fine, and if you must have a wheat product, purchase one with organic whole-wheat flour. Nuts and seeds are good, as are certain fruits, such as cherries. These dietary changes could bring about a reduction in weight, which is going to be helpful not only for the gout but for any associated health problems mentioned above. Taking a 1,500 mg vitamin C supplement is thought to help in cases of gout, as is folic acid, bromelain, and vitamin E.

Dyspepsia (Indigestion)

Dyspepsia is a term used to describe indigestion or different conditions that affect the stomach or upper abdominal gastrointestinal organs. Indigestion is painful, and it can strike at any time. It can be brought on by a variety of things, including alcohol, eating spicy or greasy foods, rushing food and not chewing, sensitivity to foods, and what I call "emotional indigestion," brought on by nerves and emotional stress. Other, more serious causes include ulceration, gallstones, and pancreatitis. Persistent indigestion should be discussed with your doctor.

Herb teas can often help, such as lemon balm, chamomile, fennel, dill, aniseed, peppermint, and ginger. Herbal tinctures such as artichoke can be helpful, as can supplements containing turmeric powder or banana powder — which are traditionally used in Asia to treat dyspepsia.

If you eat slowly and chew thoroughly to the point of boredom, this in itself is often all that's needed to help reduce bouts of indigestion and the flatulence that often accompanies it. Massage your upper abdomen area between meals with the following oils or blends, chosen from whichever category is most appropriate, and using 15–20 drops per 2 tablespoons (30 mL) of carrier oil.

General Indigestion Oils

Aniseed (*Pimpinella anisum*)
Coriander seed (*Coriandrum sativum*)
Peppermint (*Mentha piperita*)
Cardamom (*Elettaria cardamomum*)
Dill seed (*Anethum graveolens*)
Fennel, sweet (*Foeniculum vulgare var. dulce*)
Ginger (*Zingiber officinale*)
Caraway seed (*Carum carvi*)
Spearmint (*Mentha spicata*)
Black pepper (*Piper nigrum*)
Orange, sweet (*Citrus sinensis*)
Petitgrain (*Citrus aurantium*)

Blend your chosen essential oils together, or choose from one of the blends below. Then dilute by using 20–30 drops per 2 tablespoons (30 mL) of carrier oil. Or, to make enough for an individual body oil, mix 3–5 drops of your blend in 1 teaspoon (5 mL) of carrier oil; this amount should suffice for both a morning and a night application. Rub over the upper abdomen.

Indigestion Blend 1

Coriander seed	10 drops
Ginger	3 drops
Orange, sweet	5 drops

Indigestion Blend 2

Cardamom	10 drops
Dill seed	5 drops
Peppermint	3 drops
Fennel, sweet	5 drops
Caraway seed	5 drops

Tonic Oils for Weak Upper Abdominal Muscles

Lavender (*Lavandula angustifolia*)
Rosemary (*Rosmarinus officinalis*)
Cypress (*Cupressus sempervirens*)
Fennel, sweet (*Foeniculum vulgare var. dulce*)
Cardamom (*Elettaria cardamomum*)
Spearmint (*Mentha spicata*)
Coriander seed (*Coriandrum sativum*)
Black pepper (*Piper nigrum*)

Weak Abdominal Muscle Blend 1

Rosemary	10 drops
Cardamom	10 drops
Black pepper	2 drops

Weak Abdominal Muscle Blend 2

Cypress	5 drops
Rosemary	5 drops
Coriander seed	15 drops

Blend the essential oils you have chosen, or choose one of the blends above. Then dilute 3–5 drops in 1 teaspoon (5 mL) of carrier oil, and rub a small amount over the upper abdomen morning and night.

Emotional or Nervous Indigestion

Ginger (*Zingiber officinale*)
Spearmint (*Mentha spicata*)
Aniseed (*Pimpinella anisum*)
Vetiver (*Vetiveria zizanoides*)
Lavender (*Lavandula angustifolia*)
Dill seed (*Anethum graveolens*)
Peppermint (*Mentha piperita*)
Clary sage (*Salvia sclarea*)

Emotional Blend

Clary sage	5 drops
Spearmint	15 drops
Lavender	15 drops

Nervous Blend

Vetiver	3 drops
Lavender	5 drops

| Cardamom | 5 drops |
| Orange, sweet | 10 drops |

Blend your chosen oils together, or chose from one of the blends above. Then dilute 3–5 drops in 1 teaspoon (5 mL) of carrier oil and rub a small amount over the upper abdomen, as needed.

Flatulence/Gas

Flatulence can be described as either rectal flatulence or belching, and it is sometimes associated with physical conditions such as hiatus hernia, bacterial infections such as *Helicobacter pylori*, and colon disorders including diverticular disease, colitis, and IBS. Flatulence can even be caused by certain medications. More usually, flatulence is food related, such as in cases of adverse reaction to gluten, known as *celiac disease*. Food allergies or sensitivities can also cause flatulence. Spicy foods and soft drinks are often at fault, along with foods high in unabsorbable carbohydrates, such as cabbage, cauliflower, beans, pulses, and onions. And some people just guzzle air as they eat — and swallow it along with everything else. For some people, the sugars and polysaccharides they ingest don't digest or get absorbed properly. In others, there's an overgrowth of bacteria in the small intestine. Having said all that, there are people who just seem to be more prone to having gas than others.

However the excess air or gas gets there, the result is that the lower abdomen swells as the intestines distend — usually causing the intestinal muscles to contract and push the gas along until it reaches the anus and is expelled. But sometimes the pressure is so great that the swelling extends under the rib cage, causing palpitations and shortness of breath and even, in some cases, a pain similar to angina pectoris. In a mature person, there can be a loss of tone in the intestinal muscles, which makes the expulsion process less efficient.

Foods you might consider cutting out of your diet are the sugars — fructose, glucose, lactose, and galactose — and starchy carbohydrates such as wheat, peas, pulses, onions, and carrots. Beans and cabbage are well-known culprits in the overproduction of gas.

ESSENTIAL OILS FOR GASTRIC FLATULENCE
Coriander seed (*Coriandrum sativum*)
Spearmint (*Mentha spicata*)
Dill seed (*Anethum graveolens*)
Cardamom (*Elettaria cardamomum*)
Eucalyptus peppermint (*Eucalyptus dives*)
Peppermint (*Mentha piperita*)
Caraway seed (*Carum carvi*)
Black pepper (*Piper nigrum*)
Aniseed (*Pimpinella anisum*)
Fennel, sweet (*Foeniculum vulgare var. dulce*)
Basil linalol (*Ocimum basilicum ct. linalool*)

If you're experiencing discomfort, make the following blend and rub it over the whole of the abdomen in a clockwise direction:

GASTRIC FLATULENCE BLEND
| Cardamom | 2 drops |
| Peppermint | 3 drops |

Blend the essential oils together, then dilute 3–5 drops in 1 teaspoon (5 mL) of carrier oil.

One remedy is to take 1 drop of spearmint essential oil and mix it with 1 teaspoon of honey, add to a mug of boiling water, let it cool to a comfortable warm temperature, and then sip slowly.

Constipation

The causes of constipation are many — for example, not eating enough fiber, such as that found in fruit and vegetables, dehydration, lifestyle changes, emotional upset, medication, resisting the urge to pass a stool, not taking enough exercise, disease, and intestinal disorder. The first things to address are diet, fluid intake, exercise levels, and stress reduction.

Complications can result from long-term constipation. If you see any blood in a stool or have constipation continuously, it's important to obtain a stool test from your physician. Feces left in the rectum become dried and hardened, and with time they become more difficult to pass. This can cause spurious diarrhea, a watery discharge caused by irritation of the rectum.

Dietary changes may be needed: add flax seed and bulking agents such as fiber to meals, and eat more dried or stewed fruits. Glycerin or herbal suppositories often help, as does taking a probiotic supplement designed specifically for those with constipation. Increase your vitamin C intake to 1,500 mg per day, and drink plenty of pure water. Avoid taking laxatives unless absolutely necessary because over the long term they can cause lazy bowel syndrome, in which the bowels can't do their job without some form of chemical stimulation.

Massaging around the lower abdomen, following the intestinal tract in a clockwise direction and moving your hand left to begin with, may help shift impacted feces. Before massaging, however, drink a cup of hot water to which is added a small amount of freshly grated ginger root.

CONSTIPATION MASSAGE ESSENTIAL OILS
Patchouli (*Pogostemon cablin*)
Fennel, sweet (*Foeniculum vulgare var. dulce*)
Rosemary (*Rosmarinus officinalis*)
Ginger (*Zingiber officinale*)
Sandalwood (*Santalum album*)
Cardamom (*Elettaria cardamomum*)
Black pepper (*Piper nigrum*)

Orange, sweet (*Citrus sinensis*)
Aniseed (*Pimpinella anisum*)
Marjoram, sweet (*Origanum majorana*)

CONSTIPATION BLEND

Orange, sweet	5 drops
Patchouli	15 drops
Black pepper	5 drops
Cardamom	5 drops

Blend the essential oils together, then dilute the 30 drops in 2 tablespoons (30 mL) of carrier oil and use as much as needed each time. For single massages, add 5 drops to 1 teaspoon (5 mL) of carrier oil.

Massage in a clockwise direction over the abdomen as deeply as you can without causing discomfort, then over the hips and lower back, and down the spine to just above the anus. Use this method three times a day. Alternatively, choose from the essential oils listed above, diluting 5 drops of essential oil to each teaspoon (5 mL) of carrier oil.

Hemorrhoids (Piles)

Piles are often the result of straining because of chronic constipation. Probiotic supplements can help, as do vitamins E and C. Bathe the area with a warm washcloth onto which you have put 2 drops of the following blend of oils. Apply the washcloth to the anal area for a few minutes, and repeat three or four times, twice a day.

HEMORRHOIDS APPLICATION BLEND

Patchouli	2 drops
Myrrh	10 drops
Cypress	5 drops
Geranium	5 drops

Blend together, then use 2 drops per application, avoiding the genital area.

SITZ TREATMENT AND OIL

Hemorrhoids can ache and be painful. This method of treatment involves using a sitz bath, which is basically a large bowl you can sit in. Put in enough water to cover the anal area, and add to it 4 drops of geranium essential oil. Sit in the bowl for five minutes. Then dry around the area, and apply a little of the following oil:

Geranium	15 drops
Cypress	10 drops
Lavender	5 drops

Blend the essential oils together, then dilute 10–15 drops in 1 teaspoon (5 mL) of carrier oil. Put this in a small container, an egg cup will do, and cover with plastic wrap. Apply a small amount around the anus, as required, avoiding the genital area.

Most people report that relief is felt by using this remedy twice a day, morning and night.

Care of the Feet

Taking care of the feet is important at any time of life, but never more so than during the maturing years. Foot baths followed by a foot massage are an excellent way to care for this often neglected area. First, bathe the feet in a bowl of water that contains two handfuls of sea salt, 1 tablespoon of bicarbonate of soda (baking soda), and 1 tablespoon of organic apple or cider vinegar. Essential oils that could be added to the water include lavender, chamomile roman, and geranium. For corns, place 1 drop of lemon essential oil directly onto each corn before massaging the feet with a carrier oil — jojoba and calendula macerated oil are good choices at this time, as is arnica macerated oil, which helps aching feet.

Nails and Nail Beds

Nails and nail beds often become diseased and thickened in the senior years and can become prone to fungal infections. If a fungal infection is present, use a combination of neem oil and tea tree oil. This isn't the best smelling combination, but who cares? It's not the fragrance you're after, but an end to the fungal infection. Both can be added neat to the area, a maximum of 1 drop each time.

If a fungus does not appear to be the cause of the problem, massage the following oil around the nail and nail bed once a week or so, to keep it healthy and free from infection:

BLEND FOR NAIL HEALTH

Tea tree	10 drops
Lavender	5 drops
Peppermint	2 drops
Lemon	5 drops

Blend the essential oils together, then dilute 5 drops in 1 teaspoon (5 mL) of jojoba oil, and apply over the toes and foot as needed.

11

Assertive Oils for Sports, Dance, and Exercise

Essential oils offer a terrific opportunity to athletes and dancers. The capacity of essential oils to heal wounds and injury is well established, but because they also play a part in preparing the muscles for full exertion, they can help prevent injury, allow the body to recover more quickly, and reduce the effects of fatigue. Keeping the body working at an optimum level is half the battle in sport and dance, but the other aspect of physical activity is the way the mind can influence performance, and in this, essential oils have a unique ability to positively affect the mind, mood, and emotion. This characteristic of essential oils is recognized within the field of clinical sports medicine, where essential oils and aromatherapy are increasingly being harnessed to optimize the potential of elite athletes.

Each sport has its own risks. Hockey players are prone to groin pull, and runners are susceptible to cartilage damage in their knees, while repetitive motion injuries affect golfers, swimmers, and tennis players alike. Anyone can pull a muscle or sprain an ankle, and footballers expect contusions with every game. Dancers are directed by choreographers to move in very precise ways, night after night. The potential for physical damage is ever-present with sport and dance, and when it's your profession, it can be more than a physical blow. Essential oils can heal wounds and may reduce pain, but they also keep the body in great condition by improving circulation and keeping the muscles toned.

Because running is such a popular activity and involved in so many sports, it has its own section in this chapter. Without good care and maintenance of the feet, we'll be running nowhere, so there's advice specifically for aromatherapy foot care, as well as for the muscles. An A–Z list of injuries is preceded by a section explaining the different methods of treatment, and for users of gyms and recreational facilities, there's a section at the end with advice on how essential oils can protect from unseen microbes. But first, we start with the mind, because without that on our side it can be hard to pull on the trainers, let alone get past the winning post.

Sport, Dance, and the Mind

This chapter is called "Assertive Oils for Sports, Dance, and Exercise" because essential oils, unlike anything else on this earth, can bring confidence and self-assurance while also helping to heal the physical body. They are assertive. Quiet, unobtrusive, and minuscule in size, they pervade the whole person, healing both body and mind. People who've used essential oils specifically for reasons to do with attaining a positive mental attitude are aware of this. If you are not yet a believer, there's only one way to find out what they can do for you. There's a chapter in this book called "Emotional Rescue" (see page 95) that you might want to explore, or have a look through my book *The Fragrant Mind*, especially the sections in chapter 7, "Emotional Healing," on alertness, assertiveness, concentration, confidence, focus, performance, positivity, and self-esteem. The essential oils are assertive because they're confident in what they can do, and they can bring that inner confidence to you too.

Sport is by its very nature competitive and so involves a certain amount of unavoidable stress. This is not a bad thing in itself because it gives us the impetus to push ourselves to a better performance. No matter where you are in terms of success, there's always competition stress — whether it's about avoiding being last in the race or maintaining your position as first in the race. In ages past, stress hormones were intended to produce the fight-or-flight response necessary for us humans to make a sudden dash to escape the occasional saber-toothed tiger. But today we're calling on those hormones to help us escape the person running at our heels, day after day, and the system intended for occasional use is being overextended. This is why taking steps to reduce stress is helpful — it brings the body back into balance so it's able to perform at optimum capacity when required. What follows are some suggestions for before the event and after.

PRE-EVENT BATH OR SHOWER BODY OIL

Vetiver	3 drops
Bergamot	4 drops
Juniper berry	1 drop
Orange, sweet	4 drops

First, blend the essential oils together, then dilute in 1 tablespoon (15 mL) of carrier oil. Apply enough to cover the whole body about 10 minutes before getting in a bath or shower.

PRE-EVENT BATH OR SHOWER BLEND

Rosemary	3 drops
Lemon	4 drops
Lavender	3 drops
Chamomile roman	2 drops

First, blend the essential oils together. Dilute 6 drops in an equal amount of carrier oil before putting into the bath, or put 4 drops of the blend onto the washcloth before getting into the shower.

AFTER-SPORT BATH OR SHOWER BLEND

Grapefruit	4 drops
Orange, sweet	2 drops
Clary sage	4 drops
Frankincense	2 drops

First, blend the essential oils together. Dilute 6 drops in an equal amount of carrier oil before putting into the bath, or put 4 drops of the blend onto the washcloth before getting into the shower.

Because sport, dance, and exercise are activities carried out over a long period of time, when using essential oils for a general increase in physical performance it's better to use smaller amounts than you would, for example, for an acute injury. The following essential oils can be used on their own, or combine those of your choice to make a blend. Use only 2 drops in baths, after diluting in a little carrier oil. For body oils, dilute 10 drops in 2 tablespoons (30 mL) of a carrier oil. This makes enough for several body rubs or massages. The benefits of using these essential oils in this way will be seen over a period of time.

ESSENTIAL OILS FOR IMPROVED
PHYSICAL PERFORMANCE
Grapefruit (*Citrus paradisi*)
Black pepper (*Piper nigrum*)
Thyme linalol (*Thymus vulgaris ct. linalool*)
Ginger (*Zingiber officinale*)
Basil linalol (*Ocimum basilicum ct. linalool*)
Lavender (*Lavandula angustifolia*)
Rosemary (*Rosmarinus officinalis*)
Frankincense (*Boswellia carterii*)
Cistus (*Cistus ladaniferus*)
Coriander seed (*Coriandrum sativum*)
Sandalwood (*Santalum album*)
Cedarwood atlas (*Cedrus atlantica*)
Lemon (*Citrus limon*)
Eucalyptus lemon (*Eucalyptus citriodora*)
Petitgrain (*Citrus aurantium*)

Fatigue is caused by physical exertion, but it seems to seep into the brain and so can be experienced as a mental event too. The brain cells seem to have flopped, just as you have! Paradoxical as it might seem, the oils that counter fatigue are relaxants rather than stimulants. The fatigue brought about by sport is often due to overstimulation, and a sudden rush of stimulation now might tire the body further. So use, for example, sweet marjoram instead of rosemary, lavender instead of lavandin, and sweet orange instead of lemongrass. Stick to low dilutions — 15 drops of essential oil to 2 tablespoons (30 mL) of carrier oil to make a body oil, and use a small amount each time.

Running

There's running like Usain Bolt in the 2012 London Olympics, when he ran away with three gold medals, and there's jogging gently around the park on the weekend. We'll come to competitive running later, but when starting out it's important not to overexert yourself, because pounding hard surfaces such as pavements puts great strain on muscles, ankle bones, and the skeletal frame, especially the lower back. The following blend of oils is intended for people taking up running or jogging; it is helpful for both the lungs and respiratory system, and for the muscular and skeletal frames. Before setting out for a run, rub a little of the blend below over your ankles, calves, thighs, buttocks, and lower back. Apply just enough to be absorbed by the skin, and if there's any excess, wipe it off.

BEGINNERS' RUNNING BLEND

Eucalyptus radiata	5 drops
Rosemary	10 drops
Ginger	5 drops
Peppermint	2 drops

First, blend the essential oils together. Then dilute 3–5 drops to each teaspoon (5 mL) of carrier oil; alternatively, dilute 3–5 drops in 1 teaspoon (5 mL) of aloe vera gel.

Power walking, jogging, and running cause different foot pressure and require a different foot-conditioning blend of oils. It's been found that walkers, for example, use more force when their heel hits the ground, so it's important to take care of any buildup of hard skin before it becomes split and cracks, leaving it open to infection.

GENERAL CONDITIONING FOOT OIL BLEND
FOR WALKERS, JOGGERS, AND RUNNERS

Peppermint	2 drops
Tea tree	5 drops
Basil linalol	4 drops
Rosemary	5 drops
Clove bud	2 drops
Cypress	5 drops
Lemongrass	5 drops

First, blend the essential oils together, then dilute 5 drops to each teaspoon (5 mL) of sesame, coconut, or tamanu carrier oil.

Repetitively landing on hard surfaces can hurt the joints of the feet and cause strain on the hip bones, as well as pressure on the skeletal frame. This can sometimes result in neck aches, headaches, and migraines, which in turn can lead to feeling fatigued. If the very thought of going for another run seems an insurmountable task, try a revitalizing foot bath: cover the bottom of a large bowl with as many small, smooth, round pebbles as you can find, pour in enough hot water to cover your ankles, and add 4 drops of either grapefruit, rosemary, lemon, pine, cypress, eucalyptus lemon, lavandin, or juniper berry essential oil. Sit back, inhale the vapors, and practice some positive-thought mantras while rolling your feet gently over the pebbles.

Revitalizing sprays are very useful to carry while running or power walking and are easily made using hydrolats. Use hydrolats of thyme, rosemary, basil, peppermint, or spearmint. A popular hydrolat combination is rosemary, lemon, and peppermint. And another is the combination of pine, rosemary, and juniper berry.

The following essential oil blends are designed to help the muscles in particular and can be used either before or after a run. It's useful to pre-prepare your chosen blend and have it ready in your sports bag. Apply to a specific area of the body, or use as an all-over body oil.

MUSCLE BLEND 1

Ginger	4 drops
Black pepper	2 drops
Rosemary	5 drops
Plai	5 drops
Immortelle	4 drops

First, blend the essential oils together, then dilute in 2 tablespoons (30 mL) of carrier oil, arnica gel, or aloe vera gel and use a small amount each time, rubbed into the muscles as needed.

MUSCLE BLEND 2

Eucalyptus radiata	5 drops
Rosemary (or immortelle)	10 drops
Lemongrass	5 drops

First, blend the essential oils together, then dilute in 2 tablespoons (30 mL) of carrier oil, arnica gel, or aloe vera gel and use a small amount each time, rubbed into the muscles as needed.

The runners' competition oils that follow take into account the positive effect that some essential oils can have on performance of both mind and body. The blends should be reserved for the occasion of a big race to give a competitive edge, because aroma sensitivity can become aroma insensitivity if a particular combination is overused. Before the event, rub the blend over specific areas of your body that are prone to injury.

RUNNERS' COMPETITION BLEND 1

Bergamot FCF	8 drops
Basil linalol	5 drops
Black pepper	2 drops
Rosemary	2 drops
Spearmint	2 drops

First blend the essential oils together, then dilute in 2 tablespoons (30 mL) of carrier oil, or in 2 tablespoons (30 mL) of aloe vera gel.

RUNNERS' COMPETITION BLEND 2

Plai	5 drops
Rosemary	2 drops
Bergamot FCF	2 drops
Peppermint	1 drop

First blend the essential oils together, then dilute in 1 tablespoon (15 mL) of carrier oil, or in 1 tablespoon (15 mL) of aloe vera gel.

Geranium oil provides a good remedy for "jogger's nipple," which is caused by the action of material rubbing on the nipple for long periods of time. The discomfort suffered by long-distance male runners, as well as by women in all sports, can be quite considerable. Clearly, all sportswomen should wear a good-fitting protective bra, but for all who have developed this problem the answer is to add 3 drops of geranium oil to each teaspoon (5 mL) of carrier oil and rub as much as needed around the area, especially before and after the sporting activity. Alternatively, if the nipple is already sore, blend 5 drops of lavender and 5 drops of chamomile german in 2 teaspoons (10 mL) of aloe vera gel or a good organic gel or ointment. This combination has anti-inflammatory properties and helps ease soreness.

The thrust of competition has always driven those involved with sport or exercise to find preparations to boost performance while keeping their body in peak condition. In ancient Greece, elite athletes bathed in mint to strengthen muscles and sinews, while today it's more likely to be baths to which the essential oils of sweet marjoram, immortelle, rosemary, lemongrass, ginger, or black pepper have been added. Physiotherapists and sports therapists often choose essential oils such as eucalyptus radiata, chamomile, lavender, plai, immortelle, black pepper, ginger, rosemary, or one of the mint essential oils, as well as preparations that contain small amounts of analgesics such as clove bud, sweet birch, wintergreen, camphor, or cinnamon leaf. Natural remedies go hand in hand with the standard methods of treating sports injuries and maintaining the well-being of the body — which sport pushes to the limits of endurance, stamina, and skill.

Foot Care

In each foot there are 26 bones, 20 articulated joints, a further 13 nonarticulated joints, and a multitude of tendons, ligaments, and muscles holding the whole complicated architecture together. Most people hardly give their feet a thought, but athletes and dancers know that their feet are their best friends.

To keep feet supple and flexible and to help prevent injury, massage them as often as you can. Dancers have different needs from those of athletes, and their feet take more punishment: classical ballet dancers have to cram fragile toes into blocked ballet shoes, while contemporary dancers often dance barefoot and street dancers' feet take a pounding from hard outdoor surfaces. A simple remedy for tired feet involves making a foot bath by adding 3 drops of rosemary essential oil and 1 tablespoon of Epsom salts to a bowl of warm water, and soaking the feet there for 10 minutes. If you have them, put some small, smooth, round pebbles in the bottom of the bowl and roll the soles of your feet over them to stimulate the reflex points. Here are two blends designed for specific foot needs:

GENERAL FOOT CONDITIONING OIL BLEND for DANCERS

Chamomile roman	5 drops
Rosemary	8 drops
Benzoin	5 drops
Geranium	6 drops
Lemon	6 drops

First, blend the essential oils together, then dilute 3–5 drops in each teaspoon (5 mL) of carrier oil or gel. The carrier oil you choose is important; try camellia seed oil, tamanu oil, macerated calendula oil, or arnica oil; or if the skin is dry and cracked, use brazil nut oil or sesame seed oil. For a nonoily carrier, use organic aloe vera gel or arnica in a gel, balm, or lotion.

GENERAL FOOT CONDITIONING OIL BLEND for ATHLETES

Thyme linalol	4 drops
Lavandin	9 drops
Rosemary	6 drops

| Peppermint | 2 drops |
| Manuka | 6 drops |

First, blend the essential oils together, then dilute 3–5 drops in each teaspoon (5 mL) of carrier oil — such as tamanu, hazelnut, or sesame.

Blisters can easily become infected, especially those on the toes. Applying 1 drop of neat lavender around the blister may stop it from becoming infected. Repeat twice a day until healed. See "Blisters" in the "Foot Problems" section that follows below.

If your feet feel especially battered and bruised, or if there is a problem with corns, bunions, or inflamed joints, the following two blends may help ease the soreness. Bruised or particularly sore feet benefit from 1 drop of immortelle gently applied to the bruised area. If there is any bleeding, apply 1 drop of cistus essential oil around the wound to help stem the flow. For foot injuries, see "A–Z of Sports and Dance Injuries" (page 304).

FEET TREAT BLEND

Thyme linalol	4 drops
Manuka	3 drops
Epsom salts	1 cup
Cider vinegar	1 tablespoon (15 mL)

Put all the ingredients in a large bowl of warm water and soak the feet in it for at least 10 minutes, adding warm water as required.

SOOTHING TREAT FOR FEET AND NERVES

Chamomile roman	4 drops
Lavender	2 drops
Bicarbonate of soda	1 cup

Put all the ingredients in a large bowl of warm water and soak the feet in it for at least 10 minutes, adding warm water as required.

If the feet are swollen, inflamed, or sore, substitute cold water for warm water, and use Epsom salts rather than bicarbonate of soda. With swollen feet, it's sometimes beneficial to massage a conditioning oil into the feet before putting them in the bowl of water. If the feet are still swollen after the foot bath, keep the legs elevated as much as you can. An effective method to alleviate swelling of the feet is to put 3 drops of juniper berry and 3 drops of eucalyptus radiata essential oil in a bowl of iced water and soak the feet. If you prefer not to soak the feet, make a compress by soaking the material in the same cold mixture, elevate the feet and legs, and cover the swollen area with the compress, replacing it as soon as it becomes warm. The following blend provides a wonderfully restorative general treatment for feet:

RESTORATIVE FOOT BATH BLEND

Spearmint	3 drops
Lavender	2 drops
Geranium	3 drops
Orange, sweet	5 drops
Ylang ylang	2 drops

First, blend the essential oils together. Use 5 drops in a bowl of warm water to which you've added 1 tablespoon of bicarbonate of soda or Epsom salts and 1 tablespoon of rock salt or pink Himalayan rock salt. After drying the feet, give yourself a foot massage using 3 drops of the essential oil blend diluted in 1 teaspoon (5 mL) of carrier oil.

FOOT PROBLEMS

Black toenail: Blue, purple, and black toenails are caused by bruising under the nail, which can be caused by a blow, ill-fitting shoes, or stubbing the toe. Nails that have become loose should be seen by a chiropodist if they're causing a problem. Apply 1 drop of immortelle or hyssop decumbens essential oil as far under the toenail as you can get it. Then add a small amount of arnica oil, or another carrier oil, over the nail and toe, twice a day for five days. Alternatively, prepare an oil by diluting 4 drops of immortelle and 5 drops of lavender in 1 teaspoon (5 mL) of carrier oil, and apply over the whole toe twice a day for five days.

Blisters: Dilute 2 drops of chamomile roman essential oil in 2 drops of iodine and apply to the area. If your feet are susceptible to blisters, soak them in cold black tea (this is a classical dancers' trick). Make up a pot of strong tea and add it to a bowl of water. Applying 1 drop of neat lavender around the blister may stop it from becoming infected; repeat twice a day until healed.

Ingrown toenail: If you already have an ingrown toenail and it has become sore and red, to avoid getting an infection apply 1 drop of a combination of equal parts of neat tea tree and lavender essential oil directly onto the area once a day, until the redness and soreness dissipates.

Fallen arches: There's no essential oil that can prevent fallen arches from developing. However, if the arch becomes a problem by causing aches and pain, this can be eased by massaging the instep daily, working toward the heel of the foot, with a small amount of the following blend:

Rosemary	10 drops
Black pepper	5 drops
Ginger	10 drops
Clary sage	5 drops

First, blend the essential oils together, then dilute 3–5 drops in each teaspoon (5 mL) of carrier oil.

Verrucas: See page 165.

For foot injuries, see "A–Z of Sports and Dance Injuries" (page 304).

Muscles

Think of a cramp. Aside from the pain, which can be excruciating, the immobility is inconvenient and, for an athlete or dancer, the end of the show. Muscles should be strong, supple, and flexible if they're to work at their best. One of the most effective methods of improving muscle tone involves putting drops of essential oil onto a wet, warm washcloth and rubbing that onto the muscles in the shower before exercise. The essential oils can be used neat or diluted in a little carrier oil beforehand. Use one of the following essential oils:

ESSENTIAL OILS FOR SUPPLE TONE
Black pepper (*Piper nigrum*)
Juniper berry (*Juniperus communis*)
Ginger (*Zingiber officinale*)
Thyme linalol (*Thymus vulgaris ct. linalool*)
Rosemary (*Rosmarinus officinalis*)
Lavender (*Lavandula angustifolia*)
Cypress (*Cupressus sempervirens*)
Plai (*Zingiber cassumunar*)
Basil linalol (*Ocimum basilicum ct. linalool*)
Clary sage (*Salvia sclarea*)
Immortelle (*Helichrysum italicum*)
Marjoram, sweet (*Origanum majorana*)
Lemongrass (*Cymbopogon citratus/flexuosus*)
Lavandin (*Lavandula x intermedia*)

When carrying out aerobic forms of activity, it can be helpful to consider using essential oils that not only tone muscles but also facilitate the efficient working of the respiratory and circulatory systems:

ESSENTIAL OILS FOR AEROBIC EXERCISE
Respiratory Oils
Eucalyptus radiata (*Eucalyptus radiata*)
Eucalyptus lemon (*Eucalyptus citriodora*)
Niaouli (*Melaleuca quinquenervia*)
Cajuput (*Melaleuca cajuputi*)
Rosemary (*Rosmarinus officinalis*)

Circulatory Oils
Geranium (*Pelargonium graveolens*)
Palmarosa (*Cymbopogon martinii*)

Black pepper (*Piper nigrum*)
Ginger (*Zingiber officinale*)
Cypress (*Cupressus sempervirens*)
Immortelle (*Helichrysum italicum*)
Basil linalol (*Ocimum basilicum ct. linalool*)

OVEREXERCISED MUSCLES

If your muscles have been overexercised and are now crying for help, take a long bath, apply a massage oil, and rest. If there are aches or pains that continue for more than 24 hours, you may have a muscular injury. Ice can help reduce swelling, if there is any, and pain caused by inflammation. Follow this with a hot bath into which you have put 3 drops of sweet marjoram and 2 drops of lavender essential oil and soak for as long as possible. After the bath, massage the affected area with one of the following blends:

Massage Oils for Overexercised Muscles

BLEND 1

Eucalyptus radiata	3 drops
Marjoram, sweet	5 drops
Peppermint	3 drops
Ginger	4 drops

First, blend the essential oils together, then dilute in 1 tablespoon (15 mL) of carrier oil or arnica gel. This is enough for several applications, depending on your size and the number of areas affected.

BLEND 2

Plai	5 drops
Immortelle	4 drops
Chamomile roman	3 drops
Lavender	3 drops

First, blend the essential oils together, then dilute in 1 tablespoon (15 mL) of carrier oil or arnica gel.

This is enough for several applications, depending on your size and the number of areas affected.

BATHS FOR QUICK RECOVERY

Taking a bath immediately after vigorous exercise dramatically reduces the degree of muscle pain experienced in the short and long term. The difference between hot and cold baths in terms of their effectiveness is marginal, but cold wins — by a hair — and that's enough of an advantage to make a cold bath after a performance the option of choice for professional athletes. In the world of professional sports, any advantage has to be taken, but as the difference is so small, a warm bath would probably be good enough for most people, and it's a lot more comfortable.

Methods of Treating Injury

COLD (CRYOTHERAPY)

In the case of an acute injury, apply ice as soon as possible after the incident. The application of a cold pack or ice or immersion in cold water causes contraction of the small capillaries, which reduces the amount of blood both leaving the site of damage and collecting around it. This action can limit the degree of swelling in the area. Because the ice cools the damaged tissues, it reduces inflammatory reactions and limits damage. In addition, the distraction created by the sensation of cold disturbs the progress of pain signals being sent to the brain, and the pain is felt as less extreme. Apply the cold/ice for 15–20 minutes, take a break for a similar period, and repeat as required. Ice cubes in plastic bags or bags of frozen peas should not be applied directly to the skin; ensure they are covered with a cloth before application.

HEAT

The application of heat is generally inadvisable when an injury has just occurred, as heat dilates the capillaries and increases blood flow to the damaged tissue. The application of heat immediately after an injury may cause seepage of blood and plasma to the injured area, fluid retention, and further damage, causing swelling and further pain. Heat is used for recovery after at least 12 hours have passed, and for conditions that have been ongoing for some days, weeks, or months. Heat can loosen ligaments and tendons and relax muscles that have contracted and are causing discomfort. Heat can also be used before exercise to release muscle tension and increase movement. Ensure that any heat pack is sufficiently covered so as to avoid redness of the skin.

Essential oils appropriate to the condition or injury can be used in conjunction with heat therapy, either singly or in blends. Apply neat or diluted essential oils under the heat pack.

P.R.I.C.E.

P.R.I.C.E. is an acronym for the protocol "protection, rest, ice, compression, and elevation," the advice most commonly given in cases of injury.

Protection: Protect the injured area to avoid additional damage.

Rest: The injury needs to be rested so full recovery can take place. Reduce physical activity wherever possible.

Ice: Healing time can be much reduced by the swift application of ice to the injured area. See "Cold" above. In the absence of an ice pack or cool pack, look in the freezer to see if you have a pack of frozen peas. Wrap it in a small towel to prevent ice burn on the skin, and apply to the area. If you have ice cubes, put them in a resealable plastic bag, crush the cubes, wrap the bag in

a piece of material, and apply it to the area. For larger areas, put ice cubes in a bowl of cold water and rest the injured area in it.

Ice-Cup Method: If sports injuries are a regular occurrence in your household, it's best to be prepared. One very simple method uses plastic drinking cups: they are filled with water, frozen, and then cut down at the side when needed to reveal solid ice that can be applied to the area. As the ice melts pretty quickly, ice burns are not usually a problem if you keep the ice block moving, although it can all get a bit wet.

Compression: Wrapping the area of injury in material to compress the subcutaneous tissue is known as *compression* and is aimed at preventing further swelling. A compress can be made with a bandage or a piece of material, folded to form a pad. The pressure applied needs to be fairly firm but should not be so tight that it prevents normal blood flow. If the person feels numbness developing or any kind of pain, remove the compress and reapply less tightly. Appropriate essential oils can be used under the compress.

Elevation: By raising the injured part of the body higher than the level of the heart, swelling and pain can often be prevented or lessened.

MASSAGE

Massage is extremely effective in the treatment of muscular spasm and contraction and, used in sports injuries, can help reduce fluid retention and swelling while stimulating blood circulation and lymphatic flow. Unless you're a sports massage therapist, use gentle forms of massage. Long, smooth strokes are the most useful for sports injuries. Use the flat of the hand, moving away from the injured part but always in the direction of the heart — from hand to shoulder, and foot to thigh.

MASSAGE OILS

For sports injuries, the general guide is 5 drops of essential oil to 1 teaspoon (5 mL) of carrier oil. In the acute stage of injury, however, a higher dose may be required — up to 10 drops in each teaspoon (5 mL) of carrier oil, for topical use on the injured area of the body. This is double the usual amount, so when the acute stage has passed, revert to 5 drops per teaspoon, and gradually reduce to 3 drops until full recovery.

COMPRESSES

During the acute stage of injury, only use cold compresses. Thereafter, compresses may be cold, hot, steamed, dry, or wet. Unless specific directions have been given, use a total of 8 drops of essential oil on the compress.

CABBAGE LEAF

For the cabbage-leaf method, only use cabbages of the *Brassica oleracea var. capitata* group, such as January King. Only these types of heritage cabbage produce the active compounds required. Remove a large, dark-green outer leaf and wash. When it's dry, run an iron lightly over it to break down the cells. The leaf should look velvety at this point. While the leaf is still warm, wrap it around the affected part of the body, holding it in place with a soft piece of cloth, and leave it in place for 10 minutes. Repeat the procedure using another warm leaf, as required.

CLAY POULTICE

Add 3 tablespoons of green illite clay to hot or cold water and blend until a thick paste is achieved. Then add the essential oils and mix well. There are several methods that could be used to apply the clay to the affected area. First, simply apply the clay paste directly on the area and cover with a bandage or piece of muslin. Alternatively, put the clay onto the bandage and then tie it onto the affected area. The poultice could also be pre-prepared by putting the clay mix between two pieces of bandage or muslin and allowing it to dry. When it's required, wet the poultice with hot water to return the clay to a paste form.

A–Z of Sports and Dance Injuries

ABDOMINAL WALL STRAIN

Injury to the muscles or tendons of the abdominal wall and lower abdominal area. Use the ice method for the first day. From the second day put 4 drops of rosemary on a warm compress and place over the painful area. Repeat three times a day. Gently massage the abdomen using a blend of equal proportions of immortelle, clary sage, and sweet marjoram. From this blend, dilute a total of 5 drops in each teaspoon (5 mL) of carrier oil.

ACHILLES TENDINITIS

Inflammation of the Achilles tendon. This limits movement, and the area may become hot and painful. For the first five days use the ice method or a cold clay poultice to which you have added 3 drops each of chamomile german and lavender. Thereafter alternate between hot and cold treatment days. On the hot treatment days, use a hot clay poultice to which you have added 3 drops of ginger and 2 drops of chamomile german. On the cold compress days, use 2 drops of peppermint, 2 drops of chamomile german, and 3 drops of eucalyptus radiata, placed on the cold compress. To massage the area use 1 teaspoon (5 mL) of carrier oil to which 3 drops of chamomile and 2 drops of lavender have been added. The ironed cabbage-leaf method also helps.

ANKLE AND HEEL CONTUSION

Bruising of the tissues as a result of a direct blow to the area. There is pain and swelling. Put 1 drop of undiluted immortelle directly on the bruised area. Use the ice method at least three times a day for three days, and in between massage all over the foot and ankle, three times a day, with the following:

Immortelle	10 drops
Cypress	10 drops
Geranium	8 drops
Lavender	2 drops

First, blend the essential oils together, then dilute 3–5 drops in each teaspoon (5 mL) of carrier oil.

ANKLE SPRAIN

A slight tearing or stretching of the ligaments in the ankle. Use the ice method, then massage the whole of the foot and ankle, and the leg to the calf muscle, using the following oil:

Lavandin	10 drops
Ginger	6 drops
Plai	10 drops
Clove bud	2 drops
Geranium	2 drops

First, blend the essential oils together, then dilute 3–5 drops to each teaspoon (5 mL) of carrier oil.

Keep the ankle protected to prevent further damage. Use ice packs for three days, followed by the massage, three times a day, and if the pain continues begin to apply alternate hot and cold washcloths. To the cold washcloth add 1 drop of peppermint, and to the hot one add 1 drop of sweet marjoram essential oil. Apply the washcloths alternately several times, for five minutes each time — three times a day. Protect the injury, rest, and elevate the ankle.

ARM STRAIN

A strain or injury to the muscles or tendons of the upper or lower arm. Use the ice method, followed by massage of the area with the following blend, three times a day for two days:

Ginger	5 drops
Black pepper	5 drops
Clove bud	2 drops
Marjoram, sweet	5 drops
Clary sage	3 drops

First, blend the essential oils together, then dilute 3–5 drops to each teaspoon (5 mL) of carrier oil.

BACK: PROLAPSED OR HERNIATED DISK

Damage to the outer case of a vertebral disk causing pressure on nerves. This should be treated by a physician and physical therapist, but intermittent additional care could be helpful. During the first three days use ice packs over the painful area to reduce inflammation. Then gently apply a small amount of the following diluted blend to the large latissimus dorsi muscles on either side of the spine, making sure not to touch the spine itself.

Rosemary	5 drops
Peppermint	2 drops
Marjoram, sweet	10 drops
Chamomile roman	3 drops
Basil linalol	5 drops
Lavender	5 drops

First, blend the essential oils together, then dilute in 2 tablespoons (30 mL) of carrier oil.

Depending on the type of injury, after the initial three-day period it may prove a more effective method of pain control to move on to alternate hot and cold compress (or washcloth) treatment. Put 2 drops of basil linalol and 1 drop of peppermint essential oil on the hot and cold compresses and apply each in turn several times. After each set of compress cycles, gently apply a small amount of the diluted blend above to the large latissimus dorsi muscles on either side of the spine, making sure not to touch the spine itself. Use this treatment method initially three times a day over a period of seven days.

BACK: GENERAL STRAIN

Stretched or torn muscle fibers in the back. Follow the treatment for **Back: Prolapsed or Herniated Disk**, but during the acute stage hold an ice bag wrapped in a towel against the painful area for at least 10 minutes, take a break, and apply again. Some people find that warmth is more helpful, in which case apply heat packs instead of ice.

BREAST CONTUSION

Bruising of the underlying tissue as a result of a direct blow to the breast area. Apply a cold washcloth to the area four times a day, and afterward gently smooth a few drops of the following diluted blend over the bruise. Any bruising in the breast area should be seen by a healthcare provider.

Chamomile german	5 drops
Geranium	10 drops
Cypress	10 drops
Lavender	5 drops
Immortelle	5 drops

First, blend the essential oils together, then dilute 3–5 drops to each teaspoon (5 mL) of carrier oil. After two days, cold compresses can be used on which 2 drops of chamomile roman have been placed. Afterward gently apply the oil as above.

BUTTOCK CONTUSION

Bruising of the underlying tissue as a result of a direct blow to the area or a fall. Use the ice method four to six times a day and apply 2 drops of neat immortelle essential oil over the area. After three days transfer to hot compresses. After each application, use a little of the following oil, gently applied over the affected area:

Cypress	10 drops
Geranium	5 drops
Lavender	5 drops
Rosemary	10 drops

First, blend the essential oils together, then dilute 3–5 drops to each teaspoon (5 mL) of carrier oil.

CHEST MUSCLE STRAIN

Strain and injury to the muscles in the chest area. Use the ice method four to six times a day and after 48 hours use the heat method. Twice a day, apply a little of the following oil over the affected area:

Ginger	3 drops
Marjoram, sweet	5 drops
Immortelle	4 drops
Plai	8 drops
Chamomile roman	5 drops
Lavender	5 drops

First, blend the essential oils together, then dilute 3–5 drops to each teaspoon (5 mL) of carrier oil.

Soaking in a hot bath can sometimes relieve the symptoms; add 2 drops each of lavender and chamomile roman essential oil.

ELBOW CONTUSION

Bruising of the tissues as a result of a direct blow to the area. Apply the ice method for three days, four to six times a day, and after each session gently apply a little of the following oil:

Hyssop decumbens	2 drops
Clary sage	6 drops

Cypress	5 drops
Lavender	9 drops
Cedarwood atlas	5 drops

First, blend the essential oils together, then dilute 3–5 drops to each teaspoon (5 mL) of carrier oil.

After three days, the hot compress or washcloth method with 1 drop of peppermint and 1 drop of ginger essential oil can be used.

ELBOW: LATERAL EPICONDYLITIS (TENNIS ELBOW)

Overuse of the muscles of the outer elbow area. This is another condition in which some people respond to heat treatment, while others respond to cold. First, try the cold approach; if that is ineffective, try the hot. In each case, compresses or washcloths are applied to the area. Soak the compress in 2 pints (950 mL) of (hot or cold) water to which 2 drops of peppermint and 2 drops of juniper berry essential oil have been added. Then apply the compress to the affected area three times a day, and afterward gently massage the whole of the arm from the wrist to the shoulder with a little of the following oil:

Chamomile roman	10 drops
Immortelle	5 drops
Basil linalol	5 drops

First, blend the essential oils together, then dilute 3–5 drops to each teaspoon (5 mL) of carrier oil.

ELBOW SPRAIN

Injury caused by overstretching the ligaments in the elbow joint. Rest the elbow in an ice pack, keeping it there for 15 minutes, three times a day if possible. Between times, massage with a little of the following oil:

Marjoram, sweet	10 drops
Plai	10 drops

Immortelle	5 drops
Clove bud	2 drops

First, blend the essential oils together, then dilute 3–5 drops to each teaspoon (5 mL) of carrier oil.

Hot-water elbow baths may help, as can alternate ice and heat elbow baths; use 2 drops each of rosemary and lavender essential oil in each elbow bath. Another method is to use alternate hot and cold compresses, on which 2 drops each of rosemary and lavender essential oil have been placed.

FACE CONTUSION

Bruising of the underlying tissue as a result of a direct blow to the face. Immediately apply a cold pack over the injured area, for five minutes, and repeat thereafter at least three times a day. If there's severe bruising, gently apply 1 drop of neat immortelle essential oil to the area — but *not* anywhere near the eyes. Afterward, apply the following facial oil over the affected area, trying not to rub or stretch the skin:

Immortelle	5 drops
Lavender	6 drops
Geranium	10 drops
Chamomile german	5 drops

First, blend the essential oils together, then dilute 3 drops to each teaspoon (5 mL) of carrier oil.

If the bruising is accompanied by swelling on the face, prepare a bowl of cold water to which you've added 1 drop of lavender and 1 drop of chamomile roman, soak a piece of cotton wool or cloth, wring it out, and apply over the area, twice a day. Keep the cloth away from the eyes.

FINGER SPRAIN

Injury to the ligaments and tissue surrounding the finger joints. Wrap the finger(s) in a cloth, or a glove, to avoid ice burn, then put the finger(s) in a bed of ice for at least 10 minutes after the sprain, if you can. Then apply a little of the following diluted hand and finger blend to the whole hand:

Chamomile german	5 drops
Marjoram, sweet	8 drops
Lavender	5 drops
Rosemary	4 drops
Geranium	7 drops

First, blend the essential oils together, then dilute 3–5 drops to each teaspoon (5 mL) of carrier oil.

After 24 hours, prepare a bowl of hot water and a bowl of cold water, adding 4 drops of the undiluted blend above to each bowl. Soak a compress in each. Apply each compress alternately, morning and night. After using the compresses, apply a little of the hand and finger oil to the injured finger(s).

FOOT BURSITIS

Inflammation of the soft sacs of fluid (bursa) that cushion the joints of the feet. This condition develops over a period of time, and treatment should be started as soon as it's suspected. Soak the foot in a cold foot bath morning and night. Afterward, massage the whole of the foot with a little of the following oil:

Geranium	5 drops
Peppermint	2 drops
Cedarwood atlas	5 drops
Juniper berry	5 drops

First, blend the essential oils together, then dilute 3–5 drops to each teaspoon (5 mL) of carrier oil.

Keep the feet up as much as possible and try to avoid any repetitive actions that may aggravate the condition.

FOOT CONTUSION

Bruising of the underlying tissues as a result of a direct blow to the area or a fall. Treat as for **Foot Bursitis** above, but gently apply the following oil:

Immortelle	5 drops
Cypress	15 drops
Geranium	10 drops

First, blend the essential oils together, then dilute 3–5 drops to each teaspoon (5 mL) of carrier oil.

FOOT GANGLION (SYNOVIAL CYST)

A small, hard, movable nodule in between or on top of a tendon or joint. This develops slowly and can sometimes be dispersed by persistent massage over time. Apply a hot compress on which 1 drop of thyme linalol oil has been added. Then massage the area quite firmly with a little of the following oil:

Thyme linalol	5 drops
Rosemary	10 drops
Basil linalol	2 drops

First, blend the essential oils together, then dilute 3–5 drops to each teaspoon (5 mL) of carrier oil.

GROIN STRAIN

Injury to the muscles or tendons in the lower abdominal/ groin area. Use the ice method over the tender area, and afterward use a little of the following oil to massage gently all over the lower abdominal area, thighs, and groin, but taking care to avoid the genitals:

Lavender	10 drops
Geranium	10 drops
Chamomile roman	10 drops

First, blend the essential oils together, then dilute 3–5 drops to each teaspoon (5 mL) of carrier oil.

Use the ice method followed by the diluted oil as above once a day. There are lymph glands in this area, and if they feel hard or if the area is swollen, visit a physical therapist or physician for further advice.

HAND CONTUSION

Bruising of the underlying tissue as a result of a knock or direct blow to the hand. To avoid ice burn, cover the hand in a cloth. Then place it in a bowl of ice and leave it there for 10 minutes. Do this twice a day, morning and night, for two days, and follow by applying a little of the following diluted blend to the hand:

Immortelle	15 drops
Plai	15 drops

First, blend the essential oils together, then dilute 3–5 drops to each teaspoon (5 mL) of carrier oil.

Also apply 1 drop of undiluted immortelle essential oil to the bruised area twice a day, whenever it is convenient.

HAND GANGLION

See **Foot Ganglion**, above.

HANDS AND ARMS: CARPAL TUNNEL SYNDROME

Compression of median nerve or tendons in the carpal tunnel in the wrist. Massage the wrists and forearms twice a day with a little of the following:

Marjoram, sweet	10 drops
Lavender	10 drops
Chamomile german	5 drops
Plai	5 drops

First, blend the essential oils together, then dilute 3–5 drops to each teaspoon (5 mL) of carrier oil.

HEAD INJURY

Injury from a blow or jar to the head. These injuries should always be checked by a physician. Until then, keep the head still, apply ice, and apply 2 drops of undiluted lavender to the area.

HIP STRAIN

Injury to the muscles and tendons that connect the hip joint to the thigh bone. Rest, and take a cold sitz bath three times a day to help reduce any inflammation. Apply ice or warmth to the area — depending on which best eases the immediate discomfort and that of any previous existing condition. Massage all over both hips and thighs using a little of the following:

Ginger	8 drops
Clove bud	2 drops
Marjoram, sweet	10 drops
Chamomile roman	5 drops

First, blend the essential oils together, then dilute 3–5 drops to each teaspoon (5 mL) of carrier oil.

KNEE: CARTILAGE INJURY

Damage to the cartilage in the knee. Apply ice to reduce swelling and inflammation. Initially, the knee may be strapped or taped to prevent further injury. Try to keep the knee elevated when sitting. Depending on the degree of injury, use the ice method three times a day, alternating with hot washcloths, and then massage the area with a little of the following to help ease the discomfort:

Lavender	8 drops
Chamomile roman	12 drops
Cypress	10 drops
Rosemary	5 drops

First, blend the essential oils together, then dilute 3–5 drops to each teaspoon (5 mL) of carrier oil.

KNEE SYNOVITIS (WATER ON THE KNEE)

Accumulation of excess fluid around the knee. Massage from the ankle to the knee and then from the knee to the top of the thigh four times a day with a little of the following:

Juniper berry	10 drops
Marjoram, sweet	5 drops
Thyme linalol	5 drops
Cypress	10 drops

First, blend the essential oils together, then dilute 3–5 drops to each teaspoon (5 mL) of carrier oil.

LEG SPRAIN (LOWER LEG)

Overstretching of the ligaments in the leg. Apply a warm compress and then massage over the affected part using as much of the following oil as needed. Then apply a warm compress once again. If the leg seems hot to the touch, apply cold compresses, or use the ice method, instead.

Immortelle	8 drops
Plai	8 drops
Basil linalol	5 drops
Lavender	3 drops
Lemongrass	4 drops

First, blend the essential oils together, then dilute 3–5 drops to each teaspoon (5 mL) of carrier oil.

Periodically massage the whole of the leg, from the ankle to the thigh.

LEG STRAIN (LOWER CALF MUSCLES)

Small tears or stretching in the muscle fibers of the calf. Follow the treatment for **Leg Sprain (Lower Leg)** above, but apply 1 drop of undiluted immortelle or plai essential oil to the affected muscle, then apply the following:

Ginger	4 drops
Chamomile roman	5 drops

Marjoram, sweet	5 drops
Lavender	2 drops
Black pepper	3 drops

First, blend the essential oils together, then dilute 3–5 drops to each teaspoon (5 mL) of carrier oil.

NECK SPRAIN OR STRAIN

Overstretching of ligaments or muscles in the neck. Regularly apply an ice pack around the neck area, for at least 10 minutes at a time. Or apply a warm compress for the same length of time. Cold can help reduce inflammation when the injury first occurs; warm compresses applied to the neck, shoulders, and upper back help relax tense muscles.

Massage the neck, shoulders, and upper back because often the upper back muscles also become contracted due to the injury. Apply a little of the following blend up to three times a day:

Lavender	10 drops
Ginger	3 drops
Marjoram, sweet	5 drops
Chamomile german	5 drops
Immortelle	5 drops
Peppermint	1 drop

First, blend the essential oils together, then dilute 3–5 drops to each teaspoon (5 mL) of carrier oil.

The ice-cup method can also be used to relieve pain (see page 303). If you have headaches as a result of the injury, use 1 drop each of basil linalol, peppermint, and geranium essential oil diluted in 1 teaspoon (5 mL) of carrier oil and massage around the back of the neck, up to the hairline, and the shoulders.

NOSE INJURY

Injury to the nose resulting from a fall or blow. Apply an ice pack immediately. Gauze can be placed in the nostrils to stem bleeding. If there is no broken skin, gently smooth a little of the following oil over the nose, forehead, and cheekbones, avoiding the eye area:

Chamomile roman (or chamomile german)	10 drops
Lavender	10 drops
Geranium	5 drops
Immortelle	5 drops

First, blend the essential oils together, then dilute 3–5 drops to each teaspoon (5 mL) of carrier oil.

SHOULDER STRAIN OR SPRAIN

Injury to muscles or ligaments in the shoulder. Use the ice method for 10 minutes at a time, and after 48 hours use a heat compress or the hot washcloth method. Three times a day massage the entire arm and shoulder area with a little of the following diluted blend:

Ginger	6 drops
Chamomile roman	10 drops
Black pepper	5 drops
Plai	10 drops
Clary sage	5 drops

First, blend the essential oils together, then dilute 3–5 drops to each teaspoon (5 mL) of carrier oil.

THIGH INJURY: HAMSTRINGS

Injury to a hamstring tendon or muscle at the back of the thigh. Use the ice method (ice packs or cold compresses) for at least 10 minutes, four times a day. Keep the area covered with a compression bandage to reduce swelling and further damage, and elevate the leg as much as possible. Massage the leg three times a day using a little of the following:

Rosemary	10 drops
Clary sage	10 drops
Chamomile roman	5 drops

Lavender	5 drops
Juniper berry	5 drops
Clove bud	2 drops

First, blend the essential oils together, then dilute 3–5 drops to each teaspoon (5 mL) of carrier oil.

WRIST GANGLION

See **Foot Ganglion**, above.

WRIST SPRAIN

Overstretching of one or more ligaments in the wrist. Apply an ice pack morning and night, or three or four times a day. Afterward massage with a little of the following oil:

Ginger	5 drops
Black pepper	5 drops
Clary sage	5 drops
Clove bud	2 drops
Marjoram, sweet	5 drops
Eucalyptus lemon	5 drops

First, blend the essential oils together, then dilute 3–5 drops to each teaspoon (5 mL) of carrier oil.

Sports, Dance, Home, and Recreational Facilities

SHOWERS

Taking a warm shower after a workout is one of the best things you can do, not only to make you feel refreshed but to help avoid delayed-onset muscle soreness caused when lactate and other metabolites, produced during physical exertion, initiate an inflammatory response.

Before taking a shower, rub the body all over — avoiding the genital area — with a clean wet washcloth on which you have put 1 drop of essential oil, and then shower in the normal way.

A combination of equal parts of rosemary, lemon, and eucalyptus radiata would be ideal for this purpose.

After showering, massage the muscles with a muscle relaxant or toning oil, depending on what you want to achieve. Any oil mentioned in this chapter could be used in the shower, but avoid peppermint, clove bud, camphor, cinnamon leaf, wintergreen, and sweet birch. Choose your oil depending on the outcome you want to achieve.

SAUNAS

Saunas are extremely useful, but they can leave you a little depleted unless you're able to roll in the snow afterward! Oils to use in the sauna are those that promote the elimination of waste products through the skin. As facilities vary so much, how you use essential oils in the sauna depends on their design. Essential oils are flammable, so they are never placed directly on any heat source. Clearly, they should also never be placed on any electrical appliance. The simplest method is to place in a corner of the cabin a bowl of steaming hot water with your choice of essential oils.

GENERAL ESSENTIAL OILS FOR THE SAUNA
Cypress (*Cupressus sempervirens*)
Cedarwood atlas (*Cedrus atlantica*)
Pine (*Pinus sylvestris*)
Rosemary (*Rosmarinus officinalis*)
Eucalyptus radiata (*Eucalyptus radiata*)
Lemon (*Citrus limon*)
Cajuput (*Melaleuca cajuputi*)
Palmarosa (*Cymbopogon martinii*)
Niaouli (*Melaleuca quinquenervia*)
Bergamot (*Citrus bergamia*)

Although not generally thought of as a sauna aroma, the following blend is effective, gentle, and relaxing, and it has a very nice fragrance.

RELAXING SAUNA BLEND
Sandalwood	10 drops
Lemon	5 drops
Geranium	2 drops

Blend in these proportions and use 8 drops at a time in 1 pint (475 mL) of water.

The following blend has more stimulating properties:

STIMULATING SAUNA BLEND
Pine	4 drops
Rosemary	3 drops
Niaouli	2 drops
Lemon	7 drops

Blend in these proportions and use 8 drops at a time in 1 pint (475 mL) of water.

Eucalyptus lemon and eucalyptus radiata are good oils to use, singly or combined, in the sauna — they clear the head and respiratory tract, as well as helping to eliminate toxins.

JACUZZIS AND HOT TUBS

The use of blue light to reduce fungal and bacterial growth in Jacuzzis and hot tubs is a welcome development, as badly managed tubs can become a veritable stew of nastiness quite easily. When choosing essential oils to add to the water, a good place to start is those with antibacterial, antiviral, and antifungal properties. Please refer to other sections in this book. But before using an oil, especially if sharing with other people, check the essential oil profiles, in chapter 20, to see if the essential oil has the potential to cause skin sensitivity.

If used over a long period of time, essential oils could cause a residue to build up in the pipes, so it may be worth contacting your supplier or manufacturer for advice before using essential oils. Generally, avoid the more viscous oils.

LOCKER ROOMS AND CHANGING ROOMS

Locker rooms, changing rooms, and communal showers could have been designed to ensure the survival of many species of bacteria, viruses, and fungi. I daresay none of us would even enter one if we had a microscope available to show just what a community of little microbes harbor and indeed flourish there.

The first and simplest thing a manager of communal facilities could do is routinely open the windows to allow fresh air to circulate, but so many facilities seem not to have windows! Essential oils in a diffuser could give the whole place a lovely, fresh natural aroma, and with the choice available, it would be no problem to find a blend in keeping with either masculine or feminine preferences.

Another option is to use antibacterial, antiviral, and antifungal essential oils. There are many essential oils you can use, but the ones that follow are generally acceptable in terms of their aroma and are appropriate for public changing rooms. All have antiseptic and antimicrobial properties that can be particularly useful during any cold or flu season.

LOCKER AND CHANGING ROOM ANTIMICROBIALS
Niaouli (*Melaleuca quinquenervia*)
Lavender (*Lavandula angustifolia*)
Pine (*Pinus sylvestris*)
Lemon (*Citrus limon*)
Ravensara (*Ravensara aromatica*)
Oregano (*Origanum vulgare*)
Thyme (*Thymus vulgaris*)
Cinnamon leaf (*Cinnamomum zeylanicum*)
Eucalyptus radiata (*Eucalyptus radiata*)
Clove bud (*Syzygium aromaticum*)
Bergamot (*Citrus bergamia*)
Lemongrass (*Cymbopogon citratus/flexuosus*)
Manuka (*Leptospermum scoparium*)
Tea tree (*Melaleuca alternifolia*)
Palmarosa (*Cymbopogon martinii*)

Anyone using communal facilities could wear shoes already dusted with the microbe-busting powder, below, to help avoid picking up infections.

MICROBE-BUSTING DUSTING POWDER
Powered cornstarch	200 g (7 oz.)
Ravensara	5 drops
Pine	5 drops
Eucalyptus radiata	5 drops
Bergamot	5 drops

First, blend the essential oils together. Put the cornstarch powder in a blender, add a few drops of essential oil, secure the lid, and slowly blend until no globules of essential oil remain. Repeat until all 20 drops of essential oil have been evenly incorporated. Store in a sealed container, and use as required.

Major Health Concerns

This chapter contains sections on cancer, heart issues, stroke, COPD, multiple sclerosis, and chronic fatigue syndrome. Each of these are clearly serious conditions, and medical advisers need to be informed if anyone intends to use essential oils to supplement their care.

Cancer

Current thinking is that there are three stages to cancer: genetic changes occur in one or more cells, then cells begin to proliferate and become known as *premalignant* cells, and finally there is progression, where the cells begin to overcome nearby tissue and spread to other areas of the body using blood and lymph. Metastases, when cells from the primary cancer break off and migrate to other parts of the body using the blood or lymph systems, is more usually what turns a local problem of rogue cell proliferation into a life-threatening one.

The genetic changes in cells that characterize the first stage may be caused by a miscellany of things, including chemical exposure, radioactivity, and hereditary factors. The risks can be decreased by not allowing body weight to go above normal parameters for body height, taking exercise, eating healthy foods, avoiding pollutants, and not smoking. Even hereditary risk can be lessened, because there's genetics, and then there's epigenetics — a part of the genetic system that turns genes on and off. The genetic code we're all familiar with wraps around histone proteins, and the manner of that connection determines whether the gene is available to be activated or not. This "activate" or "repress" action is triggered by DNA methylation, itself triggered by the presence of methyl groups found in some dietary sources. The mechanism of epigenetic change could start any time, from in utero or childhood through to old age, and it may also be affected by drugs and pharmaceuticals and environmental chemicals. Epigenetics is a hugely important subject, and researchers are now looking into its impact on many health processes, from cancer and autoimmune disease to mental health.

Stopping the proliferation of cells at stage two is the subject of much research today, especially with regard to inflammation. According to a number of specialists in the field, when the innate immune system (including the basic system of warrior cells, as opposed to the adaptive immune system, which involves more specific cells) identifies the genetically altered cancer cell, it rushes to the site. This can cause inflammation, a perfectly normal and usually good sign that the defense and repair system is functioning properly. But for reasons not yet understood, the cancer cell persuades the immune system cells to assist it, instead of killing it. So the very cells that are supposed to help us instead turn renegade and help the cancer cell proliferate. What researchers believe is that allowing inflammation to become chronic — to continue for too long — allows the cancer cells to hijack the immune system cells and redirect them into helping the cancer cells live and proliferate.

Many cancers are known to develop, in some people, from other conditions. For example, the *Helicobacter pylori* bacteria could lead to gastric cancer, the hepatitis B and C viruses could lead to liver cancer, and colitis could lead to colon cancer. The body deals with these original problems by providing an immune response in the form of inflammation — and the cells involved in that process can go on and become workers for a genetically damaged, or cancer, cell. So reducing inflammation becomes a priority, as it denies the cancer cell the army of workers it needs to progress. This can be seen as a preventative measure, and in this essential oils could play a part. Avoiding infection, or dealing with infection quickly, contributes to the avoidance of inflammation. And in this, the area of infection control, essential oils can be very effective as well.

Cancers can occur anywhere in the body — from a brain tumor to a subungual melanoma in the toenail or fingernail. With cancer, early diagnosis is crucial, and any unusual sign or symptom should be investigated by a physician as soon as possible. Fear shouldn't stop anyone from going to their physician, especially as most symptoms, no matter how similar to some cancer symptoms

they may seem at the time, will turn out to be an altogether more innocuous condition.

Symptoms that should not be ignored include any unexplained repeated bruising; hard lumps or hard bumps anywhere on the body; unexplained swelling in the face or neck; blood in urine, feces, phlegm, saliva, or semen; more frequent or loose bowel movements; a persistent mouth or tongue ulcer; a persistent or changing cough; an unexplained, persistent croaky voice or loss of voice; unexplained breathlessness (which can also indicate a heart problem); problems when passing urine; difficulty swallowing; a change in the shape, size, or color of a mole; an unexplained sore; a sore that is not healing; unexplained pain in the abdomen, chest, or shoulder; unexplained continual aches that are combined with other unfamiliar symptoms; repeated chest infections; unexplained weight loss; feeling more tired or exhausted than usual; and night sweats. Whew! That's a lot to think about!

These symptoms are common to many other conditions, which can make it difficult to know when something should get checked. But it is wise to get any physical changes looked at by a physician if they persist for longer than two weeks. Men additionally need to tell their physician if there's a lump in the testicles or pain on ejaculation, if they continually pass small amounts of urine during the night, if passing urine is difficult because of pain, if starting or stopping the stream is difficult, or if there is dribbling. These are just some of the symptoms of a variety of cancers, so take any physical change seriously and get professional advice quickly. Early diagnosis and prompt treatment may avoid the need for more invasive procedures.

Science has made some remarkable breakthroughs in cancer medication and treatment, but we still have a long way to go. There are many thoughts and theories as to the risk factors involved, including stress, infection, modern agricultural methods and additives, electromagnetic fields, pollution, overexposure to the sun, and of course lifestyle choices, such as smoking, and genetic factors. While the likelihood is that cancer is caused by a combination of factors, many of them are outside our control. Alcohol consumption is increasingly being discouraged for health reasons, but the question is, How much is too much? — and opinions differ. Stress certainly makes the body behave in ways that are detrimental to our health, and cancer may, in some cases, be related to that. And it's almost impossible to avoid the many pollutants in the world today — those in the air we breathe, or the water we drink, or those absorbed into food during production and processing.

All any of us can do is try to reduce our exposure to these pollutants, in every aspect of our lives, and to reduce stress. We can all try to keep our weight to a reasonable level and take exercise. "Junk food" is given that name because it's so heavily processed and clearly does not do us much good. Returning to basic food ingredients and cooking proper meals may be the first step we need to take — not only as a measure of cancer prevention but in self-care if we are facing cancer itself.

RESEARCH INTO ESSENTIAL OILS AND CANCER

Increasingly, essential oils and their phytochemical components are being researched around the world for their possible anticancer activity. The research is carried out on tissue cells or animals such as rodents, and little has as yet been carried out on living human beings. Some of the international research pertains to essential oils that have been specifically distilled from traditional indigenous healing plants to try to identify particular

compounds that may be effective. Researchers are trying to identify not only which essential oils or their individual phytochemicals can reduce cancer cell activity, but which of the multiple phases of the cell cycle are being hindered. Also, given that there are so many different types of cancer, we can begin to see that although this subject is very exciting, it is complex. And, of course, there's a huge and as yet untaken leap between recognizing that essential oils can inhibit cancer cells in a laboratory and establishing that these same essential oils can have a positive inhibitory effect on cancer inside the body of a living person.

Having said all that, essential oils on which promising cancer research has been carried out include black pepper, caraway seed, cedarwood atlas, chamomile german, chamomile roman, citronella, clary sage, copaiba, eucalyptus, frankincense, ginger, grapefruit, greenland moss, jasmine, lavender, lavender stoechas, lemon, lemongrass, mandarin, sweet marjoram, mastic, melissa, myrrh, neem, sweet orange, peppermint, rosemary, rose otto, rosewood, sandalwood, spearmint, thyme, turmeric, and vetiver.

What's interesting about the research is that so often essential oils or their phytochemicals are proving to have an inhibiting effect on cancer cells. A phrase often heard from scientists is that the particular essential oil or component they're working on "warrants further research." And as this anticancer research is still in its early stages, there are still many essential oils and components that have yet to be looked at for their cytotoxic potential.

Many, but not all, of the essential oils listed above are routinely used in aromatherapy and could be incorporated into blends for well-being, stress reduction, and alleviating symptoms. For example, lavender combined with frankincense would be a relaxing blend for anyone, and there seems to be no reason why people diagnosed with cancer should not be able to use them too, providing they're avoided during chemotherapy when drug interaction is unpredictable and inadvisable.

ESSENTIAL OIL USE AND CANCER

An integrative treatment plan might include nutrition choices, lifestyle changes, and the use of certain essential oils to ease some of the symptoms of having cancer or some of the side effects of having treatment. If you intend to use essential oils for this purpose, inform your oncologist and ensure that they know, and support, your intentions.

This chapter looks at nutrition; essential oils for the mind and emotions, including relaxation, well-being, and insomnia; specific symptoms and side effects, such as infection, pain, aching muscles, constipation, fatigue, headaches, indigestion, nausea, neuralgia, respiratory distress, lymphedema, and male and female reproductive issues; skin care; massage and cancer; and palliative care.

NUTRITION

According to the World Health Organization, being overweight is linked to cancers as varied as those of the breast, endometrium, colorectum, kidney, and esophagus. This is why any advice on cancer prevention usually starts with maintaining a healthy weight and taking regular exercise. The link between food and specific cancers is supported by international studies. For example, while female colon cancer is rare in Nigeria, where meat consumption is low, the incidence of this type of cancer is highest in New Zealand, where it is high. And there are few cases of breast cancer in Thailand, where dietary fat intake is low, but a high incidence in Holland, where it is high. Given the statistics, avoiding dairy may seem an

attractive proposition, but dairy provides calcium and vitamin D, which we all need. However, there are many plant-based sources of calcium including plant-based milks, and vitamin D is produced in the body in reaction to sunlight on the skin and can also be found in foods such as oily fish.

There are two elements to any discussion about cancer and nutrition: using food as a preventative and what foods to eat while undergoing treatment. These are two entirely different subjects because foods, herbs and spices, and nutritional supplements could possibly interfere with the working of the pharmaceuticals being given during treatment. For example, while rosemary is a potential anticancer herb that is well advised as part of a preventative diet, the phytochemicals within it might be counterproductive during treatment. The same might be said of the spice turmeric.

The first word of advice regarding nutrition is *moderation*. The second word is *variety*. And the third word is *organic*. *Moderation* means keeping a balance between all the food groups: protein, fiber, fruit, and vegetables. If you know you don't eat enough fruit and vegetables, eat more. *Variety* means being more adventurous. Walk down the fruit and vegetable aisle and pick out items depending on their color — red, orange, yellow, green, white, brown. If you can find something pink or purple, throw it in the basket and figure out what you're going to do with it when you get home! Beta-carotene, in its natural form, has been shown to have a beneficial effect on the body and is readily available through carrots and other red, yellow, and dark-green leafy vegetables.

Organic foods should have been produced without the use of pesticides, herbicides, and fungicides, and although they can sometimes be more expensive, eating these foods means a reduction in the chemicals you're taking into the body.

Because fats tend to absorb and hold chemicals, start by changing to organic fat sources. Bread is the number one basic food for many people, but today it is highly overprocessed. Seek out artisan bakers in your neighborhood, or try to bake your own.

The immune system is the means by which our body fights and destroys unwanted cells and clears debris that shouldn't be there, and a strong immune system is the best thing we can have when facing cancer. For this reason, seek out immune system boosters — like Grandma's homemade chicken soup or broth.

Foods to incorporate into the diet include the following:

Cruciferous vegetables from the Brassicaceae family: cabbage, broccoli, spinach, cauliflower, brussels sprouts, kale

Other vegetables: carrots, sweet potatoes, peppers — especially red — eggplant, squash/pumpkin, onions

Legumes/pulses: small red beans, red kidney beans, pinto beans, black beans, peas, lentils

Herbs, spices, and flavoring foods: garlic, ginger, turmeric, oregano

Fruits: blueberries, cranberries, blackberries, raspberries, strawberries, black grapes, melon, apricots, figs, goji berries, tomatoes

There are other foods and drinks that are helpful, including antioxidant-packed pecan nuts; seeds, such as chia, hemp, flax, and pumpkin; seaweed; shiitake mushrooms; good-quality green tea; olive oil — a main component of the healthy Mediterranean area diet; oatmeal; and barley. Avoid unrefined sugar, cut down on processed carbohydrates, and eat instead fiber that comes from whole grains.

CARING FOR THE MIND AND EMOTIONS

Essential oils and aromatherapy are perhaps best known for helping people cope with emotional issues, and being given a diagnosis of any type of cancer is for most people an incredibly painful emotional experience. Some people respond to the diagnosis by going to a space where there's no emotion, unable to cry or even recognize the problem. This emotional numbness is their way of coping. Other people may become completely hysterical. And anyone could feel very alone and isolated. The prospect of the treatment ahead can be daunting, even when someone is told that with this particular type of cancer, most people respond well to treatment.

Some people go into a frantic emotional overdrive, rushing to get their affairs sorted out, writing a Will, leaving messages for old friends, making a memory box for the children, and making a list of things they've always wanted to do — and doing them. Other people prefer to keep the diagnosis private, just between their oncologist and themselves, aiming to continue to have as normal a life as possible, keeping their energy for their own healing instead of having to cope with the family's emotions as well. Yes, the emotions surrounding a cancer diagnosis are without doubt one of the most emotional states a human being may have to face.

Using the fragrance of essential oils has helped many people with various types of cancer cope with emotions such as fear, grief, anger, tension, anxiety, worry, depression, and distress, and has helped with much-needed stress reduction and relaxation.

Relaxation

Learning to relax is difficult for some people at the best of times, but having periods of rest and relaxation can be almost impossible for people with cancer, as they try to juggle treatment or physician's appointments with work and family commitments, as well as having to cope emotionally with the situation they find themselves in. The essential oils that follow are generally suitable for most people:

ESSENTIAL OILS FOR RELAXATION

Bergamot (*Citrus bergamia*)
Clary sage (*Salvia sclarea*)
Petitgrain (*Citrus aurantium*)
Vetiver (*Vetiveria zizanoides*)
Chamomile roman (*Anthemis nobilis*)
Geranium (*Pelargonium graveolens*)
Frankincense (*Boswellia carterii*)
Grapefruit (*Citrus paradisi*)
Lemon (*Citrus limon*)
Orange, sweet (*Citrus sinensis*)
Lavender (*Lavandula angustifolia*)
Sandalwood (*Santalum album*)
Patchouli (*Pogostemon cablin*)
Chamomile maroc (*Ormenis multicaulis*)

These essential oils can be used individually or made into various blends. Use neat essential oil drops in diffusers or other room methods, but always dilute when using in baths or showers or in body oils. Look through the other chapters in this book for information regarding which essential oils might be best suited to you, and make your own exclusive blend. Change the blend as you increase in emotional strength so each blend you create is a move forward into wellness.

Well-Being

The following essential oils make a very helpful multipurpose blend intended for general well-being and to keep the emotions on an even keel. This is a synergistic blend that can be used in a variety of ways. First, blend the essential oils together and bottle so the appropriate number of drops can be taken for the various methods of use. No matter how it's applied, keep a small bottle handy, as emotional moments can occur at any time.

THE GENERAL WELL-BEING SUPPORT BLEND

Sandalwood	20 drops
Frankincense	30 drops
Niaouli	4 drops
Lavender	4 drops
Chamomile roman	3 drops
Geranium	8 drops
Palmarosa	3 drops
Lemon	10 drops
Lemongrass	5 drops
Orange, sweet	4 drops

For inhalation: use 1 drop on a tissue and inhale as required.

For a body oil: Dilute 1–3 drops per 1 teaspoon (5 mL) of carrier oil.

In baths: Dilute 1–3 drops in a small amount of carrier oil before adding to the bathwater, and swish around well.

In showers: Put 1 or 2 drops on a wet washcloth.

For room diffusion: Use 4–6 drops in the usual room methods.

This is a professional type of formula, with large amounts that allow for the incorporation of the smaller elements in the correct proportions required, so there is synergy between all the essential oils in the blend.

When preparing the blend, add the drops of essential oil in the order in which they appear on the list. Then, while rolling the bottle between your hands to integrate the blend, think positive, beautiful thoughts — injecting positive energy into the bottle.

If surgical intervention is required, use a little of the General Well-Being Support Blend every day leading up to the day of surgery as a body oil, diluting 1 or 2 drops per 1 teaspoon (5 mL) of carrier oil. During treatment itself, use the blends in the following sections for specific symptom relief, if approved by your oncologist.

This General Well-Being Support Blend is also what I call an *accord* — it's something you can add, if you wish, to other blends: add 1 or 2 drops per blend.

Making Personal Well-Being Blends

Aroma preference is a very individual thing, and the list of oils that follows contains essential oils that could be used to make a personal blend.

CALMING AND SOOTHING ESSENTIAL OILS
Lavender (*Lavandula angustifolia*)
Frankincense (*Boswellia carterii*)
Chamomile roman (*Anthemis nobilis*)
Orange, sweet (*Citrus sinensis*)
Lemon (*Citrus limon*)
Petitgrain (*Citrus aurantium*)
Geranium (*Pelargonium graveolens*)
Rose otto (*Rosa damascena*)
Neroli (*Citrus aurantium*)
Sandalwood (*Santalum album*)
Mandarin (*Citrus reticulata*)
Cedarwood atlas (*Cedrus atlantica*)
Clary sage (*Salvia sclarea*)
Rosewood (*Aniba rosaeodora*)
Coriander seed (*Coriandrum sativum*)
Chamomile german (*Matricaria recutita*)
Spikenard (*Nardostachys jatamansi*)
Cardamom (*Elettaria cardamomum*)
Palmarosa (*Cymbopogon martinii*)
Vetiver (*Vetiveria zizanoides*)

Some of the essential oils in the list above can also be found in the list below. The two lists have been separated, as the calming and soothing oils are more about relaxation and emotional strength, while the oils below are more about a general, all-round well-being boost. Use the essential oils singly, on their own, or in blends using three essential oils. From your chosen blend, use 1–3 drops in any of the usual methods.

WELL-BEING BOOSTER ESSENTIAL OILS
Frankincense (*Boswellia carterii*)
Lemon (*Citrus limon*)
Melissa (*Melissa officinalis*)
Lemongrass (*Cymbopogon citratus/flexuosus*)
Vetiver (*Vetiveria zizanoides*)
Rose otto (*Rosa damascena*)
Grapefruit (*Citrus paradisi*)
Orange, sweet (*Citrus sinensis*)
Sandalwood (*Santalum album*)
Ravintsara (*Cinnamomum camphora ct. cineole*)
Geranium (*Pelargonium graveolens*)
Immortelle (*Helichrysum italicum*)
Patchouli (*Pogostemon cablin*)
Rosemary (*Rosmarinus officinalis*)
Ginger (*Zingiber officinale*)
Copaiba (*Copaifera officinalis*)

Insomnia

When anyone is given a cancer diagnosis or is undergoing treatment, bedtime can become the time when the brain goes into overdrive, crowded with thoughts about the future. Yet everyone feels more able to cope with the day ahead after a good night's sleep.

The following essential oils will not suit everyone but are worth a try. They provide a pleasant and gentle method of trying to get to sleep. Use small amounts to begin with — 1 or 2 drops under the corner of a pillow or in one of the room methods.

ESSENTIAL OILS TO AID SLEEP
Lavender (*Lavandula angustifolia*)
Melissa (*Melissa officinalis*)
Clary sage (*Salvia sclarea*)
Neroli (*Citrus aurantium*)
Mandarin (*Citrus reticulata*)
Spikenard (*Nardostachys jatamansi*)
Frankincense (*Boswellia carterii*)
Petitgrain (*Citrus aurantium*)
Chamomile roman (*Anthemis nobilis*)
Vetiver (*Vetiveria zizanoides*)
Orange, sweet (*Citrus sinensis*)
Valerian (*Valeriana officinalis*)

ALLEVIATING SYMPTOMS AND SIDE EFFECTS

The following symptoms, along with corresponding essential oil suggestions, appear in other places throughout this book, but this section suggests choices that are more appropriate at this time. Where a guide is provided on the amounts to use — for example, a range of 1–3 drops — the lower figure is the better choice if a person is particularly fragile, while for most people 2 drops would be a good starting point.

Infection Control
INFECTION CONTROL ESSENTIAL OILS
Thyme linalol (*Thymus vulgaris ct. linalool*)
Ravensara (*Ravensara aromatica*)
Ravintsara (*Cinnamomum camphora ct. cineole*)
Tea tree (*Melaleuca alternifolia*)
Manuka (*Leptospermum scoparium*)
Fragonia (*Agonis fragrans*)
Lavender (*Lavandula angustifolia*)
Palmarosa (*Cymbopogon martinii*)

INFECTION CONTROL BLEND

Thyme linalol	20 drops
Ravintsara	10 drops
Manuka	10 drops
Lavender	10 drops
Tea tree	5 drops

First, blend the essential oils together. Then dilute 1–3 drops per 1 teaspoon (5 mL) of carrier oil for body application; or dilute into a gel using 12–18 drops of the blend to 1 fl. oz. of aloe vera gel. For a water spray, add 18 drops per 1 fl. oz. of water, and shake well before use. Use neat for inhalation. Use neat in room diffusers, depending on their style — follow manufacturer's instructions.

Pain Relief
ESSENTIAL OILS FOR PAIN RELIEF
Plai (*Zingiber cassumunar*)
Immortelle (*Helichrysum italicum*)
German chamomile (*Matricaria recutita*)
Chamomile roman (*Anthemis nobilis*)
Geranium (*Pelargonium graveolens*)
Lavender (*Lavandula angustifolia*)
Peppermint (*Mentha piperita*)
Marjoram, sweet (*Origanum majorana*)
Spikenard (*Nardostachys jatamansi*)
Ginger (*Zingiber officinale*)
Rosemary (*Rosmarinus officinalis*)
Cypress (*Cupressus sempervirens*)

Pain is clearly a personal experience, dependent on many factors. The following blend is for general aches and pain relief, and could be applied anywhere on the body.

PAIN RELIEF BLEND

Immortelle	12 drops
Chamomile roman	5 drops
Marjoram, sweet	5 drops
Lavender	6 drops
Peppermint	2 drops

[handwritten margin note: avoid prolonged use]

First, blend the essential oils together. Then dilute 1–3 drops per 1 teaspoon (5 mL) of carrier oil for body application; or dilute 12 drops of the blend

30ml

to 1 fl. oz. of aloe vera gel. Use a small amount of the oil or gel over the affected area.

Aching Muscles
Essential Oils for Aching Muscles
Plai (*Zingiber cassumunar*)
Immortelle (*Helichrysum italicum*)   *avoid prolonged use*
Chamomile roman (*Anthemis nobilis*)
Geranium (*Pelargonium graveolens*)
Lavender (*Lavandula angustifolia*)
Peppermint (*Mentha piperita*)
Marjoram, sweet (*Origanum majorana*)
Rosemary (*Rosmarinus officinalis*)
Ginger (*Zingiber officinale*)
Cypress (*Cupressus sempervirens*)

Aching Muscle Blend
Plai	10 drops
Rosemary	5 drops
Lavender	8 drops
Peppermint	1 drop
Ginger	1 drop
Immortelle	10 drops

First, blend the essential oils together. Then dilute 1–3 drops per 1 teaspoon (5 mL) of carrier oil for body application; or dilute 12 drops of the blend to 1 fl. oz. of aloe vera gel. Use a small amount of the oil or gel over the affected area.

Constipation
Drink plenty of water to keep hydrated, and eat lots of fresh fruits and vegetables to increase fiber in your diet.

Essential Oils for Constipation
Black pepper (*Piper nigrum*)
Patchouli (*Pogostemon cablin*)
Grapefruit (*Citrus paradisi*)
Orange, sweet (*Citrus sinensis*)
Basil linalol (*Ocimum basilicum ct. linalool*)

Constipation Blend
Grapefruit	5 drops
Orange, sweet	5 drops
Black pepper	2 drops
Basil linalol	3 drops

First, blend the essential oils together. Then dilute 1–3 drops per 1 teaspoon (5 mL) of carrier oil and massage over the lower abdomen in a clockwise direction.

Fatigue
Essential Oils for Fatigue
Lavender (*Lavandula angustifolia*)
Melissa (*Melissa officinalis*)
Marjoram, sweet (*Origanum majorana*)
Rosemary (*Rosmarinus officinalis*)
Thyme linalol (*Thymus vulgaris ct. linalool*)
Eucalyptus radiata (*Eucalyptus radiata*)
Palmarosa (*Cymbopogon martinii*)
Vetiver (*Vetiveria zizanoides*)
Sandalwood (*Santalum album*)
Pine (*Pinus sylvestris*)
Peppermint (*Mentha piperita*)
Orange, sweet (*Citrus sinensis*)
Grapefruit (*Citrus paradisi*)

Fatigue varies in intensity, and the purpose of using an essential oil for people suffering fatigue is not to increase vitality but to create equilibrium. When someone is suffering from fatigue it's not wise to overstimulate the system, but rather the aim is to give support to the body and mind.

General Fatigue Blend
Lavender	5 drops
Marjoram, sweet	3 drops
Eucalyptus radiata	2 drops
Grapefruit	2 drops

First, blend the essential oils together. Then dilute 1–3 drops per 1 teaspoon (5 mL) of carrier oil and apply a small amount over the solar plexus area, lower back, and feet.

Headaches

ESSENTIAL OILS FOR HEADACHES

Lavender (*Lavandula angustifolia*)
Melissa (*Melissa officinalis*)
Peppermint (*Mentha piperita*)
Spikenard (*Nardostachys jatamansi*)
Basil linalol (*Ocimum basilicum ct. linalool*)
Orange, sweet (*Citrus sinensis*)
Chamomile roman (*Anthemis nobilis*)
Rosemary (*Rosmarinus officinalis*)

HEADACHE BLEND

Chamomile roman	4 drops
Peppermint	2 drops
Eucalyptus radiata	3 drops
Basil linalol	1 drop
Lavender	5 drops

First, blend the essential oils together and dilute the total amount in 4 teaspoons (20 mL) of carrier oil, or alternatively, in 20 mL of aloe vera gel. For each application, rub a small amount over the back of the neck or over the soles of both feet.

Indigestion

ESSENTIAL OILS FOR INDIGESTION

Frankincense (*Boswellia carterii*)
Marjoram, sweet (*Origanum majorana*)
Black pepper (*Piper nigrum*)
Lime (*Citrus aurantifolia*)
Lemon (*Citrus limon*)
Cardamom (*Elettaria cardamomum*)
Ginger (*Zingiber officinale*)
Coriander seed (*Coriandrum sativum*)

Please don't think that this remedy for indigestion should be taken orally — that should never be assumed for essential oil use. The following blend is for external use only.

INDIGESTION BLEND

Cardamom	10 drops
Coriander seed	5 drops
Ginger	2 drops
Frankincense	1 drop

First, blend the essential oils together. Dilute 1–3 drops per 1 teaspoon (5 mL) of carrier oil and massage over the whole abdomen, as required.

Nausea

Nausea is a common side effect of treatment, and inhaling certain essential oils may offer some relief. Each person will experience differing degrees of nausea and may find that inhaling certain essential oils helps more than others; you will need to experiment. Here are three suggestions:

1. Peppermint and lemon in equal parts
2. Ginger and lemon in equal parts
3. Cardamom and sweet orange in equal parts

Other suitable oils are frankincense, peppermint, spearmint, ginger, black pepper, and lemon. Use by adding 1 drop to a tissue and inhaling as needed.

Neuralgia

Neuralgia is a pain caused by damage to a nerve, or by some form of physical irritation, and it is felt as a pain that seems to follow the nerve pathway.

ESSENTIAL OILS FOR NEURALGIA

Chamomile roman (*Anthemis nobilis*)
Geranium (*Pelargonium graveolens*)
Marjoram, sweet (*Origanum majorana*)
Ginger (*Zingiber officinale*)
Black pepper (*Piper nigrum*)
Lavender (*Lavandula angustifolia*)
Immortelle (*Helichrysum italicum*)
Plai (*Zingiber cassumunar*)

NEURALGIA BLEND

Marjoram, sweet	5 drops
Black pepper	3 drops
Geranium	6 drops
Plai	6 drops

First, blend the essential oils together. Dilute 1–3 drops per 1 teaspoon (5 mL) of carrier oil; or mix 12 drops of the blend in 1 fl. oz. of aloe vera gel. Massage a small amount of the oil or gel over the affected area.

Skin Care

External radiation therapy can lead to radiation dermatitis and leave the skin feeling sunburned and looking red and swollen. The skin can become dry and itchy and get flaky and peel, and blisters can occur, as can infection. If radiation is planned, it is beneficial to prepare the skin with a nourishing oil in the weeks leading up to the therapy. This will help the skin to both cope with the radiation therapy and recover more quickly afterward.

Inform the radiologist of all the products you're using on your skin at this time, and take advice from them, or the nurse specialist, about when any skin products can be applied. Each case is different, obviously. During treatment the skin may need to be kept dry and clear of all products, so wash off any residue oil before therapy. It is probably inadvisable to apply any products to the skin in the 12 hours prior to therapy, unless advised otherwise.

There are three stages to skin care:

1. Prior to radiation therapy
2. During therapy cycles
3. After the therapy cycle is complete

Prior to radiation therapy: It may help soften and strengthen the skin to apply good, nourishing organic carrier oils, such as the following:

Almond, sweet (*Prunus amygdalus var. dulcis*)
Argan (*Argania spinosa*)
Apricot kernel (*Prunus armeniaca*)
Avocado (*Persea americana*)
Hemp seed (*Cannabis sativa*)
Jojoba (*Simmondsia chinensis*)
Camellia seed (*Camellia japonica*)
Kukui (*Aleurites moluccana*)
Macadamia (*Macadamia ternifolia*)
Rosehip seed (*Rosa rubiginosa*)
Sesame (*Sesamum indicum*)

And certain macerated or infused oils such as organic calendula / marigold (*Calendula officinalis*) and carrot (*Daucus carota*) may also help.

During therapy cycles: Good organic aloe vera gel can be applied to the skin following radiation therapy. On days when there is no therapy, the skin oils listed above could be used.

After the therapy cycle is complete: Essential oils can be used once the entire therapy cycle is complete. Listed below are essential oils that would be suitable at this time, as well as a blend, and both options should be diluted in your choice of the nourishing carrier oils listed above. Alternatively, aloe vera could be used — either on its own, or blended with one of the nourishing carrier oils above, or with essential oil added.

After radiation therapy when the skin is so sensitive, it's important that any essential oils you use be carefully chosen and organically produced. From the list below use no more than 2–3 drops diluted in 2 teaspoons (10 mL) of organic carrier oil (see the list above).

AFTER-THERAPY ESSENTIAL OILS FOR SKIN CARE
Chamomile roman (Anthemis nobilis)
Chamomile german (Matricaria recutita)
Lavender (Lavandula angustifolia)
Petitgrain (Citrus aurantium)
Neroli (Citrus aurantium)
Geranium (Pelargonium graveolens)
Cajuput (Melaleuca cajuputi)
Niaouli (Melaleuca quinquenervia)
Mandarin (Citrus reticulata)
Ho wood (Cinnamomum camphora ct. linalool)

AFTER-THERAPY SKIN CARE BLEND
Lavender   10 drops
Chamomile german   10 drops
Chamomile roman   5 drops
Petitgrain   3 drops
First, blend the essential oils together. Dilute 1–2 drops per 1 teaspoon (5 mL) of carrier oil; or dilute 12 drops of the blend to 1 fl. oz. of aloe vera gel. Use a small amount of oil or gel over the affected area. A good carrier combination would be one comprised of equal amounts of three oils: camellia seed oil, avocado oil, and marigold/calendula macerated oil. Or use a single oil such as jojoba oil, sweet almond oil, kukui oil, or argan oil.

Respiratory Distress
Respiratory distress or respiratory problems are often experienced by those with life-limiting illness — either as a result of the illness itself or as a side effect of the treatment. The following is a list of essential oils that could be used when treatment is finished to ease and comfort those suffering from respiratory problems:

ESSENTIAL OILS FOR RESPIRATORY DISTRESS
Cypress (Cupressus sempervirens)
Frankincense (Boswellia carterii)
Benzoin (Styrax benzoin)
Cajuput (Melaleuca cajuputi)

Ravensara (Ravensara aromatica)
Rosemary (Rosmarinus officinalis)
Thyme linalol (Thymus vulgaris ct. linalool)
Ravintsara (Cinnamomum camphora ct. cineole)
Eucalyptus radiata (Eucalyptus radiata)
Niaouli (Melaleuca quinquenervia)
Rosalina (Melaleuca ericifolia)
Elemi (Canarium luzonicum)

The essential oil used very much depends upon the type of respiratory problem being experienced. So following is a general help blend that can be used as an accord (that is, add 1 or 2 drops to other blends), if needed.

RESPIRATORY BLEND
Frankincense   10 drops
Ravensara   10 drops
Niaouli   10 drops
Blend the essential oils together. Use in a room diffuser, or put 1–2 drops on a tissue for inhalation, or use 2–4 drops in 1 teaspoon (5 mL) of carrier oil for a back and chest rub, using a small amount each time.

Lymphedema
Lymphedema is localized fluid retention and tissue swelling due to removal of the lymph glands or other forms of treatment. This is best treated by someone trained in medical lymphatic drainage; however, that option is not always available. So a really gentle massage — more like stroking — of the area may be the best help at hand.

Always stroke upward. For example, if the swelling is in the arm, stroke upward toward the armpits. If the swelling is in the leg, stroke upward toward the groin area. Often the affected area is tender to the touch and the skin is fragile due to being overstretched. For this reason, it's important to try to use a skin-nourishing carrier oil (see the list on page 325 in "Skin Care" above). The following essential oils or blends could be diluted in such a carrier oil and used in this way with the approval of your healthcare practitioner.

If choosing from the list below, dilute 1 drop of essential oil in 1 teaspoon (5 mL) of carrier oil and use only as much as required.

LYMPHEDEMA ESSENTIAL OILS

Grapefruit (*Citrus paradisi*)
Juniper berry (*Juniperus communis*)
Orange, sweet (*Citrus sinensis*)
Cypress (*Cupressus sempervirens*)
Cedarwood atlas (*Cedrus atlantica*)
Immortelle (*Helichrysum italicum*)
Manuka (*Leptospermum scoparium*)
Plai (*Zingiber cassumunar*)

For those who want to use a blend of oils, the following suggestions could be used. Blend 2 would be more appropriate if the area appears red and inflamed.

LYMPHEDEMA BLEND 1

Juniper berry	5 drops
Grapefruit	2 drops
Cypress	2 drops
Orange, sweet	5 drops

First, blend the essential oils together. Then dilute 1–3 drops per 1 teaspoon (5 mL) of carrier oil. Use only as much as required, and apply as directed above.

LYMPHEDEMA BLEND 2

Lavender	6 drops
Juniper berry	3 drops
Chamomile german	6 drops

First, blend the essential oils together. Then dilute 1–3 drops per 1 teaspoon (5 mL) of carrier oil. Use only as much as required, and apply as directed above.

MALE AND FEMALE REPRODUCTIVE ISSUES

The object of this section is to alleviate a concern many people have regarding the products they use while they have cancer, such as body oils, bath products, and air fragrances. A cursory look at the ingredients in a range of commercial products can include many about which we know little. Some people would like to take more control over the products they use, and there is no time more appropriate than now.

Many women rely on body products to keep their skin supple, and without them their sense of well-being would be much reduced. We all need a bit of spoiling, and someone with cancer needs it more than most. Essential oils are already present in many shop-bought preparations, but some — such as sweet fennel, sage, anise, and caraway seed — may best be avoided because it's thought they contain phytohormones (or plant growth regulators, PGRs). Although there's no evidence that these phytohormones are actually harmful from a hormone-disrupting point of view within an actual living human being, it's probably sensible in this instance to seek alternatives. Of course PGRs are a natural part of plants and are found in foods we eat every day.

The World Health Organization (WHO) published a report in 2012 titled *State of the Science of Endocrine Disrupting Chemicals*, which examined the evidence for harmful effects to human health from close to 800 synthetic chemicals found in personal care products, pesticides, metals, and additives or contaminants in food. It might come as a surprise to know that, according to the WHO, "the vast majority of chemicals in current commercial use have not been tested at all." There is a plethora of endocrine-disrupting chemicals all around us, and it seems only reasonable that someone with an endocrine-related cancer will want to look into natural alternatives.

Uterine Cancer

Several distinct cancer types are put under the umbrella category "uterine," and these are sometimes referred to as "endometrial cancers" because they often originate in the lining of the womb — the endometrium — although the surrounding muscles can also be involved. Premenopausal women are less often affected, but any woman with symptoms such as nonmenstrual bleeding or an offensive discharge needs to consult their physician as soon as possible.

If a diagnosis of uterine cancer has been given, the essential oils can be used as an emotional support and for an overall sense of well-being. They could be used in any of the environmental methods, such as diffusion, as well as in baths and in body oils. As a carrier use one of the nourishing carrier oils listed in the "Skin Care" section earlier in this chapter (see page 325). In room or bath methods, use the usual amount, which can be found in the "Methods of Use" section in chapter 1 (see page 13). For body oils, use only 1–3 drops in 1 teaspoon (5 mL) of carrier oil. This amount will be enough for a body application; simply apply to areas you can reach, such as the upper chest, abdominal area, and lower back. Avoid using the body oil when undergoing chemotherapy or radiation therapy unless approved by your cancer care team.

Geranium (*Pelargonium graveolens*)
Rose otto (*Rosa damascena*)
Neroli (*Citrus aurantium*)
Frankincense (*Boswellia carterii*)
Myrrh (*Commiphora myrrha*)
Lemon (*Citrus limon*)
Chamomile roman (*Anthemis nobilis*)
Lavender (*Lavandula angustifolia*)
Petitgrain (*Citrus aurantium*)
Orange, sweet (*Citrus sinensis*)
Mandarin (*Citrus reticulata*)

Cervical Cancer

All women are encouraged to get a regular Pap test, whether they are sexually active or not, because when it's caught at the early, premalignant stage, the chances of cervical cancer developing can be much reduced. The Pap test can include investigation for infection by the papillomaviruses (HPV), thought to be responsible for around 70% of cervical cancer cases. Symptoms range from irregular bleeding or spotting between periods to bladder problems and pain on intercourse. Some women just report "feeling uncomfortable" inside. Anything unusual always indicates a visit to your physician is required.

Because cervical cancer has been associated with high levels of stress that can deplete the immune system, using essential oils is focused on reducing stress generally.

Geranium (*Pelargonium graveolens*)
Rose otto (*Rosa damascena*)
Carrot seed (*Daucus carota*)
Niaouli (*Melaleuca quinquenervia*)
Benzoin (*Styrax benzoin*)
Lavender (*Lavandula angustifolia*)
Lemon (*Citrus limon*)
Ginger (*Zingiber officinale*)
Orange, sweet (*Citrus sinensis*)
Cedarwood atlas (*Cedrus atlantica*)
Frankincense (*Boswellia carterii*)
Cypress (*Cupressus sempervirens*)
Sandalwood (*Santalum album*)
Jasmine (*Jasminum grandiflorum/officinale*)
Ylang ylang (*Cananga odorata*)
Petitgrain (*Citrus aurantium*)
Mandarin (*Citrus reticulata*)

Make an uplifting blend using essential oils from the list above, or use one essential oil. Add 1–3 drops to your bathwater. For a body oil, mix 2–3 drops of essential oil in each teaspoon (5 mL) of nourishing carrier oil (see page 325). There are some delightful oils on the essential oil list above, and with a little experimentation you'll be able to make yourself a blend that appeals to your personality and helps you relax. Here are some suggestions for blends you might like to try:

FOR BATHS

Geranium	10 drops
Lavender	5 drops
Frankincense	5 drops
Benzoin	7 drops
Lemon	10 drops

First, blend the essential oils together, then dilute 1–3 drops in a little carrier oil for each bath.

FOR BODY OIL

Cypress	5 drops
Sandalwood	10 drops
Geranium	10 drops
Ginger	2 drops
Carrot seed	2 drops

First blend the essential oils together, then dilute 2–3 drops to each 1 teaspoon (5 mL) of carrier oil. Alternatively, dilute the entire blend in 2 fl. oz. (60 mL) of carrier oil, and use a small amount each time. Use as you would any body oil, or just cover areas you can reach such as the upper chest, abdominal area, and lower back. Avoid using the body oil when undergoing chemotherapy or radiation therapy unless approved by your cancer care team. Adopt as positive an attitude as you can, and help your immune system by avoiding stress and eating good, healthy organic food.

Breast Cancer

It doesn't matter if you've lived an exemplary lifestyle, eaten all the right foods, avoided alcohol and nicotine, and had plenty of exercise: breast cancer can affect any woman. For this reason, checking the breasts and underarm area for any hard pea-like lumps, or any other kind of change in the tissue or nipple, should be part of every woman's regular healthcare regime.

A diagnosis of breast cancer or of precancerous cells, or even the knowledge that there is a genetic predisposition, can lead to a labyrinth of questions and options that can leave a woman feeling confused, stressed, and out of control. Incorporating some integrative medicine methods into your care may help you gain back some sense of control. The stress and anxiety so often associated with a diagnosis might be alleviated by using essential oils in room methods, baths, and body oils. Good options would be one, or a blend, of the following:

Frankincense (*Boswellia carterii*)
Lemon (*Citrus limon*)
Lemongrass (*Cymbopogon citratus/flexuosus*)
Myrrh (*Commiphora myrrha*)
Rosemary (*Rosmarinus officinalis*)
Lavender (*Lavandula angustifolia*)
Chamomile roman (*Anthemis nobilis*)
Chamomile german (*Matricaria recutita*)
Sandalwood (*Santalum album*)
Cedarwood atlas (*Cedrus atlantica*)
Petitgrain (*Citrus aurantium*)
Neroli (*Citrus aurantium*)
Juniper berry (*Juniperus communis*)
Mandarin (*Citrus reticulata*)

Use an essential oil on its own, or make a blend that you enjoy using two or three essential oils. Use the essential oils listed above in diffusers or any other room method, or add 2–3 drops to a bath — diluted first in a small amount of carrier oil. To make a body oil, use 2–3 drops in 1 teaspoon (5 mL) of carrier oil. If having radiation therapy, refer to the "Skin Care" section earlier in this chapter. Avoid using the body oil when undergoing chemotherapy or radiation therapy unless approved by your cancer care team. If electing to have surgery, you might find the following blend useful:

PRESURGERY BLEND

Lavender	5 drops
Chamomile german	2 drops
Petitgrain	4 drops
Rosemary	2 drops

The blend above can be used every day leading up to surgery to keep the skin in good condition. First, blend the essential oils together, then dilute 2–3 drops to each 1 teaspoon (5 mL) of rosehip seed oil or a macerated calendula oil, or choose from one of the nourishing carrier oils listed in "Skin Care" earlier in this chapter (see page 325). (An alternative carrier could be aloe vera gel, preferably preblended with a little nourishing oil.) Apply a small amount of this blend over the abdomen and upper chest, avoiding the breast area. After surgery, avoid using any carrier oil until the scars have healed. If infection appears to be a problem after surgery, inform your cancer care team if intending to use essential oils.

Prostate Cancer

Most men with prostate cancer have no symptoms at first, but, in fact, prostate cancer is very common and the chances of developing it rise with age. When symptoms do occur, they're usually related to urination or sex. Signs to watch for are the frequent sensation of wanting to urinate and then passing small amounts, pain on passing urine, blood in the urine, lower back pain, pain during ejaculation, or unfamiliar sensations. There are several other conditions that can have these same symptoms. The risk of having prostate cancer increases if a brother or father has had it or if there is African American heritage. In any event, if one or more of the symptoms occur, a physician should be consulted.

There's been huge debate about the benefits and risks of prostate-specific antigen (PSA) screening, with opinions currently varying among doctors, and even countries. For example, the charity organization Cancer Research UK attributes the drop in deaths to testing, while the U.S. Preventive Services Task Force does not recommend testing because it can lead to false-positive results, complications from biopsy, and side effects from treatment, risks that can be avoided in many cases where the cancer grows slowly and is nonfatal. It can be difficult to know what to do — especially as prostate cancer is the second leading cause of death from cancer in men in both the UK and the United States. This is a subject on which every man needs consultation and advice — which is where the physician comes in.

The stress of prostate cancer, whether arising from the symptoms or from the treatment, is understandable, given that the condition affects a potential loss of control over the basic human functions of urination and sex. The essential oils listed below address this stress and can be used in a variety of ways. The oils can be used singly, on their own, or use two or three in a blend that suits you. Use them in all the usual room methods, in baths or showers, and in body oils. For body oils use 2–3 drops in 1 teaspoon (5 mL) of carrier oil.

Geranium (*Pelargonium graveolens*)
Cedarwood atlas (*Cedrus atlantica*)
Frankincense (*Boswellia carterii*)
Lemongrass (*Cymbopogon citratus/flexuosus*)
Chamomile german (*Matricaria recutita*)
Chamomile roman (*Anthemis nobilis*)
Sandalwood (*Santalum album*)
Lavender (*Lavandula angustifolia*)
Niaouli (*Melaleuca quinquenervia*)
Fragonia (*Agonis fragrans*)
Juniper berry (*Juniperus communis*)
Petitgrain (*Citrus aurantium*)

If you have elected to have surgery, the following blend can be used on the days leading up to it. Apply over the lower abdomen and the lower back, into the crease between the buttocks but not as far as the anus:

Sandalwood	5 drops
Cedarwood atlas	5 drops
Frankincense	5 drops
Juniper berry	5 drops
Chamomile german	5 drops

First, blend the essential oils together, then dilute 2–3 drops in 1 teaspoon (5 mL) of organic calendula macerated oil or in 1 teaspoon (5 mL) of aloe vera gel. Alternatively, choose a carrier from the list in "Skin Care" earlier in this chapter.

If infection appears to be a problem after surgery, inform your cancer care team if you intend to use essential oils. Avoid essential oil use on the day of surgery itself.

MASSAGE AND CANCER

Massage is a very comforting process for the person being massaged — a loving and healing experience in itself. To a person with cancer, it also shows support and understanding and brings reassurance. People with cancer sometimes have a disconnected relationship with their body — a feeling that their body has been invaded or that it has let them down. Massage helps a person reconnect with themselves, and the loving touch of another person reconnects them to the larger world in a positive way.

In addition, massage combined with an appropriate essential oil blend can bring relaxation, reduce physical pain in the muscles or limbs, assist in the regulation of digestive problems, improve sleep, and increase flexibility around scar tissue. Using the right essential oils combined with massage can help decrease the side effects of chemotherapy and help increase the physical tolerance level when faced with further treatment.

The psychological effects of using massage and essential oils include reducing anxiety, lifting depressive states, and easing any negative thoughts, including the sadness of potentially leaving loved ones behind. The positive emotional effects are many, and it is good for the person with cancer to feel they are part of the healing process rather than disconnected from it.

When massaging someone with cancer, the key is to forget about all the various massage techniques you have learned or watched being carried out by other people. When massaging someone with cancer, the strokes are made without applying any pressure, yet are gentle and firm. The words *gentle* and *firm* in this context mean touching the skin in a way that is not weak or floppy and can be felt as a positive supporting touch by the person receiving the massage.

Professional therapists have the training and skill to understand the physiological processes involved and are able to massage according to the type of cancer and the treatment that has been given or is being given. A nonprofessional person should take care to avoid any areas of recent surgery and any area receiving radiotherapy. When giving massage to someone with cancer, less is often more. Always provide the opportunity for the person being massaged to say, "That's enough for now" by asking, "Is that OK?" or "Shall I continue?" This opens the door for the expression of feelings about the experience.

First, pour a little of the essential oil and carrier oil blend into the palm of one hand, and spread it over both of your hands. Then apply by using only gentle movements. Think of the movements as more like stroking or gentle rubbing, rather than like movements more usually thought of as massage. Depending on the person and their situation, apply the oil over either just one section of the body or the whole body. If it's accessible, the back is always a good place to start.

There are also ways to touch the body using diluted essential oils that involve no massage as such. These include placing one hand gently over the affected area, using no pressure, just holding the hand there for a few seconds or minutes. The hand may feel as if it's getting warm, and this can indicate the transference of positive energy. If a person is bedridden, hooked up to an intravenous drip, or for whatever reason difficult to reach, simply hold one foot between two hands, and then do the same thing with the other foot.

Over the years there have been many myths regarding the use of massage in cases of cancer, but these have now been dispelled. There is no need to feel hesitant about it so long as you use appropriate and pure organic essential oils, avoid their use during chemotherapy or radiation therapy, inform the cancer care team, and apply in the way outlined above.

PALLIATIVE CARE

Essential oils and aromatherapy are being used in palliative care all over the world — in hospices, hospitals, nursing homes, and, of course, in people's own homes. Aromatherapy is now recognized as a welcome adjunct to the care being given. The premise behind palliative care is that it's helpful to provide a place where people who have had a life-limiting diagnosis can be supported, and it may involve multiple disciplines, in both physiological and psychological care, or none. Whatever the individual's particular needs, the entire focus is on support and making this time less difficult than it might otherwise be. That is the case primarily for the person edging toward the end of life, but the needs and feelings of their family can be taken into consideration too.

Up to this point in an individual's care, medical teams may have had all the control and the family or loved ones may have felt overcome with helplessness. After all, hospital treatments have had to focus on the physical body rather than paying attention to the person's emotional or spiritual self. Being able now to prepare exquisite essential blends with care and love, or to give gentle massage, gives the family or close friends the

opportunity to transfer the love they feel. Caring for someone by using the fragrances of essential oils is a way to help everyone get through this most difficult of times.

Good palliative care is concerned with attending to the wishes and needs of a person while trying to keep them as comfortable as possible. The fragrance of pure essential oils adds an extra dimension, because in this context the aroma is being used to bring calm to the emotional and spiritual aspects of a person. This is one of those times when it's the fragrance of the essential oil and its ability to uplift a person that is at the fore, rather than its use as a therapeutic agent. This is not to say that essential oils should not also be used for their therapeutic properties, such as for pain relief, infection control, or helping to relieve specific symptoms. Rather, it is an awareness that there are other emotional and spiritual needs that could be taken into consideration at the same time. Because essential oils are so multifaceted, it's possible to find essential oils that have more than one effect and even very different purposes.

Essentially, the aim now is to improve the quality of life. Choose essential oils that help reduce stress and tension, help ease fear and distress, and bring relaxation and a sense of well-being. Many people find that certain fragrances have great spiritual meaning for them, and indeed fragrance plays a part in the spiritual practices of a majority of cultures, providing a link between the human realm and the spiritual world.

Aroma is a hugely personal thing. A particular aroma can link deep into the memory and bring back feelings long lost. These are subtle realities, and we have no idea what lies deep inside the subconscious mind of even our closest relative. So this is the time to be as sensitive as possible, to ensure that anyone we care for actually wants the particular aroma we're using around them. So being sensitive means making time for the person to give some indication of whether they like a particular aroma or not. Of course, if you know someone loves neroli or rose or cedarwood, that's another matter, and even if they can't communicate their preference, you already have an idea that they will like it.

Well-chosen essential oils that someone enjoys can have a very liberating effect. They can release fear of the unknown and worry about leaving loved ones behind, and bring comfort, reassurance, and acceptance. There can be a profound improvement in a person's self-image. These are deep claims, but there's nothing in this world that affects people on the deepest level in the same way that aroma can.

Aroma has another quality: it can open the door of communication. The person you're caring for may have thoughts that you're unaware of. They may be thinking not of themselves, but of others, or they may be concerned that they can't protect the family from pain. Perhaps they feel unable to express their needs because it might upset someone. The natural fragrances of essential oils are like conduits providing two-way communication, and they can be used to facilitate the most important conversations anyone is likely to have.

Because aroma can remind people of places and experiences, using them may give a person the opportunity to talk about their past. Our role in this is to be the listener, to just be still and listen. Let them express their wishes, their regrets, their love. Even if the person receiving palliative care seems unaware, tell them you love them. This is the time to forgive, or to ask for forgiveness.

Essential Oils Most Used in Palliative Care
Rose otto (*Rosa damascena*)
Neroli (*Citrus aurantium*)
Sandalwood (*Santalum album*)
Frankincense (*Boswellia carterii*)
Cedarwood atlas (*Cedrus atlantica*)
Bergamot (*Citrus bergamia*)
Lemon (*Citrus limon*)
Orange, sweet (*Citrus sinensis*)

These essential oils can be used in room diffusion, in washing or bathing, and in body oils; they can be put under the corner of a pillow or simply sniffed from a tissue whenever needed.

Room Fragrance

Essential oils can be used in all the usual room diffusion methods to create a more peaceful atmosphere, one that is soothing and calming all round. Aside from nullifying other odors that may be present, a pleasant fragrance can reduce stress and lift the atmosphere for family and other visitors, as well as for nursing staff and care providers.

Massage in Palliative Care

Massage in palliative care is rarely about body massage per se. It's about touch, care, comfort, communication, and in some cases, helping to alleviate pain in a particular area. Generally, palliative care massage is carried out on small areas of the body: the face, hands, feet, or shoulders. The key words are *gentle*, *thoughtful*, and *caring*. Make sure the person receiving the massage is in a comfortable position before beginning and that they actually want to be massaged. The massage could last just a minute, or maybe 15 minutes. Use a light touch, being careful with delicate skin.

Touch can be wonderfully reassuring and can convey the love felt between two people better than words. And there is nothing on this earth more beneficial than the energy of a loving touch. Use a low dilution of essential oils, and a small amount each time:

For adults: 2 drops of essential oil in 1 teaspoon (5 mL) of carrier oil

For children: 1 drop of essential oil in 1 teaspoon (5 mL) of sweet almond oil

The Family

When someone passes on, they leave beloved family and friends behind. These are the people shedding tears. Some may want to tell everyone how the loss has affected them, while others react by going silent and can seem unmoved. With so much to do in practical terms at this time, keeping busy is some people's coping mechanism, and for them the shock may hit some time later. Everyone reacts differently (see "Bereavement" in chapter 5, "Emotional Rescue").

Aromatherapy affects the mind, body, and spirit at all times, including during the last days of someone's life, and for this reason essential oils can provide a unique and profound comfort. Planning to use essential oils during palliative care is helpful if the aromatic likes or dislikes of the person being cared for are already known. So a little preplanning can save a lot of uncertainty later because a blend can be prepared. That same blend can be diffused later, to bring back memories of the loved one who has passed. This aromatic link may make the sadness of losing someone a little less difficult to bear.

The Spiritual Connection

Fragrance has always been a key feature in many cultures' spiritual practice throughout known history. This is a subject I have explored in my book *Aromatherapy for the Soul: Healing the Spirit with Fragrance and Essential Oils.* Each culture has specific fragrances that it uses in spiritual practice to connect this life with that of the divine. And even an atheist may have an aroma or aromas that they find link them with their spiritual core.

Using essential oils for their spiritual connection is a dimension of the subject of palliative care that also needs sensitivity. That said, the person leaving this life may be grateful to have as an accompaniment a fragrance that forms an ethereal bridge between the two worlds. Using an appropriate oil at this time brings a dignity that little else can provide when someone is facing that most mysterious journey we shall all, eventually, take.

Heart Issues

Poets and composers have forever linked the heart with love: "They made my heart sing," "My heart leapt when he/she walked into the room," "My heart aches for love," "My heart is broken," "I'm following my heart." I wonder how this extraordinary organ became the symbol of love and affection, but it clearly is. And there's no doubt in my mind that the energy of the heart, if not the actual heart itself, does play a significant role in our emotional and spiritual self.

This incredible muscle, the heart, beats 100,000 times each day, continuously pumping and circulating blood around our bodies, every moment of our lives. Day in, day out, the heart pumps oxygen-laden blood to every part of our body. It is without doubt the most important and hardest working muscle in the body; and when it stops functioning properly, the scariest. In today's world it is no surprise that heart disease is on the increase and is now one of the leading causes of death in the Western world. An uneasy heart is made worse by our sedentary lifestyles and automatic methods of transport, the tendency to sit for long hours in front of a computer at work and at home, the use of household gadgets to take the effort out of doing things, and an ever-increasing mountain of daily stress. A higher risk of heart disease is thought to be attributable to being overweight — particularly around the middle and abdomen — to smoking, drinking too much alcohol, eating too much red meat and too many junk foods high in saturated fats, salt, and sugar, and not eating enough fresh vegetables and fruit, as well as not taking enough daily exercise.

The heart does warn us when we are taking liberties with it. Signs of a weakening heart can include blood pressure that is too high or too low, discomfort or pain in the center of the chest, mild or strong, a sudden unexplained ache in the left arm, an aching jaw, neck, and upper back, shortness of breath, nausea, heartburn, constant fatigue, coughing, heart palpitations, and loss of appetite. Many people begin to worry about their heart only when there's a problem. Suddenly they appreciate that their heart is their best friend. A regularly beating heart becomes the most reassuring sound.

A variety of problems can affect this most important of organs, and in many cases there is not much we can do about them. But where we can help ourselves is by thinking about the arteries that supply the heart muscle, moving the life-giving oxygen-rich blood around. These arteries can be subject to a buildup of fatty material, called *plaque*. This process is called *atherosclerosis*, and over time, the arteries could become too narrow to allow enough blood to reach the heart.

As far as self-help is concerned, it's all about prevention. We know what we should be doing — preventative measures include not smoking, reducing "bad" cholesterol, bringing down blood pressure so it's within normal range, avoiding being overweight, and being physically active. If at all possible, work fewer hours and reduce stress on all fronts. Consider a lifestyle change that takes the pressure off you, concentrate on developing a healthy pattern of eating, with plenty of exercise, and have some fun.

HEART CARE

Using essential oils, we can help reduce stress and tension, which may thereby improve the health of the circulation and nervous system.

HEART CARE BLEND 1

Chamomile roman	5 drops
Geranium	10 drops
Bergamot	3 drops
Lavender	10 drops
Lemon	2 drops

First, blend the essential oils, then use 2–3 drops in a bath, or 1–2 drops in the shower method.
Or:
Blend the essential oils, then dilute 2–5 drops to each 1 teaspoon (5 mL) of carrier oil, and use as a body oil.

HEART CARE BLEND 2

Geranium	8 drops
Peppermint	1 drop
Rosemary	2 drops
Ginger	5 drops
Eucalyptus radiata	2 drops

First, blend the essential oils, then use 2–3 drops in a bath, or 1–2 drops in the shower method.
Or:
Blend the essential oils, then dilute 2–5 drops to each 1 teaspoon (5 mL) of carrier oil, and use as a body oil.

Preventative health care for the heart involves keeping cholesterol levels low and blood pressure in check. Diet plays a major role in preventative heart care — overconsumption of fatty foods, sugar, and salt are all thought to lead to an unhealthy heart. Eating enough whole-food fiber has been clearly shown to reduce the incidence of heart-related problems. Also, eating plenty of fresh vegetables and fruits plays a major role in keeping the heart healthy. Try to consume less red meat and processed meats, eat more fatty, oily fish, and ditch the junk food. Supplements can be helpful, such as essential fatty acids, in particular omega 3, and vitamins C, E, and D.

People who have had heart attacks or suffer from angina have been shown to have less essential fatty acids in their body than people with no heart trouble. It's a question of choice, and in preventative heart care it makes more sense to go for fish and vegetables rather than steak and fries.

Those who already have a heart problem should not only follow all the dietary advice available but also try to take time out for themselves to have an aromatherapy treatment once a month. If this isn't possible, try self-massage once a week and use the essential oils in your bath or shower at least twice a week. In Asia, ginger has been known as a heart strengthener for thousands of years, and oil of ginger happens to be one of the essential oils recommended for use in heart care.

Choose your preferred essential oils from the two lists below, using the oils singly or in combinations. Use up to 3 drops in the bath or shower method, or 2–5 drops in 1 teaspoon (5 mL) of carrier oil for a body oil. When applying essential oils always massage in upward strokes toward the heart. For the purposes of heart care, concentrate on the back between the shoulders, the shoulders themselves, the back of the neck, and both sides of the arms.

Heart Care Essential Oils
Geranium (*Pelargonium graveolens*)
Frankincense (*Boswellia carterii*)
Rosemary (*Rosmarinus officinalis*)
Black pepper (*Piper nigrum*)
Rose otto (*Rosa damascena*)
Cardamom (*Elettaria cardamomum*)
Rose maroc (*Rosa centifolia*)
Ginger (*Zingiber officinale*)
Niaouli (*Melaleuca quinquenervia*)

To Alleviate Stress and Strain
Bergamot (*Citrus bergamia*)
Cypress (*Cupressus sempervirens*)
Clary sage (*Salvia sclarea*)
Basil linalol (*Ocimum basilicum ct. linalool*)
Vetiver (*Vetiveria zizanoides*)

Cedarwood atlas (*Cedrus atlantica*)
Rosewood (*Aniba rosaeodora*)
Sandalwood (*Santalum album*)

Heart Care Blend 3
Cardamom	2 drops
Geranium	1 drop
Clary sage	2 drops
Bergamot	1 drop
Ginger	1 drop

First, blend the essential oils. Then use 3–4 drops in a bathtub, diluted in a little carrier oil, or put 1–2 drops on a washcloth and use in a shower.
Or:
Blend the essential oils, then dilute 3–5 drops to each 1 teaspoon (5 mL) of carrier oil.

ATHEROMA AND ARTERIOSCLEROSIS

These two conditions affect the arteries and are often associated. Arteriosclerosis, or the thickening and hardening of arterial walls, is often due to atheroma, which is the deposit of cholesterol and other fatty matter on the lining of an artery. These have the potential to be life-threatening conditions, affecting arterial blood flow efficiency and increasing the chances of fatty deposits breaking away from the arterial wall and causing a blockage in the artery. Coronary thrombosis is brought about by a clot in the arteries supplying the heart, and a stroke can result from a thrombosis in the arteries supplying the brain. Loss of efficiency in the blood flow may also cause all manner of other serious problems, from angina to kidney failure.

Ideally, an individual essential oil blend would be prepared for you by a qualified aromatherapist or essential oil therapist, but there are things you can do to help yourself. Carry out some gentle daily exercise. Swimming is ideal. Do some deep, yoga-style breathing each day, and take up tai chi or qi gong or another energy-balancing form of exercise.

ESSENTIAL OILS FOR ATHEROMA
AND ARTERIOSCLEROSIS
Juniper berry (*Juniperus communis*)
Ginger (*Zingiber officinale*)
Rosemary (*Rosmarinus officinalis*)
Lemon (*Citrus limon*)
Black pepper (*Piper nigrum*)
Rose otto (*Rosa damascena*)
Geranium (*Pelargonium graveolens*)

ATHEROMA AND ARTERIOSCLEROSIS BODY OIL

Ginger	8 drops
Rosemary	5 drops
Grapefruit	5 drops
Geranium	8 drops
Black pepper	2 drops

First, blend the essential oils together, then dilute 2–5 drops in 1 teaspoon (5 mL) of carrier oil.

Stroke

The word *stroke* describes two quite different events, both of which affect the routine blood supply to the brain. By far the most usual event, known as a *cerebral infarction* or a *brain ischemia*, happens when there is a reduction in the supply of blood to the brain. The less usual form of stroke occurs when there is too much blood in the brain, and this can have several causes. Strokes of this sort have the word *hemorrhage* in them, which gives a graphic picture of what has happened. This type of stroke can result from a head injury or an aortic vein rupture, or from damage to a blood vessel on the surface of the brain or inside the brain. Headaches can be a symptom. But most strokes occur when a blood clot forms within the vein — known as a *thrombosis* — or when there is an obstruction caused by atherosclerosis, in which a piece of fiber and plaque breaks away (an embolism) and obstructs the flow of blood to the brain.

Strokes affect people both physically and mentally, ranging along a very wide spectrum. Transient ischemic attacks (or TIAs) are mini-strokes that can last from minutes to hours; these are caused by a brief interruption of blood and oxygen but appear at the time to pose the same problems as a full-blown stroke. It's only in retrospect, after a quick recovery, that a TIA can be seen to be a passing event. A silent cerebral infarct (SCI) has no noticeable signs and can happen without the person even realizing it's occurring, but it can have long-lasting effects, often causing psychological changes. Another type of brain condition linked to strokes, called *lacunar infarction* or *small vessel disease*, is caused by tiny blockages in the small arterial blood vessels in the brain and leaves a person more susceptible to TIA.

Immediate signals that a stroke has occurred might be seen in the face, which tends to be lop-sided; also, perhaps the arms can't be held up for long, or speech is slurred or makes no sense. People can become paralyzed, usually on one side of the body, which indicates which area of the brain is affected and what symptoms may be presented. It's important to get the person to the hospital as quickly as possible because there's a short window of possibility when clot-busting drugs can be administered.

Advice given for avoiding any type of stroke is much the same as that given for avoiding a heart attack — and that is to try and avoid the buildup of fatty material in the arteries that can break off and cause an embolism. So don't smoke, take exercise, eat a well-balanced fresh-food diet, avoid sugar and salt in the diet, and don't allow yourself to get overweight. High blood pressure causes up to 50% of strokes, so clearly that is something to watch and control, as are fasting blood sugar levels — which may be indicative of diabetes — your cholesterol level, and alcohol consumption. Young people playing around with so-called recreational drugs like cocaine and amphetamines need to know they are at higher risk of having a stroke. A few days volunteering on a stroke ward may be more effective in getting them off drugs than months in rehab.

Essential oils used alongside physical therapy could help people who have been made somewhat immobile by a stroke. Professional massage may help keep the muscles flexible and help the stroke victim recover more quickly.

The essential oils used in body oils for stroke victims are very much symptom-dependent. Look through the book to find blends that relate to the symptoms being experienced. Rehabilitation can be a slow process, and massage with essential oils can be part of that process. Gentle massage of any affected limbs is useful, as are back massage and foot massage. If the face is affected, gentle massage can be applied if care is taken to avoid getting essential oils in the eye. If planning to use essential oils during the rehabilitation process, your physician should be consulted as an individual's particular condition and medications will need to be taken into account.

TABLE 10. ESSENTIAL OILS FOR STROKE REHABILITATION

CONCERN	OILS
STRENGTH	Black pepper (*Piper nigrum*) Cedarwood atlas (*Cedrus atlantica*) Pine (*Pinus sylvestris*) Cardamom (*Elettaria cardamomum*) Immortelle (*Helichrysum italicum*) Star anise (*Illicium verum*) Niaouli (*Melaleuca quinquenervia*) Basil linalol (*Ocimum basilicum ct. linalool*)

CONCERN	OILS
MUSCLES	Ginger (*Zingiber officinale*) Black pepper (*Piper nigrum*) Clary sage (*Salvia sclarea*) Thyme linalol (*Thymus vulgaris ct. linalool*) Pine (*Pinus sylvestris*) Basil linalol (*Ocimum basilicum ct. linalool*) Rosemary (*Rosmarinus officinalis*) Marjoram, sweet (*Origanum majorana*) Clove bud (*Syzygium aromaticum*) Star anise (*Illicium verum*) Immortelle (*Helichrysum italicum*) Peppermint (*Mentha piperita*)

CONCERN	OILS
INFLAMMATION	Chamomile german (*Matricaria recutita*) Chamomile roman (*Anthemis nobilis*) Lavender (*Lavandula angustifolia*) Peppermint (*Mentha piperita*) Immortelle (*Helichrysum italicum*)
DIGESTION	Ginger (*Zingiber officinale*) Peppermint (*Mentha piperita*) Orange, sweet (*Citrus sinensis*) Coriander seed (*Coriandrum sativum*) Lemon (*Citrus limon*) Star anise (*Illicium verum*) Eucalyptus radiata (*Eucalyptus radiata*) Cardamom (*Elettaria cardamomum*) Basil linalol (*Ocimum basilicum ct. linalool*)

CONCERN	OILS
CIRCULATION	Geranium (*Pelargonium graveolens*) Ginger (*Zingiber officinale*) Rosemary (*Rosmarinus officinalis*) Thyme linalol (*Thymus vulgaris ct. linalool*) Rose otto (*Rosa damascena*) Rose maroc (*Rosa centifolia*) Black pepper (*Piper nigrum*) Cedarwood atlas (*Cedrus atlantica*) Marjoram, sweet (*Origanum majorana*)
EMOTIONAL SUPPORT	Rose otto (*Rosa damascena*) Rose maroc (*Rosa centifolia*) Lavender (*Lavandula angustifolia*) Neroli (*Citrus aurantium*) Ylang ylang (*Cananga odorata*) Grapefruit (*Citrus paradisi*) Lemon (*Citrus limon*) Sandalwood (*Santalum album*)

Although a paralyzed limb is often thought to have no sensation, this may not always be the case in people who have experienced strokes. If they've lost the power of communication, make sure that any pressure being applied is not causing muscular discomfort or soreness, and that the patient actually wants to be massaged. Not all people respond positively to being touched — particularly by a stranger or someone they do not like. If they didn't like a family member before they had a stroke, they won't like them afterward. Massage should be given with loving, caring, and understanding energy.

When applying a massage oil to someone affected by stroke, the oil and the method used really depend upon the type of stroke someone has had. One of the best ways toward recovery is to use specific-area aromatherapy massage every day. This may apply to the limbs, the side of the body, the face, or the back. For the first few months, full-body massage doesn't appear to be as successful as concentrating on one specific area every day. The best times to carry out massage are in the morning — when stiffness is sometimes worse — and in the evening before bed. If the person is in the hospital, massage can still be applied on an arm or a leg, a hand or a foot. If you're uncertain how to start helping the person who has suffered a stroke, a good place to begin would be a gentle foot rub. Face massage is always good for those whose face is affected and can improve mobility surprisingly quickly — massage upward and outward toward the ears. When massaging limbs, use gentle movements to start with and with time, gradually increase the pressure applied. If the person cannot speak, remember to watch their face to see if they grimace, which will tell you that the pressure is too hard or that they have had enough. Aim for movements that are gentle but firm, always massaging toward the direction of the heart. This means that on the leg, movements are upward toward the groin,

and on the arm, work upward from the wrist to the shoulder. Don't give up on the massage; persevere even if it seems progress is not being made.

When making your own blend, choose oils from the lists above, blend the essential oils together, and then dilute them using 3–5 drops in 1 teaspoon (5 mL) of carrier oil for an individual massage. If making up a bottle of massage oil for multiple uses, use no more than 18–30 drops of essential oil diluted in 1 fl. oz. (30 mL) of carrier oil. The strength of dilution should be on the lower end of the scale during the first few sessions, and then gradually increase the number of drops used as time goes on — but only up to the maximum number as outlined above. Always be aware of the medications that are being taken, and inform the care team that you intend to carry out massage.

STROKE BODY MASSAGE BLEND

Orange, sweet	5 drops
Immortelle	5 drops
Marjoram, sweet	2 drops
Lavender	3 drops
Geranium	10 drops
Rosemary	5 drops

First, blend the essential oils together, then dilute between 18 and 30 drops in 1 fl. oz. (30 mL) of carrier oil. For the first few massage sessions, use the lower dosage of 18 drops and gradually increase to 30 drops over time. Use a small amount for each massage. Do not use on the face. For face massage, see below.

STROKE FACIAL MASSAGE

Geranium	1 drop
Lavender	1 drop
Rosewood	1 drop

Dilute the essential oil in 2 teaspoons (10 mL) of rosehip seed oil, and use a small amount each time.

With stroke, using essential oils appropriate to each person is important, as it is with other major health problems in this section, and many things need to be considered. As well as the condition itself, other factors to think about are the person's particular symptoms and needs, their general well-being, and whether there has been any bacterial infection or a recent severe viral infection. It's always helpful to include in the blend an essential oil or oils that can help out in terms of the mood and emotions. Having a stroke often takes control away from the person, and that is always upsetting. I find that geranium essential oil is valuable in any blend for people who have experienced a stroke, and other choices may include bergamot or rosemary — both of which have been used with success on stroke victims.

Essential oils can also be applied directly to the soles of the feet, either in dilution or neat. If using the essential oil neat, first check the essential oil profiles in chapter 20 to ensure that the particular essential oil will not cause skin sensitivity. Neat or diluted, start by using just 1 drop of essential oil on each foot.

Chronic Obstructive Pulmonary Disease (COPD)

Difficulty in breathing could be caused by a wide variety of conditions — some of which are serious — so acute or chronic shortness of breath needs to be diagnosed correctly. Chronic obstructive pulmonary disease (COPD) is the name given to several conditions of the lung, all of which lead to shortness of breath. These include emphysema and chronic bronchitis, but not asthma or pneumonia. Asthma and pneumonia are classified differently because they can be treated, whereas COPD is a condition that often gets worse with time. As the name suggests, COPD is characterized as being chronic, or ongoing. *Obstructive* and *pulmonary* mean that lung function is impaired. All this is very different from the shortness of breath (dyspnea) caused by, for example, congestive heart failure, anemia, or pulmonary embolism. Any shortness of breath should be taken seriously.

There are probably as many people going around with undiagnosed COPD as there are with the condition diagnosed as such. Underreporting of breathing problems is surprisingly high. Symptoms of COPD include difficulties in breathing, such as breathlessness or the inability to take a deep breath, a chronic cough with or without sputum, a tight feeling in the chest, wheezing, and fatigue. Simple everyday movements such as walking up stairs can become difficult.

The lungs are fed with air through bronchial tubes, which branch out into thousands of smaller tubes called *bronchioles*, at the end of which are 300 million tiny air sacs called *alveoli*. When air gets to the alveoli there's an exchange of gases — with oxygen passing into the bloodstream through the tiny capillaries and carbon dioxide coming out. The tiny alveoli are stretchy, like balloons, filling out when you breathe in and deflating when you breathe out. The breathlessness that is characteristic of COPD is caused by one or more dysfunctions in this process. When looking at a lung damaged by COPD, it can often be seen that the walls between the air sacs have been damaged so there are fewer of them, and they are larger — making the whole gas exchange process less efficient. The normal elasticity of the air sacs, or the airways, might be reduced. Or there could be inflammation in the walls of the airways, making them thicker. An additional problem is that the airways can become clogged with mucus.

This damage could have been caused by several factors, and the origin of the problem may have been decades ago and now be hard to identify. The number one suspect is smoking, but many people with COPD have never smoked a cigarette in their lives. That brings us to suspect number two — passive smoking. And that brings us to suspect number three — tiny particles in the air that we breathe in. This might include something natural, such as pollen, mildew, or mold spores. But it's more likely to be environmental pollutants we have little control over, such as car exhaust fumes and industrial particulates, and pollutants over which we have total control, such as chemical products in the home, including air fresheners and aerosol cleaners. Another culprit could be the working environment, from too much flour in the atmosphere in a bakery to dust on the factory floor. And some people have COPD because of a genetic condition known as alpha-1 antitrypsin (AAT) deficiency.

The minuscule little airways and alveoli were not designed to handle the plethora of chemicals and particles that float in the modern airspace. Particles in the air, in the form of dust or fumes, encourage the mucous glands lining the bronchial tubes to overproduce mucous. When the alveoli are working well they fill with air and expand, and then spring back and push the air out again when the gas exchange has taken place. But when the alveoli have been damaged, they fill up but can't spring back. So the air just sits there, trapped, in a process called *hyperinflation*. If the walls of the alveoli become damaged and broken, the sacs combine into fewer and larger ones instead of many small, elastic air sacs. If this happens, the gas exchange process becomes far less efficient.

There are so many different types of working environment that can pose a problem for our respiratory systems that it can seem hard to avoid them all during a long working life. The key is to be aware of them and take appropriate action if possible. Face masks might look wimpy, but 20 years from now you might be glad you used them. Where we have most control is in our own home, and here the person with COPD can

take a full evaluation of any risk factors. These might include carpets and furnishings that harbor dust, heating and air conditioning systems, and the chemical fragrances found in a multitude of household products, from candles to the softener sheets put in clothes dryers. Mold is a suspect in the exacerbation of COPD, if not the cause, so look behind every cupboard to seek it out and remove it. Essential oils can be used to deal with mold, and as so many people have had success with a wide variety of oils it's worth a try. Start with those you might otherwise throw away because they're out of date for use on the body. Try lemongrass, thyme, citronella, oregano, clove bud, or cinnamon leaf.

Whenever someone consults me after receiving a diagnosis of COPD, my first question is "What preceded the diagnosis?" Although COPD is attributed to certain respiratory problems such as chronic bronchitis or emphysema, it can occur alongside other conditions — asthma, for example. I have also known the starting point to be pneumonia, pleurisy, heart conditions, and other health problems that can also involve respiratory trauma.

So deciding which essential oils to use very much depends on a person's current overall health and specific health history. The object is to find an essential oil or blend that makes symptoms more manageable and helps the person lead a fuller life than before. Another factor to consider is a person's emotional reactions. You only have to remember that an emotional event can spark an attack in someone with asthma to realize how much the mind affects the body. With COPD, likewise, the degree of difficulty can be exacerbated by stress, tension, anxiety, or depression.

Using essential oils with some degree of anti-inflammatory activity alongside those oils traditionally known to assist respiratory conditions often helps ease COPD. If the breathing difficulties include chronic bouts of coughing, essential oils attributed with antispasmodic activity may also be helpful. Some essential oils are expectorants and assist the body in removing phlegm. If there has been, or is at present, a bacterial or viral infection, consider using essential oils with antimicrobial activity. Please cross-reference with chapter 3, "The Self-Defense Kit." Each case of COPD is unique, so although the essential oil lists and blends that follow have been shown to help generally, there may be throughout this book other suggestions more specifically appropriate to a particular person's symptoms and psychological state.

COPD General Respiratory Essential Oils
Frankincense (*Boswellia carterii*)
Eucalyptus lemon (*Eucalyptus citriodora*)
Cajuput (*Melaleuca cajuputi*)
Niaouli (*Melaleuca quinquenervia*)
Fragonia (*Agonis fragrans*)
Benzoin (*Styrax benzoin*)
Thyme linalol (*Thymus vulgaris ct. linalool*)
Elemi (*Canarium luzonicum*)
Eucalyptus radiata (*Eucalyptus radiata*)
Ravensara (*Ravensara aromatica*)
Cardamom (*Elettaria cardamomum*)
Ravintsara (*Cinnamomum camphora ct. cineole*)
Cypress (*Cupressus sempervirens*)
Myrtle (*Myrtus communis*)
Damiana (*Turnera diffusa*)
Manuka (*Leptospermum scoparium*)
Orange, sweet (*Citrus sinensis*)

COPD Expectorant Essential Oils
Eucalyptus radiata (*Eucalyptus radiata*)
Cajuput (*Melaleuca cajuputi*)
Ravintsara (*Cinnamomum camphora ct. cineole*)
Niaouli (*Melaleuca quinquenervia*)
Elemi (*Canarium luzonicum*)
Copaiba (*Copaifera officinalis*)
Cedarwood atlas (*Cedrus atlantica*)
Clove bud (*Syzygium aromaticum*)
Eucalyptus globulus (*Eucalyptus globulus*)

Cubeb (*Piper cubeba*)
Fragonia (*Agonis fragrans*)
Hyssop decumbens (*Hyssopus officinalis var. decumbens*)

COPD Warming Essential Oils
Cinnamon leaf (*Cinnamomum zeylanicum*)
Black pepper (*Piper nigrum*)
Cardamom (*Elettaria cardamomum*)
Clove bud (*Syzygium aromaticum*)
Ginger (*Zingiber officinale*)
Cubeb (*Piper cubeba*)
Marjoram, sweet (*Origanum majorana*)

COPD Anti-inflammatory Oils
Chamomile german (*Matricaria recutita*)
Chamomile roman (*Anthemis nobilis*)
Peppermint (*Mentha piperita*)
Lavender, spike (*Lavandula latifolia*)
Immortelle (*Helichrysum italicum*)
Spikenard (*Nardostachys jatamansi*)
Fragonia (*Agonis fragrans*)

GENERAL TWO-PART BLENDS

The following two-part blends are to be used on alternate days. Use for no more than two weeks, then take a week off. This is the first cycle. When using for a second cycle, increase the number of days off by two days. In other words, instead of taking seven days off, take nine days off. In this way, gradually increase the number of days you're not using the essential oil blends until the length of time without using essential oils is longer than the time they are used. Continue in this way until the number of days that the essential oils are used is zero — the purpose of this is to avoid becoming reliant on essential oils.

The Day One COPD General Blend is designed to ease breathing difficulties. The Day Two COPD General Blend is to assist in the reduction of inflammation, as well as reducing the level of anxiety or stress. Both can be used as a massage oil applied over the whole of the lung area — the upper chest, ribs, and upper back. If there's nobody around to apply it to the back, simply apply to that part of the area you can reach yourself.

Day One COPD General Blend

Eucalyptus lemon	6 drops
Niaouli	3 drops
Cajuput	4 drops
Fragonia	5 drops
Thyme linalol	5 drops

First, blend the essential oils together, then dilute in 1½ fl. oz. (45 mL) of carrier oil. Use no more than ½ teaspoon (2½ mL) for each application.

Day Two COPD General Blend

Geranium	6 drops
Cardamom	2 drops
Chamomile german	6 drops
Frankincense	4 drops
Orange, sweet	4 drops

First, blend the essential oils together, then dilute in 1½ fl. oz. (45 mL) of carrier oil. Use no more than ½ teaspoon (2½ mL) for each application.

COPD Blend for Chronic Cough

Immortelle	5 drops
Marjoram, sweet	5 drops
Benzoin	3 drops
Myrtle	5 drops
Niaouli	3 drops
Ravintsara	4 drops

This blend could be tried if there is a chronic cough. First, blend the essential oils together. For a body oil, dilute in 1½ fl. oz. (45 mL) of carrier oil and use ½ teaspoon (2½ mL) each time, applied to the chest, ribs, and upper back. Alternatively, blend the essential oils and use in the steam inhalation or room spray methods. Steam inhalation

involves dropping 2–4 drops of essential oil into a bowl of steaming hot water placed in the corner of the room or on a table, and allowing the aroma molecules to rise into the atmosphere.

COPD Environmental Blend

Eucalyptus radiata	8 drops
Chamomile roman	2 drops
Cajuput	4 drops
Geranium	2 drops

First, blend the essential oils together. The blend can be used in the steam inhalation or room spray methods outlined above or as a room spray. Dilute 12 drops of essential oil to 4 fl. oz. (120 mL) of warm water in a new spray bottle, and then shake well. This volume is enough for several days' use. Each time, add a little hot water, and shake the spray bottle before use. Spray the room and then exit for around five minutes.

Some COPD sufferers might find this method helpful before sleep, when a couple of drops of lavender may also combine well with the blend. The room spray method could be used with any combination of essential oils on the COPD General Respiratory list on page 343, diluting 12 drops in 4 fl. oz. (120 mL) of warm water and using a small amount each time.

Essential oils are volatile compounds and these could be inhaled. Clearly, someone with COPD may have a sensitivity to some types of volatile compounds, so it's important to bear this in mind when considering whether to use essential oils.

Multiple Sclerosis

No one is sure what causes multiple sclerosis (MS) or why some people may be more predisposed to it than others. Several theories have been proposed, including environmental factors, bacterial or viral infection, and nutritional deficiency. Perhaps it's a combination of several factors. Whatever the cause, MS is a disorder of the central nervous system, made up of the brain and spinal cord from which radiates a body-wide system of nerves communicating back and forth to the brain. The area affected by MS is very specific — it is the membrane known as the *myelin sheath*, which protects the nerve fibers of the central nervous system. In MS the myelin sheath degrades, which makes effective nerve communication difficult. This causes a variety of symptoms, depending on where the damage has occurred and on a person's own individual physiology. There might be the sensation of pins and needles in the skin, tingling, burning, or numbness. This loss of sensitivity is accompanied by muscle weakness and loss of muscular control or spasm, which makes moving about difficult. Coordination and balance can be hard to control. There may be difficulty with vision, speech, or swallowing. With these possible symptoms to deal with, it's understandable that a person with MS might experience extreme emotions, mood swings, deep depression, mental fatigue, and exhaustion.

The *multiple* in the name *multiple sclerosis* refers to the multiple sites of damage, and *sclerosis* refers to the scarring, thickening, and hardening that happens to the myelin sheath. No two people have the exact same set of symptoms.

Clearly, people have been looking for ways to alleviate the symptoms of MS for decades, and each person no doubt has advice they can offer fellow sufferers. One idea to emerge in recent years is to make sure you have enough vitamin D, which we usually get through exposure to the sun. But in some people, getting enough sun is not the problem; the problem is being unable to process the vitamin D.

Vitamin B1 (thiamine) is very important to cell function. In its natural form, thiamine is water soluble and passes easily through the body, which is why a good daily nutritional program for MS sufferers is so important. Fatigue in people with MS is said to be reversed by thiamine, even when the patient already has a normal level of B1. Some researchers think people with MS might have an as-yet-unidentified problem with their enzyme function or the movements within their cells. Natural sources of thiamine include yeast and yeast extract; spirulina and seaweed; nuts, including pistachios, macadamias, pecans, and pine nuts; sunflower and sesame seeds and sesame butter, also known as *tahini*; fish, including salmon and tuna; some meats, such as pork; certain herbs and spices; brown rice; beans, including black, pinto, and lima beans and fresh or dried peas; and sun-dried tomatoes.

Studies have shown a correlation between a diet high in fats and the progression of MS, so anyone with MS should seriously consider reducing fat intake and using the unsaturated variety. Switch from meat to fish wherever possible, and try to incorporate into your diet foods high in lecithin, such as wheatgerm, avocadoes, soybeans, and eggs — particularly egg yolk. The advantages of having a diet made up of organic, non-GM, natural, unprocessed foods cannot be overstated.

Essential oils can help with many of the symptoms of MS, including muscular spasms, muscular fatigue, insomnia, pain, and the emotional aspects, including depression. Throughout this book you will find many suggestions for essential oils to use to suit an individual's unique set of symptoms. If taking large quantities of medication it is always wise to inform your physician that you intend to use essential oils to help alleviate some of your symptoms. What follows is a list of essential oils that are generally beneficial for MS sufferers and address many of the symptoms they experience:

Essential Oils for MS

Geranium (*Pelargonium graveolens*)
Chamomile roman (*Anthemis nobilis*)
Lavender (*Lavandula angustifolia*)
Juniper berry (*Juniperus communis*)
Immortelle (*Helichrysum italicum*)
Plai (*Zingiber cassumunar*)
Orange, sweet (*Citrus sinensis*)
Grapefruit (*Citrus paradisi*)
Cypress (*Cupressus sempervirens*)
Peppermint (*Mentha piperita*)
Rosemary (*Rosmarinus officinalis*)
Basil linalol (*Ocimum basilicum ct. linalool*)
Eucalyptus radiata (*Eucalyptus radiata*)
Fragonia (*Agonis fragrans*)
Lemon (*Citrus limon*)
Petitgrain (*Citrus aurantium*)
Lemongrass (*Cymbopogon citratus/flexuosus*)
Niaouli (*Melaleuca quinquenervia*)
Marjoram, sweet (*Origanum majorana*)
Cardamom (*Elettaria cardamomum*)
Clary sage (*Salvia sclarea*)
Thyme linalol (*Thymus vulgaris ct. linalool*)
Palmarosa (*Cymbopogon martinii*)
Cedarwood atlas (*Cedrus atlantica*)
Sandalwood (*Santalum album*)
Eucalyptus lemon (*Eucalyptus citriodora*)
Black pepper (*Piper nigrum*)
Cistus (*Cistus ladaniferus*)

MS Muscular Fatigue Body Blend

Rosemary	10 drops
Peppermint	2 drops
Black pepper	4 drops
Geranium	8 drops
Basil linalol	6 drops
Myrtle	5 drops

First, blend the essential oils together, then dilute 3–5 drops in 1 teaspoon (5 mL) of carrier oil. Apply over any area that feels fatigued, and over the lower back.

MS Muscular Pain Body Blend

Immortelle	10 drops
Plai	8 drops
Lavender	7 drops
Marjoram, sweet	5 drops
Clary sage	5 drops
Eucalyptus lemon	5 drops

First, blend the essential oils together, then dilute 4–5 drops in 1 teaspoon (5 mL) of carrier oil. Use whenever and wherever the pain occurs.

MS Loss of Physical Sensitivity Body Blend

Geranium	8 drops
Clary sage	3 drops
Niaouli	10 drops
Black pepper	3 drops
Eucalyptus lemon	8 drops
Lemongrass	8 drops

First, blend the essential oils together, then dilute 3–5 drops per 1 teaspoon (5 mL) of carrier oil. Apply over the areas where you feel a loss of sensation as soon as those feelings appear.

MS Tired or Exhausted but Cannot Sleep Blend

Marjoram, sweet	6 drops
Vetiver	2 drops
Clary sage	4 drops
Lemon	2 drops
Basil linalol	2 drops
Orange, sweet	9 drops

First, blend the essential oils together. Use 1–2 drops to inhale from a tissue, or 3–5 drops in a room diffuser. If applying to the body, use 5 drops per 1 teaspoon (5 mL) of carrier oil. The blend can also be used in a bathtub — 4 drops of the blend into the tub, slightly diluted beforehand in a little carrier oil.

Chronic Fatigue Syndrome

Chronic fatigue syndrome (CFS), or myalgic encephalomyelitis (ME), confounds medical practitioners who strive to explain the cause of this group of symptoms, which includes debilitating muscular pain and inflammation resulting in disabling, extreme, and long-term daily fatigue, accompanied by any one or a combination of the following: muscle pain, soreness or pain when applying pressure to the tissues, overly sensitive bodily tissues, inflammation, irritable bowel syndrome, headaches, migraine, pain in the jaw, insomnia, loss of concentration and memory, mental confusion, irritability, depression, and impaired balance, sight, and hearing. Many sufferers develop CFS after a severe viral infection that invoked an immune response. Instead of getting better, the sufferer becomes profoundly tired after the slightest activity and develops a unique set of other symptoms, which change over time — confusing both the sufferer and their physician.

Before accepting a diagnosis of CFS, physicians usually rule out anything that can also cause pronounced fatigue. These include anemia, diabetes, chemical sensitivity, hyperthyroidism, and psychiatric issues arising usually from extreme and prolonged stress.

Emotional stress seems to exacerbate CFS symptoms, but avoiding stressful situations is not easy for any of us, and CFS sufferers have more challenges to deal with. The daily aggravations we all have to deal with affect people with CFS deeply, often leading to extreme physical sensitivity, exhaustion, and a flare-up of symptoms. CFS can be a long-term condition and lead to loss of livelihood and economic security, concern about raising children, and relationship difficulties.

Using aromatherapy and essential oils can help alleviate symptoms and increase general well-being, enabling a person to cope better with the condition. Take each day's symptoms as they come and use the appropriate essential oils as required. Several of the main symptoms of CFS are discussed separately in this section; for those that are not here, you'll find other suggestions throughout the book. The following list of essential oils contains those that will cover many of the symptoms experienced by CFS sufferers:

CFS ESSENTIAL OILS

Geranium (*Pelargonium graveolens*)
Chamomile roman (*Anthemis nobilis*)
Lavender (*Lavandula angustifolia*)
Juniper berry (*Juniperus communis*)
Immortelle (*Helichrysum italicum*)
Plai (*Zingiber cassumunar*)
Orange, sweet (*Citrus sinensis*)
Grapefruit (*Citrus paradisi*)
Cypress (*Cupressus sempervirens*)
Peppermint (*Mentha piperita*)
Rosemary (*Rosmarinus officinalis*)
Basil linalol (*Ocimum basilicum ct. linalool*)
Eucalyptus radiata (*Eucalyptus radiata*)
Lemon (*Citrus limon*)
Petitgrain (*Citrus aurantium*)
Lemongrass (*Cymbopogon citratus/flexuosus*)
Niaouli (*Melaleuca quinquenervia*)
Marjoram, sweet (*Origanum majorana*)
Cardamom (*Elettaria cardamomum*)
Clary sage (*Salvia sclarea*)
Thyme linalol (*Thymus vulgaris ct. linalool*)
Ravensara (*Ravensara aromatica*)
Cedarwood atlas (*Cedrus atlantica*)
Sandalwood (*Santalum album*)
Eucalyptus lemon (*Eucalyptus citriodora*)
Myrtle (*Myrtus communis*)

MUSCULAR FATIGUE

If you've ever seen a cartoon of someone so exhausted they fall asleep in their soup, it was probably a CFS sufferer. Few of us, unless we have run a marathon or spent many nights awake with a sick and crying baby, can truly understand the profound nature of CFS muscle fatigue. It can come and go quite suddenly, and people experience it in different ways, and in different ways on different days. It may be like having lead weights for limbs, or an ache in the muscles like a bad flu attack, or aching bones, or just a general weakness.

If you have had CFS for a long time you may have noticed a pattern to your fatigue; if so, use this information to your advantage and treat yourself with the appropriate oils before an attack is due. If you are unfortunate enough to be one of those who has continuous muscle fatigue, choose a time when you have nothing to do except apply the oils. Keep the oils handy so that you can use them when the best opportunity presents itself.

CFS Muscle Fatigue Essential Oils
Grapefruit (*Citrus paradisi*)
Plai (*Zingiber cassumunar*)
Rosemary (*Rosmarinus officinalis*)
Peppermint (*Mentha piperita*)
Eucalyptus lemon (*Eucalyptus citriodora*)
Cardamom (*Elettaria cardamomum*)
Cypress (*Cupressus sempervirens*)
Juniper berry (*Juniperus communis*)
Niaouli (*Melaleuca quinquenervia*)

CFS Muscle Fatigue Blend
Cypress	2 drops
Orange, sweet	8 drops
Cardamom	10 drops
Niaouli	5 drops
Eucalyptus lemon	6 drops
Peppermint	3 drops

First, blend the essential oils together. This blend can be used in several ways. Dilute 3–5 drops in 1 teaspoon (5 mL) of carrier oil to make a muscle rub. Too tired to contemplate using the blend? Just sniff the blend from a tissue, and/or apply onto the soles of your feet. The blend can also be used in the bath — use 2–4 drops diluted in a small amount of carrier oil.

INSOMNIA

Paradoxical as it may seem, insomnia is one of the problems people with severe fatigue can encounter. To be terribly tired yet unable to sleep is one of the worst aspects of CFS.

CFS Insomnia Essential Oils
Valerian (*Valeriana officinalis*)
Clary sage (*Salvia sclarea*)
Marjoram, sweet (*Origanum majorana*)
Sandalwood (*Santalum album*)
Chamomile roman (*Anthemis nobilis*)
Lemon (*Citrus limon*)
Spikenard (*Nardostachys jatamansi*)
Vetiver (*Vetiveria zizanoides*)

The oils can be applied to the body before having an essential oil bath. For individual massages, dilute 5 drops of your chosen essential oil blend in 1 teaspoon (5 mL) of carrier oil, or pre-prepare enough for two massages by diluting 10 drops of your essential oil blend in 2 teaspoons (10 mL) of carrier oil. Massage over the whole body, including the shoulders and neck. You can do this while the bath is running. Then add 4 drops of your chosen essential oil or blend into the bath, which should be neither too hot nor too cold. Get in the water and relax. If you have the energy, read a novel that doesn't make you think too much — but make sure you don't fall asleep in the bath.

CFS Insomnia Blend
Vetiver	8 drops
Valerian	2 drops

Spikenard	2 drops
Orange, sweet	10 drops
Bergamot FCF	6 drops

First, blend the essential oils together. Use 1 drop in a bathtub, or dilute 2–3 drops in 1 teaspoon (5 mL) of carrier oil and rub a small amount over the chest and back. This is a very aromatically intense blend and may not appeal to everyone, but it does seem to help those who cannot sleep in spite of being extremely tired. See also the "MS Tired or Exhausted but Cannot Sleep Blend" described in the "Multiple Sclerosis" section on page 346.

DEPRESSION

The cause of the depression that often accompanies CFS is as difficult to identify as the cause of the condition itself. The complexity of CFS, especially with regard to the frustrations surrounding its source, is enough to make anyone depressed because the route ahead is so unclear. Conflicting opinions are nowhere more apparent than with CFS. However, there are so many physical factors involved in this multi-organ condition that it is very likely that any one of them could produce a change in brain chemistry that leads to a depressed state of mind. So it is not simply experiencing the symptoms of the condition that causes depression, but also the physiological outcomes of this multi-system condition.

CFS DEPRESSION ESSENTIAL OILS
Grapefruit (*Citrus paradisi*)
Rose otto (*Rosa damascena*)
Tangerine (*Citrus reticulata*)
Geranium (*Pelargonium graveolens*)
Neroli (*Citrus aurantium*)
Petitgrain (*Citrus aurantium*)
Bergamot FCF (*Citrus bergamia*)
Patchouli (*Pogostemon cablin*)
Sandalwood (*Santalum album*)
Cedarwood atlas (*Cedrus atlantica*)

Because CFS affects each person differently, and each person differently each day, experiment with the oils listed, using them singly or in blends of your choice in all the usual methods.

LOSS OF MEMORY

Foggy brain is one of the things CFS sufferers hate the most — feeling as if your mind is stuffed full of clay and you cannot think straight, let alone remember anything. You can never be sure when this symptom will kick in, but it is usually after a prolonged bout of stress and it calls for immediate adjustments, particularly if you are at work with a great long to-do list. Of course it's frustrating and irritating to watch the simple things of the past become a series of little uphill struggles, but you can learn to adjust. Try to become aware of your daily rhythms in terms of mental and muscular fatigue, along with the other lows and highs, and see if a pattern emerges. As this is a disorder with individual sets of symptoms, what helps one person may not help another. And essential oils that are effective for a particular person on one day may not be effective on another day.

CFS GENERAL CONCENTRATION
AND MEMORY ESSENTIAL OILS
Rosemary (*Rosmarinus officinalis*)
Grapefruit (*Citrus paradisi*)
Bergamot FCF (*Citrus bergamia*)
Lavender (*Lavandula angustifolia*)
Peppermint (*Mentha piperita*)
Lemon (*Citrus limon*)
Basil linalol (*Ocimum basilicum ct. linalool*)

Try to always have a small bottle of diluted oils in your desk drawer or wherever you work, and inhale as needed or apply a small amount to the temples and nape of the neck. You could also keep a small atomizer for personal use handy in your desk. You decide how best to use the oils

— perhaps in a shower in the morning or inhaled on the way to work.

CFS Concentration and Memory Blend

Basil	8 drops
Grapefruit	10 drops
Peppermint	7 drops
Rosemary	5 drops

Blend the essential oils together using these proportions and bottle. Use as needed.

OTHER SYMPTOMS

There are many possible symptoms associated with this condition. CFS is so individual, you will probably have to design your own essential oil treatment. For some, stress is a factor that should be managed. Try the various relaxation techniques, including meditation. Breathe correctly, get plenty of fresh air, and eat fresh organic food. If what you eat swims, flies, walks, or grows — fine; if it comes out of a package, box, or can — forget it. Increase your vitamin and mineral intake: vitamins B, D, and C are all useful, as are zinc, selenium, and germanium. The UK government body that issues health guidelines, the National Institute for Health and Care Excellence, recommends that people with CFS have screening blood tests for gluten sensitivity. The connection between celiac disease and CFS is worth exploring, if only by omitting wheat, rye, and barley from the diet for a period of time to see if symptoms improve.

13

The Fragrant Way to Beauty

If eyes are the window to the soul, the face is a mirror, reflecting the ups and downs of an internal life. It shows the joy and happiness, as well as the disappointment and pain. There may be laughter lines, or a worried brow. The mouth may have an upturned smile, or lines going down from the corners, showing years of discontent or melancholy. Love brings a glow to the face, but stress and tension can make the skin dry and taut. Lack of sleep can result in dull skin, patches of redness, enlarged pores with increased sebum production, and dark rings around the eyes. The skin reflects what we eat, as well as what we feel and think, and ill health can likewise be detected on the surface of our face. They say the face is like a book, and that book is the book of our life.

Psychodermatology is the field of study examining the mind-skin connection. As skin is the largest organ in the human body, there are many areas of the face and body on which emotional issues can manifest. The skin is the target organ for stress in some people, while in others stress tends to express itself in the form of headaches or gastrointestinal problems, for example. The connection between the brain, nervous system, and skin is so close that scientists can confirm a diagnosis of the brain disorder Parkinson's disease by looking for proteins such as alpha-synuclein in a person's skin.

The body works as an integrated whole. Women know very well that their skin can react to the release of hormones at different times of their menstrual cycle. One hormone that affects the skin of women and men alike is cortisol, the fight-or-flight hormone that's released by the adrenal glands when a person feels stressed. That stress calls into action the fight-or-flight system, and because it anticipates trouble to come, it diverts blood from the skin to more vital internal organs, making them ready for any emergency. If the stress continues, the cortisol builds up in the body and histamine is released, which causes the skin to react more easily to any pressures and to become more sensitive generally. Stress leads to a slowdown in the production of collagen and elastin, which is why the skin becomes less smooth and elastic and loses its youthful appearance. The body treats sleep deprivation as a form of stress, producing more cortisol and negative effects on the skin.

Glycation occurs when too much sugar is eaten, leading to excess glucose molecules that cross-link, or form a bridge, with proteins such as collagen and elastin, which in turn leads to a molecular rearrangement making them rigid, less able to function as strong, bouncy fibers, and less able to regenerate. The end result is a loss of smooth texture and bounce, thinning of the skin, dullness, sagging, wrinkles, and skin that looks prematurely aged. The advanced glycation end products produced by too much sugar, fat, or processed foods not only affect the skin but are implicated in a huge range of health issues, including those of the eyes and liver.

Taken in excess, caffeine increases blood sugar levels, which in turn increases the production of sebum from the sebaceous glands, leading to inflammation and an uneven skin tone. Additionally, it stimulates the production of cortisol, which also damages collagen and elastin. So what we eat and drink most definitely affects how our skin looks, as well as our health.

Tap water can have a bad effect on skin, depending on where you live and the chemicals that have been used to process it. In some places, washing the face is better done with cleansers or micellar waters. Electrosmog is the new threat, bombarding our skin with unseen frequencies from electronic devices that can turn the face red, which we can see, and having a deeper effect, which we can't. Pollution from traffic never improved skin, and never will. Sunny, hot weather can produce lumps and bumps on the face, as well as dryness and wrinkles, but moist, damp air can give the skin a dewy texture.

There are so many factors to consider when looking at your face in the mirror; it's no wonder every cosmetic company searches high and low for ingredients. And they, like us, turn to essential oils and nourishing plant oils for "actives" to help the skin recover from all the hazards it faces in a modern daily life.

The skin has three main layers. The layer we see is the epidermis, and it's the thinnest layer — thinnest over the eyelids and thickest under the feet. It's part of the body's immune system, protecting us from harm. Below that is the thickest layer, the dermis, which contains blood and lymphatic vessels, sweat glands and pores, hair roots, and sebaceous glands. The lower level is comprised of subcutaneous fat, which protects the internal tissues, regulates temperature, transports the blood, lymph, and nerve cells and provides the connecting tissue that holds the skin to the muscles and bones. In a square inch of skin there could be approximately 100 sebaceous oil glands, 60 hairs, 620 sweat glands, 1,200 nerve endings, 20 blood vessels, approximately 60,000 melanocytes — melanin-producing cells that give skin its color — and around 9 million cells. If that sounds like a lot, consider the fact that the face may contain 500 million bacteria per square inch! The connective tissue contains two elements that are hugely important to the look of skin — collagen, which is sometimes described as the skin's scaffolding, and elastin, which gives everything its bounce.

Essential oils affect the skin in various ways. Most are antiseptic to a certain degree, and some are antibacterial, able to keep bacteria under control. The inflammation caused by blemishes of any kind can be soothed by certain anti-inflammatory essential oils. Inflammation in the short term is a normal body response, but when the skin is subjected daily to a multitude of environmental chemicals and pollutants, a form of perpetual inflammation occurs, and this can lead to sensitivity and irritation, which age the skin. The circulation-stimulating properties of some essential oils ensure that the oxygen required for skin repair and regeneration is being supplied, and essential oils also have proven antioxidant activity, which is important in helping prevent the damage that can be caused by free radicals. When essential oils are used to relieve general stress and tension, even in any of the methods available that are not specifically for the face, the results can be seen on the face in terms of relaxation and anti-aging effects.

One of the extraordinary aspects of working with essential oils is that if a patient comes to me for treatment for a physical condition — back pain, for example — they'll look about 10 years younger after about six weekly sessions. Partly this is due to the reduction in pain, but there's more to it than that. The texture of the skin all over the body, including the face, seems to go through a fundamental change, and I am, again and again, reminded of how comprehensive the benefits of essential oils can be. When treatment is designed specifically for the face, over time — enough time for cell renewal — the results are often nothing short of miraculous.

The most expensive skin preparations in the world contain plant extracts in one form or another — essential oils, plant stem cells, plant oils, and other plant components — as their principal active ingredients, but because the product will have to endure a long period of storage, transportation, and shelf life, they invariably contain preservatives. Some of these have been recognized as harmful and are, thankfully, being phased out. However, many cosmetic lines still contain these and other chemical preservatives, even though nature-based preservatives are available. Many hydrolats, hydrosols, and floral waters are used in this chapter and for a full explanation of the distinction between these water-based products, please see chapter 19, "Carrier Oils and Hydrolats." The quantities of essential oils used in this chapter have been amended from professional treatments for home use. The professional may also wish to refer to my book *Aromatherapy for the Beauty Therapist*, used for aesthetician training in various countries including the United Kingdom, France, and Japan.

This chapter starts with a luxury facial serum, an indispensable item in anyone's skin care regime that nourishes and balances the skin, helps prevent the signs of aging, and gives a beautiful tone to the skin. The serum has been designed to be either used on its own or augmented with essential oils, if you so choose. It can be used by people of all ages, both men and women. When preparing the serum ensure you add the ingredients in the order in which they are listed.

Luxury Facial Serum

Camellia seed oil	3 teaspoons (15 mL)
Avocado oil	1 teaspoon (5 mL)
Argan oil	2 teaspoons (10 mL)
Olive squalane	1 teaspoon (5 mL)
Borage seed oil (or evening primrose seed oil)	20 drops
Rosehip seed oil	20 drops
Sea buckthorn oil	10 drops

Cleansers

"Once upon a time, there was a beautiful princess who washed her lovely face in the sparkling water of the river running fresh and pure near her castle." Those days are long gone! The water coming out of the average tap today has been piped for hundreds of miles, recycled several times, and treated with chemicals to make it safe to drink. Chlorine is used as an antibacterial disinfectant, and in areas where a lot of pesticides are used there may be residues of mercury and arsenic. The quality of water very much depends on the locality someone happens to live in, and these qualities vary tremendously. This may account to some extent for the fact that while some people find tap water doesn't negatively affect their skin, others find it makes their skin dry, probably as a result of the protective fats and lipids being stripped from it by highly treated water.

Which brings us to cleansers. It's very common to see as the first and largest ingredient in many cleansing and cosmetic products the word *aqua* — water. Glacial water — water that's been filtered through volcanic rock — and mineral waters are sterilized or distilled before being included in commercial products to make them inert, or not chemically active. At home, we can use filtered tap water or distilled water to wash our faces. But this section outlines alternative cleansers that don't use water, and they have the advantage of being easily adjusted to suit not only your own skin type, but the variation in climate and environmental conditions over the course of the year.

CLEANSING OILS AND BALMS

It's easy to make oil and balm cleansers at home — all you need are a good selection of carrier oils and the ingredients to make a balm. The important thing is to choose rich carrier oils that are light, yet can remove what needs to be removed and are not so heavy that they clog the pores and skin. Surprisingly, perhaps, a good cleansing oil will not make the skin oilier, nor blemished skin more prone to spots, including acne. Conversely, many people have found that some water-based cleansers or soaps, and tap water, can cause an increased oiliness and more blemishes. Some people find that when they swap soap and water for cleansing oils, the skin doesn't feel as fresh; however, by using a hydrolat or floral water after cleansing, it can be just as refreshing and not so drying.

ESSENTIAL OILS USED IN CLEANSING OILS
Rosemary (*Rosmarinus officinalis*)
Eucalyptus radiata (*Eucalyptus radiata*)
Chamomile roman (*Anthemis nobilis*)
Lavender (*Lavandula angustifolia*)
Cedarwood atlas (*Cedrus atlantica*)
Clary sage (*Salvia sclarea*)
Tea tree (*Melaleuca alternifolia*)
Manuka (*Leptospermum scoparium*)
Caraway seed (*Carum carvi*)
Jasmine (*Jasminum grandiflorum/officinale*)
Bergamot FCF (*Citrus bergamia*)
Geranium (*Pelargonium graveolens*)
Lemongrass (*Cymbopogon citratus/flexuosus*)
Sandalwood (*Santalum album*)

Palmarosa (*Cymbopogon martinii*)
Ylang ylang (*Cananga odorata*)
Spearmint (*Mentha spicata*)
Coriander seed (*Coriandrum sativum*)

The following carrier oils can be used as facial cleansers. The more waxy oils such as jojoba, which is technically a liquid wax, will remove heavy makeup and heavy pollutants from the skin.

PLANT OILS TO USE IN CLEANSING OILS
AND BALMS
Coconut (*Cocos nucifera*)
Almond, sweet (*Prunus amygdalus var. dulcis*)
Hazelnut (*Corylus avellana*)
Apricot kernel (*Prunus armeniaca*)
Peach kernel (*Prunus persica*)
Sunflower (*Helianthus annuus*)
Jojoba (*Simmondsia chinensis*)
Grapeseed (*Vitis vinifera*)
Rice bran (*Oryza sativa*)
Safflower (*Carthamus tinctorius*)

BASIC NOURISHING CLEANSING OIL
FOR ALL SKIN TYPES

Almond oil, sweet	1 fl. oz. (30 mL)
Apricot kernel oil	1 fl. oz. (30 mL)
Coconut oil	2 teaspoons (10 mL)
Sunflower oil	1 tablespoon (15 mL)
Jojoba	1 tablespoon (15 mL)

Combine all the oils together, and blend well. This can be used on its own, or you could add essential oils if you wish (see below).

To Use a Cleansing Oil

To use a cleansing oil, apply as you would your normal cleanser. Remove it from the face using a hot, wet cloth or cotton wool pads. Apply a hydrolat or floral water tonic after cleansing.

Essential Oil Blends for Use in Cleansing Oils

INVIGORATING MORNING BLEND

Rosemary	4 drops
Spearmint	1 drop
Lemongrass	1 drop
Manuka	1 drop
Lavender	2 drops

Blend the essential oils together before adding to 3½ fl. oz. (100 mL) of cleansing oil.

RELAXING EVENING CLEANSING BLEND

Lavender	3 drops
Orange, sweet	3 drops
Chamomile roman	1 drop
Rosewood	2 drops
Geranium	3 drops

Blend the essential oils together before adding to 3½ fl. oz. (100 mL) of cleansing oil.

Cleansing Pastes

Cleansing pastes are cleansing and exfoliating treatments for the face, neck, and décolletage. They contain dry ingredients that smooth, cleanse, and gently exfoliate the skin. Generally, cleansing pastes are used once a week as a skin treatment.

To make a cleansing paste, first combine the essential oil and plant oil blends together, ensuring even distribution. Then place all the dry ingredients in a blender, or blend by hand, and mix well. Slowly incorporate the essential oil and plant oil blend into the dry ingredients until a smooth paste is obtained. If the ingredients separate at any time, stir well to remix them. If the paste is stored in a sealed jar in the fridge, it will keep up to three months.

To use: Scoop out about 2 teaspoons of the paste for each application and apply over the face, avoiding the eye area. Remove with a rolling movement of the fingers, then use a hot wet cloth to remove any residue. Apply a hydrolat or floral water tonic after cleansing.

Essential oils to use in cleansing pastes include geranium, lavender, sweet orange, lemon, rose otto, jasmine, and ylang ylang.

ALMOND CLEANSING PASTE

Essential oil or blend of your choice	10 drops
Almond oil	10 teaspoons (50 mL)
Almonds, ground	60 g (2.12 oz.)
Pink clay (optional)	5 g (0.18 oz.)
Cider vinegar	5 teaspoons (25 mL)
Spring water	5 teaspoons (25 mL)

APRICOT EXFOLIATING CLEANSING PASTE

Essential oil or blend of your choice	10 drops
Apricot kernel oil	10 teaspoons (50 mL)
Apricot powder	½ teaspoon
Almonds, ground	60 g (2.12 oz.)
White clay (optional)	5 g (0.18 oz.)
Cider vinegar	5 teaspoons (25 mL)
Spring water	5 teaspoons (25 mL)

JOJOBA CLEANSING AND EXFOLIATING PASTE

Essential oil or blend of your choice	10 drops
Jojoba	10 teaspoons (50 mL)
Almonds, ground	60 g (2.12 oz.)
Jojoba wax peeling grains (natural)	1 teaspoon
White clay (optional)	5 g (0.18 oz.)
Cider vinegar	5 teaspoons (25 mL)
Spring water	5 teaspoons (25 mL)

Cleansing Balms

Cleansing balms are mixtures of waxes, plant oils, and essential oils. Cleansing balms have a slightly soft consistency, rather like a stiff ointment.

SIMPLE BASIC CLEANSING BALM

Almond oil	4 teaspoons (20 mL)
Apricot kernel oil	4 teaspoons (20 mL)
Beeswax	5 g (0.18 oz.)
Essential oil or blend of your choice	5 drops

Use the bain-marie or double boiler method to make cleansing balms. First, melt the beeswax, then slowly add the plant oils, while mixing all the time. Remove from heat, add the essential oils, and mix in well, then pour into a storage container and leave to cool. If a harder, more solid balm is preferred, add to the basic blend above a small amount of beeswax and cocoa butter. Keep away from heat sources that may cause the balm to melt.

Exfoliants and Face Polishes

Exfoliators are used to remove dead skin cells, leaving the face looking fresh and dewy. Only a small amount is needed — about 1 teaspoon is enough for each application. Several foodstuffs found in the kitchen cupboard could be used as the basic raw ingredient, as well as products used by professionals such as natural jojoba wax beads — spherical granules made of jojoba oil. Oatmeal is still used in many cosmetic products as it has a soothing effect on the skin and can be combined with ground almonds for a facial polish.

OAT AND ALMOND FACE POLISH

This is a polish suited for normal to oily skin types. It incorporates basil linalol and lemon essential oils that enliven the skin tone.

Essential oil blend	1 drop
Almonds, ground	5 g (0.18 oz.)
Oatmeal, fine ground	5 g (0.18 oz.)
Almond oil, sweet	½ teaspoon (2½ mL)
Cider vinegar	½ teaspoon (2½ mL)

Salt (sea or Himalayan pink)	1 pinch

To make the essential oil blend, combine 1 drop of lemon essential oil with 1 drop of basil linalol essential oil, and use just 1 drop of this combination. Blend the ground almonds and oatmeal and put to one side. Mix the almond oil and 1 drop of essential oil together, then add the vinegar and salt, and finally stir in the almond/oat mix. Blend everything together well. Use damp fingers to gently roll the polish over the surface of your skin. Remove by rinsing with water or by using a hot, wet washcloth. Then, if you wish, apply a hydrolat, tonic, or face oil.

INGREDIENTS THAT COULD BE USED IN FACIAL POLISHES

When deciding which essential oils or plant oils to incorporate into facial polishes, choose those that are suitable for your skin type, as listed elsewhere in this chapter. These are some of the other exfoliating products that could be used:

- Ground flower petals: for example, rose, jasmine, lavender, orange blossom
- Fruit powders: for example, apricot, pineapple, cranberry, pomegranate, cupuaçu
- Fig seeds
- Jojoba wax grains
- Fine sugar
- Salt, various types

Face Masks

Face masks are known for improving the color and tone of the skin, but if they're well formulated with a specific person in mind — that's you! — they can accomplish much more. For example, a mask can be made to nourish, rejuvenate, and stimulate the skin; cleanse and refine the skin; soothe and calm inflammation; treat blemishes; or act as an anti-wrinkle treatment and natural face-lift.

The active ingredients of face masks can include vitamins and minerals, clays, fruit and flower extracts, food extracts, exotic gels, gold, silver, and rare essential oils. Dry ingredients can be blended using flower waters, hydrolats, or plain mineral or spring water, and plant oils are added for their fatty acid content. Although the merits of using just one essential oil are many, if you prepare a blend of oils and leave it to stand for a couple of days so the oils have a chance to energize each other, so much the better. The basic recipes outlined in this section can be adapted to accommodate the essential oil(s) chosen for your particular skin type.

CLAY FACE MASKS

Clays have taken thousands of years to become infused with minerals from the earth, nutrients from plant materials, and energy from the sun. There are white, pink, red, orange, yellow, green, brown, black, and even blue clays from all over the world, but not all are suitable for facial skin care. Each clay has a distinct mineral profile, with differing effects on the skin, and only the most gentle should be used in skin care. Clays have long been widely used for beauty treatments and are much valued for their rejuvenating and anti-aging effects.

Facial clay masks can be made by mixing clay with hydrolats, floral waters, herbal distillates, plain waters of various types, aloe vera, or milk. Additional powdered ingredients could include fruit powders, milk powder, honey powder, and seaweed. Clays are not generally oil soluble; however, plant oils can be included after a smooth paste has been made. Essential oils work very well in clay masks and are incorporated into the plant oils before being added to the clay mixture.

White cosmetic clay (kaolin) is suitable for most skin types, including delicate and sensitive skin. The powder is a fine, soft clay and used in many cosmetics for its soothing and refining properties. It has a slight astringent and tightening effect, and like most clays, it helps remove impurities from the skin while cleansing and improving circulation.

Pink French clay (rose clay) is suitable for most skin types, including sensitive, dry, or normal complexions. It has a toning and softening effect, can brighten dull and tired-looking skin, and can be used as a gentle exfoliating agent.

Green French illite clay is rich in calcium, magnesium, potassium, and sodium and can be used on most skin types except those that are sensitive, fragile, or dry. It has a revitalizing effect on more mature skin, and used in face masks it can be helpful in cases where the skin has been disturbed by blemishes or acne. It is also used to balance combination skin and reduce the harmful effects of pollution on the skin. French green clay is emollient, antiseptic, and healing and leaves the skin silky smooth. It gently stimulates the flow of blood and lymph, enabling oxygen to speed up the elimination of waste products.

Rhoussel clay from Morocco can be used on most skin types. It has beneficial effects on the skin and is often used in facial treatments. Rhoussel clay can be used in combination with other products for specialized skin care purposes as it combines well with other powdered clays, as well as various other powders.

Fuller's earth can overstimulate the skin, which is why it's not advised for use on any skin that's sensitive, delicate, or dry and is more suitable for normal and oily skins. It is a soft brown clay, renowned for its absorbent and skin-lightening effects. It's cleansing, and also has a desquamation action — that is, it removes dead cells.

All around the world there are long traditions of clays being used for medicinal purposes, the best-known methods being healing compresses and poultices applied to specific areas of the body to alleviate a multitude of conditions. For the more serious mud-lover, there's only one thing that will satisfy — full-body immersion in a bath full of mud. Luckily we're not running a spa so we don't need vast amounts of the stuff, just a little dried powder to get us closer to beautiful skin.

If the clay hasn't been adulterated in any way, it has a practically unlimited shelf life. As with essential oils, quality is important. In general, when you start making and applying clay masks, less is more — there's no need to use too much.

Combinations of clay can work very well for specific facial types, for example:

For sensitive, dry, or mature and aging skin: Combine white and pink clays (some pink clays are already a blend of red and white clay).

For a soothing anti-aging mask: Combine rhoussel clay with white and pink clay.

For a cleansing and purifying effect: Combine rhoussel clay with green clay.

For oily or combination skin: Combine green and white clay.

For acne: Often there's an element of inflammation that can get overlooked when the focus is on the zits themselves. Initially, combine white and pink clay, then progress to a combination of green and white. To help avoid scarring, gentle treatments are preferred to the harsh products often marketed to teenagers.

A homemade face mask will take you no more than a few minutes to put together, even for those with little time to pamper themselves who are looking for an instant fix. Once the basic ingredients are ready in a jar, the face pack is almost ready to use, tailor-made to suit your own skin type requirements. And depending on how the skin feels at any particular moment, additional ingredients can be added.

Ready-for-Action Mask

What follows is a combination of clays and powders that can be used as the basis of a mask, ready for your chosen additional ingredients that have more specialized therapeutic purposes. Clay is light, so for clarity's sake, the following suggestions are given in tablespoons rather than in weight measurements. The quantities are enough for several masks, depending on how thickly you like to apply them. The ingredients provide a gentle, purifying, smoothing, and toning base for clay-based facial masks, and this basic mask is included in the formulations for the more specialized clay face masks.

BASIC CLAY FACE MASK INGREDIENTS

French green clay	2 tablespoons
White cosmetic clay	4 tablespoons
Pink clay (or rhoussel clay for anti-aging purposes)	4 tablespoons
Corn flour powder, organic	2 tablespoons

Combine the clays together, then add the corn flour powder.

How much of the Basic Clay Face Mask you blend together depends on the thickness of the final mask you prefer, the size of the face, the skin type, and the volume of other ingredients that will be added later. The basic dry ingredients above can be prepared and stored in a lidded jar for quite a long time.

To make a face mask using only the above ingredients, add either water or a hydrolat to 1 tablespoon of the Basic Clay Face Mask, until you reach your preferred consistency. If you make too much of the final mask, cover it well and refrigerate. Clay has natural antibiotic properties and many essential oils do too, and this helps preserve the face mask for up to a week.

Making a Specialized Clay Face Mask

Always mix all dry ingredients from the following suggestions together well before combining them with the liquid ingredients. This is to ensure that each ingredient can be evenly mixed into the mask. Add 1 tablespoon of this mixture to sufficient liquid, as shown below, to form a paste. How much liquid is needed will depend to some extent on the quality of the clays, as well as on how thick or thin a consistency you want the mask to be. If it's too thick, add more of the liquid; if too fluid, add more clay. Clay masks are best applied to damp skin; to dampen the skin choose a hydrolat from the mask's formulation. Clay face masks are best used no more than once a week, unless otherwise indicated.

NORMAL SKIN REVITALIZING MASK

Dry ingredient:

Basic Clay Face Mask	4 teaspoons

Liquid ingredients:

Vegetable glycerin	1 teaspoon (5 mL)
Orange blossom hydrolat or floral water	1 teaspoon (5 mL)
Rose hydrolat or floral water	1 teaspoon (5 mL)
Rosemary hydrolat or floral water	1 teaspoon (5 mL)
Essential oil blend (see below)	1 drop

Make the essential oil blend by combining:

Geranium	2 drops
Ho wood	1 drop

DRY SKIN CLAY MASK

Dry ingredients:

Basic Clay Face Mask	4 teaspoons
Pink clay	3 teaspoons
Oatmeal, fine ground	1 teaspoon

Liquid ingredients:

Vegetable glycerin	1 teaspoon (5 mL)
Jojoba oil	1 teaspoon (5 mL)
Evening primrose seed oil	1 teaspoon (5 mL)
Rose hydrolat or floral water	1 tablespoon (15 mL)
Essential oil blend (see below)	1 drop

Make the essential oil blend by combining:

Chamomile roman	1 drop
Rose otto	1 drop

OILY SKIN FACE MASK

Dry ingredients:

Basic Clay Face Mask	1 teaspoon
Green French clay	1½ tablespoons
Brewer's yeast, powdered	¼ teaspoon

Liquid ingredients:

Rosemary hydrolat	1 tablespoon (15 mL)
Lavender hydrolat	2 teaspoons (10 mL)
Essential oil blend (see below)	1 drop

Make the essential oil blend by combining:

Rosemary	1 drop
Lavender	1 drop
Lemon	1 drop

ANTI-AGING REVITALIZING MASK

Dry ingredients:

Basic Clay Face Mask	1 tablespoon
Rhoussel clay	1 tablespoon
Slippery elm powder	1 teaspoon
Brewer's yeast	¼ teaspoon

Liquid ingredients:

Rosehip seed oil	1 teaspoon (5 mL)
Carrot root oil, macerated	1 teaspoon (5 mL)

Orange blossom hydrolat	1 tablespoon (15 mL)
Rose hydrolat	1 tablespoon (15 mL)
Frankincense essential oil	1 drop
Immortelle essential oil	1 drop
Rose otto essential oil	1 drop

Brewer's yeast contains B vitamins and trace elements; slippery elm is soothing and calming. Use the face mask no more than once every seven days for a six-week period, then use once a month.

Acne-Prone Skin Face Mask

Dry ingredients:

Basic Clay Face Mask	1 tablespoon
Green clay	2 tablespoons
Brewer's yeast	1 teaspoon

Liquid ingredients:

Aloe vera liquid	1 tablespoon (15 mL)
Thyme hydrolat	1 tablespoon (15 mL)
Lavender hydrolat	1 tablespoon (15 mL)
Colloidal silver liquid	1 teaspoon (5 mL)
Chamomile german essential oil	1 drop
Palmarosa essential oil	1 drop
Ho wood essential oil	1 drop

To begin with, this mask can be applied every five days for a period of six weeks, then reduced to once every 15 days, or once a month. After the mask is removed, apply a mixture of thyme and lavender hydrolat to the face.

GEL FACIAL MASKS

Gel facial masks are suitable for all skin types and skin conditions, depending on the ingredients incorporated into the gel. Commercially sold gels are often sophisticated concoctions with active cosmetic ingredients that can include anything from hyaluronic acid to coral collagen. Reproducing these at home is difficult, but simple versions of face gels are easy to make. The facial mask gels outlined in this section should be kept in a refrigerator and will keep for at least a week even if no preservatives have been used.

Some food items that can be used in gel facial masks include tapioca starch from cassava (*Manihot esculenta*), pectin obtained from a variety of fruits, quince seeds, and xanthan gum produced from the bacteria *Xanthomonas campestris*. Carrageen and agar agar gelling agents are made from sea vegetables — carrageen (also known as Irish moss) is produced from *Chondrus crispus*, while agar agar is produced from *Gelidium amansii* and *Gracilaria verrucosa*. If purchasing seaweed, only buy the natural, unadulterated flakes used in food production as thickening agents.

However, a simple organic aloe vera gel can also be used as a base into which essential oils and hydrolats can be incorporated to make a gel facial mask. The choice of essential oils is yours, but I would suggest you refer to the lists of essential oils and blends appropriate to different skin types in the "Skin Care Oils" section, starting on page 365.

Simple Aloe Vera Gel Mask

Aloe vera gel	2 fl. oz. (60 mL)
Plant oil	1 tablespoon (15 mL)
Essential oils	2 drops

Simple Aloe Vera Hydrolat Gel Mask

Aloe vera gel	2 fl. oz. (60 mL)
Hydrolat	1 tablespoon (15 mL)
Plant oil	1 teaspoon (5 mL)
Essential oils	2 drops

To choose which hydrolat would be appropriate, look at those suggested for various skin types in the "Facial Sprays and Tonics" section, starting on page 362. Blend the aloe vera gel and hydrolat together, then blend the plant oil and essential oils together, and then mix both together well.

Facial Steaming

Facial steaming has long been an integral part of professional beauty treatments and is especially valued in highly polluted city locations. Gentle puffs of steam are directed at the face, sometimes combining ozone and ions to help the facial pores open and excrete dirt, toxins, and environmental pollutants, with the cleansing leading to a more refined skin surface.

Steam treatments are extremely easy to do at home — all you need is a bowl of boiling purified water, a towel, and any ingredients you wish to add such as essential oils, hydrolats, floral waters, or herbal extracts. Put your chosen essential oils or other additions on the surface of the water, stir well, then cover your head with the towel, making sure that the sides are closed. You'll need to come up for air every so often, but basically plan to be under the towel, with your eyes closed, for about five minutes.

This method should be avoided by those with broken facial capillaries, acne, rosacea, sunburn, or highly sensitive skin. It does suit very well those with all kinds of seborrhea and blemished skins, and with normal skin it often improves the texture and tonality of the skin. The following are suggestions for different skin types:

ESSENTIAL OILS FOR NORMAL SKIN
Fennel, sweet (*Foeniculum vulgare var. dulce*)
Lavender (*Lavandula angustifolia*)
Lemon (*Citrus limon*)
Orange, sweet (*Citrus sinensis*)
Neroli (*Citrus aurantium*)
Rosemary (*Rosmarinus officinalis*)
Juniper berry (*Juniperus communis*)
Cedarwood atlas (*Cedrus atlantica*)
Geranium (*Pelargonium graveolens*)
Jasmine (*Jasminum grandiflorum/officinale*)

Suggestion: 2 drops of lavender and 1 drop of lemon
Use 2–4 drops on a bowl of steaming water. Follow the steam treatment with deep facial cleansing and then use a facial spray or tonic.

ESSENTIAL OILS FOR DRY SKIN
Chamomile roman (*Anthemis nobilis*)
Rose otto (*Rosa damascena*)
Chamomile german (*Matricaria recutita*)
Neroli (*Citrus aurantium*)
Geranium (*Pelargonium graveolens*)
Clary sage (*Salvia sclarea*)
Lavender (*Lavandula angustifolia*)
Sandalwood (*Santalum album*)

Suggestion: 2 drops of geranium and 1 drop of clary sage
Use 2–4 drops on a bowl of steaming water. Follow the steam treatment with deep facial cleansing and then use a facial spray or tonic.

ESSENTIAL OILS FOR OILY SKIN
Bergamot (*Citrus bergamia*)
Chamomile roman (*Anthemis nobilis*)
Cypress (*Cupressus sempervirens*)
Eucalyptus radiata (*Eucalyptus radiata*)
Juniper berry (*Juniperus communis*)
Ylang ylang (*Cananga odorata*)
Frankincense (*Boswellia carterii*)
Lemongrass (*Cymbopogon citratus/flexuosus*)
Grapefruit (*Citrus paradisi*)
Rosemary (*Rosmarinus officinalis*)
Palmarosa (*Cymbopogon martinii*)
Immortelle (*Helichrysum italicum*)

Suggestion: 1 drop of bergamot and 2 drops of rosemary
Use 2–4 drops on a bowl of steaming water. Follow the steam treatment with deep facial cleansing and then use a facial spray or tonic.

Essential Oils for Acned Skin

Chamomile roman (*Anthemis nobilis*)
Chamomile german (*Matricaria recutita*)
Cistus (*Cistus ladaniferus*)
Clary sage (*Salvia sclarea*)
Thyme linalol (*Thymus vulgaris ct. linalool*)
Lavender (*Lavandula angustifolia*)
Palmarosa (*Cymbopogon martinii*)
Juniper berry (*Juniperus communis*)
Cypress (*Cupressus sempervirens*)
Grapefruit (*Citrus paradisi*)
Immortelle (*Helichrysum italicum*)

Suggestion: 1 drop juniper berry, 1 drop clary sage, and 1 drop palmarosa

Use 2–4 drops on a bowl of steaming water. Follow the steam treatment with deep facial cleansing and then use a facial spray or tonic.

Facial Sprays and Tonics

Gentle facial sprays can have many purposes; for example, they can cool, calm, and give the skin an all-round boost. Some are tonic, some astringent — all are refreshing. They can help refine open pores and smooth unevenly textured skin. Facial sprays are generally applied after cleansing to ensure the complete removal of any residue left from creams or lotions, and they can also be used during the day or evening to refresh the skin. For a facial spray, use a single hydrolat or a combination of hydrolats, or combine a hydrolat and a floral water, or aloe vera liquid, with a quality non-tap water.

For a facial tonic, use a hydrolat combined with essential oil. Combine the hydrolats, glycerin or aloe vera, and essential oil together in a bottle, shake really well, and leave to stand for at least 24 hours. Shake the bottle again, filter through an unbleached paper coffee filter to remove any essential oil globules, and store in the fridge.

Hydrosol/Hydrolat and Other Waters* for Face Tonics

Normal Skin

Waters: hydrolats, hydrosols, essential oil waters, or floral distillates

Lavender (*Lavandula angustifolia*)
Geranium (*Pelargonium graveolens*)
Immortelle (*Helichrysum italicum*)
Spearmint (*Mentha spicata*)
Lemon (*Citrus limon*)
Cornflower (*Centaurea cyanus*)
Orange flower (*Citrus aurantium*)
Rose (*Rosa damascena/centifolia*)

Face Tonic for Normal Skin

Geranium water	3 fl. oz. (90 mL)
Lavender water	1 fl. oz. (30 mL)
Vegetable glycerin	1 teaspoon (5 mL)
Geranium essential oil	2 drops
Spearmint essential oil	1 drop
Lavender essential oil	1 drop

To create a fusion, combine the hydrolats, glycerin, and essential oils together in a bottle, shake really well, and leave to stand for at least 24 hours. Shake the bottle again, filter through an unbleached paper coffee filter to remove any essential oil globules, and store in the fridge.

Normal to Dry Skin

Waters: hydrolats, hydrosols, essential oil waters, or floral distillates

Rose (*Rosa damascena/centifolia*)
Lavender (*Lavandula angustifolia*)
Chamomile roman (*Anthemis nobilis*)
Chamomile german (*Matricaria recutita*)
Cornflower (*Centaurea cyanus*)
Geranium (*Pelargonium graveolens*)

Face Tonic for Normal to Dry Skin

Rose water	2 fl. oz. (60 mL)
Chamomile water	2 fl. oz. (60 mL)

Vegetable glycerin   1 teaspoon (5 mL)
Sandalwood essential oil   4 drops
Ho wood essential oil   2 drops
To create a fusion, combine the hydrolats, glycerin, and essential oils together in a bottle, shake really well, and leave to stand for at least 24 hours. Shake the bottle again, filter through an unbleached paper coffee filter to remove any essential oil globules, and store in the fridge.

Normal to Sensitive Skin
Waters: hydrolats, hydrosols, essential oil waters, or floral distillates
Chamomile roman (*Anthemis nobilis*)
Lavender (*Lavandula angustifolia*)
Chamomile german (*Matricaria recutita*)
Cornflower (*Centaurea cyanus*)
Clary sage (*Salvia sclarea*)
Yarrow (*Achillea millefolium*)
Marigold (*Calendula officinalis*)

FACE TONIC FOR NORMAL TO SENSITIVE SKIN
Chamomile roman water   2 fl. oz. (60 mL)
Lavender water   2 fl. oz. (60 mL)
Aloe vera liquid   1 teaspoon (5 mL)
Chamomile german
   essential oil   1 drop
Lavender essential oil   2 drops
To create a fusion, combine the hydrolats, aloe vera, and essential oils together in a bottle, shake really well, and leave to stand for at least 24 hours. Shake the bottle again, filter through an unbleached paper coffee filter to remove any essential oil globules, and store in the fridge.

Normal to Blemished or Acned Skin
Waters: hydrolats, hydrosols, essential oil waters, or floral distillates
Pine (*Pinus sylvestris*)
Rosemary (*Rosmarinus officinalis*)
Thyme (*Thymus vulgaris*)

Manuka (*Leptospermum scoparium*)
Tea tree (*Melaleuca alternifolia*)
Bay laurel (*Laurus nobilis*)
Lavender (*Lavandula angustifolia*)
Sage (*Salvia officinalis*)
Melissa (*Melissa officinalis*)

FACE TONIC FOR NORMAL TO BLEMISHED OR ACNED SKIN
Rosemary water   3 fl. oz. (90 mL)
Lavender water   1 fl. oz. (30 mL)
Aloe vera liquid   1 teaspoon (5 mL)
Juniper berry essential oil   2 drops
Geranium essential oil   2 drops
To create a fusion, combine the hydrolats, aloe vera, and essential oils together in a bottle, shake really well, and leave to stand for at least 24 hours. Shake the bottle again, filter through an unbleached paper coffee filter to remove any essential oil globules, and store in the fridge.

Normal to Oily Skin
Waters: hydrolats, hydrosols, essential oil waters, or floral distillates
Cypress (*Cupressus sempervirens*)
Spearmint (*Mentha spicata*)
Clary sage (*Salvia sclarea*)
Lemon (*Citrus limon*)
Rosemary (*Rosmarinus officinalis*)
Pine (*Pinus sylvestris*)
Myrtle (*Myrtus communis*)
Rose (*Rosa damascena / centifolia*)
Orange flower (*Citrus aurantium*)
Petitgrain (*Citrus aurantium*)

FACE TONIC FOR NORMAL TO OILY SKIN
Orange flower water   3 fl. oz. (90 mL)
Rose water   1 fl. oz. (30 mL)
Aloe vera liquid   1 teaspoon (5 mL)
Petitgrain essential oil   4 drops
Orange, sweet,
   essential oil   2 drops

To create a fusion, combine the hydrolats, aloe vera, and essential oils together in a bottle, shake really well, and leave to stand for at least 24 hours. Shake the bottle again, filter through an unbleached paper coffee filter to remove any essential oil globules, and store in the fridge.

Mature to Aged Skin

Waters: hydrolats, hydrosols, essential oil waters, or floral distillates
Cistus (*Cistus ladaniferus*)
Geranium (*Pelargonium graveolens*)
Rose (*Rosa damascena/centifolia*)
Mastic (*Pistacia lentiscus*)
Frankincense (*Boswellia carterii*)
Melissa (*Melissa officinalis*)

FACE TONIC FOR MATURE TO AGED SKIN

Rose water	2 fl. oz. (60 mL)
Melissa water	1 fl. oz. (30 mL)
Frankincense water	1 fl. oz. (30 mL)
Vegetable glycerin	1 teaspoon (5 mL)
Aloe vera liquid	1 teaspoon (5 mL)
Frankincense essential oil	1 drop
Palmarosa essential oil	1 drop

To create a fusion, combine the hydrolats, glycerin, aloe vera, and essential oils together in a bottle, shake really well, and leave to stand for at least 24 hours. Shake the bottle again, filter through an unbleached paper coffee filter to remove any essential oil globules, and store in the fridge.

Suggestion: Cotton-wool pads can be soaked in a tonic or aloe vera liquid and then divided into thinner sections before being put in a tightly sealed box with an extra couple of teaspoons of tonic passed over them — and, hey presto, you've got your own brand of natural, instant, freshen-up facial pads.

Astringents

Sometimes a stronger facial tonic is required, one with more astringent values. These incorporate vinegars and can be used on skins that are normal, oily, blemished, or acned. Combine the liquid ingredients, then add the essential oils, shake well, leave for 24 hours, shake again, pass through an unbleached paper coffee filter to remove any essential oil globules, and keep the fusion in the fridge.

GENERAL ASTRINGENT TONIC

Witch hazel	1 fl. oz. (30 mL)
Orange flower water	3 fl. oz. (90 mL)
Cider vinegar, organic (optional)	½ teaspoon (2½ mL)
Juniper berry essential oil	3 drops
Lemon essential oil	1 drop
Grapefruit essential oil	1 drop

STIMULATING ASTRINGENT TONIC

Witch hazel	1 fl. oz. (30 mL)
Rose water	3 fl. oz. (90 mL)
Cider vinegar, organic (optional)	½ teaspoon (2½ mL)
Rosemary essential oil	2 drops
Spearmint essential oil	1 drop
Bergamot FCF essential oil	1 drop

SKIN VINEGAR FOR BLEMISHED, OILY, AND OPEN-PORED SKIN

Spring water	3½ tablespoons (50 mL)
Orange flower water	5 teaspoons (25 mL)
White wine vinegar, organic	3 teaspoons (15 mL)
Palmarosa essential oil	2 drops
Spearmint essential oil	1 drop

Skin Care Oils

Skin care oils are one of the best ways to take care of your skin and can easily be adapted to take into account changes in circumstances, such as stress levels, health, lifestyle, and general well-being. These factors often change from month to month, and by blending your own skin care oils you can accommodate your ever-changing skin care needs, which reflect physical, environmental, and emotional factors.

The first step in deciding which particular skin care regime to choose is to establish which basic skin type you have. Then, if you're experiencing emotional difficulties, cross-reference the list of essential oils for your skin type against those in chapter 5, "Emotional Rescue," and see if there are essential oils appropriate for both your skin and your emotional needs.

Many people believe their skin is a combination of skin types. Combination skin is a patchwork of normal, oily, and dry skin, with the oil patches usually occurring on the forehead, nose, and chin. This type of skin can develop at any time from changes in health, lifestyle, working conditions, and, of course, stress levels. Treat combination skin as you would normal skin, and if the oily patches become a problem use the face oils for oily skin on those areas. As the skin starts to balance you can adjust the treatment accordingly. Our skins can change quite rapidly, so do take notice of the changes and be ready to switch oils as and when needed.

EVENLY BALANCED — NORMAL SKIN

Really, there's no such thing as normal skin. Or, more correctly, children have normal skin, and the rest of us aspire to it! The perfect skin of pre-puberty is plump, in that the cells are firm and solid, neither dry nor oily, finely textured with no visible pores, spots, or blemishes, soft and velvety to the touch, and unwrinkled. Adults can only yearn for this perfection, and we call skin "normal" if it reaches somewhere near it — about halfway is close enough. The term *normal* is so inappropriate in this context that I prefer to call this type of skin *evenly balanced*.

If you have skin that falls into this category you could use almost any essential oil in your skin preparations. Avoid those intended to treat acne or disturbed and blemished skin unless needed for those hormonal days when the odd pimple makes its appearance.

BALANCED NORMAL SKIN: CARRIER OILS
Almond, sweet (*Prunus amygdalus var. dulcis*)
Apricot kernel (*Prunus armeniaca*)
Hazelnut (*Corylus avellana*)
Jojoba (*Simmondsia chinensis*)
Argan (*Argania spinosa*)
Camellia seed (*Camellia japonica*)

SPECIALIST PLANT OIL ADDITIONS FOR BALANCED NORMAL SKIN
Evening primrose seed (*Oenothera biennis*)
Rosehip seed (*Rosa rubiginosa*)
Borage seed (*Borago officinalis*)
Carrot, macerated (*Daucus carota*)
Cucumber seed (*Cucumis sativus*)
Pomegranate seed (*Punica granatum*)
Sea buckthorn (*Hippophae rhamnoides*)
Passion flower seed (*Passifloria incarnata*)
Kiwi seed (*Actinidia chinensis*)

ESSENTIAL OILS FOR BALANCED NORMAL SKIN
Chamomile german (*Matricaria recutita*)
Lemon (*Citrus limon*)
Palmarosa (*Cymbopogon martinii*)
Neroli (*Citrus aurantium*)
Geranium (*Pelargonium graveolens*)
Jasmine (*Jasminum grandiflorum/officinale*)
Lavender (*Lavandula angustifolia*)

Rose otto (*Rosa damascena*)
Frankincense (*Boswellia carterii*)
Chamomile roman (*Anthemis nobilis*)

DAY CARE OIL FOR BALANCED NORMAL SKIN

Rose otto	14 drops
Geranium	3 drops
Chamomile roman	2 drops
Lavender	3 drops
Lemon	3 drops

Optional additions to 1 fl. oz. (30 mL) of carrier oil:

Rosehip seed oil	20 drops
Carrot macerated oil	10 drops

First, blend the essential oils together, then dilute 2–3 drops in each teaspoon (5 mL) of hazelnut or sweet almond carrier oil. Apply a small amount to damp skin, massage into the face and neck, avoiding the eye area, and then dab the face with a tissue to remove excess oil.

NIGHT CARE OIL FOR BALANCED NORMAL SKIN

Geranium	9 drops
Palmarosa	5 drops
Rosewood	5 drops
Orange, sweet	3 drops
Lavender	5 drops

Optional additions to 1 fl. oz. (30 mL) of carrier oil:

Rosehip seed oil	20 drops
Sea buckthorn oil	10 drops

First, blend the essential oils together, then dilute 2–3 drops in each teaspoon (5 mL) of camellia seed oil to which you've added 5 drops of evening primrose seed oil. Apply a small amount to damp skin, massage into the face and neck, avoiding the eye area, and then dab the face with a tissue to remove excess oil.

NORMAL TO DRY SKIN

The cells on the outer surface of the skin are essentially at the last stage of the shedding process, known as *desquamation*, and are held together by the hydrolipidic film. This consists of amino acids and lactic acid from sweat, fatty acids from sebum, and moisturizing by-products of keratinization — which is the process by which skin cells are shed from the top layer and replaced by those underneath. When the hydrolipidic layer is disturbed for some reason, the skin feels dry. This may be because the normal pH balance is disturbed, not enough sebum is being produced, the skin is being dried out by central heating, there are hormonal changes, medications have upset the normal balance of the skin protection system, or for many other reasons.

When the skin becomes dry it's less supple and more prone to wrinkles, and it can even become flaky. In time it can become sensitive, prone to inflammation, and easily dehydrated by wind and sun. This type of skin is prone to peeling and itching during periods of stress. It generally feels taut after washing. Sometimes dry skin is caused by hormonal changes and menopause.

NORMAL TO DRY SKIN: CARRIER OILS

Almond, sweet (*Prunus amygdalus var. dulcis*)
Avocado (*Persea americana*)
Apricot kernel (*Prunus armeniaca*)
Argan (*Argania spinosa*)
Hemp seed (*Cannabis sativa*)
Meadowfoam (*Limnanthes alba*)
Rice bran (*Oryza sativa*)
Macadamia (*Macadamia ternifolia*)
Camellia seed (*Camellia japonica*)

SPECIALIST PLANT OIL ADDITIONS FOR NORMAL TO DRY SKIN

Evening primrose seed (*Oenothera biennis*)
Borage seed (*Borago officinalis*)
Red raspberry seed (*Rubus idaeus*)
Acai berry (*Euterpe oleracea*)
Olive squalane (*Olea europaea*)
Rosehip seed (*Rosa rubiginosa*)

Sea buckthorn (*Hippophae rhamnoides*)
Cranberry seed (*Vaccinium macrocarpon*)
Carrot, macerated (*Daucus carota*)

ESSENTIAL OILS FOR NORMAL TO DRY SKIN
Chamomile german (*Matricaria recutita*)
Chamomile roman (*Anthemis nobilis*)
Lavender (*Lavandula angustifolia*)
Sandalwood (*Santalum album*)
Geranium (*Pelargonium graveolens*)
Rose otto (*Rosa damascena*)
Palmarosa (*Cymbopogon martinii*)
Carrot seed (*Daucus carota*)
Ho wood (*Cinnamomum camphora ct. linalool*)
Neroli (*Citrus aurantium*)
Clary sage (*Salvia sclarea*)
Frankincense (*Boswellia carterii*)

DAY CARE OIL FOR NORMAL TO DRY SKIN
Chamomile german	3 drops
Sandalwood	15 drops
Mandarin	3 drops
Ho wood	4 drops

Optional additions to 1 fl. oz. (30 mL) of carrier oil:
Olive squalane oil	20 drops
Raspberry seed oil	10 drops

First, blend the essential oils together, then dilute 2–3 drops in each teaspoon (5 mL) of camellia seed oil, to which you've added 2 drops of evening primrose seed oil. Apply a small amount to damp skin, massage into the face and neck, avoiding the eye area, and then dab the face with a tissue to remove excess oil.

NIGHT CARE OIL FOR NORMAL TO DRY SKIN
Carrot seed	5 drops
Sandalwood	8 drops
Lavender	3 drops
Clary sage	3 drops
Palmarosa	4 drops

Optional additions to 1 fl. oz. (30 mL) of apricot kernel or sweet almond carrier oil:

Olive squalane oil	20 drops
Rosehip seed oil	30 drops

NORMAL TO OILY SKIN

Oily skin is caused by overactive sebaceous glands. These are subject to hormonal changes, which is why oily skin can be a problem during puberty. Overactive sebaceous glands can lead to seborrhea, but more often the problem presents as oily patches that leave the skin shiny. Ironically, an oily skin can result from overcleanliness — from scrubbing the face with harsh cleansers and soaps or using astringents that contain alcohol. Many commercial lotions designed to degrease the skin actually stimulate the sebaceous glands to produce more sebum. Thankfully, essential oils have the capacity to balance the skin without prompting the glands to produce more sebum and can provide the perfect solution to this seemingly intractable problem.

NORMAL TO OILY SKIN: CARRIER OILS
Hazelnut (*Corylus avellana*)
Grapeseed (*Vitis vinifera*)
Safflower (*Carthamus tinctorius*)
Hemp seed (*Cannabis sativa*)
Sunflower (*Helianthus annuus*)
Jojoba (*Simmondsia chinensis*)
Argan (*Argania spinosa*)

SPECIALIST PLANT OIL ADDITIONS FOR NORMAL TO OILY SKIN
Borage seed (*Borago officinalis*)
Carrot, macerated (*Daucus carota*)
Rosehip seed (*Rosa rubiginosa*)
Kiwi seed (*Actinidia chinensis*)
Sea buckthorn (*Hippophae rhamnoides*)
Blueberry seed (*Vaccinium corymbosum*)
Echium seed (*Echium plantaginoum*)
Strawberry seed (*Fragaria ananassa*)

ESSENTIAL OILS FOR NORMAL TO OILY SKIN

Chamomile german (*Matricaria recutita*)
Lavender (*Lavandula angustifolia*)
Geranium (*Pelargonium graveolens*)
Frankincense (*Boswellia carterii*)
Juniper berry (*Juniperus communis*)
Cypress (*Cupressus sempervirens*)
Palmarosa (*Cymbopogon martinii*)
Petitgrain (*Citrus aurantium*)
Bergamot (*Citrus bergamia*)
Patchouli (*Pogostemon cablin*)
Niaouli (*Melaleuca quinquenervia*)
Orange, sweet (*Citrus sinensis*)
Lemon (*Citrus limon*)
Marjoram, sweet (*Origanum majorana*)
Lime (*Citrus aurantifolia*)
Rosemary (*Rosmarinus officinalis*)
Jasmine (*Jasminum grandiflorum/officinale*)
Ylang ylang (*Cananga odorata*)

DAY CARE OIL FOR NORMAL TO OILY SKIN

Juniper berry	8 drops
Geranium	10 drops
Petitgrain	10 drops
Rosemary	2 drops

Optional additions to 1 fl. oz. (30 mL) of carrier oil:

Kiwi seed oil	10 drops
Borage seed oil	10 drops

First, blend the essential oils together, then dilute 2–3 drops in each teaspoon (5 mL) of jojoba or sunflower oil, to which you've added 10 drops of carrot macerated oil. Apply a small amount to damp skin, massage into the face and neck, avoiding the eye area, and then dab the face with a tissue to remove excess oil.

NIGHT CARE OIL FOR NORMAL TO OILY SKIN

Juniper berry	10 drops
Petitgrain	15 drops
Frankincense	5 drops
Marjoram, sweet	5 drops
Orange, sweet	10 drops

Optional additions to 1 fl. oz. (30 mL) of carrier oil:

Rosehip seed oil	10 drops
Blueberry seed oil	10 drops
Evening primrose seed oil	5 drops

First, blend the essential oils together, then dilute 2–3 drops in each teaspoon (5 mL) of hazelnut oil. Apply a small amount to damp skin, massage into the face and neck, avoiding the eye area, and then dab the face with a tissue to remove excess oil.

SENSITIVE SKIN

Anyone's skin can become sensitive at any time. Even skin previously considered normal can become prone to sensitivity after contracting a virus, eating certain foods, coming into contact with synthetic perfumes or synthetic cosmetic ingredients, including preservatives, and so on. Some skins become sensitive only during extremes of weather — when it's too cold, hot, or windy. Sometimes skin changes can be linked to an emotional situation, such as the loss of a loved one, moving or changing jobs, stress, or even just a change in lifestyle. It could be too that the skin can no longer deal with environmental pressures such as overheating at the workplace, too much electrosmog, or pollution. Sensitive skin can also be inherited. Allergies can develop suddenly, and for clues as to what's causing the trouble it may be useful to have patch testing carried out.

If you've become sensitive to skin care products in general, it could be that you'll be sensitive to certain plant oils or essential oils too. This is why it's important for you to carry out a skin test before using anything on the face. Apply a small amount of oil, or diluted essential oil, in the crook of an elbow or behind the ear, and leave it for 24 hours. If there's no reaction such as itchiness, redness, soreness, or swelling, then that oil might suit you.

The best choices for highly sensitive skins are water-based products such as hydrolats, hydrosols, plant distillates, floral waters, and the like. Only use essential oils in very low dosages, increasing the amount used as you become confident there's no skin reaction, and use carrier oils that are known to be gentle on the skin. As this is such an individual situation — everyone is different in terms of their sensitivities and reactions — not all the suggestions below might be appropriate for you. Always choose organic products.

HYDROLATS FOR SENSITIVE SKIN
Chamomile roman (*Anthemis nobilis*)
Chamomile german (*Matricaria recutita*)
Lavender (*Lavandula angustifolia*)
Rose (*Rosa damascena/centifolia*)

ESSENTIAL OILS FOR SENSITIVE SKIN
Lavender (*Lavandula angustifolia*)
Chamomile german (*Matricaria recutita*)
Chamomile roman (*Anthemis nobilis*)
Geranium (*Pelargonium graveolens*)
Sandalwood (*Santalum album*)
Neroli (*Citrus aurantium*)

CARRIER OILS FOR SENSITIVE SKIN
Almond, sweet (*Prunus amygdalus var. dulcis*)
Rice bran (*Oryza sativa*)
Jojoba (*Simmondsia chinensis*)
Calendula, macerated (*Calendula officinalis*)
Grapeseed (*Vitis vinifera*)
Camellia seed (*Camellia japonica*)

Wrinkles and the Aging Skin

We don't always notice ourselves aging, nor perhaps do our close friends and family, yet when we meet someone we haven't seen for several years, we notice they've aged, and they notice that we have too. That's often when we're struck by the thunderbolt of recognition that age has crept up on us silently.

The search for the elixir of youth is as old as the hills. Ancient texts abound with tales of alchemists striving to satisfy that demand from their rulers. Today, exclusive clinics offer natural cosmetic treatments to those who can afford them, and celebrity clients keep the source of their youthful appearance a closely guarded secret. After all, if everyone looks as great as they do, it defeats the purpose of looking better than the rest! Cosmetic surgery is almost commonplace, and injectable treatments are so ubiquitous they're something people now have done at home. Investment bankers know that if they can find the fledgling company with the latest answer to the ancient question — how to stay young? — they'll be flying high!

Behind the scenes of all this frenetic activity, nature's essential oils have been quietly playing their part. Aromatherapy began in Europe, where it's widely incorporated into all aspects of life, including at the ritzy Swiss clinics reserved for *les clients privée*. Cellular regeneration is the key to youthful skin, and because skin cells renew themselves all the time, there's hope for improvement. Cells need oxygen, which some essential oils may encourage with their circulation-stimulating properties. They also have antioxidant activity, which is needed to deal with free radicals that can easily destroy molecules, including those of all skin layers. Also, some essential oils contain phytohormones, hormonal-like properties that may account for their being able to give skin a firmer and more youthful appearance when used over time.

ESSENTIAL OILS FOR AGING SKIN

Many essential oils have properties that can help prevent the onset of the telltale signs of aging. The following are used in various combinations by aromatherapists to treat the effects of declining skin tone. Some essential oils have more potent effects than others, and these are often used in combinations. However, some — such as neroli, spikenard, rose, and jasmine — are used singly in luxury anti-aging products.

ANTI-AGING ESSENTIAL OILS
Rose otto (*Rosa damascena*)
Rose absolute (*Rosa centifolia*)
Juniper berry (*Juniperus communis*)
Marjoram, sweet (*Origanum majorana*)
Violet leaf (*Viola odorata*)
Mastic (*Pistacia lentiscus*)
Clary sage (*Salvia sclarea*)
Neroli (*Citrus aurantium*)
Spikenard (*Nardostachys jatamansi*)
Cardamom (*Elettaria cardamomum*)
Rosewood (*Aniba rosaeodora*)
Chamomile german (*Matricaria recutita*)
Carrot seed (*Daucus carota*)
Frankincense (*Boswellia carterii*)
Immortelle (*Helichrysum italicum*)
Magnolia flower (*Michelia alba*)
Geranium (*Pelargonium graveolens*)
Palmarosa (*Cymbopogon martinii*)
Petitgrain (*Citrus aurantium*)
Ylang ylang (*Cananga odorata*)
Lavender (*Lavandula angustifolia*)
Sandalwood (*Santalum album*)
Orange, sweet (*Citrus sinensis*)
Cistus (*Cistus ladaniferus*)
Jasmine (*Jasminum grandiflorum/officinale*)
Patchouli (*Pogostemon cablin*)
Rosemary (*Rosmarinus officinalis*)
Coriander seed (*Coriandrum sativum*)

In this section you'll find special combination formulas for face treatments for four age groups, because the skin has different requirements at different stages of life. Using the correct essential oil for your facial skin serum or oil can be more than just taking into account the skin condition and the hoped-for outcome. Before blending a personal anti-aging facial oil, a holistic aesthetician specializing in essential oil skin care will examine the skin and take into account your well-being, overall health, stress levels, and any emotional factors that might be affecting your skin's condition and rate of aging. So before you choose your oils, cross-reference with other sections of this book to see which would be the most appropriate for you. And because you're making these products yourself, you can adapt them over time to take account of changes in your personal circumstances.

Each essential oil has its own particular qualities. For example, geranium can help with specific skin conditions such as drying or dry patches on the face, increased oiliness, enlarged pores, wrinkles and lines, dark circles under the eyes, and lack of elasticity — all of which can result from going through difficult emotional experiences. But it can also help with the underlying trauma by reducing stress, tiredness, and anxiety — the sort of anxious feelings that can keep a person awake at night and contribute to an aging skin.

Life presents many hurdles, and even on a day-to-day basis, most of us are juggling a career, personal relationships, and child care, not to mention maintaining financial security. Any resulting anxieties could inhibit the action of the immune, digestive, and lymphatic systems — all of which can have an effect on the skin. Despite all this, forget about aging gracefully. No one wants to look their age, and I've never met anyone — male or female — who doesn't want to age as well as they can. So fight it every step of the way.

SKIN-ENHANCING OIL EXTRACTS FOR USE IN FACE OILS

You've heard of the Gold Rush? Well, welcome to the Oil Rush! Patent offices all over the world are receiving applications from cosmetic company research labs trying to corner the market on processing methods for and commercial uses of plant oils — with any variation thereof you could possibly imagine! Fortunately, this drive for monopoly doesn't affect the normal user of these oils — you and me — so we can still take advantage of them.

Before getting to the antiwrinkle oils for the various age groups, we'll look at some of the most beneficial additions you could incorporate in small quantities into your oil blends. These can be used on the face, neck, and décolleté area of the upper chest:

Acai berry oil (*Euterpe oleracea*): Emollient, nourishing skin oil used in anti-aging preparations; has moisturizing and anti-inflammatory properties; suits damaged, extra-dry skin types; conditions the skin; includes omegas 6 and 9 and vitamin E; antioxidant

Blackberry seed oil (*Rubus fructicosis*): Skin nourishing and conditioning oil; suits mature, dry, and sensitive skins; includes omegas 3, 6, and 9 and vitamin E; antioxidant

Black raspberry seed oil (*Rubus occidentalis*): Helps retain elasticity; suits most skin types; anti-aging; includes omegas 3, 6, and 9 and vitamin E; antioxidant

Blueberry seed oil (*Vaccinium corymbosum*): Skin protecting oil with antioxidant properties; suits most skin types; including those with acne or blemishes

Borage seed oil (*Borago officinalis*): Moisturizing and nourishing; effective for skin maintenance oils; suits most skin types; high in gamma-linolenic acid (GLA)

Chia seed oil (*Salvia hispanica*): High in omega 3

Cranberry seed oil (*Vaccinium macrocarpon*): Good moisturizing and nourishing properties for anti-aging; suits damaged, irritated, or prematurely aged skin; includes omega 3 and vitamin E; antioxidant

Cucumber seed oil (*Cucumis sativus*): Good moisturizing and skin protective properties; cell regenerating; revitalizing; improves the elasticity and strength of the skin; anti-aging; suitable for most skin types

Evening primrose seed oil (*Oenothera biennis*): Skin conditioning and skin strengthening; useful in anti-aging skin care and scar-reducing facial oils; can be used on most skin types; high in GLA

Gotu kola (*Centella asiatica*): Macerated oil; skin regenerative; stimulates synthesis of collagen

Hemp seed oil (*Cannabis sativa*): Nourishing and skin conditioning; helps retain moisture and skin elasticity in troubled and distressed skin

Olive squalane extract (*Olea europaea*): Skin soothing and softening; suits most skin types; suits extra-dry skin; anti-aging

Pomegranate seed oil (*Punica granatum*): Nourishing and moisturizing; improves skin elasticity; rejuvenating; conditioning; high in omega 5 fatty acid (conjugated linoleic acid, or CLA)

Red raspberry seed oil (*Rubus idaeus*): Skin protective; anti-inflammatory; nourishing and conditioning for damaged and dry skin; includes omegas 3 and 6 and vitamin E; antioxidant

Rosehip seed oil (*Rosa rubiginosa*): Cell regenerating and cell stimulating; improves the appearance of scarring; improves texture and elasticity of the skin; anti-aging; suits mature and sun-damaged skin types

Sea buckthorn berry oil (*Hippophae rhamnoides*): Nourishing and revitalizing; cell regenerating; suits most skin types including prematurely aged skin; anti-aging

Strawberry seed oil (*Fragaria ananassa*): Moisturizing and texture improving; suits most skin types including oily skin types; blemishes

THE ANTIWRINKLE NIGHT OILS

The following blends are suggestions for general applications and should suit most people. The blends take into account the various health and well-being issues usually associated with the different age groups.

ANTIWRINKLE NIGHT OIL
FOR THE OVER-TWENTIES

Petitgrain	4 drops
Lavender	5 drops
Rosemary	5 drops
Chamomile german	2 drops
Chamomile roman	2 drops
Lemon	4 drops
Geranium	7 drops
Plus the plant oils:	
Rosehip seed oil	20 drops
Evening primrose seed oil	10 drops

First, blend the essential oils together. Then add the plant oils into the essential oils. Dilute this blend of oils by adding 1 or 2 drops to each teaspoon (5 mL) of your chosen carrier oil — such as hazelnut, almond, or apricot kernel oil. Lightly apply a small amount of the fully diluted oil over the face, neck, and décolletage.

ANTIWRINKLE NIGHT OIL FOR THE OVER-THIRTIES

Sandalwood	4 drops
Palmarosa	5 drops
Lavender	4 drops
Rosewood	5 drops
Orange, sweet	4 drops
Chamomile roman	2 drops
Carrot seed	3 drops
Plus the plant oils:	
Rosehip seed oil	20 drops
Sea buckthorn oil	10 drops

First, blend the essential oils together. Then add the plant oils into the essential oils. Dilute this blend of oils by adding 1 or 2 drops to each teaspoon (5 mL) of your chosen carrier oil — such as hazelnut, almond, or apricot kernel oil. Lightly apply a small amount of the fully diluted oil over the face, neck, and décolletage.

ANTIWRINKLE NIGHT OIL FOR THE OVER-FORTIES

Neroli	6 drops
Lavender	4 drops
Frankincense	5 drops
Rosemary	2 drops
Cistus	3 drops
Lemon	3 drops
Immortelle	2 drops
Carrot seed	3 drops
Plus the plant oils:	
Evening primrose seed oil	10 drops
Rosehip seed oil	10 drops
Sea buckthorn oil	15 drops

First, blend the essential oils together. Then add the plant oils into the essential oils. Dilute this blend of oils by adding 2–3 drops to each teaspoon (5 mL) of your chosen carrier oil — such as hazelnut, almond, or apricot kernel oil. Lightly apply a small amount of the fully diluted oil over the face, neck, and décolletage.

ANTIWRINKLE NIGHT OIL FOR THE OVER-FIFTIES

Cistus	3 drops
Immortelle	3 drops
Geranium	5 drops
Rose absolute	5 drops
Lavender	3 drops
Ho wood	4 drops
Plus the plant oils:	
Rosehip seed oil	30 drops
Sea buckthorn oil	30 drops
Evening primrose seed oil	10 drops

First, blend the essential oils together. Then add the plant oils into the essential oils. Dilute this blend of oils by adding 2–3 drops to each teaspoon

(5 mL) of your chosen carrier oil — such as hazelnut, almond, or apricot kernel oil. Lightly apply a small amount of the fully diluted oil over the face, neck, and décolletage.

Problem Skin

FRAGILE OR BROKEN CAPILLARIES

The most usual areas on the face where broken capillaries are found are the cheeks, chin, and around the nose, although anywhere on the face can be affected. The tiny vessels that supply blood to the face can be damaged by physical trauma, too much sun or wind, inflammation of the skin, and alcohol. Anyone can develop broken capillaries; sometimes they're a consequence of genetics or age. Although no essential oil treatment can remove them once they've appeared, certain essential oils may help prevent them from getting any worse. These are the oils to use:

CARRIER AND ESSENTIAL OILS TO USE
IN CASES OF FRAGILE CAPILLARIES
Carrier Oils
Almond, sweet (*Prunus amygdalus var. dulcis*)
Avocado (*Persea americana*)
Apricot kernel (*Prunus armeniaca*)
Hazelnut (*Corylus avellana*)
Jojoba (*Simmondsia chinensis*)
Peach kernel (*Prunus persica*)
Hemp seed (*Cannabis sativa*)
Grapeseed (*Vitis vinifera*)

Oils That Could Be Added to Carrier Oils
Borage seed (*Borago officinalis*)
Carrot, macerated (*Daucus carota*)
Evening primrose seed (*Oenothera biennis*)
Rosehip seed (*Rosa rubiginosa*)
Kiwi seed (*Actinidia chinensis*)
Cranberry seed (*Vaccinium macrocarpon*)

Essential Oils
Rose otto (*Rosa damascena*)
Chamomile german (*Matricaria recutita*)
Geranium (*Pelargonium graveolens*)
Cypress (*Cupressus sempervirens*)
Juniper berry (*Juniperus communis*)
Cedarwood atlas (*Cedrus atlantica*)
Chamomile roman (*Anthemis nobilis*)
Spearmint (*Mentha spicata*)
Mastic (*Pistacia lentiscus*)
Immortelle (*Helichrysum italicum*)

NIGHT TREATMENT OIL FOR
BROKEN CAPILLARIES

Geranium	9 drops
Cypress	5 drops
Immortelle	3 drops
Lemon	5 drops
Juniper berry	3 drops

Optional additions to 1 fl. oz. (30 mL) of carrier oil:

Rosehip seed	10 drops
Evening primrose seed	5 drops

First, blend the essential oils together. Then add the plant oils into the essential oils. Dilute this blend of oils by adding 1–2 drops to each teaspoon (5 mL) of equal amounts of jojoba and hemp seed oils. Apply a small amount over the face and neck, avoiding the eye area. Use gentle, light, smooth movements, trying not to overstimulate the skin.

WHITEHEADS (MILIA)

Milia, commonly called whiteheads, are tiny cysts on the skin, filled with a hard, milky-white protein called keratin. They can appear singly or in clusters, usually on the cheeks or around the eye but anywhere on the face or body. If they've been on the skin for some time, it's best to have the contents removed by a professional aesthetician, but recently found milia can be dispersed by massage. Before massaging in the following blend, steam the face using 2 drops of palmarosa and 1 drop of niaouli (or eucalyptus radiata) in the water. While the pores are still open from the steam, apply 1 drop of the following blend of essential oils directly on the milia only, using a cotton swab, and then massage with one finger in a circular movement over the hardened lump. It may take a few attempts before the milia are easy to remove.

BLEND FOR MILIA

Black pepper	1 drop
Eucalyptus lemon	3 drops

Dilute in 2 teaspoons (10 mL) of jojoba oil.

A very small amount of the oil can be used to massage the milia twice a day, in the morning and at night. Try not to get the oil blend on the rest of the face.

BLACKHEADS (COMEDONES)

When oil and sebum, and debris such as cellular fragments from the skin, get blocked in an open pore, oxidation occurs and turns the debris black. The problem with blackheads, aside from their unwelcome appearance, is that removing the material can cause inflammation and more blockage. Blackheads can appear practically anywhere on the body, but they're mostly found on the face, especially around the nose.

Steaming opens the pores and provides an excellent way to loosen blackheads on the face. Put hot, steaming water in a bowl and add 1 drop of eucalyptus lemon oil on the water. Then cover your head with a towel, close your eyes, and steam your face until it feels warm. Rinse the face or apply a hot, wet compress using 1 teaspoon of cider vinegar added to hot, but not boiling, water. If the blackhead is softened, gently squeeze, taking care not to damage the skin. Then splash the face with this tonic.

BLACKHEAD TONIC

Mineral water	3½ tablespoons (50 mL)
Cider vinegar	2 teaspoons (10 mL)
Witch hazel	2 teaspoons (10 mL)

Bergamot FCF	2 drops
Cypress	2 drops

After dabbing the skin dry, apply the following blend on the skin. It may help prevent blackheads from recurring while also loosening any that are already established.

BLACKHEAD PREVENTION BLEND

Lemongrass	5 drops
Lavender	2 drops
Clary sage	2 drops
Thyme linalol	5 drops

Blend the essential oils together, dilute 1 or 2 drops in each teaspoon (5 mL) of jojoba oil, and massage a small amount into the area morning and night.

BLEMISHED SKIN

Have you ever noticed how blemishes or spots seem to break out when they're least wanted? I know a woman who didn't have a single blemish on her skin until her wedding day, when a big spot appeared on the end of her nose! A spot can only "know" when it will be least welcome if it's picking up emotional signals from us, so instead of expressing negative fear — "I hope I won't get a spot" — try some positive certainty: "My skin is going to look great." If you already have a spot or one that's on its way, apply the formula below while saying, "This spot is going to go" — and try to believe it!

Just smear a little of the Spot Mix, undiluted, directly on the affected area twice a day, using a cotton swab. Try not to get any of the mix on other parts of the skin. Allow three days for it to clear.

SPOT MIX

Lavender	2 drops
Palmarosa	5 drops
Basil linalol	1 drop
Spearmint	2 drops
Chamomile german	2 drops
Manuka	1 drop

Blend all the above in 6 drops of jojoba oil.

ACNE

Beauty is more than skin deep, but that can be hard to remember when you have acne. Acne usually appears as an oily skin with a lot of blackheads, whiteheads, pimples, inflammation, and possibly scarring. It can occur not only on the face but on the neck, back, and chest as well. Sometimes the problem is exacerbated by the proliferation of a bacteria that normally lives on skin without causing problems, *Propionibacterium acnes*. Acne can cause discomfort as well as being unsightly. The temptation to squeeze the spots and remove the pus can be difficult to resist, but squeezing could cause scarring. Acne is often hormone related and associated with puberty, but it can appear at any time of life.

The bactericide and anti-inflammatory properties of essential oils are extremely useful in helping the healing process. Adopt a diet of fresh, home-cooked food and avoid processed foods, sugar, and fats. If antibiotics have been prescribed, also take a probiotic supplement to counteract the reduction of "good" bacteria.

The acne treatment outlined in this section comes in four stages, and the carrier oils, rich plant oil additions, and essential oil suggestions are listed below. There are no sun protective factors in the Day Treatments that follow.

CARRIER OILS FOR ACNE
Almond, sweet (*Prunus amygdalus var. dulcis*)
Jojoba (*Simmondsia chinensis*)
Grapeseed (*Vitis vinifera*)
Argan (*Argania spinosa*)
Safflower (*Carthamus tinctorius*)

PLANT OIL ADDITIONS FOR ACNE
Borage seed (*Borago officinalis*)
Carrot, macerated (*Daucus carota*)
Evening primrose seed (*Oenothera biennis*)
Blueberry seed (*Vaccinium corymbosum*)
Echium seed (*Echium plantaginoum*)
Calendula, macerated (*Calendula officinalis*)

STAGE ONE ESSENTIAL OILS FOR ACNE
Chamomile german (*Matricaria recutita*)
Palmarosa (*Cymbopogon martinii*)
Chamomile roman (*Anthemis nobilis*)
Frankincense (*Boswellia carterii*)
Lavender (*Lavandula angustifolia*)
Geranium (*Pelargonium graveolens*)
Bergamot FCF (*Citrus bergamia*)
Juniper berry (*Juniperus communis*)
Eucalyptus radiata (*Eucalyptus radiata*)
Peppermint (*Mentha piperita*)

STAGE TWO ESSENTIAL OILS FOR ACNE
Bergamot FCF (*Citrus bergamia*)
Clary sage (*Salvia sclarea*)
Lavender (*Lavandula angustifolia*)
Thyme linalol (*Thymus vulgaris ct. linalool*)
Eucalyptus radiata (*Eucalyptus radiata*)
Geranium (*Pelargonium graveolens*)
Carrot seed (*Daucus carota*)
Palmarosa (*Cymbopogon martinii*)
Lemongrass (*Cymbopogon citratus/flexuosus*)
Grapefruit (*Citrus paradisi*)

STAGE THREE ESSENTIAL OILS FOR ACNE
Violet leaf (*Viola odorata*)
Juniper berry (*Juniperus communis*)
Lemon (*Citrus limon*)
Carrot seed (*Daucus carota*)
Lavender (*Lavandula angustifolia*)
Orange, sweet (*Citrus sinensis*)
Geranium (*Pelargonium graveolens*)
Petitgrain (*Citrus aurantium*)
Bergamot FCF (*Citrus bergamia*)

STAGE FOUR ESSENTIAL OILS FOR ACNE — MAINTENANCE
Ylang ylang (*Cananga odorata*)
Cypress (*Cupressus sempervirens*)
Geranium (*Pelargonium graveolens*)

Cedarwood atlas (*Cedrus atlantica*)
Patchouli (*Pogostemon cablin*)
Palmarosa (*Cymbopogon martinii*)
Chamomile roman (*Anthemis nobilis*)
Lavender (*Lavandula angustifolia*)

Stage One

Stage One aims to promote healing and reduce inflammation. Start the rebalancing process by using this skin care regime over a 14-day period. It will take patience and more time for the acne to clear and the skin to completely rebalance.

Use a gentle cleansing routine — with organic cleansing products, or make your own — making sure that every scrap of cleanser is removed by a tonic or water. In the final rinse water put 1 teaspoon (5 mL) of thyme hydrolat or cider vinegar, then pat the skin dry. During the day, wear a small amount of the following face oil. Try to avoid wearing any concealer or foundation, if at all possible.

Stage One: Day Treatment

Geranium	4 drops
Palmarosa	10 drops
Chamomile german	8 drops
Lavender	8 drops

Blend the essential oils together, then dilute 2–3 drops in each teaspoon (5 mL) of jojoba oil and 3 drops of macerated carrot root oil. Apply a small amount to damp skin by pressing the oil into the face and neck, avoiding the eye area. Leave the oil to soak into the skin for a few minutes if you have time and then dab off the excess oil with a tissue. The macerated carrot oil is orange and can give the skin a healthy look.

In the evening, after gently cleansing, rinsing, and toning the face, apply 5 drops of Foundation Night Oil over the whole of the affected area. (This foundation oil will be used throughout the three stages of the treatment program).

Then apply a small amount of Stage One: Night Treatment. Leave to soak into the skin, then dab off any excess oil before going to sleep. Don't use any other nighttime skin care cream, lotion, or potion.

Foundation Night Oil

Carrot macerated oil	30 drops
Borage seed oil	30 drops
Chamomile german essential oil	10 drops

Blend the oils together, and use 5 drops each evening. Apply by gently pressing into the skin rather than rubbing. Leave for a few minutes, then apply the appropriate night treatment:

Stage One: Night Treatment

Palmarosa	10 drops
Chamomile roman	5 drops
Lavender	10 drops
Frankincense	5 drops

Blend the essential oils together, then dilute 3 drops in each teaspoon (5 mL) of jojoba oil. Apply by pressing into the skin over the top of the Foundation Night Oil shortly before going to bed, and remove any excess before sleeping by gently pressing a tissue to the face.

During these 14 days get into the fresh air as much as possible. Eat only "live" food — fresh vegetables, fruit in moderation, grains, pulses, carbohydrates, and fish. Drink herbal teas and plenty of mineral water. Increase your intake of vitamins C and B and zinc with a supplement that contains all three. Use no face masks or steam treatments during this time.

Stage Two

Stage Two continues with the rebalancing program. Cleanse as in Stage One, except this time make up a bottle that contains the following ingredients and use 1 teaspoon in the final rinse, patting dry afterward:

Cider vinegar	3½ fl. oz. (100 mL)
Lavender	20 drops
Eucalyptus radiata	20 drops

STAGE TWO: DAY TREATMENT

Eucalyptus radiata	5 drops
Clary sage	5 drops
Thyme linalol	5 drops
Lavender	15 drops
Carrot seed oil	5 drops

Blend the essential oils together, then dilute 1 or 2 drops in each teaspoon (5 mL) of jojoba oil and 3 drops of macerated carrot root oil. Apply a small amount to damp skin by pressing the oil into the face and neck, avoiding the eye area. Leave the oil to soak into the skin for a few minutes if you have the time, and then dab off the excess oil with a tissue.

STAGE TWO: NIGHT TREATMENT

Juniper berry	20 drops
Bergamot FCF	10 drops
Lavender	5 drops
Geranium	5 drops
Eucalyptus radiata	10 drops

Blend the essential oils together, then dilute 4 drops to each teaspoon (5 mL) of jojoba oil to which 5 drops of evening primrose seed oil have been added. Before using this oil, apply 5 drops of the Foundation Night Oil by gently pressing it into the skin rather than rubbing. Leave for a few minutes before then applying the Stage Two: Night Treatment, which is gently pressed into the skin over the top of the Foundation Night Oil shortly before going to bed. Before sleep, press a tissue over the face to remove any excess oil.

Follow the dietary advice outlined in Stage One and continue Stage Two treatment for 14 days.

Stage Three

Stage Three is the last stage. Hopefully, by now your skin has responded and may look so much better you might decide not to continue the treatment. But if you want to see further improvements, continue you must for another 14 days. Use the cleansing rinse outlined in Stage Two, both morning and night, pat the face dry, and use the relevant day or night treatments below.

STAGE THREE: DAY TREATMENT

Geranium	10 drops
Juniper berry	4 drops
Lavender	6 drops
Cypress	6 drops

Blend the essential oils together, then dilute 2 drops in each teaspoon (5 mL) of jojoba oil and 3 drops of macerated carrot root oil. Apply a small amount to damp skin by pressing the oil into the face and neck, avoiding the eye area. Leave the oil to soak into the skin for a few minutes if you have the time, and then dab off the excess oil with a tissue.

STAGE THREE: NIGHT TREATMENT

Petitgrain	10 drops
Bergamot FCF	5 drops
Ylang ylang	4 drops
Frankincense	5 drops
Patchouli	2 drops

Blend the essential oils together, then dilute 3 drops in each teaspoon (5 mL) of jojoba oil to which 5 drops of rosehip seed oil have been added. Before using this oil, apply 5 drops of the Foundation Night Oil by gently pressing it into the skin rather than rubbing. Leave for a few minutes before then applying the Stage Three: Night Treatment, which is gently pressed into the skin over the top of the Foundation Night Oil shortly before going to bed. Before sleep, press a tissue over the face to remove any excess oil.

When the six weeks are up, continue to use the essential oils either from the maintenance lists or, depending on how your skin feels, from the Stage One through Stage Three lists. Use only organic 100% pure soaps, and avoid harsh acne preparations.

ROSACEA

Rosacea is often mistaken for acne vulgaris, as in some respects it's very similar. Rosacea is a permanent inflammatory skin condition, most usually occurring over the cheeks and nose area, that in some cases may be caused by a *Demodex* mite. This condition seldom affects anyone under 30 years of age, and it can be distressing when it develops.

The affected areas appear flushed and can look lumpy and uneven, although generally any spots (pustules) do not produce pus unless infected. The treatment is similar to that for acne, except that the essential oils used are different. Follow the dietary and vitamin advice in the **Acne** section on page 375, and carry out the cleansing and rinsing routine given there. Treatment comes in two stages, each of 14 days' duration.

CARRIER OILS FOR ROSACEA
Jojoba (*Simmondsia chinensis*)
Apricot kernel (*Prunus armeniaca*)
Calendula, macerated (*Calendula officinalis*)
Gotu kola (*Centella asiatica*)
Tamanu (*Calophyllum inophyllum*)
Hazelnut (*Corylus avellana*)

STAGE ONE ESSENTIAL OILS FOR ROSACEA
Chamomile german (*Matricaria recutita*)
Lavender (*Lavandula angustifolia*)
Chamomile roman (*Anthemis nobilis*)
Geranium (*Pelargonium graveolens*)
Bergamot FCF (*Citrus bergamia*)
Rosemary (*Rosmarinus officinalis*)

Manuka (*Leptospermum scoparium*)
Ho wood (*Cinnamomum camphora ct. linalool*)
Patchouli (*Pogostemon cablin*)
Immortelle (*Helichrysum italicum*)

STAGE TWO ESSENTIAL OILS FOR ROSACEA
Cypress (*Cupressus sempervirens*)
Geranium (*Pelargonium graveolens*)
Eucalyptus radiata (*Eucalyptus radiata*)
Juniper berry (*Juniperus communis*)
Chamomile german (*Matricaria recutita*)
Manuka (*Leptospermum scoparium*)
Chamomile roman (*Anthemis nobilis*)
Ho wood (*Cinnamomum camphora ct. linalool*)

Follow the instructions for acne, Stage One, but using the following formulas. Use only a small amount of oil on the skin, making sure the oil has been well absorbed. There is no sun protective factor in the Day Treatment that follows.

STAGE ONE: DAY TREATMENT
Chamomile german	15 drops
Manuka	10 drops

Blend the essential oils together, then dilute by adding 2 drops to 1 teaspoon (5 mL) of jojoba oil.

STAGE ONE: NIGHT TREATMENT
Chamomile german	5 drops
Ho wood	5 drops
Lavender	10 drops

Blend the essential oils together, then dilute by mixing 2–3 drops in 1 teaspoon (5 mL) of tamanu oil.

After 14 days, follow the instructions for acne, Stage Two, using the following formulas. There is no sun protective factor in the Day Treatment.

STAGE TWO: DAY TREATMENT
Chamomile roman	5 drops
Geranium	5 drops
Patchouli	5 drops

Blend the essential oils together, then dilute 1–3 drops in 1 teaspoon (5 mL) of argan oil.

STAGE TWO: NIGHT TREATMENT

Cypress	5 drops
Eucalyptus radiata	15 drops
Chamomile roman	5 drops

Blend the essential oils together, then dilute 1–3 drops in 1 teaspoon (5 mL) of tamanu oil.

The Neck

The neck is one of the first parts of the body to show its age, but thankfully for many people this area responds well to essential oil treatments — cleansing and oiling especially. The shape of the neck is very much an inherited feature, and in this some are luckier than others. If your mother or grandmother had a neck that sagged over time, you can be pretty sure that yours will benefit from a little forward planning in terms of care and attention.

ESSENTIAL OILS FOR USE IN NECK CARE

Rose otto (*Rosa damascena*)
Lemon (*Citrus limon*)
Palmarosa (*Cymbopogon martinii*)
Patchouli (*Pogostemon cablin*)
Geranium (*Pelargonium graveolens*)
Cedarwood atlas (*Cedrus atlantica*)
Clary sage (*Salvia sclarea*)
Petitgrain (*Citrus aurantium*)
Orange, sweet (*Citrus sinensis*)
Vetiver (*Vetiveria zizanoides*)

CARRIER OILS

Jojoba (*Simmondsia chinensis*)
Avocado (*Persea americana*)
Camellia seed (*Camellia japonica*)
Rice bran (*Oryza sativa*)
Apricot kernel (*Prunus armeniaca*)
Argan (*Argania spinosa*)

ADDITIONS TO CARRIER OILS

Borage seed (*Borago officinalis*)
Evening primrose seed (*Oenothera biennis*)
Rosehip seed (*Rosa rubiginosa*)
Red raspberry seed (*Rubus idaeus*)

The neck area is delicate and should be cleansed with the same quality of preparation that you use on your face. If you wish, you can simply add 1 drop of one of the above essential oils to each tablespoon (15 mL) of your usual cleansing cream, or make your own cleansing oil. Each night apply a small amount of the following oil, leave it for a few minutes, and then dab off the excess with a tissue:

NECK NIGHT OIL

Petitgrain	6 drops
Orange, sweet	3 drops
Carrot seed	5 drops
Palmarosa	5 drops
Lemon	5 drops

Blend the essential oils together, then dilute in the following carrier oil:

Almond oil, sweet	1 tablespoon (15 mL)
*Rosehip seed oil	1 tablespoon (15 mL)

*Rosehip seed oil is deep orange and may stain clothing.

NECK SPECIAL TREATMENT BLEND

Jasmine	5 drops
Lemon	5 drops
Carrot seed	20 drops

For special treatments, blend the essential oils above and dilute 4 drops in 1 teaspoon (5 mL) of evening primrose seed oil, every two weeks or as and when needed. Massage well into the skin and leave it there for at least 10 minutes, rather like using a neck mask, before wiping off any excess.

The Eyes

The eye area is extremely sensitive and, for such a small area, encounters many problems, including puffy bags under the eyes, darkened rings around the eyes, wrinkles at the outer edges of the eyes, and so forth. As a general rule, essential oils are kept well away from the eyes, and the water-based products — variously called hydrolats, hydrosols, floral waters, or herbal distillates — are always better options. There are several ways to make eye pads to relieve puffy and tired eyes.

Eye pads can be made using cotton wool pads and a hydrolat made from the blue cornflower (*Centaurea cyanus*). Cornflower is not a by-product of essential oil distillation and is produced as a hydrolat (floral water or distillate) because it's an extremely valuable product. It has long been used in Europe, not only in general facial skin care but also to soothe tired eyes or reduce bags under the eyes. Combine it with chamomile roman (*Anthemis nobilis*) hydrolat for soothing computer-stressed eyes. Soak cotton wool pads in cornflower hydrolat on its own, or in a blend of cornflower and chamomile hydrolats. Keep the pads in a sealed box in the fridge, where they will keep up to two weeks.

Alternatively, make up the following infusion:

Eye Pads for Puffy Eyes

Cornflower hydrolat	1 tablespoon (15 mL)
Witch hazel	1 tablespoon (15 mL)
Chamomile german essential oil	1 drop
Cypress essential oil	1 drop

Combine all the ingredients and mix together well. Then pour through an unbleached paper coffee filter to remove any essential oil globules, bottle, and place in the fridge. Put a couple of cotton pads onto a saucer or plate, pour some of the filtered mixture over them, and place over the puffy areas, being sure to close your eyes.

Tired eyes can also benefit from cold, used green tea bags used as eye pads. Or make a cup of green tea and keep it in the fridge to use on eye pads as needed. It should keep for about a week.

The following essential oil skin care chart is a guide to the essential oils that could be used in blends for skin care. Each individual essential oil could complement other essential oils listed in the same column. It is always advisable when creating your own personal blends of essential oils for facial skin care to use minimal amounts, between 0.5% and 1% of the whole product.

TABLE 11. ESSENTIAL OILS FOR FACIAL SKIN CARE

ESSENTIAL OIL	SKIN TYPE					
	Balanced/ Normal	Aging	Dry	Oily	Sensitive	Blemished
Bergamot				★		★
Cardamom	★	★		★		★
Carrot seed	★	★	★	★		
Chamomile german	★	★	★	★	★	★
Chamomile roman	★	★	★	★	★	★
Cistus	★	★				

ESSENTIAL OIL	SKIP TYPE					
	Balanced/ Normal	Aging	Dry	Oily	Sensitive	Blemished
Clary sage		★	★			★
Coriander seed		★				★
Cypress	★			★		★
Frankincense	★	★	★	★		
Geranium	★	★	★	★	★	
Ho wood	★	★	★			★
Immortelle		★				★
Jasmine	★	★		★		
Juniper berry		★		★		★
Lavender	★	★	★	★	★	★
Lemon	★			★		★
Lemongrass	★					★
Magnolia flower	★	★				
Mandarin	★			★		
Manuka	★			★		★
Marjoram, sweet		★		★		★
Mastic		★				
Neroli	★	★	★			★
Niaouli	★	★		★		★
Orange, sweet		★		★		★
Palmarosa	★	★	★	★		★
Patchouli		★		★		★
Petitgrain	★	★		★		
Rosemary		★		★		★
Rose otto	★	★	★			
Rosewood	★	★	★			
Sandalwood	★	★	★			
Spikenard	★	★				★
Tea tree						★
Thyme linalol				★		★
Ylang ylang		★		★		

Hydrolats and Beauty

Hydrolats are extremely valuable products for beauty purposes, used either on their own as tonics, or in compresses, or incorporated into masks. Hydrolats are gentle, which makes them particularly useful for hypersensitive skin. They can be effective in treatments for all skin types and for a variety of conditions, as outlined in tables 12–14. See the hydrolat section in chapter 19, "Carrier Oils and Hydrolats," for further information.

TABLE 12. HYDROLATS FOR FACIAL SKIN CARE

HYDROLAT	SKIN TYPE						
	Most Types	Normal	Sensitive	Dry	Oily	Aging	Sluggish
Angelica seed		★			★		★
Bay laurel					★		★
Calendula	★	★	★	★	★		★
Carrot seed		★				★	
Cedarwood					★		
Chamomile german	★	★	★	★		★	
Chamomile roman	★	★	★	★		★	
Clary sage		★			★	★	★
Eucalyptus					★		★
Fennel, sweet		★		★		★	
Geranium	★	★		★		★	
Immortelle						★	
Lavender	★	★	★	★	★	★	
Lemon verbena	★	★			★		
Linden blossom			★	★			
Melissa	★	★		★	★	★	★
Myrtle					★		★
Neroli	★	★	★			★	★
Peppermint					★		★
Rose	★	★	★	★		★	
Rosemary					★	★	★
Sage				★		★	
Thyme					★		★
Yarrow		★			★		

TABLE 13. HYDROLATS AND THEIR USES IN SKIN CARE

HYDROLAT	APPLICATION IN SKIN CARE							
	Tonic	Astringent	Stimulant	Refreshing	Regenerative	Balancing	Soothing	Softening
Angelica seed						★		★
Bay laurel		★	★					
Calendula							★	
Carrot seed				★	★			
Cedarwood		★				★		
Chamomile german					★	★	★	
Chamomile roman					★	★	★	
Clary sage			★		★	★		
Eucalyptus		★		★			★	
Fennel, sweet	★			★				★
Geranium	★				★	★		
Immortelle	★				★			
Lavender				★	★	★	★	★
Lemon verbena		★						
Linden blossom						★	★	
Melissa	★			★	★			★
Myrtle	★				★		★	
Neroli		★		★	★	★	★	
Peppermint	★		★	★			★	
Rose	★			★	★	★		★
Rosemary	★		★	★	★			
Sage					★	★		★
Thyme				★		★		
Yarrow				★	★		★	★

TABLE 14. HYDROLATS IN THE TREATMENT OF SKIN CONDITIONS

HYDROLAT	SKIN CONDITION					
	Acne & Spots	Skin Infection	Inflammation	Eczema & Psoriasis	Scars	Sore Eyes (pads on closed eyes only)
Angelica seed	★					
Calendula	★		★	★		★
Carrot seed	★				★	
Cedarwood	★	★				
Chamomile german	★	★	★	★	★	★
Chamomile roman	★		★	★	★	★
Clary sage	★	★				★
Eucalyptus	★	★				
Fennel, sweet						★
Geranium					★	★
Immortelle	★	★			★	
Laurel	★	★				
Lavender	★		★	★	★	★
Lemon verbena						★
Linden blossom			★			
Melissa	★	★				
Myrtle		★				★
Neroli					★	★
Peppermint			★		★	
Rose					★	★
Rosemary	★	★				
Sage					★	
Thyme	★	★				
Yarrow	★		★	★	★	

Hair Care

When people describe someone, they often start with the hair — "She was the one with the blond bob," or "the natural black curls," or "the long red hair." Almost immediately, we know who they're talking about. We know too that when someone describes us, they'll start with the hair, and most people are very sensitive about the condition of their hair. Even people with good hair can find something to complain about. Altogether, the hair comes in for a lot of focus.

You only have to look at the ingredient list on product packaging to know that a lot of different chemicals are being put on hair, day in and day out, not to mention year in and year out. The end result can be hair that has lost its natural sheen or is damaged in some way. The use of hair straighteners and extensions has led to a whole new set of problems.

Many of the essential oil suggestions in this section can be added to a fragrance-free shampoo made of 100% natural ingredients. Alternatively, make a soapwort shampoo, as outlined here, and use that as your base. Natural hair care also involves fabulous plant oils that nourish and condition.

SHAMPOOS

The scalp is absorbent, so it's always best to use organic, naturally derived shampoos. Many of the simple organic shampoo bases available can be mixed with essential oils or therapeutic plant oils. It's also possible to make a very simple base shampoo yourself that uses only natural ingredients; a recipe for one follows. It will clean the hair, and your choice of essential oils and herbals can be added to it, but it will not lather as impressively as a commercial shampoo with a detergent base. For those who find they have an irritated or dry scalp precisely because of the detergents in shampoos, the soapwort solution often works well and may alleviate the problem.

Whatever kind of hair you have, or want to achieve, the soapwort shampoo or other natural, organic, fragrance-free shampoo can be supplemented with therapeutic plant oils, essential oils, or herbal extracts, as outlined in the various hair condition sections that follow. While it's not as convenient as using a store-bought product, it can be fun to add your own individual touch to a base and find the perfect solution to any hair issue.

Soapwort Shampoo Base

Soapwort root is so named because it's the raw material that was originally used to make soaps and other personal cleaning products. The roots can be purchased either in their natural form and crushed, or in prepared powdered form. Alternatively, the plant can be grown in the garden and harvested for later use.

| Soapwort root | ½ ounce |
| Spring water | 2 pints (950 mL) |

Boil the water, pour it over the soapwort in a bowl, and mix well. Leave it to infuse for at least an hour, then filter it through a piece of fine muslin, an unbleached paper coffee filter, or a fine strainer, then bottle. When you use the soapwort base, use more than you would of commercial shampoo — 2 tablespoons (30 mL) at least. The lather will not be what you're used to with commercial products, but it still does the job of cleaning the hair.

RINSES

Some of the nicest final rinses to use after shampooing are those you've made yourself. They can be designed for your specific needs and aims, and you'll know exactly what's in them. A simple rinse can be made by using a favorite hydrolat, which can match the essential oil(s) used in other hair care steps. For example, if you use a final hair oil that contains rosemary, lemon, and lavender, you could make a post-shampoo hair rinse by mixing the hydrolats of rosemary, lemon, and lavender together — diluted in a good spring water using the proportions of 20% hydrolat to 80% water.

Alternatively, you could make and bottle a blend of essential oils, then add 2 drops of the blend to 1 pint (475 mL) of boiling water, cover, and leave to stand until cool. Either strain the mixture through an unbleached paper coffee filter, or shake the mixture well before using as a rinse.

Adding apple cider vinegar to the hair rinse can be revitalizing while also helping to maintain the natural pH level of the skin and reduce styling product buildup. Vinegar has long been known to increase the shine of hair; it's thought that the astringent effect smooths the cuticle that surrounds each hair shaft. Add 2 drops of essential oil of your choice to 1 teaspoon (5 mL) of organic apple cider vinegar, and add this to your final rinse water.

Choose which essential oils to use according to your hair type and the suggestions that follow within each section. If you want to achieve a lovely aroma, try the flower essential oils, such as ylang ylang. Keep in mind that some of the really fabulous floral essential oils, like jasmine, are absolutes and have a thicker consistency and are not easily incorporated into final rinses.

HAIR OILS

Certain therapeutic plant oils are terrific for nourishing, conditioning, and giving hair a beautiful, luxurious effect. Some are applied directly on the hair itself, while others are more of a scalp treatment — to encourage growth or to address a particular problem such as dandruff, eczema, or psoriasis. While the lighter oils are more suited to use in hair applications, some oils and plant butters have a heavier texture and are more suited to being used as overnight scalp treatments.

With oils that are applied directly on the hair itself only a small amount is needed. Rub just a drop or two between your fingers, and run the fingers through the hair to give it shine, smoothness, volume, and also in some cases, perfume.

Plant Oils for Hair Care

Abyssinian seed (*Crambe abyssinica*): Useful for very curly hair, and for those who want shiny, smooth hair

Almond, sweet (*Prunus amygdalus var. dulcis*): Good to include in general conditioning oils

Argan (*Argania spinosa*): Can be used on all hair types to protect, nourish, and condition the hair

Avocado (*Persea americana*): A nourishing, moisturizing, and conditioning oil suitable for all hair and scalp types, including dry and undernourished hair caused by ill health or stress

Baobab (*Adansonia digitata*): Protects sun damaged hair and overprocessed hair, helping to ward off further damage while nourishing the scalp

Black cumin seed (*Nigella sativa*): Useful for inflamed and irritating skin conditions

Camelina (*Camelina sativa*): Particularly useful for overprocessed hair

Camellia seed (*Camellia japonica*): A balancing oil that conditions the scalp and helps promote hair growth

Coconut (*Cocos nucifera*): Shines and strengthens hair, helps tame frizzy and unmanageable hair, and conditions the scalp

Hemp seed (*Cannabis sativa*): Useful for damaged or overprocessed hair and promotes a healthy scalp condition

Jojoba (*Simmondsia chinensis*): A conditioning and balancing oil good for all scalps, including those that are itchy or inflamed

Meadowfoam (*Limnanthes alba*): Can give shine, condition, and smoothness to the hair, and helps prevent moisture loss

Moringa (*Moringa oleifera*): A balancing and conditioning oil that strengthens hair and gives it a shiny gloss

Peach kernel (*Prunus persica*): Beneficial for most hair types, so can be included in any conditioning oil

Rice bran (*Oryza sativa*): A nourishing and strengthening oil with sun protective properties; use for sun damaged and overprocessed hair

Sesame (*Sesamum indicum*): Too heavy for some hair types, particularly fine hair, but has some sun protective properties and is useful in scalp treatments

Shea butter (*Butyrospermum parkii*): Suitable for dry, overprocessed, or sun-damaged hair and irritated scalps — solid product; has to be melted

Tamanu (*Calophyllum inophyllum*): Strengthens and conditions the hair and can be used for dry, flaky, sore, and irritated scalps

Ungurahui (pataua) (*Oenocarpus bataua*): Absorbs well, softens and conditions hair, and helps to nourish and restore balance to both distressed and undistressed scalps

Other Helpful Oil Additions

Borage seed (*Borago officinalis*): Restores balance, bringing vitality to the hair, and conditions both hair and scalp

Calendula, macerated (*Calendula officinalis*): Soothes and calms irritated scalps; this oil is deep orange in color and should be avoided for use on light-colored hair

Cranberry seed (*Vaccinium macrocarpon*): Can help soothe, nourish, and balance a scalp irritated by stress conditions

Evening primrose seed (*Oenothera biennis*): Helps soothe hair distressed by overprocessing and hair straightening

Neem (*Azadirachta indica*): Can help soothe scalp disorders such as dandruff, eczema, and psoriasis; also is an antiparasitic oil

Olive squalane (*Olea europaea*): For dry, irritated, or damaged scalps; helps reduce inflammation and scaly scalp

BASIC HAIR OIL BLEND

This blend provides a good basic all-purpose hair oil to condition and strengthen the hair.

Argan oil	4 teaspoons (20 mL)
Camellia seed oil	1 tablespoon (15 mL)
Meadowfoam oil	1 teaspoon (5 mL)
Rice bran oil	4 teaspoons (20 mL)
Jojoba oil	2 tablespoons (30 mL)

Blend the oils together, following the order in which they're listed. The hair oil can be used simply as it is, or essential oils can be added. If there's a scalp disorder such as psoriasis or eczema, add 2 teaspoons (10 mL) of tamanu oil to the blend above. Use a small amount — a few drops for each application.

Which essential oils you add to any hair oil will determine whether it will become a soothing, stimulating, or revitalizing hair oil.

SOOTHING HAIR OIL — ESSENTIAL OILS

Clary sage (*Salvia sclarea*)
Marjoram, sweet (*Origanum majorana*)
Chamomile roman (*Anthemis nobilis*)
Lavender (*Lavandula angustifolia*)
Ho wood (*Cinnamomum camphora ct. linalool*)
Rosewood (*Aniba rosaeodora*)
Bergamot (*Citrus bergamia*)
Petitgrain (*Citrus aurantium*)

Vetiver (*Vetiveria zizanoides*)
Frankincense (*Boswellia carterii*)
Geranium (*Pelargonium graveolens*)
Rose otto (*Rosa damascena*)
Neroli (*Citrus aurantium*)
Jasmine (*Jasminum grandiflorum/officinale*)
Cedarwood atlas (*Cedrus atlantica*)
Sandalwood (*Santalum album*)

Soothing Hair Oil Blend

Clary sage	2 drops
Lavender	6 drops
Frankincense	1 drop
Petitgrain	5 drops
Chamomile roman	1 drop
Bergamot	2 drops

Blend the essential oils together, then add 1 drop of the blend to each teaspoon (5 mL) of hair oil.

Stimulating Hair Oil — Essential Oils

Ginger (*Zingiber officinale*)
Rosemary (*Rosmarinus officinalis*)
Black pepper (*Piper nigrum*)
Palmarosa (*Cymbopogon martinii*)
Lemongrass (*Cymbopogon citratus/flexuosus*)
Eucalyptus radiata (*Eucalyptus radiata*)
Thyme linalol (*Thymus vulgaris ct. linalool*)
Oregano (*Origanum vulgare*)
Basil linalol (*Ocimum basilicum ct. linalool*)
Peppermint (*Mentha piperita*)
Spearmint (*Mentha spicata*)
Mastic (*Pistacia lentiscus*)

Stimulating Hair Oil Blend

Peppermint	1 drop
Ginger	2 drops
Palmarosa	3 drops
Eucalyptus radiata	1 drop
Rosemary	2 drops

Blend the essential oils together, then add 1 drop of the blend to each teaspoon (5 mL) of hair oil.

Revitalizing Hair Oil — Essential Oils

Rosemary (*Rosmarinus officinalis*)
Ginger (*Zingiber officinale*)
Cardamom (*Elettaria cardamomum*)
Basil linalol (*Ocimum basilicum ct. linalool*)
Geranium (*Pelargonium graveolens*)
Cypress (*Cupressus sempervirens*)
Clove bud (*Syzygium aromaticum*)
Bay laurel (*Laurus nobilis*)
Immortelle (*Helichrysum italicum*)
Grapefruit (*Citrus paradisi*)

Stimulating Hair Oil Blend

Basil linalol	4 drops
Cardamom	2 drops
Geranium	5 drops
Bay laurel	1 drop
Grapefruit	4 drops

Blend the essential oils together, then add 1 drop of the blend to each teaspoon (5 mL) of hair oil.

NORMAL HAIR

Even for those lucky enough to have a good head of healthy hair, it sometimes becomes troublesome. Hair can be affected by stress or emotional strain, medications or antibiotics, chlorine in swimming pools, or simply too much sea, sun, and fun. Whatever the reason, normal hair can become dry or greasy or can develop dandruff. But using gentle, nature-based shampoos and treatments will keep the hair in good condition, or if it's been depleted, bring it back to its glory.

Essential Oils for Normal Hair

Lavender (*Lavandula angustifolia*)
Cedarwood atlas (*Cedrus atlantica*)
Lemon (*Citrus limon*)
Orange, sweet (*Citrus sinensis*)
Geranium (*Pelargonium graveolens*)

Eucalyptus lemon (*Eucalyptus citriodora*)
Carrot seed (*Daucus carota*)
Rosemary (*Rosmarinus officinalis*)

PLANT OILS FOR NORMAL HAIR
Meadowfoam (*Limnanthes alba*)
Camellia seed (*Camellia japonica*)
Coconut (*Cocos nucifera*)
Argan (*Argania spinosa*)
Almond, sweet (*Prunus amygdalus var. dulcis*)
Evening primrose seed (*Oenothera biennis*)
Peach kernel (*Prunus persica*)
Borage seed (*Borago officinalis*)

Essential Oil Shampoo Blends for Normal Hair

STIMULATING
Rosemary   2 drops
Lemon   2 drops
Eucalyptus lemon   3 drops
Blend the essential oils together, then add to 3½ fl. oz. (100 mL) of a natural, fragrance-free shampoo.

MOISTURIZING
Geranium essential oil   3 drops
Carrot seed essential oil   2 drops
Lemon essential oil   2 drops
Borage seed oil   4 drops
Blend all the ingredients together, then add to 3½ fl. oz. (100 mL) of a natural, fragrance-free shampoo.

CONDITIONING TREATMENT FOR NORMAL HAIR
Lecithin (liquid)   1 teaspoon (5 mL)
Meadowfoam oil   1 tablespoon (15 mL)
Jojoba oil   2 teaspoons (10 mL)
Borage seed oil   3 drops
Then add the essential oil:
Geranium   2 drops
Sandalwood   2 drops

Using the bain-marie or double boiler method, over a low heat, blend all the ingredients until a smooth mixture is obtained. Leave the mixture to cool before applying. Apply a small amount of the conditioner all over the hair, and leave for at least 10 minutes before shampooing. These quantities are enough for several treatments.

VINEGAR RINSE FOR NORMAL HAIR
Water   5 teaspoons (25 mL)
Cider vinegar   2 teaspoons (10 mL)
*Orange, sweet, or
   lemon essential oil   3 drops
Generally orange for dark hair, lemon for blond hair.
   Mix the cider vinegar and essential oil together, then add to the water. Use 1 teaspoon (5 mL) in the final water rinse. These quantities are enough for several treatments.

DRY HAIR

When sebum, the protective lubricant provided by the sebaceous glands, is not being produced in sufficient quantity to keep the hair in good condition, dry hair can be the result. It becomes easily tangled, split, broken, and generally damaged. The hair then becomes more vulnerable if exposed to chlorine in swimming pools, chemicals in coloring or styling products, or pressure and stress through, for example, repetitive use of straightening or heating tools or the wearing of hair extensions. Overexposure to the sun and sea can exacerbate the problem and lead to brittle, unmanageable hair.

ESSENTIAL OILS FOR DRY HAIR
Lavender (*Lavandula angustifolia*)
Frankincense (*Boswellia carterii*)
Carrot seed (*Daucus carota*)
Palmarosa (*Cymbopogon martinii*)
Rosemary (*Rosmarinus officinalis*)

Sandalwood (*Santalum album*)
Geranium (*Pelargonium graveolens*)

PLANT OILS FOR DRY HAIR
Jojoba (*Simmondsia chinensis*)
Almond, sweet (*Prunus amygdalus var. dulcis*)
Evening primrose seed (*Oenothera biennis*)
Sunflower (*Helianthus annuus*)
Avocado (*Persea americana*)
Borage seed (*Borago officinalis*)
. Shea butter (*Butyrospermum parkii*)
Argan (*Argania spinosa*)
Tamanu (*Calophyllum inophyllum*)
Camellia seed (*Camellia japonica*)

Essential Oil Shampoo Blends for Dry Hair

STIMULATING
Almond oil, sweet	1 teaspoon (5 mL)
Rosemary essential oil	2 drops
Geranium essential oil	2 drops
Frankincense essential oil	3 drops

Blend all the ingredients together, then add to 3½ fl. oz. (100 mL) of a natural, fragrance-free shampoo.

MOISTURIZING
Meadowfoam oil	2 teaspoons (10 mL)
Jojoba oil	5 drops
Carrot seed essential oil	5 drops
Sandalwood essential oil	2 drops
Lavender essential oil	2 drops

Blend all the ingredients together, then add to 3½ fl. oz. (100 mL) of a natural, fragrance-free shampoo.

CONDITIONING TREATMENT FOR DRY HAIR
Lecithin (liquid)	1 teaspoon (5 mL)
Avocado oil	1 teaspoon (5 mL)
Hemp seed oil	1 tablespoon (15 mL)
Meadowfoam oil	1 tablespoon (15 mL)

Borage seed oil (or evening primrose seed oil)	2 drops
Geranium essential oil	3 drops

Using the bain-marie or double boiler method, over a low heat blend all the ingredients until a smooth mixture is obtained. Leave the mixture to cool before applying. Apply a small amount, enough to cover the hair and scalp, leave for 10 minutes, and then shampoo off. These quantities are enough for several treatments.

CONDITIONING TREATMENT FOR SUN-DAMAGED OR BLEACHED HAIR
Lecithin (liquid)	2 tablespoons (30 mL)
Jojoba oil	2 teaspoons (10 mL)
Evening primrose seed oil	1 teaspoon (5 mL)
Camellia seed oil	1 teaspoon (5 mL)
Coconut oil	2 teaspoons (10 mL)
Argan oil	1 teaspoon (5 mL)
Lemon juice	1 teaspoon (5 mL)
Ho wood essential oil	5 drops

Using the bain-marie or double boiler method, over a low heat blend all the ingredients together until a smooth mixture is obtained. Apply a small amount over the hair while the oil is still warm, but not hot. Rub in well, then cover the hair with a plastic bag. Leave for at least 10 minutes, then shampoo off. These quantities are enough for several treatments. Finish off with the vinegar rinse that follows, leaving a small amount on the hair.

Vinegar Rinse for Dry Hair
Add 1 drop of sandalwood or ho wood essential oil to 1 teaspoon (5 mL) of cider vinegar and mix together well. Add to a cup of boiled water, and then add this to a bowl of water you will be using as your final rinse. Rinse your hair thoroughly in this water, repeatedly pouring over those parts of the hair not immersed in the bowl.

OILY HAIR

Under the skin, adjacent to the hair follicles, lie the sebaceous glands. These glands produce the sebum that moisturizes the hair, but if overproductive, they can cause oiliness. Despite all efforts to deal with it, oily hair can still look unwashed, have a lanky appearance, and develop dandruff. The underlying cause may be health related, but often the impetus to wash the hair frequently, using harsh shampoos, just exacerbates the problem. The cycle can seem an endless, and a pointless, chore.

ESSENTIAL OILS FOR OILY HAIR
Rosemary (*Rosmarinus officinalis*)
Lime (*Citrus aurantifolia*)
Lavender (*Lavandula angustifolia*)
Petitgrain (*Citrus aurantium*)
Thyme linalol (*Thymus vulgaris ct. linalool*)
Grapefruit (*Citrus paradisi*)
Cypress (*Cupressus sempervirens*)
Basil linalol (*Ocimum basilicum ct. linalool*)
Lemon (*Citrus limon*)
Geranium (*Pelargonium graveolens*)
Eucalyptus lemon (*Eucalyptus citriodora*)
Juniper berry (*Juniperus communis*)
Bergamot (*Citrus bergamia*)
Cedarwood atlas (*Cedrus atlantica*)

PLANT OILS FOR OILY HAIR
Evening primrose seed (*Oenothera biennis*)
Borage seed (*Borago officinalis*)
Peach kernel (*Prunus persica*)
Almond, sweet (*Prunus amygdalus var. dulcis*)
Coconut (*Cocos nucifera*)
Hemp seed (*Cannabis sativa*)
Rice bran (*Oryza sativa*)
Sunflower (*Helianthus annuus*)

Essential Oil Shampoo Blends for Oily Hair

STIMULATING

Rosemary	3 drops
Basil linalol	1 drop
Grapefruit	3 drops
Cypress	1 drop

Blend the essential oils together, then add to 3½ fl. oz. (100 mL) of a natural, fragrance-free shampoo.

FOR MORE SHINE

Spearmint essential oil	2 drops
Lavender essential oil	2 drops
Rosemary essential oil	3 drops
Meadowfoam oil	3 teaspoons (15 mL)

Blend all the ingredients together, then add to 3½ fl. oz. (100 mL) of a natural, fragrance-free shampoo.

DRY SHAMPOO FOR OILY HAIR
The following ingredients should be thoroughly mixed together, and although this can be done by hand it's better to use a blender. Add the essential oils drop by drop through the hole in the top, with the lid on tight…you don't want to be giving the entire kitchen a dry shampoo!

Cornstarch	1 oz. (30 g)
Rosemary essential oil	2 drops
*Orange, sweet, or lemon essential oil	1 drop

Generally, orange for dark hair, lemon for blond hair.

Use about ¼ teaspoon on a real bristle brush and brush through the underside of the hair on the days when you don't wet-shampoo but when your hair still needs some attention. Make sure you brush thoroughly to remove all traces.

Vinegar Rinse for Oily Hair
Add 2 drops of thyme linalol essential oil to 1 teaspoon (5 mL) of cider vinegar and mix it well to

disperse the thyme essential oil as much as possible. Then add to ½ pint (240 mL) of distilled or filtered water. Add this amount to a sink or large bowl full of warm water, and after shampooing and rinsing as normal, use a small pitcher to run the water from the sink through the hair several times to ensure effective coverage.

FRAGILE HAIR

There are many reasons why hair becomes fragile. It could be that the person has ill health, has been on a long course of medication, or is under stress. Or it could be that a series of unhelpful products has left the hair thin, split, or just fragile to the point of breaking on touch. This type of hair has to be treated very gently to avoid further damage.

Essential Oils for Fragile Hair
Lavender (*Lavandula angustifolia*)
Clary sage (*Salvia sclarea*)
Chamomile roman (*Anthemis nobilis*)
Sandalwood (*Santalum album*)
Geranium (*Pelargonium graveolens*)
Neroli (*Citrus aurantium*)
Rose otto (*Rosa damascena*)
Petitgrain (*Citrus aurantium*)
Lemon (*Citrus limon*)
Marjoram, sweet (*Origanum majorana*)

Plant Oils for Fragile Hair
Jojoba (*Simmondsia chinensis*)
Peach kernel (*Prunus persica*)
Borage seed (*Borago officinalis*)
Almond, sweet (*Prunus amygdalus var. dulcis*)
Evening primrose seed (*Oenothera biennis*)
Coconut (*Cocos nucifera*)
Argan (*Argania spinosa*)
Avocado (*Persea americana*)
Hemp seed (*Cannabis sativa*)

Essential Oil Shampoo Blend for Fragile Hair

Stimulating
Lavender	2 drops
Rosemary	2 drops
Clary sage	2 drops

Blend the essential oils together, then add to 3½ fl. oz. (100 mL) of a natural, fragrance-free shampoo. Use no more than once a week. In general, try to reduce the number of times you wash the hair.

Conditioner for Fragile Hair
Lecithin (liquid)	1 teaspoon (5 mL)
Borage seed oil	1 teaspoon (5 mL)
Jojoba oil	2 teaspoons (10 mL)
Geranium essential oil	1 drop

Using the bain-marie or double boiler method on a low heat, blend all the ingredients together well. Leave the mixture to cool before applying a small amount, and leave it on the hair for at least 10 minutes before shampooing off.

Richer Conditioner for Fragile Hair
Shea butter	5 teaspoons (25 mL)
Meadowfoam oil	5 teaspoons (25 mL)
Borage seed oil	1 teaspoon (5 mL)
Avocado oil	1 teaspoon (5 mL)
Evening primrose seed oil	10 drops
Lecithin (liquid)	2 teaspoons (10 mL)
Chamomile roman essential oil	3 drops

Using the bain-marie or double boiler method on a low heat, first melt the shea butter and then add the plant oils, stirring all the time. Then add the liquid lecithin and chamomile roman essential oil. Stir continually until well blended together. Remove from the heat, and pour into a covered container until required. Only use a small amount, and leave it on the hair for at least 10 minutes before shampooing off.

AFRO-TEXTURED HAIR

Due to its structure, afro-textured hair is often fine, and because of the tightness of the curls, the hair can easily break unless it's moisturized. Keeping the scalp in good condition protects hair growth, and this is best accomplished by using natural oils that are similar to the skin's own sebum and have good moisturizing properties and omega fatty acid profiles.

PLANT OILS FOR AFRO-TEXTURED HAIR
Jojoba (*Simmondsia chinensis*)
Argan (*Argania spinosa*)
Avocado (*Persea americana*)
Kukui (*Aleurites moluccana*)
Meadowfoam (*Limnanthes alba*)
Baobab (*Adansonia digitata*)
Brazil nut (*Bertholletia excelsa*)
Hemp seed (*Cannabis sativa*)
Moringa (*Moringa oleifera*)
Borage seed (*Borago officinalis*)
Evening primrose seed (*Oenothera biennis*)

ESSENTIAL OILS FOR AFRO-TEXTURED HAIR
Rosewood (*Aniba rosaeodora*)
Cedarwood atlas (*Cedrus atlantica*)
Marjoram, sweet (*Origanum majorana*)
Rosemary (*Rosmarinus officinalis*)
Petitgrain (*Citrus aurantium*)
Frankincense (*Boswellia carterii*)
Ho wood (*Cinnamomum camphora ct. linalool*)
Ylang ylang (*Cananga odorata*)
Chamomile roman (*Anthemis nobilis*)
Geranium (*Pelargonium graveolens*)

Essential Oil Shampoo Blends for Afro-Textured Hair

MOISTURIZING
Avocado oil	5 drops
Argan oil	10 drops
Kukui oil	5 drops
Hemp seed oil	5 drops
Geranium essential oil	4 drops
Frankincense essential oil	2 drops
Ylang ylang essential oil	1 drop

Blend the ingredients together, then add to 3½ fl. oz. (100 mL) of a natural, fragrance-free shampoo.

STIMULATING
Jojoba oil	10 drops
Hemp seed oil	5 drops
Camellia seed oil	10 drops
Rosemary essential oil	3 drops
Marjoram, sweet, essential oil	1 drop
Palmarosa essential oil	3 drops

Blend the ingredients together, then add to 3½ fl. oz. (100 mL) of a natural, fragrance-free shampoo.

CONDITIONING TREATMENT FOR AFRO-TEXTURED HAIR
Lecithin (liquid)	4 teaspoons (20 mL)
Shea butter	4 teaspoons (20 mL)
Avocado oil	2 teaspoons (10 mL)
Argan oil	4 teaspoons (20 mL)

Then add:
Borage seed oil	1 teaspoon (5 mL)
Clary sage essential oil	3 drops
Lavender essential oil	2 drops
Ho wood essential oil	2 drops
Geranium essential oil	3 drops

Using the bain-marie or double boiler method over a low heat, melt the shea butter. Then remove from the heat and add all the other ingredients, one at a time, continuing to stir well. Pour into a covered container until required. This conditioning treatment can be applied to the hair either warm or cool. Use enough to cover the hair, then cover with a towel and leave for at least 10 minutes before shampooing off, with a natural shampoo. These quantities are enough for several treatments.

Hair Rinses for Afro-Textured Hair

SWEET HAIR RINSE

Organic cider vinegar	1 teaspoon (5 mL)
Spring water (or geranium hydrolat)	½ pint (240 mL)
Ylang ylang essential oil	3 drops
Orange, sweet, essential oil	4 drops

REFRESHING HAIR RINSE

Organic cider vinegar	1 teaspoon (5 mL)
Spring water (or geranium hydrolat)	½ pint (240 mL)
Geranium essential oil	3 drops
Rosemary essential oil	4 drops

With both rinses: Add the essential oils to the cider vinegar and mix well to disperse the essential oil as much as possible. Then add to the ½ pint (240 mL) of spring water. Add this to warm water in a sink or large bowl, and after shampooing and rinsing as normal, run it through the hair several times to ensure effective coverage.

FALLING HAIR

Hair goes through a cycle of growing (the anagen phase), which lasts up to three years, then a static period of around 3–4 months (the catagen phase), before a period when the hair falls out (the telogen phase). This growth-rest-shedding cycle is usually unnoticed, as more hair grows to replace the old. But when more hair than usual can be seen after combing or brushing, and there seem to be more hairs than normal shed on the pillow, the hair may be classed as "falling hair," and it's best to address the problem early. For suggestions on other essential oils and plant oils that could be used for falling hair, see the section below, "Hair Loss and Alopecia"

Shampoos for Falling Hair

There are two shampoo options here; use whichever you prefer. But try not to wash the hair more than once a week for the time being, as the action of rubbing the head does nothing to help the immediate problem.

SHAMPOO 1

Jojoba oil	10 drops
Chamomile roman essential oil	2 drops
Cedarwood essential oil	1 drop

Blend the ingredients together, then add to 3½ fl. oz. (100 mL) of a natural, fragrance-free shampoo.

SHAMPOO 2

Jojoba oil	5 drops
Camellia seed oil	1 teaspoon (5 mL)
Avocado oil	½ teaspoon (2½ mL)
Rosemary essential oil	1 drop
Petitgrain essential oil	2 drops

Blend the ingredients together, then add to 3½ fl. oz. (100 mL) of a natural, fragrance-free shampoo.

Conditioners for Falling Hair

Of the two conditioner options below, choose which you prefer and use it before shampooing, leaving it on the hair for 10 minutes before rinsing off. Blend the ingredients using the bain-marie or double boiler method. These quantities are enough for several treatments.

CONDITIONER 1

Shea butter	2 teaspoons (10 mL)
Almond oil, sweet	2 tablespoons (30 mL)
Clary sage essential oil	5 drops

Using the bain-marie or double boiler method over a low heat, melt the shea butter. Then remove from the heat, add the other ingredients, and stir well. Pour into a covered container until required. Using a small amount each time, apply to the hair and leave it on for at least 10 minutes before shampooing off, using a natural shampoo. These quantities are enough for several treatments.

CONDITIONER 2

Lecithin (liquid)	1 teaspoon (5 mL)
Almond oil, sweet	2 tablespoons (30 mL)
Jojoba oil	5 drops
Evening primrose seed oil	10 drops

Using the bain-marie or double boiler method over a low heat, gently warm all the ingredients at the same time, stirring well. Remove from the heat and allow to cool, then pour into a covered container until required. Use a small amount each time. Leave for at least 10 minutes before shampooing off, using a natural shampoo. These quantities are enough for several treatments.

Rinses for Falling Hair

RINSE 1

Cider vinegar	1 teaspoon (5 mL)
Spring water	4 fl. oz. (120 mL)
Clary sage essential oil	5 drops

RINSE 2

Cider vinegar	1 teaspoon (5 mL)
Spring water	4 fl. oz. (120 mL)
Rosemary essential oil	3 drops
Lavender essential oil	2 drops

With both rinses: Add the essential oils to the cider vinegar and mix well to disperse as much as possible. Then add to 1 pint (475 mL) of boiled or filtered water. Add this to warm water in a sink or large bowl, and after shampooing and rinsing as normal, run it through the hair several times to ensure effective coverage.

HAIR LOSS AND ALOPECIA

Hair loss and alopecia are very often the result of medical problems, stress, or hereditary factors. The first thing to do is check with your physician to see if there's any underlying reason for the hair loss. If eczema or psoriasis of the scalp is suspected, see the corresponding section on page 398, and if ringworm is suspected, see that section in chapter 7 (page 166). A vitamin or mineral deficiency can sometimes cause hair loss, such as low levels of iron, zinc, and vitamins B12 and D. Overexercise and weight-loss diets can cause hair loss. Hair extensions and tight braids look pretty but can have pretty awful effects on the hair in some cases. Hair loss can also be the result of hormone imbalance, not only in terms of the male and female hormones we're familiar with but also with those of the thyroid, parathyroid, thymus, adrenals, pituitary, and pineal gland. For women, menopause or PCOS can sometimes lead to hair loss. Medications for acne and depression are other possible reasons for hair loss.

Alopecia has been categorized as an autoimmune problem, where the immune system attacks the hair follicles. When the hair is lost in patches all over the head it's called *diffuse alopecia areata,* when the whole head is affected it's *alopecia totalis,* and when hair is lost from the entire body, it's *alopecia universalis.* Any degree of alopecia is upsetting because there's often no apparent cause and it's difficult to find a solution to it. Hair might seem a superficial subject, but when things go wrong it can be utterly devastating and life changing. With any degree of hair loss, the key is to try to address the problem as soon as it's identified.

Use the essential oils listed below for both hair loss and alopecia. Some essential oils could stimulate the hair follicle and increase circulation sufficiently to bring about regrowth of hair in some cases, although this may resemble vellus, or baby hair. While encouraging growth with the essential oil treatments, use only purified water (boiled or filtered) to wash your hair. Avoid chlorinated swimming pools, or at least wet the hair before getting in the pool so less chlorine is absorbed, and avoid polluted lakes and rivers.

Essential Oils for Hair Loss
Rosewood (*Aniba rosaeodora*)
Lemon (*Citrus limon*)
Mastic (*Pistacia lentiscus*)
Thyme linalol (*Thymus vulgaris ct. linalool*)
Cedarwood atlas (*Cedrus atlantica*)
Rosemary (*Rosmarinus officinalis*)
Lavender (*Lavandula angustifolia*)
Ylang ylang (*Cananga odorata*)
Ginger (*Zingiber officinale*)
Spikenard (*Nardostachys jatamansi*)
Palmarosa (*Cymbopogon martinii*)
Black pepper (*Piper nigrum*)
Cypress (*Cupressus sempervirens*)
Clary sage (*Salvia sclarea*)
Chamomile german (*Matricaria recutita*)
Rose otto (*Rosa damascena*)
Chamomile roman (*Anthemis nobilis*)
Sandalwood (*Santalum album*)
Clove bud (*Syzygium aromaticum*)
Geranium (*Pelargonium graveolens*)

Plant Oils for Hair Loss
Ungurahui (pataua) (*Oenocarpus bataua*)
Hemp seed (*Cannabis sativa*)
Camellia seed (*Camellia japonica*)
Jojoba (*Simmondsia chinensis*)
Coconut (*Cocos nucifera*)
Tamanu (*Calophyllum inophyllum*)
Carrot, macerated (*Daucus carota*)
Avocado (*Persea americana*)
Evening primrose seed (*Oenothera biennis*)
Borage seed (*Borago officinalis*)

Plant Oil Additions
(Include in small volumes.)
Cranberry seed (*Vaccinium macrocarpon*)
Cucumber seed (*Cucumis sativus*)
Lemon seed oil (*Citrus limon*)

Hair Loss Essential Oil Blend
Cedarwood atlas	10 drops
Sandalwood	10 drops
Cypress	5 drops
Clary sage	5 drops
Chamomile roman	1 drop
Fennel, sweet	1 drop

First, blend the essential oils together, then dilute 2 drops in 1 teaspoon (5 mL) of a plant oil such as avocado. Gently apply onto the affected areas of the scalp, either during the day or at night.

Shampoo
Jojoba oil	12 drops
*Carrot oil, macerated	6 drops
Rosemary essential oil	6 drops
Lavender essential oil	4 drops

Carrot macerated oil is deep orange and may stain clothing.

Blend the ingredients together, then add to 3½ fl. oz. (100 mL) of a natural, fragrance-free shampoo. Alternatively, instead of the rosemary and lavender essential oils, substitute 10 drops of essential oil from the Hair Loss Essential Oil Blend, above.

Hair Loss Preshampoo Oil
Jojoba oil	½ teaspoon (2½ mL)
Evening primrose seed oil	10 drops
Hemp seed oil	20 drops
Avocado oil	1 teaspoon (5 mL)
Argan oil	1 teaspoon (5 mL)
Palmarosa essential oil	1 drop

Blend the ingredients together, and massage into the scalp before shampooing. Leave for at least 30 minutes before washing off. These quantities are enough for several treatments.

DANDRUFF

Dandruff can affect any hair type and is very common. It can be caused by a diverse range of things, from simple dry skin on the scalp to psoriasis or eczema, hair products, or a fungal infection. There are many essential oils that can be incorporated into dandruff treatments, so it should be easy to find a combination to suit any suspected cause and aroma preference. As with all dandruff treatments, it takes a little while for the scalp to recover and stop shedding those annoying little white flakes.

ESSENTIAL OILS TO TREAT DANDRUFF
Tea tree (*Melaleuca alternifolia*)
Manuka (*Leptospermum scoparium*)
Rosemary (*Rosmarinus officinalis*)
Cypress (*Cupressus sempervirens*)
Lemon (*Citrus limon*)
Lavender (*Lavandula angustifolia*)
Basil linalol (*Ocimum basilicum ct. linalool*)
Ylang ylang (*Cananga odorata*)
Mastic (*Pistacia lentiscus*)
Bay, West Indian (*Pimenta racemosa*)
Clove bud (*Syzygium aromaticum*)
Cedarwood atlas (*Cedrus atlantica*)
Clary sage (*Salvia sclarea*)
Oregano (*Origanum vulgare*)
Myrrh (*Commiphora myrrha*)
Chamomile german (*Matricaria recutita*)
Geranium (*Pelargonium graveolens*)
Patchouli (*Pogostemon cablin*)
Sandalwood (*Santalum album*)
Palmarosa (*Cymbopogon martinii*)

PLANT OILS TO TREAT DANDRUFF
Evening primrose seed (*Oenothera biennis*)
Borage seed (*Borago officinalis*)

Jojoba (*Simmondsia chinensis*)
Neem (*Azadirachta indica*)
Argan (*Argania spinosa*)
Camellia seed (*Camellia japonica*)
Tamanu (*Calophyllum inophyllum*)
Black cumin (*Nigella sativa*)
Meadowfoam (*Limnanthes alba*)
Coconut (*Cocos nucifera*)
Calendula, macerated (*Calendula officinalis*)
Carrot root, macerated (*Daucus carota*)

Essential Oil Shampoo Blends for Dandruff
There are two shampoos in this treatment plan. The first loosens the crusty layer of dead skin cells, which are often removed during the washing process. Blend 1 may encourage the healing mechanisms of the skin to prevent a further buildup of dandruff scales. Use this shampoo, avoiding the harsher types of shampoo on the market, before moving on to Blend 2.

BLEND 1
Rosemary essential oil	10 drops
Eucalyptus radiata essential oil	3 drops
Manuka (or tea tree) essential oil	2 drops
*Neem oil	5 drops

*The aroma of neem oil is not universally liked.

Blend the ingredients together, then add to 3½ fl. oz. (100 mL) of a natural, fragrance-free shampoo.

BLEND 2
Ho wood	3 drops
Basil linalol	3 drops
Peppermint	1 drop
Geranium	4 drops

Blend the essential oils together, then add to 3½ fl. oz. (100 mL) of a natural, fragrance-free shampoo.

VINEGAR RINSE FOR DANDRUFF
Dandruff responds well to vinegar rinses.

Cider vinegar	4 fl. oz. (120 mL)
Thyme linalol essential oil	5 drops
Peppermint essential oil	2 drops
Tea tree (or manuka) essential oil	5 drops

Blend the ingredients together, then add to ½ pint (240 mL) of spring water and bottle. Using about a teaspoon (5 mL) each time, massage into the scalp (not the hair) every night before going to bed, taking care not to get any in the eyes.

DANDRUFF NIGHT HAIR OIL

*Neem oil	5 drops
Jojoba oil	15 drops
Evening primrose seed oil	15 drops
Cypress essential oil	3 drops
Juniper berry essential oil	5 drops

The aroma of neem oil is not universally liked.

Blend the ingredients together, and massage a small amount directly into the scalp. Leave on overnight, and shampoo off in the morning.

ECZEMA AND PSORIASIS OF THE SCALP

Eczema and psoriasis have so many potential causes that finding a solution to them is often difficult, and no more so than when it is on the scalp and difficult to reach under the hair. The following suggestions for essential oils and plant oils might be able to help. Incorporate them into all the usual methods outlined in this hair section.

ESSENTIAL OILS FOR ECZEMA OR PSORIASIS OF THE SCALP
Rosewood (*Aniba rosaeodora*)
Tea tree (*Melaleuca alternifolia*)
Geranium (*Pelargonium graveolens*)
Clary sage (*Salvia sclarea*)
Bergamot (*Citrus bergamia*)
Juniper berry (*Juniperus communis*)
Spikenard (*Nardostachys jatamansi*)
Chamomile german (*Matricaria recutita*)
Chamomile roman (*Anthemis nobilis*)
Lavender (*Lavandula angustifolia*)
Ho wood (*Cinnamomum camphora ct. linalool*)
Sage (*Salvia officinalis*)

PLANT OILS FOR ECZEMA OR PSORIASIS OF THE SCALP
Avocado (*Persea americana*)
Moringa (*Moringa oleifera*)
Chaulmoogra (*Hydnocarpus laurifolia*)
Rosehip seed (*Rosa rubiginosa*)
Evening primrose seed (*Oenothera biennis*)
Tamanu (*Calophyllum inophyllum*)
Argan (*Argania spinosa*)
Borage seed (*Borago officinalis*)
Calendula (*Calendula officinalis*)
Neem (*Azadirachta indica*)
Camellia seed (*Camellia japonica*)

BLEND

Chamomile german	5 drops
Bergamot	5 drops
Juniper berry	1 drop
Rosewood	5 drops
Lavender	2 drops

Add to:

Borage seed oil	3 teaspoons (15 mL)
Tamanu oil	3 teaspoons (15 mL)
Camellia seed oil	4 teaspoons (20 mL)

First, blend the essential oils together, then the plant oils, then combine the two. Apply a small amount to the scalp, as required. Often, camellia seed oil used on its own can ease irritation and itching when applied to the scalp.

14

The Home Spa — Body Beautiful

The word *spa* comes from a town in Belgium, called Spa, that is famous for its healing cold-water springs — the ancient Romans called it Aquae Spadanae — *aquae* meaning "water." All over the world, spa towns and resorts have been built up around healing mineral-rich springs, either hot or cold, with many still thriving today. The oldest in the United States is Jefferson Pools, near Warm Springs, Virginia, which dates from at least 1761. It's thought that people have been flocking to healing springs since prehistoric times because ancient artifacts, thought to be offerings, have been found at them. Today, although spas do often offer water-based treatments, the whole concept has moved from healing toward relaxation and beautifying. So we arrive at the point where there are holiday resort spas, spa hotels for short and long stays, day spas, and spa rooms in gyms.

Five-star spas struggle to find that exclusive treatment range that makes them stand out from the crowd. I get invited to create many wonderful body treatments based on science and high-quality organic ingredients — including spa treatments and product lines based on nature. Products made lovingly by hand take into account the healing ability of each ingredient, its energetics and

exclusivity, and they can be expensive to produce when I use real diamonds, emeralds, sapphires, rubies, gold, and silver that have been energized by healers and formulated to produce positive effects not only on the body but on the mind and spirit too.

But large-scale commercial production calls for a long shelf life and preservatives, and fewer active ingredients so profit can be maximized. The client may be led to believe they are getting one thing when they may be getting something else altogether. Some commercial body balms, scrubs, and polishes used by spas are being produced without the ingredients the product designer originally intended. For example, the original formula may have been reproduced using cheaper, lower-grade starting materials, fewer active ingredients, a lower percentage of an active ingredient, or essential oils other than those intended. It could be that the only thing not being changed is the price!

This is where the home spa enters, because at home, or when making products for friends, you can include the high volume of active ingredients required, and since everything is fresh, there's no need for synthetic preservatives. Instead of something therapeutically dead, you can make something vital and alive and highly effective. Homemade spa products might not be as foamy or soapy as commercial products containing detergents, and the texture may not be as smooth, but they'll do the job required of them and be much better for your overall well-being.

Most of the following suggestions are plant oil–based, as bacteria don't generally grow in oil so there's little need for synthetic antimicrobials. However, plant oils do have a limited shelf life and some of the finest active ingredients are prone to oxidization, so do follow the guidelines of your ingredient suppliers when making home spa treatments.

When you make your own spa products, you're not concerned about profit or shelf life and can create something using time-honored ingredients that are known to work. Some of the raw ingredients are not actually that expensive, even when they're the highest quality available; it's all about knowing which particular ingredients do which particular job. When it comes to the essential oils, as I never tire of saying, quality is everything if you expect a therapeutic job to be done. Aromatherapy is just that, a therapy; it's not just about aroma.

In the long millennia before distillation was invented, people extracted the active ingredients from plants by a process known as *maceration*. The flower petals or herbs were crammed into a receptacle, covered in oil, and left in the sun while the active ingredients diffused into the oil; then the plant material was replaced with fresh, and the whole process repeated over and over again until the oil was thoroughly infused. Today, some macerated plant oils are still made in much the same way. And for centuries, plant oils have been extracted from a wide variety of plants, not only for cooking but for beautifying purposes as well. Some of these plant oils leave a golden gleam on the skin that no other substance can reproduce, and used regularly, they can give the skin a soft

and conditioned sheen that makes heads turn — forget artificial body glimmers, next to the real thing they look dry and fake.

Nature has always provided human beings with luxurious delights to make them look good, and feel good too. Many exciting things are happening in the world of raw product development. For example, many fruit seeds, including lemon, are being made into oils. With this ever-increasing diversity in ingredients that can be incorporated in spa products, clarity becomes ever more important. For example, the word *lemon* in beauty preparations could mean lemon essential oil, lemon juice, ground lemon peel, lemon wax, or lemon seed oil.

There's so much choice with both plant oils and essential oils that you'll be able to find a perfect combination that not only conditions skin and makes it look and feel great but also appeals to your aesthetic judgment. The essential oils give great delight when used for pampering the body, and you can rest assured that used and combined correctly in body care, their effect will be experienced not only on the body but on the mind and spirit too. So please enjoy this chapter. It's our right to feel good, and apparently Mother Nature agrees because she makes it happen.

Body Polishes and Scrubs

The main purpose of the body polish or scrub is to remove any dead skin cells that remain after simply using a washcloth or body brush in the shower or bath. Skin renews itself, with the uppermost level shedding over a period of up to 30 days, depending on a person's age, skin type, health, and even the time of the year. Older skin cells are non-reflective and can give the skin a dull, dry look. By removing the dead skin cells, a fresher, more light-reflective look is given to the skin, and body products — whether used for health or beauty — can penetrate the skin better.

A good-quality body polish should consist of an ingredient that can help remove the dead skin cells. This is blended with other skin-protective ingredients that can protect the newly revealed skin, and these can be oil-based or water-based, depending on which central polishing ingredient has been chosen. A body scrub, on the other hand, usually consists of mainly dry ingredients that are often infused with fragrance or herbs. Some people prefer body polishes, some prefer scrubs — so which is chosen is just a matter of personal choice.

The key with any product aimed at removing dead skin cells is that it shouldn't damage the underlying, newly revealed skin. Unfortunately, some commercially prepared body scrubs are more focused on the scrub than on protecting the skin. Both, however, are equally important, and given the number of raw materials now available, there's no need to skimp on either.

Exfoliating materials can include ground and powdered seeds, nuts, grains, roots, even semiprecious and precious gems. The choice of material depends on the desired final effect. Broadly speaking, polishes and scrubs can be sweet or salty. Sweet, or "sweetness," body polishes most often utilize sugar as the exfoliating material, while salt-based exfoliates often incorporate herbs or seaweed. But there are endless combinations that could be used, providing endless possibilities. Here are some suggestions:

Basic body-exfoliating materials: Sugar, both refined and unrefined, salt of various kinds, ground almond, rice, pomegranate and cranberry seed, lotus root, hibiscus

Best reserved for feet: Loofah, pumice stone, bamboo, cocoa shells, walnut shells, apricot kernels

Useful plant oils in body exfoliates: Jojoba oil, avocado oil, moringa oil, argan oil, coconut oil, rice bran oil, sweet almond oil, safflower oil

Useful additions: Olive squalane, evening primrose seed oil, borage seed oil, cranberry seed oil, blackcurrant seed oil, sea buckthorn oil, rosehip seed oil, raspberry seed oil, natural vitamin E in oil-soluble form

ESSENTIAL OILS

Essential oils can be chosen for their aroma or for specific therapeutic properties. The following, for example, could be used in a cellulite or detoxification product.

Peppermint (*Mentha piperita*)
Lemongrass (*Cymbopogon citratus/flexuosus*)
Rosemary (*Rosmarinus officinalis*)
Elemi (*Canarium luzonicum*)
Basil (*Ocimum basilicum*)
Grapefruit (*Citrus paradisi*)
Cardamom (*Elettaria cardamomum*)
Coriander seed (*Coriandrum sativum*)
Niaouli (*Melaleuca quinquenervia*)
Saro (*Cinnamosma fragrans*)
Lemon (*Citrus limon*)
Palmarosa (*Cymbopogon martinii*)
Cypress (*Cupressus sempervirens*)
Juniper berry (*Juniperus communis*)
Pine (*Pinus sylvestris*)
Cabreuva (*Myrocarpus fastigiatus*)
Manuka (*Leptospermum scoparium*)

And the following, for example, could be used in relaxation or general body conditioning products:

Ylang ylang (*Cananga odorata*)
Jasmine (*Jasminum grandiflorum/officinale*)
Rose absolute (*Rosa centifolia*)
Neroli (*Citrus aurantium*)
Petitgrain (*Citrus aurantium*)
Geranium (*Pelargonium graveolens*)
Palmarosa (*Cymbopogon martinii*)
Orange, sweet (*Citrus sinensis*)

Lavender (*Lavandula angustifolia*)
Magnolia leaf (*Michelia alba*)
Mandarin (*Citrus reticulata*)
Sandalwood (*Santalum album*)
Bergamot (*Citrus bergamia*)
Cedarwood atlas (*Cedrus atlantica*)
Spikenard (*Nardostachys jatamansi*)
Frankincense (*Boswellia carterii*)
Rosewood (*Aniba rosaeodora*)
Chamomile roman (*Anthemis nobilis*)

SWEETNESS BODY POLISHES

A wide range of sugars are available. For the following recipe I would suggest using an unrefined organic brown sugar because it contains properties that are good for the skin such as vitamins B1, 2, 3, and 6 and trace minerals such as calcium, zinc, and magnesium. Turbinado brown sugar (cane sugar) could be used or, if a whiter product is required, white refined sugar. Other sugars that could be used for exfoliating are palm sugar and sanding sugar, which is a white sugar that has light-reflecting properties.

Sweetness Body Polish

Unrefined organic sugar	9 oz. (250 g)
Jojoba oil	3½ fl. oz. (100 mL)
Mandarin essential oil	10 drops
Orange, sweet, essential oil	2 drops
Geranium essential oil	5 drops

There are 17 drops of essential oil in this formula, but you could add other oils of your choice — using no more than 25 drops — blended into the jojoba (or another carrier oil of your choice), before adding to the sugar. Mix the sugar and oil together well, then store in a container with a lid. To retain the slightly sweet note of the sugar, it's best to use a carrier oil that is fragrant-neutral. If you don't want to incorporate essential oils, use coconut oil instead of the jojoba oil or, for a chocolatey aroma, use melted unrefined cocoa butter.

Both options work well with the sweetness of the sugar.

SALTY BODY SCRUBS

Genuine Dead Sea salt retains some of the oiliness that can be found in the Dead Sea. This is the best salt option for polishes and scrubs but can be difficult to find. It comes in fine and coarse salt grades, as do many of the other salt options available.

Salty Basil and Mint Body Scrub

Dead Sea salt, fine (or sea salt)	9 oz. (250 g)
Jojoba oil	3½ fl. oz. (100 mL)
Peppermint essential oil	4 drops
Basil linalol essential oil	4 drops
Spearmint essential oil	7 drops
Lemon essential oil	6 drops

There are 21 drops of essential oil in this formula, and you could add 4 drops of another essential oil of your choice. Alternatively, use any essential oils you wish, but no more than 25 drops in total. First, dilute the essential oil into the jojoba oil (or a carrier oil of your choice), then add to the salt, and mix well.

Conditioning Body Polish

Dead Sea salt, fine	1 oz. (28 g)
Almonds, ground	2 oz. (57 g)
Oatmeal	2 oz. (57 g)
Milk powder	1 oz. (28 g)
Sandalwood essential oil	10 drops
Evening primrose seed oil	1 teaspoon (5 mL)
Jojoba oil	1.7 fl. oz. (50 mL)
Avocado oil	4 teaspoons (20 mL)

Blend all the oils together. Then carefully blend the dry ingredients together and add them to the oils, a little at a time, until you get a thick paste. This is then gently rubbed over the body to loosen the skin cells. Then rinse off in the shower or bath before applying a nourishing body oil.

Conditioning Body Scrub

Ground almonds	1 handful
Oatmeal	1 handful
Sandalwood essential oil	2 drops
Evening primrose seed oil	2 drops

Bind the ingredients together and then rub the mixture all over the skin, paying particular attention to dry, scaling areas such as the elbows, knees, and backs of the heels. Then rinse off in the shower or bath before applying a nourishing body oil.

Body Scrub for Blemished Back/Chest

Sea salt	1 handful
Ground almonds	1 handful
Oatmeal	1 handful
Thyme linalol essential oil	4 drops
Lemon essential oil	4 drops
Rosemary essential oil	2 drops

Bind the ingredients together and rub the mixture over the blemished skin area, paying particular attention to the back and shoulders if these are affected. Then rinse off in the shower or bath.

THE LUXURIOUS EMPRESS BODY POLISH

One of the most luxurious and sensual body preparations used in times past is here revived to suit today's modern woman, who doesn't have a posse of handmaidens to attend to her every wish. The powders in the formula can be purchased, or they can be made at home if you have the kitchen equipment to turn dried ingredients into powder form. The Luxurious Empress Body Polish removes dead skin cells and leaves the skin glowing, fragrant, and soft as silk.

Ground, powdered citrus fruit peel	2 teaspoons (10 g)
Ground almonds	1 tablespoon (15 g)
Oatmeal, fine	2 teaspoons (10 g)
Clove powder	1 pinch
Powdered rose petals	1 teaspoon
Nutmeg powder	1 pinch
Honey powder (or honey)	2 teaspoons
Goat's milk powder	1 tablespoon
Almond oil, sweet	2 tablespoons (30 mL)
Rose absolute essential oil	5 drops
Lemon essential oil	2 drops
Sandalwood essential oil	3 drops
Jasmine essential oil	1 drop

Blend all the dry ingredients together. Then blend the essential oils into the sweet almond oil. (If you're using liquid honey, rather than honey powder, mix it in with the sweet almond oil/essential oil blend.) Now combine the dry and wet blends together until you have a paste, adding more sweet almond oil if the mixture feels too dry for you. (If you blend double the quantities of sweet almond and essential oil, you'll also have enough to apply as a body oil when the body polish treatment is complete.)

The four essential oils in this treatment have moisturizing and skin conditioning properties. There are 11 drops in total, and if you prefer, you could substitute 11 drops of essential oil of your choice. Traditional options include neroli — which is made from the exquisite-smelling flower of orange blossom — and other good choices would be jasmine, bergamot, or ylang ylang. You could also use any essential oil made from a favorite flower or exotic wood. In China, osmanthus, lotus, pine, or mandarin essential oils might be preferred; while in India, tuberose, sandalwood, jasmine, and patchouli could be favorites; and in the Middle East, rose, oud, and frankincense may be chosen.

Once you have prepared the Luxurious Empress Body Polish, take a bath or shower, dry yourself off, and, standing in the bathtub, firmly roll and massage the mixture all over your body.

Massage it well into dry areas of skin such as the elbows and knees. The aim is to cover the skin with a very fine layer of the mixture, which is why you need to roll the paste over the body.

Let the paste dry and then brush it off, starting where you first applied it. Using a dry washcloth, briskly wipe away any remaining areas of paste. Finish by applying a light body oil that complements the aroma in the body polish — this could be the one you made earlier if you made twice the amount of sweet almond and essential oil blend.

Body Masks

Body masks used in spa treatments are intended to remove impurities and detoxify, as well as to tone the skin, encourage weight loss, improve the texture of the skin, and give an overall sense of well-being. In luxury spas, body masks are often tailor-made for the client, and you too can easily personalize a body mask to suit your exact requirements.

Each ingredient can be chosen for its specific therapeutic value. Start with a clay, mud, or seaweed. Additions might be fruit, plant, or flower powders. Mixing agents can include hydrolats, essential oil waters, nut milks, or a really good mineral water. Choose which essential oils to add depending on your particular requirements, referring to the lists in this chapter or the essential oil profiles in chapter 20 and, of course, your own aroma preferences. All the chosen ingredients are simply mixed together in a bowl: start with the primary ingredient — whether clay, mud, or seaweed — mix it with spring, mineral, or distilled water, hydrolat, or another blending agent, then add your other ingredients and the essential oils.

Body masks can be quite messy to use, so always cover the area you intend to relax in while the mask does its job. Thin plastic disposable sheeting is the best, such as those used to cover newly cleaned clothes. Mix approximately 3½ oz. (100 g) of the clay of choice with enough liquid to make a paste that's easy to apply with either a brush or your hand — not too stiff but resembling the consistency of thick mud. Add any additional ingredients. Leave the body mask on for around 15 minutes, and then sponge off with lukewarm water.

CLAY — THE PRIMARY INGREDIENT

Clay is wonderfully absorbent, and some clays seem to act as a magnet for all the pollution, environmental toxins, and debris lurking on and in our skins.

Argilez, or French clay: Comes in various colors that have different therapeutic values:

> **Pink clay:** Soothing and cleansing; can be used on sensitive skin
>
> **White clay:** Gentle; can be used on all skin types
>
> **Red clay:** Rejuvenating and cleansing; stimulating — good for circulation; can stain clothing and skin
>
> **Green clay:** Cleansing and detoxifying
>
> **Yellow clay:** Invigorating and stimulating; can stain clothing and skin

Montmorillonite clay: Toning; improves skin tone and tissue elasticity

Rhoussel clay: Toning; improves skin tone and texture; detoxifying

Zeolite clay: A detoxifying clay and slimming ingredient

OTHER BODY MASK INGREDIENTS

Ground, dried seaweed or algae: Can be purchased in powder form and makes a good addition to, or alternative for, clay; valuable in treating muscular or joint conditions

Herbs: Choose for their individual therapeutic properties

Fruit and herbal powders: Can have valuable vitamins and minerals

Apricot powder: Useful for all skin types

Rose, lavender, and flower petal powders: For inclusion in luxury body masks

Seaweed powder: Slimming and detoxifying

Nut and milk powders: Nourishing and conditioning

It's quite normal for people to spend hours at the spa, moving from one treatment room to another, taking relaxation breaks during which healthy snacks and drinks are served. And you too can spend the day pampering yourself. Start with a body exfoliating treatment in the form of a body polish or scrub, then apply your choice of body mask, rinse it off and take a milk and essential oil bath, and, finally, cover yourself in a luxurious body oil. You'll have a lovely day, save yourself a fortune, and feel absolutely great!

Body Lotions

A lotion is an amalgamation of water in oil or oil in water, both containing an emulsifying agent, and it can take time and experience to achieve just the right balance using the raw materials at home. In theory essential oils can be incorporated into any pre-prepared lotion or cream, and there are many on the market that are pure and natural and could be used as a base. Add either single essential oils or blends of essential oils to the body lotion, and mix as thoroughly as possible.

Body Butters and Balms

There's a world of therapeutic butters, waxes, and oils that can be combined in countless ways to make body balms. Butters can be soft, or they can be hard — like cocoa butter. Many plant oils actually come in semisolid form and become a liquid only when in contact with some form of warmth — a hand, for example. Some plant butters, such as apricot butter, have been through processing to arrive at the butter-like consistency required. The most recognizable wax is beeswax, but many plant waxes are now being produced. And, of course, there are hundreds of plant oils — of which some are heavy, some light; some have an aroma, some are deodorized, and some have no aroma at all. Many plant oils are used only as small therapeutic additions to a blend, rather than being the main ingredient.

There's wide scope for making a variety of therapeutic body balms, and many recipes and techniques are available. The only thing I would say is that when adding essential oils or other active ingredients to body butters and balms, it's usually better to wait before adding them until the liquid has cooled but not yet solidified.

Body Splashes and Spritzers

Body splashes and spritzers can be invigorating or soothing sprays, with a variety of uses. They can stimulate or tone, uplift or relax — depending on the ingredients and the essential oils used. They're easy to make because they're so simple. Have an array of them in your bathroom ready to use whenever the mood takes you. Splashes are a favorite with men as they do a great job of making a person feel good without leaving an oily residue on the skin, especially after shaving. In times past body splashes were called *les vinaigres de toilette*, and we follow the same principle and in some cases use the same ingredients. The vinegars to use are white wine vinegar or cider vinegar, whichever you prefer. If you use alcohol, use food-grade alcohol or vodka. Avoid using splashes that contain alcohol if you have sensitive or dehydrated skin, as alcohol can be very drying; vegetable glycerin can be used instead.

DEODORANT SPLASH OR SPRITZ

White wine or cider vinegar	1 teaspoon (5 mL)
Vodka (or glycerin)	1 tablespoon (15 mL)
Lavender essential oil	5 drops
Coriander seed essential oil	5 drops
Lemon essential oil	5 drops
Rosemary essential oil	5 drops
Peppermint essential oil	2 drops
Grapefruit essential oil	5 drops
Spring water or hydrolat	1 pint (475 mL)

First blend the essential oils together. Add them to the vodka or glycerin and shake well for as long as you can. Leave the mixture to settle, then add the vinegar. Pour the whole mixture into the spring water or hydrolat and again, shake well. Finally, pass the liquid through an unbleached paper coffee filter. The longer you leave the essential oils in the vodka and vinegar mix before adding to the water, the stronger the fragrance will be.

Follow this same procedure when making all the splashes that follow.

BODY SPLASHES OR SPRITZERS:
BASE INGREDIENTS

High-proof vodka or vegetable glycerin	2 teaspoons (10 mL)
White wine vinegar or cider vinegar	1 teaspoon (5 mL)
Spring water or hydrolat	1 pint (475 mL)

INVIGORATING ESSENTIAL OIL BLEND

Lime	10 drops
Lavender	10 drops
Peppermint	5 drops
Lemon	3 drops

SOOTHING ESSENTIAL OIL BLEND

Benzoin	10 drops
Ho wood	2 drops
Sandalwood	10 drops
Geranium	5 drops

FRUITY ESSENTIAL OIL BLEND

Orange, sweet	10 drops
Lemon	5 drops
Mandarin	10 drops
Grapefruit	5 drops

TONING ESSENTIAL OIL BLEND

Lemongrass	18 drops
Basil linalol	2 drops
Black pepper	3 drops
Frankincense	5 drops
Patchouli	3 drops

Baths and Bubbles

There are several ways essential oils can be used in water treatments — in baths, showers, foot baths, and hand baths. In addition, in the professional spa they could be used in steam rooms, hot dry rooms, ice rooms, hammams, water jets, overhead body water sprinklers, hot tubs, Jacuzzis, and pools. Bathing is an integral part of any spa, and ingredients might include milk, oils, salts, and even seaweed or algae. Essential oils are used in all kinds of bath treatments, including prebath body oil treatments to soften the skin.

Essential oils can be added to naturally based bubble bath bases, up to 2%. And essential oils can also be incorporated into homemade bath crystals. These can be combinations of large sea salt crystals, Epsom salt, and baking powder. Simply measure your dry ingredients and add the essential oils of your choice: to each 9 oz. (250 g) add 20 drops of essential oil — mixing in well to evenly distribute the essential oils.

NOURISHING PLANT OIL BATHS

Most people find plain tap water drying to the skin and like a bath oil to counteract its effects. There are some plant/carrier oils that have been treated to become dispersible in water, such as jojoba, apricot kernel, sweet almond, and sunflower. However, these are treated with synthetic emulsifiers that may impede their therapeutic value.

A simple aromatic bath can be made by first diluting 3–5 drops of essential oil in a small amount of plant or carrier oil in the palm of your hand, or in any type of receptacle, before adding to the bath. Swish your hand around in the water to disperse the oils. This gives the bath a wonderful aroma, and gives you the therapeutic values of whichever oil(s) you have chosen.

One of the most favored ways to help alleviate skin dryness is to apply a plant oil onto the body before getting into a bath. While in the bath, massage the oil into the skin. Any nourishing plant oil can be used, singly or in a blend. Add 2–5 drops of essential oil per 1 teaspoon (5 mL) of plant oil, and use a teaspoon in each bath. Here is a blend that could be prepared for several baths:

NOURISHING OIL

Avocado	2 teaspoons (10 mL)
Apricot kernel	2 teaspoons (10 mL)
Almond, sweet	2 tablespoons (30 mL)

Add up to 20 drops of essential oils per 1.7 fl. oz. (50 mL) of carrier oil.

SPECIAL BATH BLENDS

GENERAL RELAXING ESSENTIAL OIL BATH BLEND

Ylang ylang	2 drops
Orange, sweet	3 drops
Lavender	1 drop
Chamomile roman	1 drop

This blend can be added to 2 teaspoons (10 mL) of carrier oil, or to fresh or dried milk, making enough for two soothing baths.

PROFESSIONAL ENERGIZING ESSENTIAL OIL BATH BLEND

Eucalyptus lemon	1 drop
Spearmint	1 drop
Grapefruit	3 drops
Rosemary	3 drops
Ginger	1 drop

This blend can be added to 2 teaspoons (10 mL) of carrier oil, or fresh or dried milk, making enough for two energizing baths.

PROFESSIONAL DETOX ESSENTIAL OIL BATH BLEND

The professional detox formula of essential oils that follows can be used in several ways. First blend the essential oils together and bottle, as there are 32 drops in the total synergistic blend. When mixed together in these proportions, the blend works as an integrated whole to achieve its purpose.

Cypress	3 drops
Juniper berry	3 drops
Frankincense	2 drops
Immortelle	2 drops
Lemongrass	4 drops
Palmarosa	4 drops
Petitgrain	10 drops
Pine	2 drops
Thyme linalol	2 drops

This special detox blend of essential oils could be used in a body oil, using 4–5 drops in 1 teaspoon (5 mL) of a suitable carrier oil. Or use 10 drops in one of the bath methods outlined below.

For the salt method, add to the bathwater 2 cups of Epsom salts and 1 cup of sea salt, combining them first. Then add 10 drops of the essential oil blend diluted in a little carrier oil, just before getting in. Soak for at least 15 minutes, massaging any oil that's floating on the surface into your upper and lower abdomen, thighs, and arms.

For a prebath treatment, dilute 10 drops of the essential oil blend into 2 teaspoons (10 mL) of acai berry oil, and apply all over the abdominal area. Add the combined salts as above, to the bath before getting in.

SEAWEED SLIMMING AND DETOX BATH

There's no getting away from the fact that seaweed baths smell like seaweed, and that's not an aroma everyone wants floating around the bathroom every day. But seaweed baths have been used in European spas for a very long time precisely because they're so effective at detoxifying, toning, and reducing stretch marks. Both bladder wrack powder (*Fucus vesiculosis*) and kelp powder (*Ascophyllum nodosum*) contain vitamins, minerals, iodine, and other valuable trace elements.

SEAWEED BATH BLEND

Sea salt	1 cup
Seaweed powder	¼ cup
Professional Detox Bath Blend (page 407)	10 drops
Acai berry oil (or other plant oil)	10 drops

First, combine the salt and seaweed, then add it to the bathwater, swishing it around well to disperse any floating powder. Then add the 10 drops of the blend and 10 drops of nourishing plant oil, swish the water around again, and get into the bath. Relax in the water for 20 minutes, adding more hot water if required. While in the water, look for any oil globules floating on the surface, scoop them up, and rub over your abdomen, thighs, and upper arms.

MILK BATHS

In spas, milk baths are often one of the more expensive treatments, valued for cooling and smoothing the skin, rejuvenating and protecting it, and for being aphrodisiacal. The main ingredient in a milk bath is generally milk powder — either cow's or goat's milk. As essential oils are oil soluble, the best powders to use are those that have full fat content. To the milk, the following ingredients could be added:

MILK BATH ADDITIONS

Essential oils
Oatmeal
Dried flower petals: Rose, jasmine, and orange blossom are favorites
Dried aloe vera powder
Honey powder
Powdered minerals or vitamins such as vitamin C
Epsom salts
Baking soda
White clay

Once you've decided on your basic ingredients, simply mix them together in a tightly lidded blender. Obviously, the petals should be excluded from this process and simply added to the bathwater along with the milk mixture.

Essential oils can be added at the blending stage; release the drops one by one into the small hole found in most blender lids. Rose otto and neroli are often used as they are clear and won't color the milk powder. If an absolute such as rose maroc or jasmine have been included in the ingredient list, these absolutes will give a yellow tinge to the product.

Often, expensive essential oils and absolutes such as rose are adulterated with synthetics, or "nature identicals," or with essential oils, accords, or aromatic chemicals — both natural and synthetic — that can be blended to give the impression of another, more expensive essential oil. Geranium and sandalwood are often involved in this game of subterfuge.

BATHS FOR BALANCED, DRY, OILY, AND BLEMISHED SKIN TYPES

Each person's skin is different, due to genetics, lifestyle, and health, and with the wide variety of essential oils available, each having its own unique properties, it's possible to design bath blends that are specific to a particular person's needs, bearing in mind their skin type, therapeutic needs, and aroma preferences.

ALL SKIN TYPES: ESSENTIAL OILS FOR BATHS

Palmarosa (*Cymbopogon martinii*)
Rose otto (*Rosa damascena*)
Geranium (*Pelargonium graveolens*)
Jasmine (*Jasminum grandiflorum/officinale*)
Ylang ylang (*Cananga odorata*)
Frankincense (*Boswellia carterii*)
Sandalwood (*Santalum album*)
Patchouli (*Pogostemon cablin*)
Lavender (*Lavandula officinalis*)
Neroli (*Citrus aurantium*)
Petitgrain (*Citrus aurantium*)
Bergamot (*Citrus bergamia*)

RELAXING ESSENTIAL OIL BATH BLEND FOR ALL SKIN TYPES

Frankincense	3 drops
Orange, sweet	5 drops
Neroli	5 drops
Petitgrain	10 drops

First, blend the essential oils together, then dilute 4–5 drops in each teaspoon (5 mL) of carrier oil, or dried milk or buttermilk powder.

DRY SKIN: ESSENTIAL OILS FOR BATHS

Benzoin (*Styrax benzoin*)
Rosewood (*Aniba rosaeodora*)
Jasmine (*Jasminum grandiflorum/officinale*)
Geranium (*Pelargonium graveolens*)
Sandalwood (*Santalum album*)
Chamomile roman (*Anthemis nobilis*)
Mandarin (*Citrus reticulata*)
Patchouli (*Pogostemon cablin*)
Petitgrain (*Citrus aurantium*)
Chamomile german (*Matricaria recutita*)
Lavender (*Lavandula officinalis*)
Rose otto (*Rosa damascena*)
Ho wood (*Cinnamomum camphora ct. linalool*)

SOOTHING ESSENTIAL OIL BATH BLEND FOR DRY SKIN

Rosewood	3 drops
Geranium	4 drops
Lavender	3 drops

First, blend the essential oils together, then dilute 4–5 drops in each teaspoon (5 mL) of carrier oil, or dried milk or buttermilk powder.

OILY SKIN: ESSENTIAL OILS FOR BATHS

Chamomile roman (*Anthemis nobilis*)
Ylang ylang (*Cananga odorata*)
Jasmine (*Jasminum grandiflorum/officinale*)
Orange, sweet (*Citrus sinensis*)
Petitgrain (*Citrus aurantium*)
Lemon (*Citrus limon*)
Lime (*Citrus aurantifolia*)
Lavender (*Lavandula angustifolia*)
Cypress (*Cupressus sempervirens*)
Clary sage (*Salvia sclarea*)
Grapefruit (*Citrus paradisi*)
Bergamot (*Citrus bergamia*)
Juniper berry (*Juniperus communis*)

BALANCING ESSENTIAL OIL BATH BLEND FOR OILY SKIN

Lemon	3 drops
Cypress	2 drops
Ylang ylang	5 drops

First, blend the essential oils together, then dilute 4–5 drops in each teaspoon (5 mL) of carrier oil, clay, seaweed, or dried milk powder.

BLEMISHED SKIN: ESSENTIAL OILS FOR BATHS
Niaouli (*Melaleuca quinquenervia*)
Chamomile roman (*Anthemis nobilis*)
Geranium (*Pelargonium graveolens*)
Clary sage (*Salvia sclarea*)
Chamomile german (*Matricaria recutita*)
Eucalyptus lemon (*Eucalyptus citriodora*)
Lavender (*Lavandula angustifolia*)
Ho wood (*Cinnamomum camphora ct. linalool*)
Palmarosa (*Cymbopogon martinii*)
Cypress (*Cupressus sempervirens*)
Cedarwood atlas (*Cedrus atlantica*)
Juniper berry (*Juniperus communis*)
Thyme linalol (*Thymus vulgaris ct. linalool*)

BALANCING ESSENTIAL OIL BATH BLEND
FOR BLEMISHED SKIN
Eucalyptus lemon	1 drop
Lavender	4 drops
Thyme linalol	2 drops
Chamomile roman	2 drops

First, blend the essential oils together, then dilute 4–5 drops in each teaspoon (5 mL) of carrier oil, adding Epsom salts or sea salt to the water.

Prebath Body Oils

Prebath body oils are treatment-based oils that are applied before getting in a bathtub, and they can be used for all manner of things — from relaxation to stimulation, increasing circulation, detoxification, toning the body, and soothing the skin. Although not that well known, this method of treatment is extremely effective and saves the necessity of applying body oil after a bath. Prebath oils have several advantages. Water is healing in its own right, and the essential oils already applied to the body will be inhaled directly, while a small amount is absorbed by the body — not only before getting in the bath but also when in the bathtub by osmosis. Body oils can be massaged into the skin after the bath too

if needed, which can complement the prebath oil. Apply the oil all over your body before stepping into the bath (this method does not have the same effect in a shower).

PREBATH BASE OIL
Almond oil, sweet	2 tablespoons (30 mL)
Jojoba oil	20 drops
Evening primrose seed oil	10 drops

DETOX PREBATH ESSENTIAL OIL BLEND 1
Lemon	2 drops
Spearmint	1 drop
Juniper berry	5 drops

Blend the essential oils together, then add 4–5 drops to each teaspoon (5 mL) of Prebath Base Oil or a light carrier oil such as sweet almond oil.

PROFESSIONAL DETOX PREBATH
ESSENTIAL OIL BLEND
Cypress	3 drops
Juniper berry	3 drops
Frankincense	2 drops
Immortelle	2 drops
Lemongrass	3 drops
Palmarosa	4 drops
Petitgrain	10 drops
Pine	2 drops
Thyme linalol	2 drops

Blend the essential oils together, then add 4–5 drops to each teaspoon (5 mL) of Prebath Base Oil or a light carrier oil such as sweet almond oil.

TONING PREBATH ESSENTIAL OIL BLEND
Ginger	2 drops
Lemongrass	4 drops
Black pepper	2 drops

Blend the essential oils together, then add 4–5 drops to each teaspoon (5 mL) of Prebath Base Oil or a light carrier oil such as sweet almond oil.

ANTICELLULITE PREBATH ESSENTIAL OIL BLEND

Grapefruit	2 drops
Cypress	2 drops
Cedarwood atlas	2 drops
Juniper berry	3 drops
Rosemary	2 drops

Blend the essential oils together, then add 4–5 drops to each teaspoon (5 mL) of Prebath Base Oil or a light carrier oil such as sweet almond oil.

REFINING PREBATH ESSENTIAL OIL BLEND

Geranium	2 drops
Orange, sweet	3 drops
Petitgrain	5 drops

Blend the essential oils together, then add 4–5 drops to each teaspoon (5 mL) of Prebath Base Oil or a light carrier oil such as sweet almond oil.

Deodorizing Body Oils

If you're prone to profuse and odorous perspiration there could be an underlying hormonal or physiological cause, but using a deodorizing body oil after a bath may help.

BODY DEODORIZING ESSENTIAL OILS

Peppermint (*Mentha piperita*)
Petitgrain (*Citrus aurantium*)
Clary sage (*Salvia sclarea*)
Eucalyptus peppermint (*Eucalyptus dives*)
Thyme linalol (*Thymus vulgaris ct. linalool*)
Palmarosa (*Cymbopogon martinii*)
Patchouli (*Pogostemon cablin*)
Cypress (*Cupressus sempervirens*)
Pine (*Pinus sylvestris*)
Cistus (*Cistus ladaniferus*)
Bergamot (*Citrus bergamia*)
Geranium (*Pelargonium graveolens*)
Mastic (*Pistacia lentiscus*)
Myrrh (*Commiphora myrrha*)
Coriander seed (*Coriandrum sativum*)

Choose from the oils listed above, or use the blend below, to make your own body oil. Use a small amount over the body after a bath or shower.

BODY DEODORIZING ESSENTIAL OIL BLEND

Clary sage	5 drops
Cypress	8 drops
Bergamot FCF	8 drops
Coriander seed	2 drops

Blend the essential oils together, then dilute 2–3 drops to each teaspoon (5 mL) of carrier oil; or dilute 2–3 drops per teaspoon of gel base. Use a small amount over the body after a bath or shower.

Dieters' Essential Helpmates

There are few people who have not at some time in their lives tried to lose weight. It's a struggle most of us can identify with. But there are some people who can eat mountains of food and stay slim, and others who just look at a muffin and put on three pounds. The scientist who figures out why human metabolisms vary so tremendously, and how to control them, will make a fortune! Until then, the message is simple: cut down on fat and sugar, eat good basic foods, drink a cup of ginger tea a day, and exercise.

There's no wonder-plant to circumvent these facts, but essential oils can certainly aid in the process of dieting by helping you avoid stretch marks and flabby skin, and massage is terrifically helpful in ridding the body of toxin debris that may have accumulated. Many of the body toning essential oils below also have a slight diuretic effect:

DIETERS' ESSENTIAL OILS

Cedarwood atlas (*Cedrus atlantica*)
Cypress (*Cupressus sempervirens*)
Orange, sweet (*Citrus sinensis*)
Ginger (*Zingiber officinale*)

Basil linalol (*Ocimum basilicum ct. linalool*)
Thyme linalol (*Thymus vulgaris ct. linalool*)
Lavender (*Lavandula angustifolia*)
Petitgrain (*Citrus aurantium*)
Grapefruit (*Citrus paradisi*)
Lime (*Citrus aurantifolia*)
Rosemary (*Rosmarinus officinalis*)
Lemongrass (*Cymbopogon citratus/flexuosus*)
Geranium (*Pelargonium graveolens*)
Lemon (*Citrus limon*)
Juniper berry (*Juniperus communis*)
Fennel, sweet (*Foeniculum vulgare var. dulce*)
Immortelle (*Helichrysum italicum*)
Spearmint (*Mentha spicata*)
Black pepper (*Piper nigrum*)
Coriander seed (*Coriandrum sativum*)

BATH OR PREBATH OILS FOR DIETERS

The following two blends can be used while trying to reduce weight and body mass. They're designed to be used in baths or in a prebath body oil.

ESSENTIAL OIL BLEND 1

Lavender	4 drops
Grapefruit	8 drops
Cypress	5 drops
Juniper berry	3 drops
Basil linalol	3 drops
Ginger	1 drop

Blend the essential oils together, then use 5 drops in 1 teaspoon (5 mL) of carrier oil, before adding to a bath, or use 4–5 drops per teaspoon (5 mL) of carrier oil for a prebath body oil.

ESSENTIAL OIL BLEND 2

Lemongrass	4 drops
Fennel, sweet	1 drop
Coriander seed	2 drops
Petitgrain	8 drops
Black pepper	4 drops

Blend the essential oils together, then use 5 drops in 1 teaspoon (5 mL) of carrier oil before adding to a bath, or use 4–5 drops per teaspoon (5 mL) of carrier oil for a prebath body oil.

TONING ESSENTIAL OIL BATHS

The following four bath blends are to help tone the body. Dilute the 5 drops of essential oil in 1 teaspoon (5 mL) of carrier oil, before adding it to the bathwater:

TONING BLEND 1

Grapefruit	3 drops
Basil linalol	2 drops

TONING BLEND 2

Rosemary	3 drops
Petitgrain	2 drops

TONING BLEND 3

Lemongrass	3 drops
Lavender	2 drops

TONING BLEND 4

Orange, sweet	3 drops
Thyme linalol	2 drops

GENERAL MASSAGE OILS FOR DIETERS

The following body massage oils can be used while trying to reduce weight and body mass. Add 30 drops of essential oil to 2 tablespoons (30 mL) of an organic carrier oil to which 10 drops of macerated carrot root oil have been added. Blend the carrier oil and carrot oil together before adding the essential oils. Use a small amount each time, concentrating on the areas of most concern.

ESSENTIAL OIL BLEND 1

Grapefruit	8 drops
Oregano	2 drops
Rosemary	10 drops
Cypress	10 drops

ESSENTIAL OIL BLEND 2

Petitgrain	10 drops
Lemon	5 drops
Juniper berry	10 drops
Black pepper	5 drops

TONING BODY MASSAGE OILS

The following body massage oils can be used while trying to tone the body. Add 30 drops of essential oil to 2 tablespoons (30 mL) of an organic carrier oil to which 10 drops of macerated carrot root oil have been added. Blend the carrier oil and carrot oil together before adding the essential oils. Use a small amount, concentrating on the areas of the body you feel require better tone.

TONING ESSENTIAL OIL BLEND 1

Basil linalol	5 drops
Lemongrass	5 drops
Cedarwood atlas	15 drops
Spearmint	5 drops

TONING ESSENTIAL OIL BLEND 2

Ginger	5 drops
Rosemary	10 drops
Orange, sweet	15 drops

MASSAGE OILS TO HELP REDUCE FLUID RETENTION

The following massage oils can be used on the body while trying to reduce fluid retention. Add 30 drops of essential oil to 2 tablespoons (30 mL) of organic sweet almond oil. Blend the essential oils together before diluting into the sweet almond oil. Apply the oil with light upward strokes: ankles and legs, toward the groin; arms toward the armpits; and clockwise circular movements around the abdomen.

ESSENTIAL OIL BLEND 1

Juniper berry	8 drops
Fennel, sweet	4 drops
Rosemary	6 drops
Grapefruit	12 drops

ESSENTIAL OIL BLEND 2

Cypress	15 drops
Lemon	10 drops
Juniper berry	5 drops

Lymphatic drainage massage helps reduce fluid retention and can assist during both general weight loss management and cellulite dispersal, but it's not easy to do without the help of a trained therapist. However, a mild form of this can be done at home by dry skin brushing or with water from a handheld shower. With the shower turned on cold to a comfortably high force (the cold contracts the blood vessels and lymph), use the impact of the water on your skin to massage up the inside of the leg, especially the thighs to the groin. Then move the water around your abdomen in clockwise circular movements, then up the inner arms to the armpit. Repeat as often as you can.

Cellulite

The characteristic sign of cellulite is puckering — dimples and nodules — in the skin, usually on the buttocks and thighs, although it can be found all over the body. Cellulite can develop for a variety of reasons and may have a genetic element. Circulation and lymphatic insufficiency are the most likely culprits, with hormonal issues, allergies, diet, and environmental toxins all playing a part.

Treatment to eliminate these unsightly fat deposits is not easy, and cellulite can always return if you have a predisposition to it. Many cases of cellulite can be reversed with no more than a change of diet, exercise, and an increased intake of vitamins and minerals. Ideally, cut out all processed and canned foods and anything that contains corn syrup or artificial sweeteners. Eat as many organic raw vegetables as possible, and cook plenty of leafy dark-green vegetables, such as kale. Use a juicer to make fresh vegetable drinks. Drink only pure mineral water — not tap water — and organic fruit juices or herb teas such as rosemary, nettle, or fennel. Drinking ginger and peppermint tea every day helps keep cellulite at bay. Take a teaspoon of fresh ginger and equal amounts of fresh peppermint leaves, pour just enough boiling water to cover the ginger and mint, and allow it to infuse for at least 10 minutes. Cover the cup with a saucer so the steam doesn't escape. You could also use frozen ginger and mint, if they come in their pure unadulterated forms. Cut down on dairy, wheat, and soy, as well as any fermented foods, including yeasts. Increase your vitamin C supplement and step up your zinc and vitamin B intake, and check supplements to make sure they're not derived from yeast.

A six-point plan of action:

1. Increase blood circulation by dry skin brushing. Using a brush made from real bristles, brush in gentle upward movements all over the body, as in the shower lymph drainage method.
2. Have an exercise plan that focuses specifically on the cellulite areas, as these are often the places that get no exercise.
3. Massage the whole body every day — not only the cellulite areas. Cellulite may show up only in certain areas, but essentially it's a whole-body problem.
4. While using essential oils in the bath, pinch and pummel cellulite areas to help break down the fatty deposits.
5. Simple as it sounds, oxygen is vital for a healthy body, so use yoga deep breathing techniques.
6. Relaxation is important for good body maintenance, while stress, on the other hand, can cause cellulite to linger, even after the stress has gone. So get plenty of sleep, and take up yoga, Pilates, tai chi, or qi gong.

ESSENTIAL OILS TO HELP REDUCE CELLULITE
Juniper berry (*Juniperus communis*)
Cypress (*Cupressus sempervirens*)
Thyme linalol (*Thymus vulgaris ct. linalool*)
Grapefruit (*Citrus paradisi*)
Rosemary (*Rosmarinus officinalis*)
Lemon (*Citrus limon*)
Sage (*Salvia officinalis*)
Cedarwood atlas (*Cedrus atlantica*)
Elemi (*Canarium luzonicum*)
Bay laurel (*Laurus nobilis*)
Basil linalol (*Ocimum basilicum ct. linalool*)
Fennel, sweet (*Foeniculum vulgare var. dulce*)
Patchouli (*Pogostemon cablin*)
Ginger (*Zingiber officinale*)
Black pepper (*Piper nigrum*)
Cistus (*Cistus ladaniferus*)
Mastic (*Pistacia lentiscus*)

ANTICELLULITE BATHS

Sea salt, Epsom salt (magnesium sulfate), and seaweed baths are often employed in spa cellulite treatments. If using at home, follow the proportions of 2 handfuls of Epsom salt to 1 handful of sea salt. Put in the bath with the water before the essential oils are added.

There are several bath blend options below because everyone's cellulite is different in that it has slightly different causes.

ESSENTIAL OIL BATH BLEND 1
Juniper berry	6 drops
Lemon	10 drops
Grapefruit	10 drops
Basil linalol	8 drops

Blend the essential oils together, then dilute 5 drops to each teaspoon (5 mL) of carrier oil before adding to the bath. While in the bath, if any oil is floating on the surface, scoop it up and massage into the cellulite-affected areas.

The following four anticellulite bath blends can be made up in larger quantities for future use — just keep to these proportions. The amounts here are sufficient for two baths. In either case, use 6 drops per bath, diluted in 1 teaspoon of carrier oil:

ESSENTIAL OIL BATH BLEND 2
Thyme linalol	8 drops
Lemon	4 drops

ESSENTIAL OIL BATH BLEND 3
Clary sage	8 drops
Patchouli	4 drops

ESSENTIAL OIL BATH BLEND 4
Rosemary	6 drops
Juniper berry	6 drops

ESSENTIAL OIL BATH BLEND 5
Juniper berry	6 drops
Lemon	6 drops

ANTICELLULITE MASSAGE OIL BLENDS

The following body massage oil blends are diluted by adding them to 2 tablespoons (30 mL) of sweet almond oil, 1 teaspoon (5 mL) of carrot root macerated oil, 1 teaspoon (5 mL) of macerated gotu kola (*Centella asiatica*) oil, and 1 teaspoon (5 mL) of jojoba oil. Blend these 45 mL of carrier oil together well before adding the essential oils. If you only have sweet almond oil, make sure it's organic.

People's bodies respond differently to both single essential oils and blends, depending on their physical constitution, and this is why most often a choice of options is provided.

ANTICELLULITE MASSAGE OIL BLEND 1
Juniper berry	12 drops
Lemon	5 drops
Geranium	6 drops
Cypress	7 drops

Blend the essential oils together, dilute in 45 mL of carrier oil, and apply enough to cover the areas of most concern on the body, before sleep.

ANTICELLULITE MASSAGE OIL BLEND 2
Rosemary	8 drops
Grapefruit	11 drops
Ginger	4 drops
Black pepper	3 drops
Elemi	4 drops

Blend the essential oils together, dilute in 45 mL of carrier oil, and apply enough to cover the areas of most concern on the body, before sleep.

ANTICELLULITE MASSAGE OIL BLEND 3
Basil linalol	8 drops
Thyme linalol	6 drops
Grapefruit	10 drops
Juniper berry	4 drops
Geranium	2 drops

Blend the essential oils together, dilute in 45 mL of carrier oil, and apply enough to cover the areas of most concern on the body, before sleep.

The full anticellulite program is as follows: Before bathing, brush the skin as described in point 1 of the anticellulite plan of action above. Baths should be taken once a day using one of the blends in warm to hot water. Afterward use the cold shower lymph drainage system as described above. Massage over the areas of cellulite with one of the massage blends, before exercise and before sleeping. Avoid exposing to direct sunlight areas where a blend containing a citrus oil has been applied.

Arms

As a consequence of weight loss or aging, the upper arms can become prone to sagging. Cellulite also tends to affect this area. Sensible arm exercise helps keep the arms toned and firm. The undersides of the upper arms benefit from dry skin brushing, which should be carried out upward toward the armpit, before applying the arm blend oil below:

Essential Oil Arm Blend

Cypress	5 drops
Lavender	8 drops
Ginger	5 drops
Black pepper	2 drops
Juniper berry	7 drops
Carrot seed	3 drops
Spearmint	2 drops

First, blend the essential oils together. Then, to make a massage oil, dilute 5 drops in each teaspoon (5 mL) of carrier oil; to make an upper arm splash or spritz, use 8 drops in a bottle containing 2 teaspoons (10 mL) of vegetable glycerin and 3 fl. oz. (90 mL) of water.

Hold one arm straight in the air above your head and with the other hand massage firmly toward the armpit. Do this at least 10 times with each arm. Now repeat the whole procedure but this time using a washcloth that's been soaked in the essential oil and water splash. Dry, then massage the whole of one arm toward the armpit, and repeat with the other arm, using the essential oil blend, as described above. Avoid getting oil in the armpit area.

Hands

Our hands are like our faces — always on show. There's no hiding them behind fabulous clothing unless we wear gloves all day, and that just isn't going to happen. Our hands work tirelessly to get us through life. And even though we know that rubber gloves should be worn to protect them when carrying out wet or dirty jobs, how many of us forget? I have my hand up, for one!

Thankfully, essential oils and some plant oils can help to keep hands looking their best. If you have a favorite hand cream, you could simply blend the essential oils or plant oils into that. It's simple to make your own hand balms and oils from scratch, but don't be surprised if you find that you're supplying the whole family — essential oil hand creams tend to disappear very quickly!

Essential Oils for Hands
Rose otto (*Rosa damascena*)
Rosemary (*Rosmarinus officinalis*)
Geranium (*Pelargonium graveolens*)
Lemon (*Citrus limon*)
Sandalwood (*Santalum album*)
Lime (*Citrus aurantifolia*)
Patchouli (*Pogostemon cablin*)
Carrot seed (*Daucus carota*)
Lavender (*Lavandula angustifolia*)
Neroli (*Citrus aurantium*)

Essential Oils for Dry Hands
Rose otto (*Rosa damascena*)
Patchouli (*Pogostemon cablin*)
Geranium (*Pelargonium graveolens*)
Carrot seed (*Daucus carota*)
Sandalwood (*Santalum album*)
Ho wood (*Cinnamomum camphora ct. linalool*)

Essential Oils for Neglected Hands
Rose otto (*Rosa damascena*)
Geranium (*Pelargonium graveolens*)
Neroli (*Citrus aurantium*)
Patchouli (*Pogostemon cablin*)
Lemon (*Citrus limon*)
Sandalwood (*Santalum album*)

BASIC HAND BUTTER BALM

Cocoa butter	½ oz. (14 g)
Jojoba oil	2 tablespoons (30 mL)
Almond oil, sweet	2 teaspoons (10 mL)
Beeswax	½ oz. (14 g)
Evening primrose seed oil	10 drops
Carrot root macerated oil	10 drops
Essential oil of your choice	10 drops

Melt the cocoa butter and the beeswax in a double boiler or bain-marie, then add the jojoba oil, evening primrose seed oil, and carrot oil. You now have a basic hand balm that can be made thinner by adding more sweet almond oil, or thicker by putting in less jojoba or almond oil. Finally, add the essential oils of your choice. Balms are oily, so you only need to use a very small amount on your hands and nails. The butter balm can be amended to suit personal requirements. For example, 2 teaspoons (10 mL) of the jojoba oil can be substituted with tamanu oil if the hands are particularly sore and irritated, or with avocado oil if you want something more nourishing.

In the oil blend below, monoi and coconut oils are solid oils that melt in warmth.

LUXURIOUS HAND AND NAIL OIL

Macadamia oil	2 teaspoons (10 mL)
Camellia seed oil	2 teaspoons (10 mL)
Monoi oil (or coconut oil)	2 teaspoons (10 mL)
Jojoba oil	1 teaspoon (5 mL)
Evening primrose seed oil	20 drops

Blend these oils together well, then add the essential oils:

Rose otto (or jasmine)	3 drops
Geranium	1 drop
Lemon	1 drop
Sandalwood	2 drops

As this is an oil, not a cream or balm, you only need a drop or two to cover both hands. Rub it into the cuticles, and use before going to sleep. If you've poured out more than you need, use it to rub into the elbows and arms.

SORE AND IRRITATED HANDS

Hands are exposed to all manner of germs in the form of bacteria, viruses, and fungi. The hands are also sensitive to long-term bouts of stress, which may show up as excessive dryness, eczema, or psoriasis. The following plant oils can be used to counteract the soreness and irritation hands can feel at times, and they can be incorporated into your favorite hand cream or used on their own at night.

Contact dermatitis — localized inflammation that occurs when the skin reacts to irritants — is becoming more common. This could be due to many factors, including people becoming more sensitive to the environment around them. If you have contact dermatitis it's best to avoid using most essential oils at this time.

PLANT OILS FOR SORE AND IRRITATED HANDS

Tamanu (*Calophyllum inophyllum*)
Sea buckthorn (*Hippophae rhamnoides*)
Cucumber seed (*Cucumis sativus*)
Black cumin seed (*Nigella sativa*)
Plum kernel (*Prunus domestica*)
Olive squalane (*Olea europaea*)
Andiroba (*Carapa guianensis*)
Castor (*Ricinus cummunis*)

Use the plant oils above singly, or in combination, up to a minimum of 25% when incorporated into an oil, cream, or balm. It really is a matter of trial and error as each person will have a different response to each oil. However, the following seems to help most people:

PLANT OIL BLEND FOR SORE AND IRRITATED HANDS

Camellia seed oil	2 tablespoons (30 mL)
Tamanu oil	1 tablespoon (15 mL)
Andiroba oil	1 teaspoon (5 mL)
*Sea buckthorn oil	½ teaspoon (2½ mL)

Sea buckthorn oil can stain clothes and skin.

Blend all the oils together, and massage a small amount into the hands — at night or after any activity that seems to irritate the skin. The oil can be used under a pair of white fine cotton gloves for nighttime use, or in the day if required.

Nails

If you go to a traditional doctor in China or India, he or she will examine your nails to see if they're fragile, flat, deformed, too soft, too big, too thick, have depressed grooves or horizontal threads, or are too white or yellow. And this is just the beginning of the nail analysis that forms part of their diagnosis of a person's health condition. To some extent, then, nails, like hair, are an outward sign of what's going on inside the body. Having said that, there's still a lot we can do to improve the condition of our nails.

ESSENTIAL OILS TO STIMULATE STRONG HEALTHY NAIL GROWTH

Lemon (*Citrus limon*)
Lavender (*Lavandula angustifolia*)
Grapefruit (*Citrus paradisi*)
Cypress (*Cupressus sempervirens*)
Cistus (*Cistus ladaniferus*)
Rosemary (*Rosmarinus officinalis*)
Geranium (*Pelargonium graveolens*)
Ylang ylang (*Cananga odorata*)
Orange, sweet (*Citrus sinensis*)
Clary sage (*Salvia sclarea*)

PLANT OILS FOR NAILS

Jojoba (*Simmondsia chinensis*)
Evening primrose seed (*Oenothera biennis*)

Borage seed (*Borago officinalis*)
Carrot root, macerated (*Daucus carota*)
Moringa (*Moringa oleifera*)
Baobab (*Adansonia digitata*)
Andiroba (*Carapa guianensis*)
Rice bran (*Oryza sativa*)
Olive squalane (*Olea europaea*)
Ungurahui (pataua) (*Oenocarpus bataua*)
Apricot kernel (*Prunus armeniaca*)
Avocado (*Persea americana*)
Argan (*Argania spinosa*)
Rosehip seed (*Rosa rubiginosa*)

NAIL STRENGTHENER BLEND

Rice bran oil	2 teaspoons (10 mL)
Jojoba oil	1 teaspoon (5 mL)
Evening primrose seed oil	10 drops
Moringa oil	1 teaspoon (5 mL)
Lemon essential oil	8 drops
Rosemary essential oil	2 drops

CUTICLE SOFTENER

Jojoba oil	10 drops
Camellia seed oil	5 drops
Olive squalane oil	10 drops
Ho wood essential oil	2 drops

Massage well into the cuticle. If you're unfortunate enough to have a fungal infection of the nails, replace the 2 drops of the ho wood essential oil in the blend with all 5 drops of essential oil in the blend below:

Lavender	2 drops
Oregano	1 drop
Tea tree	2 drops

ESSENTIAL OILS TO TREAT NAIL INFECTIONS

Tea tree (*Melaleuca alternifolia*)
Thyme linalol (*Thymus vulgaris ct. linalool*)
Eucalyptus radiata (*Eucalyptus radiata*)
Ravensara (*Ravensara aromatica*)
Myrrh (*Commiphora myrrha*)
Lavender (*Lavandula angustifolia*)

Patchouli (*Pogostemon cablin*)
Oregano (*Origanum vulgare*)
Ravintsara (*Cinnamomum camphora ct. cineole*)
Saro (*Cinnamosma fragrans*)
Manuka (*Leptospermum scoparium*)
Clove bud (*Syzygium aromaticum*)
Lemongrass (*Cymbopogon citratus/flexuosus*)
Cinnamon leaf (*Cinnamomum zeylanicum*)

GENERAL NAIL INFECTION ESSENTIAL OIL BLEND
Tea tree   10 drops
Eucalyptus radiata   5 drops
Manuka   10 drops

Blend the essential oils together, then dilute in 2 tablespoons (30 mL) of tamanu or gotu kola (*Centella asiatica*) oil. Apply around the nail bed three times a day. Massage in well.

ONYCHIA

Onychia is an inflammation of the nail bed caused by, for example, the hands being in water and detergent for long periods of time. Treat as for nail infection above, but add 10 drops of chamomile german and 5 drops of lavender essential oil to the General Nail Infection Essential Oil Blend.

Feet

Our faithful feet carry us around, day after day, not asking for anything. It's we who subject *them* to unnatural contortions caused by fashionable shoes and sporting activities, not to mention what the classical ballet dancer's feet go through, balancing on their toes. It's only when our feet begin to hurt that we look down and notice them. And feet are very modest. They are constantly at work, keeping our bodies balanced and out of harm's way.

Reflexology is a diagnostic and treatment system that works entirely by "reading" and manipulating the reflex points on the feet. In acupuncture there are at least 30 acupoints on the soles of the feet. Feet love nothing more than walking barefoot on soft grass and moss, or along a sandy beach, or being dangled in the lapping water of a lake. They want to be free! And their freedom allows a discharge of static electrical energy from us to the ground. Feet literally ground us. They are so important to us and do such a good job — they deserve a treat. First, though, let's deal with the hardened skin.

HARDENED SKIN

Hard skin that's allowed to build up on areas of the feet that are under the most pressure, such as the heels, sides of the feet, or under the toes, can cause discomfort and should be tackled as soon as the skin starts to harden. Or, better still, prevention may stop it from appearing at all. Pumice stone, in its natural volcanic rock form rather than the concrete copies, is one of the best methods to remove hardened skin, and all manner of devices are available. But exfoliating agents can prevent the buildup from occurring in the first place.

EXFOLIATION AGENTS
Pumice powder
Loofah granules
Bamboo powder
Coffee granules (use spent coffee granules that have cooled and dried)
Large brown sugar crystals
Large salt crystals: Dead Sea salt, sea salt, Himalayan pink salt

FOOT SPA TREATMENT RITUAL

1. Soak the feet in a bowl of warm water that has small round pebbles placed in the bottom — add sea salt, herbs, essential oils.
2. While the feet are soaking, roll the soles of the feet over the pebbles.

3. Dry the feet, then take an exfoliating agent and rub over the whole of the foot, paying particular attention to the areas of foot pressure where hard skin is likely to develop, such as the heels, sides of the feet, and under the toes.

4. Put the feet back into the bowl of water and soak or wash off the exfoliating agent and dead skin.

5. Apply a foot mask made from clays that are either detoxifying or soothing — such as pink, white, or green clay — to help aching or sore rheumatic conditions.

6. After 10 minutes, rinse off the clay foot mask and dry the feet.

7. Massage the feet with a cream, oil, or gel containing essential oil appropriate to the purpose of the spa treatment.

ESSENTIAL OILS FOR FEET

Lemongrass, peppermint, spearmint, rosemary, basil linalol, and grapefruit: Refreshing oils — great before a party or after a long day standing at work or walking; dilute the peppermint or spearmint in equal parts of a carrier oil if adding to a foot bath

Lavender, chamomile roman, juniper berry, sweet orange, peppermint, and cypress: Helpful for swollen feet and ankles — used alone or mixed in equal parts

Geranium: Strengthens the skin and improves elasticity; may help prevent blistering and improve circulation in the feet

PLANT OILS FOR FEET

Calendula oil and *carrot root macerated oil: Help to smooth and soften hard skin and corns
*May cause staining to clothing or skin

GENERAL PUMICE STONE HARD SKIN
PREVENTATIVE

Sea or rock salt	1 tablespoon (15 g)
Epsom salts	1 tablespoon (15 g)
Jojoba oil	1 teaspoon (5 mL)
Calendula oil (or arnica oil or comfrey macerated oil*)	1 teaspoon (5 mL)

*Especially if the feet are aching

Rub a pumice stone all over the foot, paying particular attention to the sides of the feet, the ball, and the heel. Then rub salt all over the foot, massaging it in well. Rinse off the salt and dead skin. Finally, massage with essential oil blended in the plant oils — again, rubbing it in well. If you already have a heavy buildup of dead skin, ask a chiropodist to remove it for you and then follow the treatment above.

SPECIAL FOOT TREATMENT

All feet will benefit from a soak in a bowl of warm water in which a dozen or so small, round pebbles have been placed, along with a tablespoon of salt and 4 drops of your favorite essential oil. You can inhale the aroma while rolling the soles of your feet back and forth over the pebbles, which should cover most of the reflexology points on the soles of the feet. Do it slowly — and enjoy it. After dabbing dry, massage the following oil well into the whole of the foot, taking time to massage the toes:

SPECIAL FOOT TREATMENT ESSENTIAL OIL BLEND

Palmarosa	6 drops
Lemon	4 drops
Thyme linalol	1 drop
Geranium	3 drops
Ylang ylang	2 drops

First blend the essential oil together, then dilute 5 drops in 1 teaspoon (5 mL) of jojoba oil. A few special treatments are all you'll need to get your neglected feet back into party shape.

TABLE 15. BEAUTY BODY OILS

ESSENTIAL OIL	SKIN TYPE				
	Normal	Dry	Sensitive	Oily	Blemished
Benzoin		★			
Bergamot	★			★	★
Carrot seed	★	★			
Chamomile german	★	★	★		★
Chamomile roman	★	★	★	★	★
Clary sage	★	★		★	★
Cypress	★			★	★
Eucalyptus lemon	★			★	★
Frankincense	★	★		★	★
Geranium	★	★		★	★
Ho wood	★	★		★	★
Jasmine	★	★		★	
Juniper berry	★			★	★
Lavender	★	★	★	★	★
Lemon	★			★	★
Mandarin	★	★	★		
Myrrh				★	★
Neroli	★	★		★	
Niaouli	★			★	★
Nutmeg	★			★	
Orange, sweet	★			★	★
Palmarosa	★			★	★
Patchouli	★	★			
Petitgrain	★	★		★	
Rose otto	★	★			
Rosewood	★	★		★	
Sandalwood	★	★			
Thyme linalol				★	★
Ylang ylang	★			★	

TABLE 16. TONING/SLIMMING OILS

ESSENTIAL OIL	APPLICATION IN SKIN CARE		
	General Toning	Diuretic	For Cellulite
Basil	★		★
Carrot seed	★		
Cedarwood atlas			★
Clary sage	★		
Coriander seed	★		★
Cypress	★	★	★
Fennel, sweet		★	★
Ginger	★		★
Grapefruit	★	★	★
Juniper berry	★	★	★
Lavender	★		
Lemon	★	★	★
Lemongrass	★		★
Lime	★		★
Orange, sweet	★		★
Oregano		★	★
Palmarosa	★		
Patchouli	★		★
Pepper, black	★		★
Peppermint	★		★
Petitgrain	★		
Rosemary	★		★
Spearmint	★		★
Thyme	★		★

15

Fragrant Care for Your Home

Welcome to the fragrant home! You can now throw out all those chemical home products and replace them with the natural alternative, the one that smells fabulous. The home will feel so positive and delightful, you'll be keen to spend more time in it — creating natural home fragrances and perfumes and a whole range of other aromatic delights.

We all know that the average human body now carries a heavy chemical "body burden" accumulated over a lifetime of exposure to synthetic chemicals in the air, water, food, personal care products, furniture "off gas," and a whole lot more. Much of this we can do little about. We have to work in environments adrift with volatile organic chemicals, drive down highways awash with invisible particulates, fly in planes saturated in flame-retardant chemicals, and eat food that's been grown and processed using who knows what. We're helpless to a large extent, just flotsam in the polluted sea of environmental toxins, but when we land back at home, there's very much we can do to ensure our home is an oasis of pure nature by using essential oils.

When I first wrote about putting essential oils in dish soap 25 years ago, people thought I was nuts! These days so-called aromatherapy dish soaps are on every supermarket shelf, but while they may have the word *aroma*, they certainly don't include essential oils — and so they don't have therapy. By using real, natural essential oils, however, you get the real deal.

There are hundreds of ways to use essential oils to enhance the home experience. Some of the methods outlined in this chapter are just for fun and pleasure, while others aim to reduce the need for chemical use in the home. Each essential oil has a different life span, with the citrus oils, in general, having a shorter span, while oils like cinnamon, clove, thyme, and oregano can maintain their therapeutic values for much longer. Clearly, if essential oils are being used on the skin or by inhalation for healing purposes, they need to be in date, but for many household jobs, the aroma is the important thing and out-of-date essential oils can be used. For example, for keeping moths away from clothes, an old lavender oil that you would not use for medical conditions will work well because it's the aroma that deters the insect. And for room fragrances, again, older essential oils could be used. But if you want the dish soap to lift you from depression, better use an oil that can still do that job!

Air Fresheners or Bespoke Perfume Designs?

There are three ways to look at home fragrance. One: essential oils can be used in all the usual room diffusion methods to deodorize unwanted aromas, combat bacterial or viral infection in the atmosphere, or lift the mood when people are upset or depressed. Two: essential oils can be formulated into bespoke perfume designs, appropriate to each room, for each season of the year, or to highlight a particular celebration. Three: do both at the same time.

The potential is enormous. Think of the permutations. Your teenage daughter has just broken up with her boyfriend but she's in the middle of her exams, so you design an aroma that will lift her from the unhappy state she's in and, at the same time, help her focus on her studies. Another day, another problem: your sister's staying over and she's been cooking cabbage soup — the house smells horrible! You make up a fabulous concoction of citrus fruit aromas and spray the whole place. Another day: the boys are back from playing football and they've thrown their shoes in the hallway, which is now permeated with the aroma of, well, feet. You make up a deodorizing blend and spray the whole area — just in time because you can see the visitors approaching the front door. Phew! That was a close one. Another day: your partner's coming back from a trip tonight and you want your reunion to be special. You make up a romantic blend of essential oils, spray them around the house — especially the bedroom — and wait to see what happens.

Some of the most exclusive boutique hotels in the world employ perfume designers to create subtle bespoke aromas that are used in diffusers in the luxury rooms, or put through the air conditioning system. The fragrances are changed seasonally. Chains of hotels have special "brand" aromas that are put in all their establishments to make their regular clients feel at home, wherever in the world they happen to be. Organizations spend a great deal of money on aroma signatures to create a great ambience, and this is something anyone can do in their own home, using essential oils.

Essential oils can be used in any of the room methods, including the plant-mister method: use about 10–20 drops to 2½ cups (600 mL) of water and spray as finely as possible into the air. Spraying water on fine fabrics such as velvet or silk and on polished wood and other vulnerable furniture should be avoided, as water stains could occur. By sheer force of gravity carpets will receive the aroma molecules. There's usually one room in the house that gets the brunt of breakfast's burned toast, and it would be a nice idea to keep a mister permanently there so there's an alternative to opening the windows every time there's an aroma leak from the kitchen.

Diffusers are an extremely easy and effective way of fragrancing. A bowl of hot water with drops of essential oil floating on top can leave a lingering scent all over the room. A cotton ball or tissue with 1 or 2 drops of essential oil can be tucked behind a radiator in winter, or put as many drops as you like in a nonelectric humidifier that's filled with water and hung on a radiator. Keeping the door shut will keep the fragrance in the room, and keeping it open will allow the fragrance to spread to other areas. Prepare the room method with the door closed, then leave the room and re-enter a couple of minutes later so the true level of aroma in the room can be judged; if a more heightened fragrance experience is required, just add more drops to whatever method is being used. Less is more when using essential oils in room fragrances — a delicate aroma is far better, especially as natural essential oils do have a psychological effect and can be tailored to the home environmental image you'd like to project. See the "Methods of Use" section in chapter 1 for further information.

Essential oils are flammable, which means that although you must be careful using them near flames, a log fire can be turned into an aromatic event. Use cypress, pine, sandalwood, or cedarwood and simply put 1 drop onto each log at least an hour before placing it on the fire.

Hallways

The unique aroma fingerprint of any home is experienced most keenly right by the front door, where it greets family and visitors alike. Hallways very often have no windows, so they easily accumulate the aromas coming from every room. As we live in the home all the time, we're seldom aware of the particular aroma fingerprint that greets visitors because a kind of home-aroma anosmia occurs — we're so used to the smell, we don't notice there's one at all. Changing this invisible aroma to a fresh and delightful one may take a little while to accomplish as layers of natural fragrance are laid, one upon the other, over a period of time. But you will notice the difference, as will your family arriving home from the polluted world outside, while regular visitors will be the first to know that something has changed.

Hallways are often neglected: we might put a scented candle in the living room, but do we think of placing anything scented in the hall? Hallways need something pleasant and fresh, rather than the spice and herb aromas of the kitchen or the more heavily scented oils we might use elsewhere. The citrus oils of lemon, lime, bergamot, and grapefruit are particular favorites for the hall, giving the impression of a clean, fresh, environment. Citrus aromas are uplifting at any time of the day but perhaps especially appealing in the morning, when there's so much to do. Blends with geranium, clary sage, and orange might be preferable in the afternoon when things are calming down. Geranium is always a good choice, blending well with just about anything, and when combined with a citrus oil such as lemon it makes guests feel good even before they've sat down. Lavender, on the other hand, is best before bedtime.

If someone in the house has a cold or flu, add 2 or 3 drops of either rosemary or niaouli to a citrus base. Using a total of 15 drops of essential oil in ½ pint (240 mL) of water in a plant mister (one reserved for essential oil use only) will keep the hallway fresh for several hours — even if the aroma seems imperceptible to you, it's there.

Hallways take a lot of traffic and are very prone to gathering dust and scuff marks. Washing down paintwork is a job made more enticing by the uplifting aromas of the essential oils — and it is helped along by knowing they're performing antiseptic, disinfectant, and other useful roles. Add 1 drop of essential oil to 2 teaspoons of white vinegar to disperse the essential oil before adding to the bucket or bowl of water used to wipe down the paintwork. The aroma of the vinegar will soon evaporate, leaving a freshness provided by the essential oils. The choice of oil(s) could be matched with those used in the air freshener spray.

Try to coordinate the choice of oils not only with the time of the day and occasion, but also with the season of the year. In summer use a light, refreshing essential oil or blend, adding in some of the oils that deter insects. In winter, use those essential oils that provide a warm and comforting glow. For example:

SPRING/SUMMER
Lime (*Citrus aurantifolia*)
Petitgrain (*Citrus aurantium*)
Lemon (*Citrus limon*)
Lavender (*Lavandula angustifolia*)
Geranium (*Pelargonium graveolens*)
Grapefruit (*Citrus paradisi*)

Ginger lily root (*Hedychium spicatum*)
Magnolia leaf (*Michelia alba*)
Spearmint (*Mentha spicata*)
Rosemary (*Rosmarinus officinalis*)
Basil (*Ocimum basilicum*)
Citronella (*Cymbopogon nardus*)
Lemongrass (*Cymbopogon citratus/flexuosus*)
May chang (*Litsea cubeba*)
Cypress (*Cupressus sempervirens*)
Bergamot (*Citrus bergamia*)

AUTUMN/WINTER
Orange, sweet (*Citrus sinensis*)
Ho wood (*Cinnamomum camphora ct. linalool*)
Benzoin (*Styrax benzoin*)
Clove (*Syzygium aromaticum*)
Nutmeg (*Myristica fragrans*)
Cinnamon (*Cinnamomum zeylanicum*)
Mandarin (*Citrus reticulata*)
Vanilla (*Vanilla plantifolia*)
Cedarwood atlas (*Cedrus atlantica*)
Bergamot (*Citrus bergamia*)
Tangerine (*Citrus reticulata*)
Frankincense (*Boswellia carterii*)
Ginger (*Zingiber officinale*)
Patchouli (*Pogostemon cablin*)

The following basic blends provide evocative fragrances that can be either used on their own or used as a base blend to which other essential oils can be added. For example, add a drop of spearmint to the spring/summer blend, and clove or cinnamon to the autumn/winter blend.

SPRING/SUMMER BLEND

Lemon	5 drops
Geranium	6 drops
Petitgrain	4 drops
May chang	5 drops

AUTUMN/WINTER BLEND

Orange, sweet	8 drops
Frankincense	3 drops
Benzoin	3 drops
Geranium	4 drops

Microbe Busters

Micro-organisms come in many forms, none of which are welcome in the home. Given that plants have had to deal with them throughout their evolutionary history, it's hardly surprising that some have developed an effective way of dealing with these tiny enemies — in the form of volatile aroma compounds, essential oils. These are particularly useful in microbe-busting room sprays, but most essential oils are antiseptic, and good mixers too.

Whichever method is used, essential oils can offer a degree of protection from microbes, while also making the home smell delightful. The essential oils listed below have a variety of antimicrobial properties and are included here because they're easily available and reasonably priced.

MICROBE BUSTERS
Cinnamon (*Cinnamomum zeylanicum*)
Pine (*Pinus sylvestris*)
Oregano (*Origanum vulgare*)
Saro (mandravasarotra) (*Cinnamosma fragrans*)
Clove bud (*Syzygium aromaticum*)
Niaouli (*Melaleuca quinquenervia*)
Lemon (*Citrus limon*)
Thyme (*Thymus vulgaris*)
Eucalyptus radiata (*Eucalyptus radiata*)
Grapefruit (*Citrus paradisi*)
Lavender (*Lavandula angustifolia*)
Lime (*Citrus aurantifolia*)
Bergamot (*Citrus bergamia*)
Tea tree (*Melaleuca alternifolia*)
Manuka (*Leptospermum scoparium*)
Palmarosa (*Cymbopogon martinii*)
Lemongrass (*Cymbopogon citratus/flexuosus*)
Geranium (*Pelargonium graveolens*)

Bay laurel (*Laurus nobilis*)
Clary sage (*Salvia sclarea*)

Although essential oils have a limited life in terms of their clinical use, their aroma quality lasts much longer, and in the case of eucalyptus, for example, its disinfectant qualities may actually improve with its age. This is why out-of-date essential oils need never go to waste. If you have some that are no longer suitable for health purposes or for incorporation into body or skin care formulations, keep them by the sink in the kitchen or bathroom and use 1 or 2 drops in the water used to wipe down surfaces.

It's great to have people over, but microbes love company as much as we do. It gives them a chance to spread out and multiply. And the trouble is, someone coming to our home might be carrying a little microbe or two with them, especially during flu season. This potential difficulty can be dealt with by using a blend made from the Microbe Busters essential oils list in one of the room methods. Nobody need know they're being protected from germs because the essential oils smell so very pleasant. The guests can just carry on enjoying themselves, oblivious to the realistic precautionary measures taken on their behalf. The Party Blend gives a terrific aroma while working hard to ensure that your guests have a safe and happy time:

THE BACTERIA BUSTERS PARTY BLEND

Lemon	3 drops
Bergamot	5 drops
Cinnamon	1 drop
Clary sage	1 drop
Geranium	5 drops

There are many possible combinations, but for Christmas parties try equal parts of cinnamon, clove, lemon, and orange. This provides the appropriate seasonal aroma while creating a flu-free zone in the home. Use 2–4 drops of the protective essential oil blend in any of the room methods, or 8 drops in a plant mister before the guests arrive. It can also be used when wiping around or cleaning the bathroom and toilet. This avoids the smell of disinfectant during party time while providing effective action against microbes.

Bathrooms can be kept hygienic and fresh smelling for the duration of the party if a box of essential oil paper tissues has been prepared, along with a little note asking guests to wipe the sink when they leave, as a courtesy to the next user. Place 10 drops of essential oil in different places throughout the box of tissues, and seal the box overnight so the aroma molecules can permeate all the tissues. Often in aromatherapy clinics and training schools, I've seen a small bottle of pre-blended essential oil left by the toilet to help eliminate smells. A simple drop of essential oil into the toilet bowl leaves a pleasant aroma, and you avoid the use of a chemical spray.

The Kitchen

The kitchen is probably the most odorous room in the house — some smells being fabulous, like homemade bread, and some being not so nice, like those from the garbage can. Essential oils are about cleansing and refreshing the air, rather than merely masking bad smells, and are best used after having opened the window for a while. In a kitchen without a window, essential oils are doubly valuable. Another huge advantage to using essential oils in the kitchen is that when used correctly, they're harmless. Indeed, many essential oils are used as preservatives in food, and rosemary and thyme, for example, can help prevent molds or other fungi. However, not all essential oils are suitable in the kitchen, and in any event, it's best to avoid spraying the kitchen when uncovered food has been left out.

During cooking, tiny molecules are released

into the atmosphere. Whether from vegetables, fish, or meat, these molecules carry the aromatic echo of the foods being cooked. What's needed afterward are natural fragrant molecules capable of attaching to, and deodorizing, the food molecules, leaving the atmosphere of the kitchen as fresh and as appetizing as the food prepared there. The following oils make excellent ingredients for kitchen air sprays, either used on their own or in combinations:

KITCHEN AIR SPRAY ESSENTIAL OILS
Rosemary (*Rosmarinus officinalis*)
Lemongrass (*Cymbopogon citratus/flexuosus*)
Lemon (*Citrus limon*)
Lime (*Citrus aurantifolia*)
Citronella (*Cymbopogon nardus*)
Grapefruit (*Citrus paradisi*)
Thyme (*Thymus vulgaris*)
Basil (*Ocimum basilicum*)
Oregano (*Origanum vulgare*)
Marjoram, sweet (*Origanum majorana*)
Peppermint (*Mentha piperita*)

KITCHEN BLEND
Marjoram, sweet	3 drops
Basil	4 drops
Rosemary	4 drops
Oregano	4 drops
Thyme	3 drops
Peppermint	2 drops
Lemon	15 drops

This blend can be used in all the usual room methods, or added to water to wipe down surfaces. Blend in these proportions and save for future use.

When washing out the fridge or freezer, prepare a final rinse water by adding 1 drop of essential oil to 1 teaspoon (5 mL) of white vinegar and 1 teaspoon (5 g) of bicarbonate of soda. You could try a citrus fruit essential oil such as lemon, lime, grapefruit, bergamot, mandarin, tangerine, or orange. The vinegar aroma will soon evaporate, leaving the appliance deodorized yet not permeated with the essential oil aroma. The aromas of the herb oils, on the other hand, are too powerful to use in this way.

Colloidal silver and grapefruit seed extract are interesting alternatives to commercial antibacterial surface sprays — follow the instructions that come with them. They can also be added to an essential oil kitchen surface wipe, and to air sprays. Work surfaces are made of a variety of materials, but in general avoid using essential oils neat or undiluted on them, so as to avoid any potential damage. When wiping down cupboards, sinks, tiles, or paintwork, use one of the following essential oils on their own, or in a blend. First, dilute the essential oil in a little white vinegar to help disperse the globules before adding to the bowl of water:

FOR WASHING KITCHEN SURFACES
Eucalyptus (*Eucalyptus radiata/globulus*)
Pine (*Pinus sylvestris*)
Lavender (*Lavandula angustifolia*)
Cypress (*Cupressus sempervirens*)
Lemon (*Citrus limon*)
Lemongrass (*Cymbopogon citratus/flexuosus*)
Lime (*Citrus aurantifolia*)
Thyme (*Thymus vulgaris*)
Grapefruit (*Citrus paradisi*)
Palmarosa (*Cymbopogon martinii*)
Oregano (*Origanum vulgare*)
Rosemary (*Rosmarinus officinalis*)

Bergamot is just one of several oils that could be added to the above list, and it has the added advantage of being an antidepressant...which brings us to washing the floor! This job can be made a little more pleasant by using any of the above: 2–4 drops to a bucket full of water as a final rinse.

The following blend can be made up and kept ready for use. It's extremely effective, being disinfecting and antibacterial, plus it leaves a delightful fragrance. It can be used around the kitchen and in an air spray: 4–6 drops to 2 pints (950 mL) of water.

THE CLEAN KITCHEN BLEND

Lavender	8 drops
Lemon	10 drops
Eucalyptus	5 drops
Grapefruit	8 drops
Palmarosa	5 drops
Thyme	4 drops
Cinnamon	2 drops

Blend the essential oils together using these proportions, and if you like the aroma, make up a larger amount by multiplying all the ingredients. Keep the blend for future use, stored in a clean, dark glass bottle, away from heat and light.

Aroma preferences vary not only from person to person but from country to country and from time to time. In South America commercial floor cleaning products contain many more times the amount of pine fragrance than a similar product would contain in the United States or Europe, where the aromas of lemon and floral fragrances reminiscent of perfumes are preferred. All too often, however, we think of a chemical smell as one that must be good at cleaning and dismiss as being ineffective an aroma as charming as an essential oil. If in any doubt about the effectiveness of essential oils, relax. There's a mass of scientific literature to prove it, and some commercial products have natural essences as their effective ingredient.

Dish towels used to be boiled — and not only to keep them white. Since modern washing machines rarely reach boiling point, we need another method to deal with the many microbes that accumulate on dish towels. Simply soak them in a bowl of boiling water to which 1 drop of lemongrass or thyme has been added, and leave them to soak for a while before washing in the machine as usual.

If, like so many others, you've ditched the dishwasher and wash dishes by hand, the chore can be made a little easier by using a personalized fragrant dish soap. There are eco-friendly, fragrance-free dishwashing liquids available, and they offer the opportunity to add a personalized fragrance. With lemon, we get the zing; lime or grapefruit bring a sparkle to the morning; lavender and chamomile will help you to relax midday; geranium will help create a soothing afternoon; and for real indulgence use ylang ylang dishwashing liquid last thing at night. If mosquitoes or other insects are being bothersome, use lemongrass or citronella to keep them away. Simply add 10–15 drops of the chosen essential oil to a bottle of dishwashing liquid, shake well, and allow to settle. If you find the whole business of dishwashing depressing, the obvious choice is bergamot, which has antidepressant properties. As I'm not crazy about dishwashing either, my own blend contains some of this oil:

SPECIAL BLEND DISHWASHING LIQUID

Lime	1 drop
Bergamot	2 drops
Lavender	1 drop
Orange	4 drops

Add to 1 pint (475 mL) bottle of dishwashing liquid and shake well. It's always wise to use protective gloves when using any type of dish soap as these cleansers are designed to remove fat and grease.

The fragranced dishwashing liquid can be added to wash water and used to clean many other things around the house besides dishes, including windows and trash cans, both inside and out. When carrying out any kitchen chore, essential oils make working in the kitchen a safer and altogether more pleasant experience.

The Utility Room

In the seventeenth and eighteenth centuries, our ancestors scented the laundry water with iris/orris root and dried their clothes and bed linen on rosemary or lavender bushes to infuse them with their aroma. We continue that tradition but use a multitude of fragrant essential oils to wash and store our clothes — and not only to make them smell sweet.

When hand washing, put 1 drop of essential oil in the water being used as a final rinse, swish it around, then remove any globules that might attach to material by sweeping a strong paper towel back and forth over the surface. This can be a particularly useful method if mosquitoes are around — use geranium, lavender, lemongrass, or cedarwood. Avoid the resinous essential oils, and some of the thick heavier oils and absolutes. To add a subtle fragrance to the wash, try lemon with lavender. If you prefer a more exotic perfume, try ylang ylang. If winter colds or flu have struck the household, put eucalyptus, rosemary, or niaouli in the wash. Or create your own blends, guided by the lists below:

FRESH
Lavender (*Lavandula angustifolia*)
Bergamot (*Citrus bergamia*)
Rosemary (*Rosmarinus officinalis*)
Petitgrain (*Citrus aurantium*)

FLORAL
Geranium (*Pelargonium graveolens*)
Neroli (*Citrus aurantium*)
Palmarosa (*Cymbopogon martinii*)
Rosewood (*Aniba rosaeodora*)
Ylang ylang (*Cananga odorata*)
Cananga (*Cananga odorata ct. macrophylla*)

ROMANTIC AND RELAXING
Ylang ylang (*Cananga odorata*)
Jasmine (*Jasminum grandiflorum/officinale*)

Sandalwood (*Santalum album*)
Rose (*Rosa damascena/centifolia*)
Clary sage (*Salvia sclarea*)
Cedarwood (*Cedrus atlantica/etc.*)

If you like to use ironing waters and want to try a natural fragrance instead when pressing clothes, add the essential oil to boiling water and leave it to infuse for a day or so before filtering the water through a paper coffee filter or muslin cloth. This water can then be used in a plant mister to spray clothes before ironing, or to spray a damp cloth that can be placed between the material and the iron. Use 1 drop of essential oil to 1 pint (475 mL) of water. Avoid using essential oil water on delicate fabrics, and antique or vintage clothing.

The natural fragrance of essential oils can be used to infuse clothes while they're in the drawer or closet. Put a drop on little pieces of natural material or cotton pads, wait until the drop has dried, then place them between the clothes.

CLOTHES SWEETENER
Ho wood	4 drops
Geranium	2 drops
Lemon	3 drops

Blend together in these proportions.

To keep moths away from clothes, use 2–3 drops of one of the following oils on cotton pads, or use in a spray. These are particularly useful when coats and woolens are stored away during the summer months:

MOTH REPELLENTS
Lavender (*Lavandula angustifolia*)
Rosemary (*Rosmarinus officinalis*)
Lemongrass (*Cymbopogon citratus/flexuosus*)
Citronella (*Cymbopogon nardus*)
Camphor (*Cinnamomum camphora*)
Vetiver (*Vetiveria zizanoides*)
Eucalyptus (*Eucalyptus globulus/citriodora*)

Cedarwood (*Cedrus atlantica/etc.*)
Cypress (*Cupressus sempervirens*)
Basil (*Ocimum basilicum*)

Drawer liners made with essential oils are much nicer than their chemical aroma counterparts and very simple to make. Cut the paper to the size of the drawer — blotting paper or other absorbent types of paper are best — and dot with the essential oils. Leave the paper to dry before placing in the bottom of the drawer. Which oils are used, and how much, is entirely a personal choice and depends on the size and contents of the drawer. Rose in the ladies' underwear drawer would be appropriate, for example, while a relaxing, calming fragrance like chamomile would suit children's nightwear drawers and a stimulating fragrance such as grapefruit or lemon could be used for the school clothes drawer. When colds are around, the family could use paper tissues that have been kept in a drawer where a liner incorporates a sweet-smelling antibacterial oil.

Shoes are often kept in the utility room. To freshen them, put 2 teaspoons of bicarbonate of soda into an egg cup and add 2 drops of lemon, tea tree, lavender, palmarosa, or rosemary essential oil. Mix well, sprinkle into the shoes, and leave overnight. Tap it out in the morning and the shoes should be as fresh as new. If someone has a foot fungal infection, use the same method as above but include 5 drops of tea tree and 5 drops of palmarosa.

Trainers can get pretty pungent even if there isn't a foot odor problem as such. Follow the method above but use 2 drops of the following blend of oils with each teaspoon of bicarbonate of soda. By morning, they won't seem the same wild things that were left there:

TRAINER TAMER BLEND

Cedarwood	2 drops
Rosemary	5 drops
Lavender	3 drops

Blend in these proportions.

The Living Room

Most living rooms get pampered with an assortment of fragranced products, from furniture polish to air fresheners, dusting powders for the carpets to upholstery cleaners. These products aren't aroma coordinated, and more importantly, they contain synthetic substances we would rather not inhale.

It's difficult to get windows absolutely perfectly sparkling — there always seem to be a few streaky marks left. To get rid of these, screw up an old sheet of paper, put a drop of lime, grapefruit, or lemon essential oil on it and polish the windows again. The essential oil soaks into the paper and combines to give a sparkling finish that also releases a fresh and subtle fragrance when the sun shines on the glass.

The so-called vintage furniture polishes are usually made with synthetic lavender fragrance and all manner of chemicals. The only old-fashioned thing about them is the vintage-looking packaging. Beeswax polish has always been valued for polishing fine furniture, which is why French polishers and antique restorers use it. It's really quite easy to make a special one of your own, and it's certainly well worth the trouble. These are the ingredients:

"THE REAL THING" FURNITURE POLISH

Beeswax	8 oz. (225 g)
Turpentine	2½ cups (600 mL)
Water	2½ cups (600 mL)
Pure soap flakes (or grated pure soap)	2 oz. (50 g)
Essential oil	10 drops or more

The beeswax should be plain and unrefined, not the white refined type. This can be acquired direct from beekeepers or from hardware or health food stores. Using the bain-marie method, melt the beeswax, take it off the heat, cool it a little, and then add the turpentine. This needs to be at room temperature, so if it's stored in a cold workshop bring it inside before it's required. Put this mixture to the side. In another pot, boil the water and melt the soap in it. Leave this until it's cool but still retains some of its warmth, and then add it very slowly to the pot with the beeswax and turpentine mixture. This should be done with great patience, trickle by trickle, stirring all the time. Finally, add the essential oil of choice. After blending all the ingredients together well, pack the polish in old flat tins or other small containers that have their own lids.

This type of polish requires using a cloth — any old soft material will do. Only a small amount is needed at a time, and the smell and shine will reward the effort. Try it out on a small, inconspicuous test area first. This formula can be adjusted according to the type of beeswax or soap flakes being used. A little white spirit will remove marks from some woods, including pine, before polishing.

Use a plant mister spray with water and essential oils to freshen up the living room, making sure the water does not fall on delicate fabrics or polished wood and other delicate furniture. As this is where family and friends spend most of their time, choose a nice, relaxing essential oil or blend. You could also use the diffuser, radiator, or humidifier methods. Make your own signature blend of oils or use this tried and tested combination:

THE RELAXING LIVING ROOM BLEND

Geranium	8 drops
Clary sage	3 drops
Lemon	5 drops
Bergamot	3 drops

Blend in these proportions.

And for something to rouse the family out of their Sunday afternoon lethargy, try this:

THE STIMULATING LIVING ROOM BLEND

Grapefruit	8 drops
Rosemary	4 drops
Lime	4 drops
Basil	2 drops

Blend in these proportions.

The Bedroom

The bedroom is the place to sleep or to play — that's up to you. If romance is on your mind, ylang ylang, rose, jasmine, sandalwood, clary sage, or some of the absolutes would add to the ambiance. To keep the bedroom smelling romantic at all times, create a special blend to use separately from the general house blend.

THE ROMANTIC BEDROOM BLEND

Palmarosa	8 drops
Ylang ylang	3 drops
Clary sage	2 drops
Nutmeg	1 drop
Orange	5 drops

Blend in these proportions.

For general bedroom use, ideal scents are chamomile, geranium, lavender, orange, melissa, neroli, petitgrain, clary sage, or cedarwood atlas. A diffuser will aid restful sleep when used with the relaxing oils, such as chamomile, lavender, or clary sage. If insomnia is a problem, the combinations of lavender and sweet orange, or petitgrain and chamomile, sprayed on the bed linen, may help. Sleep is a very personal time and what suits one person may not suit another, so just find what works best for each person.

Closets can benefit from fragrance too. Simply place cotton pads in the corners of the closet with your favorite blend of essential oils on them, or use one to keep the moths away; see "The Utility Room" on page 430. Fragranced drawer liners can also be put at the bottom of the closet. The aroma of the essential oils may permeate all the clothes hanging in the closet if too much is used, so aim for a subtle aroma, just to keep the air fresh.

The Bathroom

The best kind of bathrooms are like the best kind of kitchens — germ-free! Use a Microbe Buster essential oil in the final rinse water when washing surfaces in a bathroom, including the bath, sink, and toilet — not only to kill germs but to give the whole place a nice fragrance.

An easy way to fragrance the bathroom is to put a couple of drops of a neat essential oil or blend on the cardboard ring inside the toilet paper roll before placing it in the holder. The cardboard soaks up the essential oil and gently releases the aroma molecules, keeping the whole area fragrant.

Following are two disinfectant and antimicrobial blends to use throughout the bathroom:

BATHROOM BLEND 1

Bergamot	5 drops
Lavender	10 drops
Cinnamon	5 drops
Lemon	10 drops
Citronella	10 drops

Blend in these proportions.

BATHROOM BLEND 2

Oregano	5 drops
Palmarosa	10 drops
Thyme	10 drops
Lemon	20 drops

Blend in these proportions.

Hard water or calcium deposits can easily build up, along with soap residues, in certain water supply areas: on showers and screens, around taps, and on other areas of the bathroom. Lemons contain citric acid, and vinegar contains acetic acid, which when combined might help prevent this from happening. Mix 1 teaspoon (5 mL) of white vinegar and 1 teaspoon (5 mL) of fresh lemon juice with 3 tablespoons (45 mL) of water and then add 2 drops of lemon or orange essential oil. Apply regularly with a nonabrasive cloth or sponge to prevent buildup, and rinse well afterward. If a buildup has already occurred, combine bicarbonate of soda with white vinegar, fresh lemon juice, and lemon or orange essential oil to create a paste and leave it on the area for several hours before removing.

Insects and Other Unwanted Visitors

In nature, aromas play a big part in attracting, or deterring, creatures of various sizes. In our homes, specific aromas can be used to deter unwanted visitors and encourage them to move along and settle somewhere else. Everyone likes to be comfortable in their own home, including insects, and they're not comfortable around certain aromas. This is why essential oils can be so helpful, and there's no killing involved, which makes a good change from so many insect products that not only zap the insects but bring unwanted chemicals into our homes. This isn't to say chemicals don't have their place; sometimes an insect invasion is so bad there's no option but total annihilation (sorry, insects). But most of the time we don't need to go to such lengths, and as Grandma used to say, "A stitch in time saves nine" — so dealing with the problem as soon as it occurs can prevent insects from multiplying, which they do at a fast rate.

Many insects have a very short life and, like tourists, they come and go at particular times of the year, in waves. One week the place is full of wasps, and another week it's daddy longlegs. Because we can obtain a lot of information about their movements and likes and dislikes, with a little planning it's fairly easy to ensure that the insects run along and bother someone else. There are, of course, many species of particular insects: for example, 85 species of mosquito have been identified in the state of Texas alone. And all of them will have somewhat different aroma preferences and dislikes. So do experiment until the essential oil that works best against your particular unwanted visitors is found. More information can be found in the "Natural Insect Repellents" chart in chapter 18, "Gardens for the Future" and also in chapter 6, "The Basic Travel Kit." These are some of the most helpful essential oils:

INSECT AND PEST DETERRENT ESSENTIAL OILS

Catnip (*Nepeta cataria*)
Eucalyptus lemon (*Eucalyptus citriodora*)
Lavender (*Lavandula angustifolia*)
Cinnamon (*Cinnamomum zeylanicum*)
Citronella (*Cymbopogon nardus*)
Thyme (*Thymus vulgaris*)
Lemongrass (*Cymbopogon citratus/flexuosus*)
Basil (*Ocimum basilicum*)
Vetiver (*Vetiveria zizanoides*)
Black pepper (*Piper nigrum*)
Rosemary (*Rosmarinus officinalis*)
Clove (*Syzygium aromaticum*)
Spearmint (*Mentha spicata*)
Peppermint (*Mentha piperita*)
Tea tree (*Melaleuca alternifolia*)
Geranium (*Pelargonium graveolens*)
Juniper berry (*Juniperus communis*)
Eucalyptus (*Eucalyptus radiata/globulus*)
Fennel, sweet (*Foeniculum vulgare var. dulce*)
Cedarwood atlas (*Cedrus atlantica*)
Eucalyptus peppermint (*Eucalyptus dives*)
May chang (*Litsea cubeba*)

Use the essential oils in all the usual room methods, or try to focus on the pests' entry points, usually the windows and doors. To deter insects from coming in, make paper strips — from a roll of paper towel, for example — or cut lengths of cotton ribbon, put a drop of essential oil on each one, and hang them or place them in strategic positions so long as these are not in direct sunlight or near any other heat source. These methods also fragrance the rooms.

Favorite moth deterrents are vetiver, lavender, cedarwood, peppermint, lemongrass, citronella, and citrus oils generally. Mosquitoes and flies dislike catnip, vetiver, eucalyptus lemon, geranium, patchouli, and lavender. Additionally, flies try to avoid spearmint, pennyroyal, basil, clove, citronella, lemongrass, peppermint, and eucalyptus. If flies tend to congregate around rubbish bins, inside or outside the home, one of these oils might be a good option to use when washing them out. One of the most effective fly deterrents is neem oil, but it doesn't have a particularly nice aroma. Neem is a very effective essential oil to use to deter all kinds of insects, but may be best used outside — in the garage or shed — as its aroma can deter people as well as insects!

The following blends will do a good job of keeping most insects on their side of the window frame. Combine the essential oils together and use in room sprays or in any other room method, including simply dropping the essential oil onto cotton pads and placing them in unobtrusive corners of the room.

FOR GENERAL INSECT PREVENTION

BLEND I

Eucalyptus lemon	20 drops
Basil	10 drops
Lavender	10 drops
Geranium	5 drops
Peppermint	5 drops

Blend 2

Lemongrass	10 drops
Peppermint	3 drops
Lavender	5 drops

Blend 3

Eucalyptus lemon	10 drops
Basil	5 drops
Clove	3 drops
Lavender	5 drops

Ants enter the home like a tiny army determined to get where they're going, and persuading them to turn around and march somewhere else is a battle best fought with peppermint, eucalyptus peppermint, orange, and catnip. But take care as these essential oils can damage surfaces if used undiluted on painted surfaces or wooden floors. If the flooring is tiled or concrete, the battle plan is simple: create a barrier using essential oils, especially at their point of entry. Other barrier methods that could be used are lines of chalk, chili powder, or mustard powder. A combination of chalk lines and peppermint oil has worked well in many a Mediterranean home. If no damage is going to be caused to surfaces, add the essential oils to these powders. For other methods, see chapter 18, "Gardens for the Future."

MICE

Mice urinate and defecate as they run, and they need to be kept from re-entering the house as soon as any signs are seen. The aromas of peppermint, spearmint, basil, and clove have been effective in discouraging mice, but only strong dilutions will do the job. Prepare a blend to spray around the suspected point of entry: 65% water, 10% alcohol, and 25% essential oil. If thinking about plugging mouse holes, consider the rather harsh option of wire wool!

When the mice are in outbuildings or running on the roof, stronger formulations can be used. I helped someone with her mouse problem at a huge French chateau by using neat essential oil comprised of 50% peppermint, 40% basil, and 10% clove. The unwelcome visitors haven't been seen since! Place the essential oil, either neat or in a dilution strength appropriate to the area affected, in all the strategic places — where they enter, and where they run. If mouse holes are seen, and you prefer a soft option, stuff the holes with cotton balls on which essential oils have been dropped. The peppermint herb, either fresh or dried, can also be helpful when placed around where the mice are entering.

Making a Mark in a New Home

When prospective buyers or renters are viewing a property, the furnishings of the previous occupant are usually still there, hiding all the cracks behind the furniture. When we arrive at an empty property with our furniture and boxes, the place that once looked warm and inviting can feel like a cold and desolate shell. We may also become aware for the first time of the true atmosphere of the property, part of which is determined by the subtle smell that permeates a place, the unique aromatic imprint of all that went before.

A UK company that specializes in humidity issues in large buildings was asked to dehumidify a centuries-old church that had been badly water damaged from a leaking roof. After the dehumidifying equipment had been in place for a few days, a powerful aroma of incense began to pervade the church. The resinous smell was a type that had not been used in incense in that church, the pastor thought, for centuries. Like a sponge, the building's stone interior had absorbed the fragrant molecules as the incense had wound its way heavenward long ago, and was now releasing it under the effect of the specialized equipment.

A great deal of controversy surrounds the idea that buildings act as a sort of recorder of the conversations and events that have taken place in them. If the thought patterns and actions of the inhabitants were on a positive vibration, so the theory goes, this positivity will be embedded in the very walls. On the other hand, if bad thoughts and actions inhabited the place, they too will be stuck in the bricks and mortar and will be contributing to a bad atmosphere. It's going to take someone a long time to prove or disprove this theory, but while we're waiting, I tend to err on the side of caution and take the idea seriously.

It's not so easy for us to release the aromatic imprint from the property we've just moved into, but we can use a simple method that's been used by so many different cultures over many centuries that it might almost be called universal. The idea is to clear a place of the energies of former inhabitants and infuse it with our personal fragrant ambiance to reduce the impact of aromas from the past. It involves the use of salt and water. When moving into a new property, even before cleaning it or putting the furniture in place, prepare a large atmosphere-cleansing room spray with one part salt and one part white vinegar to each six parts of water. Open the windows of each room and spray the empty rooms thoroughly with the salt and water mix, spraying high in the air and if possible onto the walls — making sure, of course, that there's nothing that could get damaged. Leave the building for a while. The next part is to create a personal fragrant ambiance. Prepare a bottle of essential oil or blend of oils. Use as many drops as desired on tissues or cotton pads and place them in each corner of the rooms. Then use the room ambiance spray method, including in your mix a teaspoon of salt, and spray high and low around the house, paying particular attention to the hallways. Do this for several consecutive days until

the odor pattern of previous inhabitants has been changed and the new home begins to feel like a fresh space. I add frankincense or sage into blends used for this purpose, as well as using incense and smudging with white sage!

All that needs to be done now is to fill the place with wonderful energies, so put on loud music, invite friends over — especially those who laugh at the top of their voices, and let the walls shake with the knowledge that new occupants have arrived!

Parties and Celebrations

We've all been to parties where the hosts have gone to a lot of trouble to provide fabulous food and drink and even a terrific playlist, yet the event was flat. And we've been to parties that will go down in history as being great events even though the food was lousy, the beer was warm, and the music nonexistent. Parties seem to have a life of their own, more dependent on atmosphere and good interaction between people than on anything else. If event managers could bottle this secret ingredient to party success, they'd be very happy. But that secret ingredient is already bottled — it's called essential oils!

You'll already know from other sections of this book that the mood-inducing effects of essential oils are one of their outstanding properties, and the art of using them at parties is to match appropriate combinations of essential oils to the type of party you're having, and the people you're inviting. For example, different blends would be used if planning an exciting Saturday night dance party, a relaxed conversational Sunday get-together, or a special romantic party for two. Citrus essential oils have universal appeal and can be used in any blend to give it a lift. The following are suggestions for essential oils that could be incorporated into your own signature party blends:

For More Stimulating Blends
Grapefruit (*Citrus paradisi*)
Coriander seed (*Coriandrum sativum*)
Rosemary (*Rosmarinus officinalis*)
Black pepper (*Piper nigrum*)
Ginger (*Zingiber officinale*)
Peppermint (*Mentha piperita*)
Basil (*Ocimum basilicum*)
Lemon (*Citrus limon*)
Eucalyptus lemon (*Eucalyptus citriodora*)

For More Relaxing Blends:
Geranium (*Pelargonium graveolens*)
Jasmine (*Jasminum grandiflorum/officinale*)
Sandalwood (*Santalum album*)
Ylang ylang (*Cananga odorata*)
Clary sage (*Salvia sclarea*)
Rose otto (*Rosa damascena/centifolia*)
Frankincense (*Boswellia carterii*)
Ginger lily root (*Hedychium spicatum*)
May chang (*Litsea cubeba*)

For Romantic Touches (use in small amounts):
Benzoin (*Styrax benzoin*)
Jasmine (*Jasminum grandiflorum/officinale*)
Vanilla (*Vanilla plantifolia*)
Rose (*Rosa damascena/centifolia*)
Patchouli (*Pogostemon cablin*)
Sandalwood (*Santalum album*)
Ylang ylang (*Cananga odorata*)
Magnolia leaf (*Michelia alba*)

These lists could be very much longer as many beautiful floral absolutes and more exotic essential oils are available, but here I've included only oils that are in general use by aromatherapists and readily available for the home practitioner. Each essential oil is rather like an individual guest in that it has a unique personality to contribute to the whole, for example:

Clary sage: Euphoric, rather masculine, relaxes and encourages conversation

Geranium: Relaxes, always creates a good and happy mood

Grapefruit: Uplifting and stimulating

Lemon: Maintains the fresh appeal of cleanliness and encourages appetite

Lemongrass: Relaxing and positive

Palmarosa: Creates an easy-going atmosphere

Rose: Romantic, special, extravagant

Sandalwood: Relaxes and encourages conversation

Vanilla: Comforting and familiar, relaxing

Ylang ylang: Heady and exotic

Blending together 1 drop of clary sage, 2 drops of geranium, and 1 drop of sandalwood would provide a good basis for a warm, relaxed, and happy evening with free-flowing conversation. Add in grapefruit or lemon to refresh and stimulate. Use any of the room methods, including diffusers or room mister sprays. In each of these, use 4–6 drops of essential oil and renew as needed. The aroma will act as an olfactory reminder to guests that it's party time.

CELEBRATIONS

Aroma has the unique ability to reach back in time and remind us of past events. For example, a random whiff of fir might immediately transport a person back to childhood Christmases spent at their grandparents' house, where a big fir tree was always waiting for the children to decorate. The fir represented something to look forward to and became the stuff of happy memories. Celebrations are times of family and friends getting together, feasting, giving gifts, laughing, and having fun together.

Oftentimes the natural aromas associated with celebrations have been lost, as fir trees are replaced by artificial ones, for example. But by using essential oils those traditional aromas can be revived, and then used each year thereafter at the same time to reinforce the experience. This may be particularly important for children; for them the details of the occasion may be blurry, but the aroma is not. Nor will it ever be. The aroma-memory connection lasts long, throughout life, well into old age. So for young and old alike, aroma memory plays an important role, both in forming memories and in recalling them.

In the essential oils we have a mobile, compact, and thoroughly modern method of re-creating the aromatic traditions. When using them around the house during a celebration, aim for an aroma that's subtly evocative without being overpowering. Gently build up an aroma picture that reflects the occasion, using several methods at the same time or making one special celebratory blend. And be sure to have good times — because that's what you want people to remember!

CHRISTMAS

The aromas associated with Christmas evolved in Europe and North America, with decorated pine trees, turkey with herb stuffing, oranges studded with cloves, and so forth. Those traditions have traveled the world, so artificial Christmas trees, with tinsel representing snow, can be seen under hot Australian skies on the 25th of December, where there's not a single flake of real snow in sight.

The aroma of real fir can easily be re-created by putting fir essential oil on a piece of absorbent material and tucking it around the base of the tree. If there are electric lights on the tree, place the essential oil on some other form of decorative greenery — holly for example, or even the wreath on the front door.

Aromas associated with Christmas differ from country to country; for example, bayberry essential oil evokes the memory of early settlers in the American northeast who extracted a sweet aromatic wax from the *Myrica pensylvanica* shrub to make candles. And in Costa Rica, cypress wreaths are traditional, while in Greece, sprigs of basil are the decorative choice.

THE CHRISTMAS ESSENTIAL OILS

Spices	*Citrus*
Cinnamon (*Cinnamomum zeylanicum*)	Mandarin (*Citrus reticulata*)
Clove (*Syzygium aromaticum*)	Orange (*Citrus sinensis*)
Bay (*Laurus nobilis*)	Tangerine (*Citrus reticulata*)
Ginger (*Zingiber officinale*)	Lime
Pimento berry (*Pimenta dioica*)	(*Citrus aurantifolia*)

Trees	*Resins*
Pine (*Pinus sylvestris*)	Frankincense (*Boswellia carterii*)
Cedarwood atlas (*Cedrus atlantica*)	Myrrh (*Commiphora myrrha*)
Fir (*Albies alba*)	Benzoin (*Styrax benzoin*)
Spruce (*Picea mariana*)	

Frankincense and myrrh were presented to the baby Jesus, and today they're used in incense and burned to release their aromatic molecules in churches all around the world, along with benzoin, which is particularly favored in Russia. Most aromatherapists use frankincense as an ingredient for spiritual uplifting, and 1 drop of frankincense could be added to the following blend to give it a spiritual edge:

CHRISTMAS HOUSE SPRAY

Fir (or pine or spruce)	2 drops
Mandarin	8 drops
Cinnamon	1 drop
Clove	2 drops

Dilute in 10 fl. oz. (300 mL) of water in a plant mister.

Many combinations of oils work equally well at Christmas, and it is a matter of personal preference, so just experiment. Mandarin, tangerine, and orange are fresh smelling and reminiscent of Christmas in some European traditions, as are the spice essential oils — which are a good choice when visitors are due. Celebratory cakes and breads all contain spices, and while baking their aromas suffuse the home with a hospitable glow. The spice essential oils of cinnamon, clove, and bay will add a warm and homely hint to blends, and with even very small quantities of essential oil it's easy to build up the welcoming "story" we're trying to create.

When making Christmas logs for the fire, apply 1–3 drops of essential oil to a log, allowing enough time for the essential oil to soak into the wood and thoroughly dry before using. Use only one oil log at a time. Surprisingly perhaps, this will be enough to contribute to the Christmas ambience.

FIREWOOD OILS

Pine (*Pinus sylvestris*)
Fir (*Albies alba*)
Sandalwood (*Santalum album*)
Frankincense (*Boswellia carterii*)
Cypress (*Cupressus sempervirens*)
Myrrh (*Commiphora myrrha*)
Cedarwood atlas (*Cedrus atlantica*)
Spruce (*Picea mariana*)

Candles add a lovely touch of warmth at Christmas, and with candle-making kits easily available, they can be made aromatic very easily using essential oils. Spruce, fir, bay, and vanilla are good choices, as are orange and the spice essential oils; they all evoke the atmosphere of Christmas.

CHRISTMAS CANDLE BLEND

Orange or mandarin	4 drops
Geranium	1 drop
Cinnamon	1 drop

This blend may work well at Christmas if orange or mandarin evokes memories of Christmases past, while the geranium will put people in a good mood, and the cinnamon will whet their appetites. This blend can also be used in a room spray — add these quantities to 2½ cups (600 mL) of water. Take care not to spray on delicate fabrics such as velvet and silk, or on wooden or other water-sensitive furniture.

Decorations are an integral part of celebrations, and essential oils can be incorporated into them very easily. Today, pinecones are usually bought in stores rather than picked up fresh from the forest floor, and they can be dry and without aroma. This is easily rectified by putting 1 drop of essential oil directly on the pinecone. Or, for a more subtle effect, infuse the cones by putting them in a large plastic bag with a cotton ball or tissue to which 2–3 drops of pine, spruce, or fir oil have been added. Seal the bag and leave it overnight, and in the morning the cones will be gently suffused with their natural aroma. They can be decorated with colorfast ribbons that have been infused or sprayed with essential oils of the season. Holly and ivy decorations can be tied in ribbons infused with bay, or with another spice or citrus essential oil. These subtle notes will contribute to the overall aroma picture of Christmas.

Oranges studded with cloves are a classic Christmas decoration, and the aromatic effect can be boosted by rolling the oranges beforehand in orange and clove, or cinnamon, essential oil.

These could be hung on ribbons, or used in closets and drawers to deter moths and insects when the celebrations are over. But why stop there? Lemons and limes can be rolled in their respective essential oils and studded with cloves to add further aromatic dimensions to the celebratory decorations. Store aromatic decorations separately in sealed plastic bags and their impact will last longer. Christmas will jump out of the bags when the season rolls around again.

Traditional gifts are always welcome, and making a whole variety of essential oil presents is literally child's play, and a creative way to keep children busy in the weeks leading up to the big day. There are many suggestions for gifts later in this chapter, and the Christmas oils can be incorporated into them. To make scented wrapping paper, simply place 2 drops of essential oil on a cotton ball and leave it in a sealed bag with the wrapping paper overnight. Use a different aroma for different members of the family.

EASTER

The aromas of Easter are those of fresh spring flowers, spicy cakes and buns, and, of course, chocolate. Each country has different flowers that represent the end of winter and the start of a new season of growth, and in Britain, these are crocuses, tulips, and bright-yellow daffodils. None of them produce essential oils, but narcissus and the highly fragrant hyacinth do. In home fragrance sprays, aim for light, fresh aromas or use the following suggestion. The spicy flavor associated with Easter can be achieved by adding 1 drop of any spice oil to the blend.

Spring Flowers Blend

Palmarosa	3 drops
Geranium	1 drop
Ho wood	1 drop
Lemon	2 drops

Spicy buns, breads, and cakes seem to be traditional in many countries at Easter, including Britain, where hot cross buns are an essential part of the celebrations. Using essential oils in the cooking will add an extra dimension to their taste and a seasonal aroma to the home. Even store-bought versions of spicy cakes can be made extra special if stored in a bag or tin with a half a teaspoon of cinnamon powder to which 1 drop of orange essential oil has been added. Or the essential oil could be put on a small piece of clean, undyed natural material and popped into the container.

It's hard to think of Easter without thinking of Easter eggs, and kits for making chocolate eggs, rabbits, and chicks are widely available. These treats are made even more delicious if you take a tip from the world's leading chocolatiers and add to the melted chocolate a drop of essential oil of spearmint, peppermint, orange, lemon, grapefruit, or lime, and blend it in well.

Gifts can be made more celebratory by wrapping them in aromatic gift paper: put a few drops of essential oil on tissue paper, let it dry, then place it between the sheets of wrapping paper. Design your own unique essential oil blend and use it each Easter so the family will always associate that aroma with family time and good food during the Easter celebrations.

SPIRITUAL OCCASIONS

Oftentimes when people come together as friends and family, or in larger groups, there's a spiritual dimension to the event. Aroma certainly has a place on these occasions because we know from the earliest written records right through to present times that fragrance and spiritual practice are inextricably linked. Information about the historic and contemporary uses of aroma for spiritual connection can be found in my book *Aromatherapy for the Soul*, including over 70 profiles of essential oils used for spiritual purposes around the world.

In Christianity, frankincense and myrrh play a central aromatic role, while in Islam, rose has a special place. The smoke of white sage has long been part of sacred practice among many indigenous American cultures, while in Tibet the burning of juniper branches traditionally played a prominent role. In their spiritual practice, Indian Hindus burn incense and fragrant woods such as sandalwood. In the Jewish tradition, at the end of the Shabbat a special box of fragrant spices is brought out to remind people of the significance of this holiday.

Essential oils can provide aromas to enhance the traditional significance of a celebration, or to help focus the mind in prayer or meditation. Which essential oils are chosen will depend both on their resonance with your spiritual core and on which fragrances you feel comfortable using. Fragrances can unlock the heart and spirit, but this is a very personal experience, for which no advice can be given. However, the following are well-known fragrances widely used in spiritual practices around the world:

ESSENTIAL OILS USED IN SPIRITUAL PRACTICES
Frankincense (*Boswellia carterii*)
Myrrh (*Commiphora myrrha*)
Rose otto (*Rosa damascena*)
White sage (*Salvia apiana*)
Hyssop (*Hyssopus officinalis*)
Yuzu (*Citrus junos*)
Sandalwood (*Santalum album*)
Cedarwood atlas (*Cedrus atlantica*)
Juniper berry (*Juniperus communis*)
Basil tulsi/holy basil (*Ocimum tenuiflorum/sanctum*)

The following is a way of bringing natural fragrance into the home environment without the use of sprays or diffusers, and is an adaption of an indigenous spiritual practice. Put sand, clay, or earth into a bowl and place there, in a vertical position, a few wooden sticks that have not been treated in any way with, for example, varnish or polish. Twigs from a tree will do, or even Popsicle sticks. Drip the essential oil, or blend of oils, onto the top of the sticks so it slowly falls down and impregnates the wood. The essential oils will slowly release their molecules into the atmosphere.

SAINT VALENTINE'S DAY

The connection between the sense of smell and memory is so fundamental to human beings that it lies deep within the brain, in the limbic system, denoting its evolutionary importance. The limbic system includes the olfactory bulbs, and its functions include olfaction, emotion, motivation, behavior, and long-term memory. These connections account for the fact that a perfume worn many years previously by a lover can reignite in the partner past emotions associated with the wearer. Using essential oils during Saint Valentine's Day is about building memories that will never be forgotten.

If you secretly admire someone, send them a valentine's card, traditionally left unsigned. Your signature will be aromatic. Put essential oils on the card, and then use that same aroma as a perfume or eau de cologne when next meeting the person it was sent to; they'll know it was you. Nothing has been said, but you'll know they know. Use a special blend that can be associated with you alone, perhaps by making a unique perfume or eau de cologne, as shown later in this chapter.

If you have a partner, the foundations of your aromatic relationship could be laid down before greeting your lover in the evening, making sure romantic intentions are conveyed as soon as your partner opens the door. Have the place infused with a special romantic aroma, with candles already lit — pink for love, red for passion. For valentines with serious matters of the heart in mind, here are a few suggestions for essential oils that could be used in blends:

SENSUAL OILS FOR SAINT VALENTINE'S DAY
Rose otto (*Rosa damascena*)
Jasmine (*Jasminum grandiflorum / officinale*)
Rose maroc (*Rosa centifolia*)
Ylang ylang (*Cananga odorata*)
Geranium (*Pelargonium graveolens*)
Sandalwood (*Santalum album*)
Rosewood (*Aniba rosaeodora*)
Cistus (*Cistus ladaniferus*)
Cedarwood atlas (*Cedrus atlantica*)
Clary sage (*Salvia sclarea*)
Vanilla (*Vanilla plantifolia*)

Ylang ylang is a well-known aphrodisiac fragrance, and it can very simply be infused into chocolates or other candies to make a special gift. Purchase your lover's favorite candy — something that is not strongly flavored itself, but bland, like fudge or plain chocolate. Put the loose candy in a pretty container along with a small piece of absorbent paper on which half a drop of ylang ylang or rose essential oil has been placed. Ylang ylang and rose not only are very sensuous essential oils but are used as flavorings in confectionery and baking. Leave the paper in the container so the flavor is absorbed. Decorate the candies with crystallized flowers and package them attractively, perhaps wrapped with a big red bow.

Romantic Baths

Romantic baths and massage oils are very personal, so I suggest making your own unique blend that will say much about you and never be replicated by others. Blends are easily adapted by the simple addition, or replacement, of one or two oils.

BLEND 1
Rose	2 drops
Palmarosa	3 drops

BLEND 2
Ylang ylang	3 drops
Grapefruit	4 drops

Romantic Body Oils

Using essential oils in blends makes the giving of massage pleasurable for the giver, as well as for the receiver.

BLEND 1
Rose	10 drops
Ylang ylang	2 drops
Lemon	8 drops
Palmarosa	2 drops

First, blend the essential oils together, then dilute 3–5 drops in 1 teaspoon (5 mL) of a light carrier oil, such as sweet almond.

BLEND 2
Jasmine	5 drops
Nutmeg	1 drop
Black pepper	3 drops
Mandarin	5 drops

First, blend the essential oils together, then dilute 3–5 drops in 1 teaspoon (5 mL) of a light carrier oil, such as sweet almond.

The morning after Saint Valentine's night, send your sweetheart into the reality of the day with an aide-mémoire tucked in their pocket — an aromatic tissue suffused with the essential oils used the evening before. Or simply use rose, cistus, jasmine, ylang ylang, or your personal choice of essential oil. As your valentine reaches for their keys or phone, an aroma will waft up to meet their nose and memories of you will be conveyed by the silent aromatic molecules of love.

HALLOWEEN

The witches and spooks have their day on October 31. Children love Halloween parties — dressing up, playing games, and teasing the grown-ups brings forth peals of laughter and squeals of delight. Provided there's adequate adult supervision, electrical diffusers can fragrance the home with some of the deep and mystical-smelling essential oils, such as galbanum, cedarwood atlas, vetiver, or spikenard. Try to make a blend that's pleasant but still has a slight yucky Halloween edge. Fragrant witches' brooms can be made by tying twigs into bundles. Soak the twigs first in a strong wood or root fragrance such as cedar or vetiver, diluted in water. These make good souvenir presents for the guests, naughty and good alike.

Essential Oils for Halloween
Cedarwood atlas (*Cedrus atlantica*)
Spikenard (*Nardostachys jatamansi*)
Cypress (*Cupressus sempervirens*)
Lemon verbena (*Lippia citriodora*)
Pine (*Pinus sylvestris*)
Benzoin (*Styrax benzoin*)
Galbanum (*Ferula galbaniflua*)
Patchouli (*Pogostemon cablin*)
Orange (*Citrus sinensis*)
Sandalwood (*Santalum album*)
Mandarin (*Citrus reticulata*)
Vetiver (*Vetiveria zizanoides*)

CREATING YOUR OWN AROMATIC TRADITIONS

Many annual events — New Year's Eve, midsummer festivals, birthdays, and anniversaries — can be enhanced and made memorable by the use of essential oils. Why not establish your own aroma traditions, to enhance the occasion and act as a reminder of times spent having fun and giving thanks? On birthdays use a favorite blend in the room methods or on your body, or both, to mark out the aromatic landscape and say, "This day is mine."

The same goes for weddings and wedding anniversaries. Make a special blend for the bride and groom and give them the formula so they can use it in the future on their anniversary, when it will stimulate clear memories of the special day. On the big day itself, use the blend as a room fragrance at the reception or put it on artificial flowers for guests to take home as a memento. No doubt you can think of other ways in which to use the unique power and charm of essential oils to make celebratory days special and turn ordinary days into celebrations.

Making Gifts

In this age of easy commercialism, the very act of taking time to make someone an individual present is a gift in itself. Throughout this book there are many blends and items that would make lovely presents for friends and family, chosen for their specific likes and needs. For example, later in this chapter there is a section on making perfumes and eau de cologne. What follows now is a collection of ideas for incorporating essential oils into a miscellany of sweet-smelling presents. If you have someone in mind and know their aroma preferences, this would be the ideal place to find ways of bringing those sweet smells into their lives.

PERFUMED PILLOWS AND SACHETS

Perfumed pillows and sachets come in many sizes — from large ones to lean back on while relaxing in the day to tiny ones to tuck in clothes drawers, hang in closets, or place in shoes overnight to keep them smelling sweet. Traditionally, herbal pillows were used for medicinal reasons and to help people sleep. Today we can think of many more purposes for these cute and useful decorative items.

All that's needed is a piece of cloth, some

dried herbal material, some essential oils, and some ideas. You may have a friend who's sad and needs comforting, or another who can't sleep. Think of what your friend or family member needs, cut the cloth to size, and sow three sides (or most of the side if making a heart or circle shape, for example), stuff it with the herbal material, add the essential oils, sow the last side closed, and plump it up nicely.

Any dried herbal or floral material could be used. If making a pillow to aid sleep, choose dried hops, chamomile, or lavender flowers. And add the essential oils of chamomile, lavender, neroli, or sweet marjoram. Day pillows can be aromatically enhanced with essential oils that match your signature home fragrance, or use, for example, lemon, geranium, or clary sage. Add as many drops of essential oil to sachets and pillows as required, depending on their size.

Making fragranced pillows and sachets with essential oils increases their effectiveness and makes reviving them very easy. To revive, simply apply the oil neat onto the outer cloth or, if this is delicate, open a little of a corner seam and drop the oil onto the stuffing.

Sachets for refreshing shoes can be made with dried herbs and flowers. Crush the herbal mixture, and to each tablespoon of herbs add 1 teaspoon of bicarbonate of soda and 1 drop of essential oil. Mix well, and pack into small cloth bags made in the same way as the pillows, above.

Small sachets can be hung by ribbons in closets to keep flies and other flying insects away. Fill with dried herbs or flowers and then add the essential oils of lavender, thyme, or citronella. If particular insects are the problem, refer to the "Insect and Pest Deterrent Essential Oils" and the "Moth Repellents" lists earlier in this chapter.

FRAGRANCED WOOD

Fragranced wood can be used as a decorative feature on its own or to freshen and perfume closets or drawers. Any dried wood will soak up the essential oils, so use your imagination to create interesting, natural set-pieces. Flower arrangers will undoubtedly be able to utilize this method to make permanent shows with dried flowers, grasses, and herbs. If you live by the sea, walking by the shore at low tide may reveal some beautiful worn pieces of wood. But even very small creations can be most impressive — and with the essential oils, aromatically satisfying too.

POTPOURRIS

Potpourris have been lending fragrance to rooms since the 1750s but have fallen out of favor as naturally fragrant petals have been replaced by silk ones, and natural aroma has been replaced by unnatural synthetic smells. No wonder they're out of fashion. But potpourris can actually be beautiful, artistic, imaginative, and naturally fragrant.

Flowers often have no aroma when dried and are used for their beauty and color only. Put them together with a few drops of essential oil in a plastic bag, and leave it sealed for a few days so the aroma can penetrate the petals. The floral fragrances are obviously the ones to go for, or try one of these blends, depending on the type of flowers you have and the additional decorative items chosen to mix them with:

FLOWERY BLEND

Ho wood	2 drops
Geranium	4 drops
Grapefruit	1 drop
Petitgrain	1 drop
Palmarosa	2 drops

ORIENTAL BLEND

Sandalwood	3 drops
Patchouli	2 drops
Benzoin	1 drop
Nutmeg	2 drops
Ylang ylang	2 drops
Lime	1 drop

First blend the essential oils together; then add them to the potpourri ingredients, drop by drop, until the desired strength is reached.

Potpourri additions could include dried wood; curly wood shavings, which soak up essential oils very well; cleaned and dried fruit stones, plums and peach especially; spices like star anise, nutmeg, and cinnamon; and dried leaves and herbs. Whole nutmegs look attractive, and if a drop of nutmeg oil is put on them and they're stored in a plastic bag for a day or so, their aromatic quality will be much intensified. The same applies to cinnamon sticks and cinnamon oil, and cloves and clove oil. Other additions to a spicy potpourri could be the peel of orange, lemon, lime, or grapefruit. These can also be enhanced by adding their corresponding essential oils to the peel.

Spicy Blends

BLEND 1

Nutmeg	2 drops
Clove	1 drop
Cinnamon	2 drops

BLEND 2

Lemon	4 drops
Basil	2 drops
Orange	3 drops

FRAGRANT PAPIER-MÂCHÉ

Papier-mâché used to be thought of as child's play, but many artists employ this method to make really beautiful objects. And when essential oils are included in the process, the results can be aromatic too. If papier-mâché is made into decorative items to be worn, the heat of the body helps the aromatic molecules evaporate, giving a hint of fragrance all day long. Papier-mâché can be made into beads or pendants to be worn, or into shapes to make mobiles to hang over children's cribs and beds.

How strong the aroma is will depend on the amount of essential oil used, and there are four opportunities for adding the essential oil during the papier-mâché-making process: into the flour and water base, to the newspaper itself, on the finished object before it's left to dry, and in the paint used to decorate. By all means, use the fragrant oils in each of these steps, and add a couple of drops to refresh the item after it's been made.

SPICY BEADS

The following is based on a centuries-old recipe for making fragrant prayer or guardian beads. The ingredients are made into a paste, which is rolled to make small round beads that can be hung on a bracelet or necklace. The warmth of the body helps to activate the aroma, as the warmer they get, the more aroma molecules are released. Rose oil was traditionally used in the recipe below, but the choice is entirely up to you. Use a single essential oil or a blend of oils to create a unique fragrance.

Powdered benzoin (the gum variety)	1 oz. (30 g)
Powdered acacia (the gum variety)	1 oz. (30 g)
Powdered orris root	½ oz. (15 g)
Powdered cinnamon	½ oz. (15 g)
Powdered clove	½ oz. (15 g)
Vanilla essence	2 drops
Grated nutmeg	½ teaspoon
Glycerin	2 tablespoons (30 mL)
Rose (or other) essential oil	10–15 drops

Mix all the ingredients together except the rose oil, which should be added last. This makes a sticky paste that can be rolled into little balls or other shapes. Leave them to partially dry, and when they are dry enough to handle, pierce a hole through with a hot darning needle. Put the beads on a metal tray and leave them to dry completely before threading them onto a ribbon or string.

BOOKMARKS

All that's needed to make bookmarks is a few bits of colored or decorated paper. They can be made that much more special by placing a drop of essential oil on them before putting in a plastic bag, sealing, and leaving it overnight for the aroma to infuse the paper. A papier-mâché or spicy bead can be strung with ribbon from the top so the bookmark hangs out from the pages of the book. Bookmarks could be made using essential oils that help the studying process — such as lemon or rosemary for focus and memory.

PAPERS AND INK

Making perfumed paper is extremely easy with essential oils. If sending a letter, invitation, or card to a friend or family member, just put a drop of essential oil onto the corner before sealing it up. To infuse a whole box of paper and envelopes, cut a small piece of paper tissue, blotting paper, or piece of old cotton fabric into around six pieces, about an inch square each. Put a drop of essential oil on each piece, and scatter them between the sheets of paper or envelopes. Seal the box tightly, or put it into a plastic bag and seal, and leave for 24 hours.

Any essential oil or blend of oils could be used. Remember, though, that the aroma will henceforth be associated subconsciously not only with the sender but with the nature of the news sent. Send only good news in perfumed letters.

Friends have traditionally sent each other uplifting fragranced letters not only because it's a caring, loving gesture, but because when the fragrance is later inhaled again by the recipient it'll automatically remind them of the sender.

Perfumed inks have the same effect as perfumed paper. Just add to the bottle 10 drops of essential oil for each teaspoon of ink. Calligraphy never smelled so good!

CARDS

If making your own greeting cards, try lemon oil on lemon- or cream-colored paper, orange oil on peach-colored paper, or lavender oil on lavender-colored paper. Or coordinate the aroma used with the design of the card being made. If making Christmas cards, add the aromas listed under that section, earlier in this chapter. For birthdays, the aroma can be masculine or feminine, or designed for a child. For get-well cards, how about sending a card infused with soothing and calming oils? There are ideas all the way through this book that can be adopted to add an extra dimension to your card-making skills.

MAKING YOUR OWN SOAPS

Making soap is a bit of a messy job, but it's well worth the trouble if you have the time. It not only ensures that the purest of ingredients are used on the skin and the exact desired fragrance is obtained, but with all the permutations there are in terms of ingredients and shape, a unique product will be the reward for your efforts.

There are so many combinations of essential oils that could be used, depending on the intended use of the soap. Here are three blends that could be tried. They each contain enough essential oil for 9 oz. (250 g) of grated soap. If using melt-and-pour soaps, ask the supplier's advice for suggested amounts of essential oils to use.

MORNING FRESH

Grapefruit	4 drops
Lime	2 drops
Lemon	1 drop
Basil	1 drop
Lavender	2 drops

GENTLEMAN'S SPICE

Nutmeg	1 drop
Bay	2 drops
Lime	6 drops
Clary sage	2 drops

COUNTRY LIFE

Lavender	3 drops
Geranium	2 drops
Chamomile roman	1 drop
Rosemary	4 drops

If using the grated soap method, always use 100% pure soap. Excellent additions would be oatmeal, ground almonds, avocado oil, olive oil, jojoba, or carrot oil. Bring to a boil an amount of water that's a quarter of the volume of the grated soap you intend to use. Put this in a bowl over a pot of boiling water on the stove, or in a bain-marie, and add the grated soap. Stir until the soap is fully melted (it becomes quite sticky and sloppy). Take it off the heat and leave until it's starting to set, then add the chosen essential oils. Mix again very well. Scoop out the soap and mold it by hand to the desired shape or put it into pre-prepared molds. For the traditional shape of soap use old soap boxes or any small carton or container of your choice, so long as they're lined. Leave until well set and then turn out the soap.

FRAGRANT CANDLES

Making candles is a hobby many people enjoy, and with candle-making kits it's relatively easy to do. Essential oils and mineral waxes such as paraffin wax do not mix, so only use soy, palm, rapeseed, coconut, or other types of vegetable wax. Or, of course, the most traditional — beeswax. To perfume the candle wax, simply add 10–20 drops of essential oil to 8 oz. (225 g) of wax, depending upon the strength of the aroma you want to achieve, and follow the instructions that come with the kit.

Choose which essential oil to use not only for its fragrance but for its other effects. Use relaxing essential oils for that special evening for two, stimulating ones to get the conversation going during the predinner drinks, and soothing ones with the after-dinner mints. Later still, you might want to bring out the candles designed for romance.

All the essential oil candles have a very subtle effect and are not overpowering like synthetic candle fragrances. The ultimate in host attentiveness must be coordinating the fragrance of the candles with their color and the decor, and when you really get the hang of it, you can match the oils with the personalities of your guests — try putting a relaxing candle next to the person who always hogs the conversation and a stimulating one next to the introverted guest.

Making Your Own Perfumes and Eau de Cologne

As increasing numbers of new perfumes are being launched each season, it seems that more people are becoming overly sensitive to fragrances and perfumes. I can only assume that this development is due to the increased number of synthetically produced aromatic components being used in the newly formulated perfumes, a trend that's matched by the decline in the use of natural botanical ingredients.

The romantic image of a perfumer is someone enclosed by a "perfumer's organ," shelves containing hundreds of small bottles, mostly of essential oils, smelling each in turn on smelling strips, and spending over two years of imagination and creativity exploring the synergy that creates a masterpiece. A master perfumer is known as "The Nose," or in French, *"Le Nez."* More likely today, the perfumer turns to a computer program of 20,000+ chemical compounds, enters what they want to create — say, a "floral, woody, musk" type of perfume — and watches while lists of potentially appropriate chemicals appear on the screen. Of course there's still skill in choosing which combination of chemicals and in what proportion will make a good aroma, but it's not the lifelong craft of *Le Nez.* The new breed of perfumer might be called *"Technicien Aromatique"* as he sits at the computer, deciding whether to include dimethyl-benzyl-carbinyl-butyrate or para-tertiary-butyl-cyclohexyl-acetate in the blend.

The laboratories of companies that manufacture synthetic aromas and flavors dissect the phytochemicals in essential oils, as if they were performing an autopsy, and then use some, copy some, invent similar, and take the life out of the whole. And there's no way that putting the new constituents together is going to re-create the emotionally enhancing properties of classic perfumes that included pure essential oils among their ingredients. The only romance and imagination in synthetic perfumes has been put there by the marketing departments. And nobody seems to be asking what the long-term effect of all these chemicals is going to be, while naturals have been used for thousands of years.

So we've reached a point when many people want to know how they can make their own natural perfumes. The first step is to get to know each essential oil and absolute oil really well before considering whether they should be put in a particular perfume blend. Try different suppliers, purchasing samples to begin with. Sometimes, an oil that doesn't smell that good in a bottle can smell wonderful when it's diluted in really tiny amounts. Then decide what type of fragrance or perfume you want to create, and how you're going to dilute it. As well as water, you'll need something to dilute and disperse the essential oils, known as the *diluent.* This may be alcohol, a fixed, waxy oil such as refined jojoba, or a fractionated oil such as coconut. The type of diluent will determine the end product, which could be a perfume balm, liquid perfume, eau de parfum, eau de toilette, eau de cologne, or splash cologne.

Many of the essential oils you may already have at home for other uses are actually used in perfumery, as you'll see later in this section. Some of those traditionally associated with perfume are expensive, especially the absolutes such as jasmine, cassia, lotus, rose, champaca, boronia, carnation, hyacinth, linden blossom, mimosa, narcissus, osmanthus, and tuberose. But these are very powerful aromatic compounds, and you might need only a few drops.

The essential oils should be used neat — that's to say, they shouldn't be prediluted in any way. Perfume always contains a percentage of water, even if this is as little as 5% of the whole, and distilled water is the better option. Ideally, the alcohol should be pure pharmaceutical grade, which can't be purchased in some countries. But there are other diluent options commercially available. Kitchen perfumers may therefore choose to use vodka — the higher the proof, the better.

The strength of a fragrance depends on the ratio of the finished blend of essential oils to the diluent. Perfume is always the strongest formulation, and the essential oils and/or absolutes should comprise 15% to 30%, with the remaining 70% to 85% being the medium in which it's diluted. If using alcohol, the percentage of water to alcohol should be taken into account in working out your percentages. For example, if making a perfume using a 20% blend, your formulation would include 70% alcohol and 10% distilled water. If using jojoba oil instead of alcohol, use 80%, as you won't need the water. Eau de parfum is lighter than perfume but lasts longer than eau de toilette, which is best put in an atomizer.

A diluent usually consists of a large portion of alcohol and a small portion of water. Some people use specialist perfumery diluent products, some use alcohol on its own, and some work with a ratio of alcohol to water. Commercial alcohol products contain around 95% ethanol, with the remainder being water and a small amount of denaturant, which can't be distilled out and exempts the alcohol from taxes. Alcoholic drinks such as vodka, even at high proof, have a percentage of alcohol, say 40%, with the remainder being water. So there is an element of water within a given alcohol to take into consideration. Bear in mind too that when alcohol is released into the atmosphere it will evaporate from the skin, so that component is always transitory. The diluent is really just a vehicle for delivering the essential oil.

Many home perfumers are reluctant to add water because it can make the perfume appear cloudy. On the other hand, there are advantages to water: it extends the volume of the product and may reduce any odor produced by the alcohol, albeit slightly; it may also reduce the speed at which the fragrance evaporates. Because of the potential for clouding, water is added last, after the alcohol, and it's added slowly, so any clouding can be seen before too much damage has been done. As for what type of water to use: avoid tap water, and use distilled water.

Working out the ingredients in a fragrance always starts with the concentration of essential oils. Some essential oils are not suitable for perfumery because they contain waxes that are insoluble in alcohol or contain resin crystals that precipitate. The volume of diluent is always worked out as 100% less the percentage of essential oils. For example, in perfume, essential oils would be 15%–30% of the total and the diluent will be between 70% and 85%. If using both alcohol and water as a diluent, the percentages can vary depending on personal preference, but always work toward the lower end of the scale to begin with, even reducing the amounts shown in the chart below:

TABLE 17. RATIO OF ESSENTIAL OILS TO DILUENT IN FRAGRANCES

TYPE OF FRAGRANCE	ESSENTIAL OIL BLEND CONCENTRATION	DILUENT CONCENTRATION
Perfume	15% to 30%	70% to 85% (of which 5% to 10% is water)
Eau de parfum	8% to 15%	85% to 92% (of which 10% to 20% is water)
Eau de toilette	4% to 8%	92% to 96% (of which 10% to 20% is water)
Eau de cologne	3% to 5%	95% to 97% (of which 30% is water)
Splash cologne	1% to 3%	97% to 99% (of which 20% is water)

EQUIPMENT

You'll need some small, sterilized glass bottles to put your creations in. Plastic containers and equipment can retain aroma molecules so are never used in professional perfumery. Glass is always the material of choice, along with stainless steel.

A notebook is going to be vital to record the exact formulations, in drops or milliliters, of the essential oils used when making the concentrate. Just one extra drop of another essential oil can completely change the aroma of your creation, and when you create a masterpiece you're going to kick yourself if you can't remember whether it was 3 drops of neroli and 1 of bergamot, or 1 of neroli and 3 of bergamot. Make notes all the way, so you know your failures as well as your successes.

PERFUMERY NOTES

The language of perfumery uses a kind of musical scale comprising base notes, middle or *heart* notes, and top or *head* notes, with *fixative* or *bridging* elements between them. This system, called "the gamut of odors," was first outlined by G. W. Septimus Piesse in *The Art of Perfumery — and Method of Obtaining the Odors of Plants*, published in 1857. Piesse wrote, "In passing the eye down the gamut it will be seen what is a harmony and what is a discord of smells. As an artist would blend his colours, so must a perfumer blend his scents."

The musical analogy is highly appropriate to perfume making, for a perfume is a symphony or concerto of aromatic elements, no different in essence from the artistic blending of notes. The best perfume designers take their work as seriously as do the great musical composers or painters — with the general form, the first impact, the subtle undertones, the highlights, and the background melodies all playing their part in making

the whole a beautiful composition. There has to be contrast, light and dark, highs and lows, movement between all the contributing parts, and, above all, harmony.

Natural perfumes are dynamic and change with people and with time. Not only do they react differently on different skin, and so cannot be said to be just one, specific smell, but they also evaporate, and as they do so, the aroma changes. The speed with which a particular component evaporates is its *volatility*: if it's fast, it's generally called a top note; those with a slower evaporation rate, a middle note; and those that evaporate much slower, a base note. However, perfume ingredients do not adhere to hard and fast rules. Often, so-called top notes are found in middle notes, while aromas generally thought of as middle notes might be used by a perfumer as a top note. It all depends on which other oils are already in the mix, the order in which they've been included, which other oils are yet to be included in the mix, and the ratio between them all. Because natural essences with different rates of evaporation are incorporated into a single perfume, a fragrance will smell differently on the skin when first applied, a few minutes later, and later on in the day.

It's the harmonious blending of these three stages of volatility that makes a classic perfume. If it changes dramatically and smells quite different as time passes, the perfume is said to be not "hanging together" — it isn't integrated into one harmonious whole. This is why a perfume needs bridges or fixatives to hold it together.

ACCORDS

Accord is the perfumer's word for a perfume formulation that can be incorporated into any perfume calling for a particular note. Master perfumers and perfume houses may have, for example, a chypre accord, a green accord, an oriental accord, a floral accord, a citrus accord, a rose accord, a resinous and wood-type accord, an amber accord, or a base note accord. Accords can be incorporated into head notes, heart notes, or base notes and can be an important part of any fine fragrance design. A rose accord might not contain all rose essential oils and may instead be a collection of aromatics that smell like rose and perhaps meld other fragrance notes together in a floral-type fragrance.

As you can imagine, these accords are highly guarded secrets among master perfumers. However, some commercial fragrance ingredient companies sell accords, along with recommendations for the perfume or fragrance they would suit. Individual perfumers may always add their signature accords into their formulations, albeit in tiny amounts. When a perfume contains "amber," usually as part of an oriental type of perfume, it's generally an accord made from several base note ingredients that resemble what the perfumer personally thinks of as an amber fragrance, generally with a balsamic, resinous, warm, and sweet edge. Just one drop of an accord in a blend can change the whole personality of the perfume and can also help correct a few mistakes.

Not all the fragrance notes in a particular aromatic classification are from the type of plant or fruit a nonperfumer might expect to be included. For instance, a floral fragrance type could include a fragrance from a root, such as ginger lily. Likewise, the essential oil of galbanum, which is steam distilled from a resin, could be included among the greener fragrance notes.

Some Essential Oils That Could Be Included in an Accord

Green notes: sweet marjoram, basil, peppermint, thyme, chamomile, immortelle, juniper berry, oregano, clary sage, galbanum

Wood notes: cedarwood, cypress, fir, sandalwood, cabreuva, oud (agarwood), rosewood, ho wood

Floral notes: ylang ylang, rose, geranium, hyacinth, carnation, magnolia flower, frangipani, jasmine, lotus, lavender, ginger lily

Spice notes: ginger, black pepper, nutmeg, pimento berry, cardamom, coriander, fennel, West Indian bay

Citrus notes: bergamot, orange, yuzu, mandarin, lime, may chang, eucalyptus lemon, melissa

Amber-type or base notes: cistus, patchouli, benzoin, vetiver, vanilla, balsam de Peru, mastic, balsam de Tolu, tonka bean, cedarwood, sandalwood

Cistus, vanilla, and benzoin could be a good starting point for a base note, with a little patchouli and tonka bean.

An accord is not a modern invention. A lily of the valley accord was suggested by Piesse in *The Art of Perfumery* in 1857. I've halved the amounts he suggested in the following: tuberose, ¼ pint; jasmine, ½ oz.; orange flower, 1 oz.; vanilla, 1½ oz.; cassia, approximately 1 oz.; rose, 1 oz.; bitter almond, 1½ drops.

You can create many other types of accords from your favorite blends, and these accords — even just one drop — can be used as a perfume signature if added to other blends.

EXAMPLES OF PERFUME NOTES

It is often helpful to know some of the ingredients that successful perfumes contained in terms of their top, middle, and base notes, and when looking for guidance we have to return to the glory days of perfume, when the ingredients were those we can recognize and appreciate. Sadly, the original versions of many wonderful perfumes are no longer available. These first two classic perfumes are from the long-standing popular French perfume house, Guerlain:

Jicky, 1889

Top: lemon, bergamot, mandarin, rosewood

Middle: jasmine, patchouli, rose, orris root, vetiver

Base: vanilla, benzoin, amber, tonka bean, **civet, *leather, frankincense

L'heure Bleue, 1912

Top: bergamot, lemon, neroli, coriander seed, sage, tarragon

Middle: clove, jasmine, rose de mai, ylang ylang, orchid

Base: sandalwood, vetiver, cedarwood, vanilla, benzoin, **musk

Leather was an accord.

**Civet and musk were animal products.*

One early perfume house, Caron, included the following essential oils in its classic 1911 perfume, Narcisse Noir:

Top: bergamot, mandarin, petitgrain, lemon

Middle: narcissus, jasmine, jonquil, orange blossom

Base: sandalwood, **civet, **musk

Perfumery may be as simple as using a natural essence and mixing it with alcohol and water to make a liquid that carries the perfume of just one flower. But the grand symphonies of perfumery come into play when creating a picture not of one flower but of a person in a field of flowers. Let your imagination conjure up aromatic images of vitality and complexity and interaction. It could be that you have in mind an alpine mountain in spring, or an English garden in summer, or a New England autumnal wood, or perhaps a Balinese flower festival, or a moonlit Caribbean night. All these images and the sensations that accompany them can be conjured up with the vast array of essential oils. Above all, be creative, and enjoy the challenges and sheer pleasure of making your own perfumes.

When making a perfume, first establish your base note, or combination of base notes, then your middle note(s), then the top notes. Put the base note essential oils into a bottle, making sure they're well combined by swirling them around, and leave for several days. Then add the middle notes and do the same thing, and finally add the top notes, again swirling the bottle well. Tightly close the lid and leave the blend in the bottle to mature, swirling it around each time you pass, for at least five days, before opening the bottle again to test the blend. A professional perfumer might leave it for four to six weeks.

Then add the essential oil concentrate to your chosen volume of diluent. Start by adding really small amounts of your concentrate to your diluent until you reach your desired fragrance strength. Make notes as you go. Swirl the mixture around gently until it's extremely well diffused and leave it to stand for at least a week before bottling.

In the lists that follow, the natural oils used in feminine fragrances are separated from the oils generally used in masculine fragrances, although you should in no way feel constrained by these traditional guidelines, as most essential oils are on both lists.

FEMININE NOTES

These notes were found in traditional perfumes and eau de cologne intended as female fragrances:

FEMININE BASE NOTES

Balsam de Peru	Cistus
Balsam de Tolu	Frankincense
Benzoin	Guaiacwood
Cedarwood atlas	Heliotrope
Cinnamon	Melilot

Myrrh
Olibanum
Opoponax
Patchouli
Sandalwood

Styrax
Tonka bean
Vanilla
Vetiver

The following oils, which are found in either base or middle notes, could be used as bridges between the two — depending on the overall formula.

FEMININE BASE OR MIDDLE NOTES

Cedarwood atlas
Cinnamon
Frankincense
Heliotrope
Myrrh

Patchouli
Sandalwood
Styrax
Vetiver

FEMININE MIDDLE NOTES

Carnation
Cassia
Clary sage
Clove
Geranium
Ginger
Ho wood
Hyacinth
Jasmine
Lemongrass
Linden blossom
Marjoram, sweet
Mimosa

Narcissus
Neroli
Nutmeg
Palmarosa
Pimento berry
Pine needle
Rose
Rosewood (bois de rose)
Thyme
Tuberose
Violet flower
Ylang ylang

FEMININE MIDDLE OR TOP NOTES

Bay
Cassia
Clary sage
Hyacinth
Marjoram, sweet
Mimosa

Neroli
Nutmeg
Palmarosa
Rosewood
Thyme

Top notes are the most volatile — that's to say, they evaporate the most quickly and are therefore the ones you smell first of all. They gradually evaporate and leave the middle notes, which eventually fade and reveal the base notes. This order is reversed when actually making the perfume, so that the top notes are your final flourish, so to speak. Use several essences, or just one, from each list to formulate your own perfume.

FEMININE TOP NOTES

Angelica seed
Anise
Basil
Bergamot
Chamomile roman
Coriander seed
Cumin
Galbanum
Juniper berry
Lavender

Lemon
Lime
Mandarin
Neroli
Orange
Petitgrain
Rosemary
Spearmint
Tarragon

Perfumes are usually composed of many ingredients, and their base, middle, and top notes are themselves quite complex concoctions. Here are some of the components of the base, middle, and top notes of some classic perfumes to give you an idea of what makes that most mysterious product, a perfume, a success:

Base Notes

vetiver + vanilla + sandalwood + balsam de Peru + benzoin + balsam de Tolu: In perfumer's terms this would be called a "sweet balsamic" note.

Middle Notes

jasmine + orris root + rose maroc + carnation + ylang ylang + tuberose: a "sweet, floral, spicy" note

jasmine + rose + narcissus + carnation + jonquil + tuberose: a "narcotic, floral" note

rosewood + cinnamon + rose + ylang ylang + jasmine + ginger + carnation: an "exotic, floral" note

Top Notes

lemon + mandarin + bergamot + rosewood: a "citrus fresh" note

bergamot + mandarin + lemon + neroli: a "fresh" note

hyacinth + narcissus + galbanum + lemon + bergamot: a "green and fresh" note

Although no perfumers will give away any part of the formula for their perfume blends, they are prepared to offer a few clues for marketing purposes while keeping the exact proportions hidden away in their vaults. Here are some of the ingredients of two famous perfumes:

Perfume 1

Top note (fresh, citrus type): lemon + bergamot + mandarin + rosewood + lavender

Middle note (floral, wood type): patchouli + rose + jasmine + vetiver

Base note (balsamic, soft type): benzoin + vanilla + balsam de Peru + frankincense

Perfume 2

Top note (spicy, warm type): orange + pimento berry + bay + petitgrain

Middle note (floral, warm, spicy type): carnation + cinnamon + jasmine + ylang ylang + cardamom

Base note (warm and soft type): vanilla + patchouli + benzoin + frankincense

MASCULINE NOTES

These notes were found in traditional perfumes and eau de cologne intended as male fragrances. When making colognes for men, follow the same procedures as for making perfume, although the concentration of essences is generally much less.

MASCULINE BASE NOTES

Bay	Olibanum
Benzoin	Sandalwood
Cedarwood	Styrax
Cinnamon	Tonka bean
Frankincense	Vanilla
Myrrh	Vetiver

The following oils, which are found in either base or middle notes, could be used as bridges between the two — depending on the overall formula.

MASCULINE BASE TO MIDDLE NOTES

Bay	Patchouli
Cedarwood	Pimento berry
Cinnamon	Sandalwood
Myrrh	Vetiver

MASCULINE MIDDLE NOTES

Angelica seed	Mandarin
Anise	Marjoram, sweet
Basil	Neroli
Caraway seed	Nutmeg
Cardamom	Oregano
Carnation	Orris root
Carrot seed	Pepper, black
Clary sage	Peppermint
Clove	Petitgrain
Coriander seed	Pine
Cumin	Rose
Galbanum	Rosemary
Geranium	Rosewood
Ginger	Sage
Jasmine	Tarragon
Juniper berry	Thyme
Lavender	Ylang ylang

MASCULINE MIDDLE TO TOP NOTES

Angelica seed	Nutmeg
Basil	Oregano
Bay	Pepper, black
Caraway seed	Pimento berry
Clary sage	Rosemary

Coriander seed	Rosewood
Lavender	Tarragon
Marjoram, sweet	Thyme

MASCULINE TOP NOTES

Anise	Lemon verbena
Bergamot	Lime
Cedar	Mandarin
Cumin	Neroli
Galbanum	Orange
Juniper berry	Peppermint
Lemon	Petitgrain
Lemongrass	Sage

The following combinations occur in some famous male colognes:

Base Notes

tonka bean + cedarwood: In perfumer's terms, this would be called a "light" base note.

vanilla + heliotrope: a "sweet" base note

cedarwood + vetiver + tonka bean + oakmoss + cistus: a "warm and woody" base note

Middle Notes

lavender + carnation + juniper berry + jasmine + pine: a "green, resinous" note

jasmine + carnation + vetiver + geranium + patchouli + orris root + cinnamon: a "floral, woody" note

clary sage + basil + orange + geranium + jasmine: a "fresh" note

jasmine + pine + carnation + thyme + cinnamon: a "spicy, resinous" note

Top Notes

lavender + anise + lemon + lime + petitgrain + mandarin + bergamot: a "citrus, fresh, herbaceous" note

lavender + bergamot + rosemary + lemon: a "lavendaceous, fresh" note

bergamot + lavender + petitgrain + basil + lemon: a "fresh, herbaceous" note

You can see from the preceding lists that fragrance ingredients that might be considered exclusively feminine actually feature very strongly in masculine preparations, and vice versa. The lines between the two are arbitrary, and they change with time. Yet the perception persists that a strong line divides masculine and feminine fragrances when the differences may have less to do with the ingredients than with the proportion of each oil used. Preconceived ideas about what is, or is not, a masculine perfumery ingredient is a barrier to delving into the entire fragrance palette and arriving at a fragrance that truly reflects a particular male character. For example, common ingredients in male products include lavender, bergamot, lemon, orange, jasmine, carnation, and geranium, more usually thought of as "feminine" fragrance ingredients.

MAKING EAU DE COLOGNE–TYPE BLENDS

The volumes in the blends below are sufficient for up to 3.4 fl. oz. (100 mL) of diluent:

BLEND 1

Bergamot	10 drops
Rosemary	2 drops
Orange	20 drops
Lemon	10 drops
Neroli	2 drops

BLEND 2

Basil	1 drop
Rose	4 drops
Petitgrain	1 drop
Bergamot	2 drops
Lemon	2 drops
Orange	2 drops
Neroli	1 drop

BLEND 3

Geranium	1 drop
Palmarosa	10 drops
Petitgrain	3 drops
Orange	8 drops
Lime	2 drops

After blending the essential oils together, slowly add them to 2.4 fl. oz. (70 mL) of 100% proof vodka or other alcohol, stirring gently but long enough to ensure complete dispersal. Seal and leave it to stand for 48 hours. Then add 2 tablespoons (30 mL) of distilled water, and again stir slowly but enough to ensure a thorough mixing is taking place.

The mixture should be bottled and left to stand for at least another 48 hours in a cool, dark place. Professional perfumers often leave the liquid for four to six weeks to *evolve*, or mature. After letting the liquid evolve, pour it through an unbleached paper coffee filter before final bottling. If you find the aroma too strong, the eau de cologne can be further diluted by adding more water and mixing well. If you find it too weak, add a further quantity of essential oils.

Making Your Own Essential Oil Waters and Hydrolats

Essential oil waters can be used as the water source for producing hydrolats, and hydrolats can be used in the production of essential oil waters. By combining these two methods of extracting the active ingredients of plants, more opportunities for therapeutic, cosmetic, or fragrance preparations become available. (See chapter 19, "Carrier Oils and Hydrolats," for the distinction between hydrolats, hydrosols, herbal distillates, essential oil waters, and a whole range of other water-and-plant products.)

ESSENTIAL OIL WATERS

Essential oil waters are waters infused with essential oil. They're not hydrolats, because they don't contain the hydrophilic plant compounds that become infused in the water used in the distillation process. Nor are they watered-down essential oils, because the action of boiling the water and filtering it through paper removes some of the essential oil components.

Essential oil waters can be used in the following ways: in compresses, saunas, steam rooms, and baths, and as an ingredient in beauty products. They are *not* a substitute for hydrolats.

MAKING ESSENTIAL OIL WATER

Your chosen essential oil	10–30 drops (or more)
Boiling water	6.8 fl. oz. (200 mL)

1. Add up to 10–30 drops of your chosen essential oil (or more for a stronger aroma) to 6.8 fl. oz. (200 mL) of boiling water. Put the lid on the pot to keep the steam in.
2. Continue boiling for around 60–120 seconds and then turn off the heat, keeping the lid on all the time.
3. Move the pot to a heat-resistant surface, and allow to cool.
4. Allow to stand for 24 hours without removing the lid. Then, slowly pour the liquid through a slightly damp unbleached paper coffee filter. This will remove most of the essential oil, leaving fragranced water behind that can be used in many ways.

Depending on which essential oil you have used, the coffee filter will be highly fragranced and, once dry, can be used to perfume drawers, closets, or rooms if left on a source of heat such as a radiator. Remember, though, that essential oils are flammable, even when dried on paper, so avoid placing the discarded filters near candles or fires.

One of the advantages of making essential oil waters is that there's no need to be limited by a single essential oil because they can be made using a number of different essential oils. For example, lavender, mint, and lemongrass work well together. There's no end to the potential combinations or to their therapeutic, cosmetic, and perfumery applications.

MAKING HYDROLATS

Hydrolats are produced in two ways: plant material is processed expressly to produce a hydrolat; and hydrolats are produced as a by-product of essential oil production. Traditionally, hydrolats are the water remaining after essential oils have been produced by steam distillation, which still contains small traces of essential oils plus the hydrophilic elements from the plant material itself. Some hydrolats smell like the plant material that the essential oils were distilled from, but many do not. Their aroma may be bland or even unpleasant. The advantages of making your own hydrolat is that you can ensure that it's fresh, and you can use a plant material from which no other hydrolat is available. Several tabletop stills are on the market that are intended for home use.

Take great care to ensure you know the exact plant species to distill. Many plants, flowers, or plant parts are poisonous. If a plant is growing in your garden and you have been in the habit of eating it raw or using it in a tea, then it should be fine made into a hydrolat or distillate. Never purchase flowers or herbs to use in a home still, as these may have been sprayed. Remember that there are hundreds of geranium plants, and only a couple of varieties are made into essential oil. So don't think that any similar-sounding or -looking plant will substitute for one used in aromatherapy. Only use organically grown plant materials. This is especially important if you plan to use your finished products therapeutically. Making your own hydrolats gives you tremendous scope for concocting your own cosmetic lotions and potions.

It might surprise you to know that essential oils and hydrolats can be and often are distilled from some dried plant material. Dried lavender, for example, is sometimes used to produce both essential oils and hydrolats. A stronger therapeutic strength can be gained by using the same water and repeating the distillation several times. Whether buying fresh or dried plant material or using your own homegrown, rinse well before making the hydrolat.

The water used must be pure water — no tap water. Use distilled water or mineral water — the latter may have the benefit of trace minerals. Essential oil waters can be used in the place of water to distill a hydrolat. The color of a hydrolat, hydrosol, or distillate can vary, depending on the plant and the amount of plant material used. It's most always very light and hardly visible, with more a tinge or hint of color than an actual color. The color also depends on the time of year and even the time of day that the plant material was cut, and also on whether the plant was flowering or not, and whether the plant material is fresh or dried.

The conditions of making, packing, and storage have to be well thought out — the packing has to be sterile and airtight. Store in a cool place, such as in the fridge. Any water-based solution is a breeding ground for bacteria, and avoiding them is your top priority. Although hydrolats include traces of essential oils, these are not at a high enough concentration to prohibit the growth of bacteria or fungi. Without any form of preservative, hydrolats will deteriorate. So make fresh batches periodically, store them in the fridge, and use them as soon as possible. If making a large amount, decant into several small bottles, rather than one large one, so you can access exactly the amount you require at any one time and don't have to open a bottle more than once, to avoid oxidation. Hydrolats can be used undiluted for therapeutic purposes, in cosmetics, and in cooking, as well as being useful in many home care methods.

Cooking with Essential Oils

Using essential oils in home cooking is easy and convenient, opening up a whole new world of possibilities and delights. The American food and drinks industry has been using essential oils for well over 130 years, with peppermint and spearmint having a particularly long history. Today, the United States produces almost 10 million pounds of peppermint and spearmint, with about 55% of that amount going into toothpaste, about 30% into chewing gum, 10% into candy, and 5% into pharmaceuticals, soaps, and shampoos. The aromatherapy market represents only a tiny proportion of mint use.

As well as adding essential oils to food and drink for their flavor, today the industry is placing great emphasis on the antioxidant and antimicrobial properties of essential oils, with particular reference to their ability to extend shelf life, and on their role in "active," or "smart," packaging. The U.S. Food and Drug Administration publishes a list of essential oils that are "generally recognized as safe" (GRAS) to use in foods and drinks, on the proviso that they're used in a quantity described as a reasonable dietary intake, and that the essential oil is solvent-free.

Food producers often proclaim that "real fruit essences" or "real oils" are included in a product,

knowing perhaps more than anyone that modern large-scale commercial production methods require the replacement of the natural aroma and flavor that manufacturing has taken out. They also appreciate that essential oils can easily be combined into totally new flavors, and that this can be a unique selling point.

But anyone can create unique flavors in the kitchen by combining essential oils and using them in imaginative ways. All that's needed are good-quality organic essential oils and good fresh raw materials. The other key point is that essential oils should be used in moderation — only as much or less than a recipe calls for. Even a simple pepper steak can be made into a gastronomic great by mixing the pepper with a tiny drop of lemon or bergamot essential oil in the cooking oil and a little fresh thyme before spreading it on the steak. Store-bought vanilla ice cream can be transformed into a delicious fantasy by adding essential oil — try a combination of ginger and lime, spearmint and geranium, or rose and bergamot. Some flavorings and essential oils that are not commonplace in the United States are very widely used in their countries of origin — for example, yuzu is extensively used in cookery in Japan.

Essential oils for the kitchen come in four

main groups: herbs, spices, citrus fruits, and flowers. They can be used in soups and starters, in marinades, salad dressings and sauces, with red and white meat dishes, with fish or vegetables, and in breads, biscuits, cakes, desserts, and confectionery.

The herb essential oils make a tasty contribution to casseroles, either used in a marinade for the meat before cooking or simply added to the pot. Added to a bread or roll mixture, the herb essential oils can create marvels — try sage and rosemary with fresh garlic, or lemon essential oil with fresh sage and onion. Or try a savory biscuit made with almonds, sun-dried raisins, and rosemary essential oil.

The citrus essential oils may be used in salad dressings, marinades, sauces, and desserts. They also work very well with both fish and poultry. Added to a wine marinade, lemon, bay laurel, or basil add excellent flavor to beef. Citrus butter works well with vegetables and fish, giving the food a special zing. And talking of butters, try ginger butter on green beans or spearmint butter on peas.

The purity and clarity of flavor obtained with essential oils is, however, just one of their advantages. They help in the digestion of meats, act as antioxidants and antimicrobials when used in food, and although their nutritional value is largely unknown, they're pure natural products that will certainly do you more good than artificial flavorings. The value of using a calming aroma doesn't diminish — it will still have a calming effect if used in uncooked food. Make some geranium frozen yogurt to cheer yourself up — geranium leaves have been used in cooking for hundreds of years, and besides giving you a lift, this simple dessert tastes good.

Not least among the advantages of the essential oils is the fact that they're very economical to use. And as you will probably have some of the essential oils at home already, you can experiment with new culinary ideas without going to any extra expense. Never use too much essential oil: the idea is to enhance the natural flavors of real food, add a flavor twist, or put flavor back into bland packaged foods. Essential oil bottles have a dropper in them, and these vary in size with each supplier. However, the dropper inserts can be purchased separately and a small size chosen to reduce the size of the drop.

THE TOOTHPICK METHOD

Sometimes less than a drop is required to achieve the right flavor balance, and the toothpick method is a good way to control the amount of essential oil you use. It involves putting a small amount of essential oil on the end of a toothpick, and using this to stir flavor into the food. Dip the toothpick into the food little by little, until the desired strength is reached, stirring through as usual.

Less is always more when using essential oils in the kitchen; the idea is to achieve subtle aroma enhancement. This chapter aims to give you some suggestions to get started on cooking with essential oils. The flair and imagination are left to you!

Aromatic and Flavored Oils and Vinegars

Flavored oils are easy to make at home and are a good way to dilute the strength and aroma of an essential oil. There are no hard and fast rules as to how much essential oil to add. With the more powerfully aromatic essential oils such as thyme, marjoram, lavender, and ginger, you'll need to add less essential oil to reach the desired effect than with a citrus essential oil. Aromatic, flavored oils are used as a complementary aroma and flavor and should not overpower the other ingredients. Start by adding 1 drop per 2 fl. oz. (60 mL) of oil and gradually increase the amount, adding the essential oil drop by drop until reaching your personal desired strength.

Choosing the right fine cooking carrier oil is the start to creating good aromatic culinary oil. Any organic salad or fine cooking oil can be used, and the flavor and aroma of the chosen salad or cooking oil will influence the final product. Olive oil, for example, is a highly flavorsome oil that's complemented by the aroma of the herb and citrus essential oils.

The citrus oils of lemon, sweet orange, mandarin, tangerine, lime, grapefruit, bergamot, and yuzu make interesting additions to salad dressings. Try them in a combination with ginger, spearmint, sweet marjoram, basil, or lavender. Use 1–2 drops of essential oil per 6 ounces of salad oil to start, shake well, and if possible leave to infuse for a few hours. Try a blend of lime and spearmint, or yuzu and tangerine. Yuzu can have a tendency to overpower other citrus essential oils, so if using that, start with 1 drop per 6 oz.

For spicy food, you'll only need to add 1 or 2 drops per 6 oz. of a fine cooking oil to start: choose from black pepper, cardamom, coriander seed, cinnamon, ginger, nutmeg, or turmeric. Try a blend of black pepper and lime, or cardamom and sweet orange — or all four!

The flavors of meat and fish dishes combine well with the herb essential oils: basil, sweet fennel, sweet marjoram, oregano, rosemary, sage, and thyme. You might want to try spearmint with lamb.

If using fine cooking oils such as almond oil in desserts, try the floral oils such as geranium, lavender, rose, neroli, ylang ylang, or cananga. Always give the oil a shake before use.

Fragrant vinegars play an important part in essential oil cuisine. Essential oils could be incorporated into vinegars at the rate of 1 or 2 drops per 2 fl. oz. (60 mL) of vinegar. Use rose, bergamot, geranium, or coriander vinegar in dips, vinaigrettes, sauces, and salad dressings; try lemongrass, grapefruit, or yuzu vinegar with fish or fatty meat dishes.

Vinegars store well, but shake them before use. New ideas will come to you; for example, the basic mayonnaise recipe below can easily be converted into countless dips, sauces, garnishing, or dressings by blending it with flavored oils or vinegars.

Dips

BASIC MAYONNAISE
1 large egg yolk
1 teaspoon wine vinegar
½ teaspoon Dijon mustard
¼ teaspoon salt
¼ teaspoon ground pepper
3 ounces (approximately 100 mL) of organic olive, sunflower, rapeseed, nut oil, or oil of choice; or a 50:50 blend; or a flavored oil. The type of oil you use will determine the final flavor.
Put the egg yolk in a bowl along with the vinegar, mustard, and salt and pepper; mix well together. Trickle the plain or flavored oil in very slowly, whisking the mixture continuously with your other hand. Use a fork or hand whisk, mixing gently, and always in the same direction, or follow your blender's instructions. How much oil you use will depend on the size of the egg and the amount and consistency required.

GARLIC AND LIME DIP
2 cloves crushed garlic
1 or 2 drops lime essential oil
8 tablespoons Basic Mayonnaise (above)
Crush the garlic with the drops of lime essential oil on a board, then mix well with the mayonnaise.

TOMATO, LEMON, AND GRAPEFRUIT DIP
6 tablespoons Basic Mayonnaise (above)
1 teaspoon tomato puree

1 drop lemon essential oil
1 drop grapefruit essential oil

Whisk the mayonnaise, tomato puree, and essential oils until the mixture is an even orange-pink color. To make the dip spicy, add 2 drops of Tabasco sauce or a chopped chili and freshly ground pepper.

CITRUS AND CORIANDER DIP

6 tablespoons Basic Mayonnaise (page 461)
Combine:
> 1 drop coriander seed essential oil with 1 drop lemon or lime essential oil, and from this use
> 1–2 drops

1 teaspoon of chopped tarragon herb

Mix the ingredients together well. This is an excellent sauce for all fish, but especially oily fish such as herring. It can easily be adapted to make a fish pâté by mixing with any flaked fish, finely chopped caper, and cucumber dill pickle. Garnish and serve with whole-grain toast.

Butters, Spreads, and Cheeses

Essential oils can be incorporated into butter to top potatoes, meat, and pastas. The butter stores well and can be frozen.

Leave about ½ cup (100 g) of butter to soften at room temperature. Place butter in a bowl, add ½ to 1 drop of your chosen essential oil, and stir well. Refrigerate and use when needed.

Use 1 drop of essential oil in 8 ounces of fromage frais, quark, or cream cheese. Try rose and mandarin fromage frais over strawberries in summer, or sweet orange and grapefruit cream cheese on a watercress salad.

Savory Sauces

Savory sauces can be used to enhance a plain dish or disguise leftovers, or they may just be eaten on their own with fresh chunks of whole-grain bread. Once again, the versatility of essential oils can be used to advantage.

BLENDER HOLLANDAISE SAUCE

3 large egg yolks
1 or 2 drops lemon essential oil
½ teaspoon salt
½ teaspoon pepper
4 ounces warm melted butter (or substitute)

Put the egg yolks into the blender along with your chosen essential oil, salt, and pepper. Blend. Slowly add the hot butter and continue blending for about 10 minutes. Grapefruit or lime essential oil could also be used.

GREEN SAUCE

2 tablespoons finely chopped parsley
2 tablespoons finely chopped watercress
1 tablespoon finely chopped onion (or scallion)
1 teaspoon finely chopped capers
1 clove garlic, finely crushed
1 small potato, boiled
1 tablespoon olive oil
1 or 2 drops grapefruit essential oil
1 drop sweet orange essential oil
1 teaspoon vinegar
Salt and pepper to taste

Combine all the chopped ingredients and the garlic together. Mash the potato in another bowl, and to it add all the oils and the vinegar, salt, and pepper. Stir into a smooth paste. Now add the combined chopped mixture and continue stirring until all the ingredients are combined. Serve with cold meats, vegetables, and pasta. Green sauce can be added to yogurt and served over boiled or baked potatoes.

LIME AND MINT SAUCE

The combination of lime and mint adds a fresh flavor to summer vegetables, pulses, and rice dishes.
4 tablespoons olive oil
1 or 2 drops lime essential oil

1 teaspoon mustard
1 teaspoon finely chopped parsley
1 teaspoon finely chopped chives
1 tablespoon finely chopped mint

Mix the olive oil and lime essential oil together. Add the remaining ingredients, and blend well. Warm slowly over a low heat if required hot. Grapefruit or tangerine essential oil could be substituted for the lime.

Appetizers

RUSSIAN EGGS

6 hard-boiled eggs
1 teaspoon chopped green olives
1 teaspoon chopped chives
3 tablespoons Basic Mayonnaise (see page 461)
1 teaspoon chopped onion
Dash of Tabasco sauce
¼ teaspoon freshly ground pepper
1 or 2 drops lemon essential oil
½–1 drop grapefruit essential oil
1 teaspoon chopped parsley

Cut the eggs in half and remove the yolks. Put yolks into a bowl and add all the other ingredients except the parsley. Mix well until it forms a paste and spoon back into the egg whites. Arrange on a bed of lettuce and sprinkle the eggs with parsley.

ORANGE, YUZU, AND GINGER PRAWNS

1 pound uncooked prawns (king if possible)
Marinade:
2 tablespoons soy sauce
2 tablespoons cooking sherry
2 tablespoons fine cooking oil
1 clove garlic, crushed
Juice of 1 small orange
2 drops ginger essential oil
1 drop yuzu essential oil
1 drop sweet orange essential oil

Mix all the marinade ingredients together and pour over the uncooked prawns. Leave for 1–2 hours in the fridge. Remove the prawns from the marinade and heat the marinade until it starts to reduce. Lightly stir-fry the prawns until cooked, using 1 teaspoon of the marinade, then add the remaining marinade to the prawns. Serve on a bed of watercress and decorate with orange slices or nasturtium flowers.

CHICKEN MINT BALLS

1 drop spearmint essential oil
1 egg, beaten
1 small onion, chopped
1 tablespoon chopped parsley
¼ teaspoon powdered cinnamon
¼ teaspoon powdered allspice
Salt
Freshly ground pepper
¾ pound minced chicken meat or nonmeat
    substitute
2 tablespoons crumbed bread

Thoroughly mix the spearmint oil into the beaten egg. Then add the onion, parsley, cinnamon, allspice, salt, and pepper and blend together well. Finally add the minced chicken or vegetarian option and the bread and mix all the ingredients to an even consistency. Place in the fridge until needed. Roll into bite-size balls and fry in a small amount of fine cooking oil. Serve with black olives and the following dip:

Dip:
2 tablespoons chopped cucumber
1 cup plain yogurt
1 drop spearmint (or coriander seed) essential oil
1 drop lime essential oil

Combine ingredients and serve in a bowl in which you dip the chicken balls.

Marinades

In the days before refrigeration, spicing meats was a way of preserving food in preparation for the long cold winter ahead. These days, marinating meat is no longer a necessity, but it is used to add flavor and to tenderize cheaper cuts of meat.

RED MEAT MARINADE

Enough for 2 pounds of beef.

1 drop thyme essential oil
1 drop sweet marjoram essential oil
1 drop bay laurel essential oil
1 drop sweet orange essential oil
2 tablespoons olive oil
1 cup red wine or nonalcoholic cooking wine
2 cloves garlic
2 clove spice buds
1 chopped onion
Good pinch of salt
¼ teaspoon whole peppercorn

Blend the essential oils together, then add in the olive oil and mix well. Pour the red wine into a dish large enough to hold your meat, and add the garlic, clove buds, onion, salt, and pepper. Gently rub 1–2 teaspoons of the blended oils into the meat, then place the meat in the red wine marinade. (The remaining blended oils will keep for another time.) Leave the meat covered for eight hours or overnight, turning once or twice. Cook in your favorite way, using the marinade to make a sauce.

FRESH TUNA MARINADE

Makes enough for 1 pound of fresh tuna.

1 cup dry white wine or nonalcoholic cooking wine
1 clove garlic
1 small onion, sliced
Pinch of salt
¼ teaspoon whole black peppercorns
1 drop lime essential oil
1 drop sweet fennel essential oil
1 tablespoon olive oil

Pour the wine into a dish large enough to hold the tuna and add the garlic, onion, salt, and pepper. Mix the lime and fennel oils with the olive oil and rub a small amount into the tuna, then place the tuna in the wine. Leave covered for 3–6 hours. Grill or poach the tuna and use the marinade for a sauce.

Soups

AVOCADO AND LIME SOUP

2 ripe avocados
1 small onion, finely chopped
5 ounces plain yogurt
5 fl. oz. milk (or dairy alternative)
1 clove garlic, crushed
2 drops lime essential oil
1 vegetable stock cube
2½ cups water
Pinch of salt
Freshly ground pepper

Blend, by hand or in a blender, the avocados, onion, yogurt, milk, garlic, and lime essential oil. Dissolve the stock cube in the water and bring to a boil. Reduce to a simmer and slowly add the blended mixture and salt and pepper, stirring all the time. Bring gently back to a boil and serve.

BASIL, TOMATO, AND POTATO SOUP

2 ounces butter
2 onions, finely chopped
1 pound tomatoes, chopped
2½ cups water
1 pound cooked, diced potatoes
Salt and pepper
2 teaspoons yogurt
½ drop basil essential oil

Melt the butter in a pan, add the onion, and cook until soft. Add the tomatoes and cook down until soft; sieve to remove skins if preferred. Add the water and bring to a boil. Now add the potatoes, salt, and pepper. Simmer for 15 minutes. Combine the yogurt and basil essential oil. Stir in the soup and serve.

MANDARIN AND CARROT SOUP

1 ounce butter

1 pound grated carrot

1 small onion, finely chopped

1 large potato, grated

Salt and pepper

2½ cups vegetable stock

1 or 2 drops mandarin essential oil

Melt the butter in a heavy pan, add the carrot, onion, potato, salt, and pepper and cook until softened, stirring occasionally. Add the stock and bring to a boil. Now add the mandarin essential oil and reduce to a simmer for 10 minutes.

An easy way to use essential oils in soups is to combine them with the oil, butter, or butter alternative used to sauté meats or vegetables before turning them into soup, or blend them with yogurt or cream before adding to the soup.

Vegetables

Vegetables benefit from the addition of essential oils in vinegars, oils, butters, and sauces. The Basic Mayonnaise recipe (see page 461) can be adapted for many uses by the addition of purees and essential oils.

POTATO SALAD

2 pounds new potatoes

4 tablespoons Basic Mayonnaise (page 461)

1 tablespoon chopped chives

1 small onion, finely chopped

1 dessertspoon finely chopped pickled cucumber or dill pickle

1 or 2 drops lemon essential oil

½–1 drop spearmint essential oil

Boil the potatoes and leave to cool. Blend the rest of the ingredients before adding to the potatoes. Chill and serve. Leave out the pickle if not to your taste.

STEAMED GREEN BEANS

2 pounds green beans

4 tablespoons Basic Mayonnaise (page 461)

¼ drop ginger essential oil

1 tablespoon flaked almonds

Steam the beans. Combine the mayonnaise with the ¼ drop of ginger essential oil using the toothpick method and blend well. Pour over the beans and decorate with the almonds.

STEAMED VEGETABLES

Steam vegetables over water to which an essential oil of your choice has been added. Nutmeg, mace, cumin, caraway seed, and the citrus oils are particularly good for cabbage and greens, but try the flower oils too, such as geranium and lavender, with other vegetables.

SWEET VEGETABLES

Sweet potatoes, beets, and root vegetables can all be used with essential oils to make interesting and unusual dishes. Tangerine or yuzu essential oils blend particularly well with sweet potatoes in desserts.

TANGERINE SWEET POTATO

1 pound sweet potatoes

2 ounces butter (or substitute)

3 tablespoons brown sugar or coconut blossom/ nectar sugar

2 drops tangerine essential oil

Pinch of ground pepper

2 tablespoons rum or nonalcoholic alternative

1 tablespoon chopped walnuts

Boil and mash the sweet potatoes. Cream the butter and sugar and add the tangerine essential oil, the ground pepper, and the rum if desired. Pour over the potatoes and mash together. Place in an ovenproof dish and sprinkle with walnuts. Heat in an oven at 325°F for between 10 and 15 minutes, and serve. You could replace the essential oil of tangerine with that of mandarin if you prefer. This also makes a filling for sweet potato flan.

Lemon or Orange Pepper

Lemon pepper is a delicious substitute for conventional pepper. Use it in any dish that you feel would be enhanced by a zing of lemon — fish and salads, for example.

Put 1 oz. of coarsely ground pepper into a small bowl and add 1 drop of lemon, or lemongrass, essential oil. Mix together, bottle, and store for at least three days before use. Orange pepper is made in exactly the same way, using sweet orange essential oil instead of lemon. There is practically no end to the unique flavors that can be created: summer berries such as strawberries can be given an interesting twist by adding a sprinkle of pepper fragranced with geranium oil.

Fish

White fish steaks can be brushed with a prepared cooking oil before grilling. Lemon, fennel, dill, coriander seed, grapefruit, and lime essential oils are all interesting additions to the flavor of white fish. Use 1 drop of essential oil to 1 tablespoon of fine cooking oil. Then simply brush your fish steak with the oil and grill in the normal way. Turn the steaks and repeat the process. Any unused oil can be stored for future use.

Oily fish such as salmon, trout, mackerel, herring, and sardines are exceptionally good with citrus essential oils such as lemon and lime.

BAKED MACKEREL
1 apple, grated
1 teaspoon chopped parsley
2 drops sweet orange or lemon essential oil
1 tablespoon fresh bread crumbs
2 large mackerel, cleaned and prepared
1 small onion, cut in rings
1 cup unfiltered apple juice
Preheat the oven to 325–350°F. Combine the apple, parsley, and sweet orange essential oil with the bread crumbs. Stuff the mackerels with equal amounts of stuffing and place the onion rings on top of the stuffing. Put the fish in an ovenproof dish and pour the apple juice over the fish. Bake for 20 minutes.

LEMON SOLE WITH ALMONDS
1 tablespoon fine cooking oil
1 drop lemon essential oil
Salt and pepper
2 fillets of sole
1 tablespoon flaked almonds
Blend the cooking oil with the lemon essential oil, salt, and pepper, then brush a small amount over the fillets on both sides. Sprinkle with almonds, and grill.

Meat

When cooking red meat, the essential oil should be combined with a fine cooking oil before being brushed over the meat: 1 drop of essential oil to 1 tablespoon (15 mL) of cooking oil is sufficient. The essential oils of rosemary, basil, thyme, sage, summer savory, black pepper, juniper berry, bay laurel, coriander seed, cardamom, and sweet marjoram can all be used for this purpose. Meat substitutes can replace meat in all the recipes.

GARLIC LAMB
Soak 4 cloves of garlic in 1 teaspoon of olive oil and 1 drop of rosemary essential oil for 30 minutes. Using a sharp pointed knife, pierce the meat and insert the cloves of garlic. Depending on the cut, the meat can be roasted, grilled, or braised.

SPICED GARLIC BEEF

Soak 4 cloves of garlic in 1 teaspoon of olive oil and 1 drop each of orange, nutmeg, and cinnamon essential oils. Prepare as for the garlic lamb, above.

MINCED BEEF OR LAMB

Minced beef or lamb dishes can incorporate various types of essential oils, as can meat substitute dishes. Use 1 drop per 1 pound of meat, adding the essential oil to the cooking oil.

HONEYED CHICKEN

1 or 2 drops lemon essential oil
1 or 2 drops orange essential oil
4 tablespoons honey
1 glass white wine, cider, or nonalcoholic alternative
1 small orange
1 lemon
1 medium chicken
2 ounces butter (or substitute)
4 ounces plain yogurt

Preheat the oven to 425°F. Add the lemon and orange oils to the honey, then mix into the wine or cider and store until needed. Place the washed whole orange and lemon inside the cleaned chicken. Smear the butter over the chicken and place in the oven. Then reduce the temperature to 350°F and roast for around 45 minutes. Remove the chicken and brush the honey mixture all over the chicken. Return to the oven until cooked, basting frequently. After removing the chicken from the roasting dish, strain the remaining liquid into a small saucepan and place over a low heat. Stir in the yogurt and add salt and pepper to taste.

GRILLED CHICKEN

4 tablespoons honey
2 teaspoons French Dijon mustard
1 or 2 drops lemon or orange essential oil

Stir all the ingredients into a smooth paste and brush over the chicken before grilling. The unused honey paste can be stored.

Desserts

Flower essential oils such as neroli, cananga, ylang ylang, geranium, rose, lavender, and jasmine can do much to enhance the taste and aroma of desserts, but they can overpower desserts if not used in minimal amounts — a subtle aroma addition is all that is required. The toothpick method is a simple way to slowly increase the amount of essential oil until the desired strength is reached: place a tiny amount of essential oil onto a toothpick and stir into the dessert. The amount of sugar being used in recipes can be reduced because the aroma of certain flower essential oils tricks the brain into thinking the dish contains more sugar.

Rice Puddings: By the addition of essential oils you can lift a traditional rice pudding out of the ordinary and into the extraordinary. Try adding ¼ to ½ drop of ylang ylang essential oil to the milk or cream in your favorite recipe, using 1 pound or more of rice.

Baked Egg Custards: Baked egg custards and other sweet egg dishes respond particularly well to the flavors of orange, bergamot, tangerine, and mandarin, and to the flower essential oils of rose, neroli, and lavender. Add ¼ to 1 drop per 2 cups of liquid. This could also make a good filling for custard tarts.

Chocolate Mousse: By adding essential oils you can create different chocolate mousse flavors simply using a basic unflavored chocolate mousse recipe or a store-purchased mousse. Simply add ¼ to 1 drop of either peppermint, lime, mandarin, lemon, orange, or ylang ylang essential oil to 2 cups of mousse. For a romantic mousse, use rose essential oil.

Soufflés: The beauty of using essential oils in soufflés is that you can achieve the flower fragrance without the risk of the soufflé sinking. Use ¼ to 1 drop of your chosen oil per 2 cups of liquid.

Crepes: Add ¼ to 1 drop of an essential oil — fruit or flower — per 2½ cups of batter.

Dessert Sauces: Use ¼ to 1 drop of essential oil per 1 cup of liquid for a sauce to transform any dessert.

Custards: Use ¼ to 1 drop of essential oil per 2 cups of custard.

Fruit Purees: Use ¼ to 1 drop of essential oil per 1 cup of puree. The essential oils of geranium, rose, and sweet orange complement the flavor of apple.

FROZEN DESSERTS

Sorbets

The following citrus sorbet makes a wonderful addition to a hot summer's day.

CITRUS SORBET
2½ cups water
6 ounces sugar
2 drops lemon essential oil
1 drop grapefruit essential oil
1 drop lime essential oil
1 egg white
Fruit as desired
You can include fruit in this recipe or leave it out. Fruit is used for its taste and texture — it could be any fruit you happen to have. Strawberries are excellent, as are raspberries, black currants, red currants, or blueberries.

Boil the water, sugar, and essential oils for 10 minutes. Cool, then partially freeze. Beat the egg white until stiff. Remove the sugar mix from the freezer and beat it until soft and mushy, then add your fruit, if required. Now fold in the stiff egg white and refreeze. Take out after a couple of

hours, quickly agitate for a moment, and return to the freezer. Any essential oil can be used in a basic sorbet mix. When using the flower oils, try decorating with petals. Tangerine or mandarin sorbet is delicious served in its own fruit peel shells.

Ice Cream

Making your own ice cream ensures that you get exactly what you want. You can cheat if you wish by buying ready-made ice cream and mixing in the essential oil of your choice: to 20 ounces add 1 or 2 drops of essential oil. Tangerine or mandarin make an interesting combination with chocolate ice cream. And how about peppermint or spearmint?

An old-fashioned ice cream mix was made from a custard, using large amounts of cream, eggs, and sugar — too rich for many of us today. Here are two recipes, one traditional and one modern:

TRADITIONAL ICE CREAM
6 eggs
1 cup castor (finely granulated) sugar
2½ cups cream
2 drops essential oil
3 ounces fruit or chocolate
Beat the eggs with the sugar and add a little of the cream. Heat the remaining cream, but do not boil. Take off the heat and gently stir in the egg mix. When thoroughly mixed, return to the lowest heat and continue stirring until the mixture begins to thicken. Remove from heat and allow to cool. Now add the essential oil and the fruit or chocolate, as well as nuts, coffee, and anything else you'd like to include at this point, and freeze.

MODERN ICE CREAM
4 egg yolks
¼ cup castor (finely granulated) sugar
1 cup milk
5 ounces cream

2 drops essential oil

2 ounces fruit or chocolate

Beat the egg yolks with the sugar and add a little of the milk. Heat the remaining milk, but do not boil. Take off the heat and gently stir in the egg mix. When thoroughly mixed, return to the lowest heat and continue stirring until the mixture begins to thicken. Remove from heat and allow to cool. Gently fold the cream into the mixture when cool. Now add the essential oil and the fruit or chocolate, as well as nuts, coffee, and anything else you'd like to include at this point, and freeze.

GERANIUM CREAM

1 cup cream

4 tablespoons sugar

1 drop geranium essential oil

8 ounces cream cheese or fromage frais

Gently heat the cream, sugar, and geranium oil together; leave to cool. When the mixture is cold, beat into it the cream cheese or fromage frais, then freeze. This cream may be eaten on its own or used to top cheesecakes or fruit.

Frozen Yogurt

Essential oils can be added to the yogurt before freezing. Use 1 drop per 2 cups of yogurt.

CAKES AND FROSTINGS

Since the essential oils will not clash with any of the ingredients, they can be incorporated into any cake recipe. A plain sponge cake can be turned into an extravagant and exotic cake just by adding essential oils during the preparation. During cooking much of the fragrance escapes, leaving a very subtle flavor. If you want a stronger fragrance or flavor, use essential oils in the creams or toppings and they will permeate the whole cake. This recipe can be used with white or whole-grain flour:

VERA'S SPONGE CAKE

1 cup soft butter (or substitute)

1 cup sugar

4 eggs

2 tablespoons warm water

2 drops sweet orange essential oil

1 cup organic self-rising flour

Preheat the oven to 350°F. Cream the butter and sugar. Add the eggs one at a time and beat well until the mixture is stiff and uniform. Add the water and sweet orange essential oil. Fold in the flour with a spoon. Divide the mixture and pour into two greased and floured 8-inch (20 cm) sponge cake pans. Bake in the center of the oven for 25 minutes.

BUTTERCREAM FROSTING

4 ounces soft butter (or substitute)

6 ounces sifted icing sugar

3–4 drops essential oil of your choice

Beat the butter and sugar to a soft cream. Add the essential oil and beat well. The cream may be used for filling and topping cupcakes. Try neroli, rose, sweet orange, lemon, grapefruit, lemongrass, lavender, geranium, cardamom, cananga, peppermint, or spearmint essential oil.

CHOCO-MINT CAKE

6 ounces soft butter (or substitute)

6 ounces sugar or coconut blossom/nectar sugar

3 eggs

1 tablespoon warm water

4 ounces organic self-rising flour

½ teaspoon natural vanilla extract

4 drops peppermint essential oil

2 ounces chocolate or carob powder

Preheat the oven to 350°F. Cream the butter and sugar, and beat in the eggs. Add the water slowly, then the flour. Blend in the vanilla, peppermint oil, and chocolate or carob powder. Divide and pour into two sponge cake pans. Bake for 25 minutes. Use peppermint or spearmint filling and topping, with grated chocolate.

EMMA'S CARROT CAKE

3 eggs

3 large carrots, grated

1 cup brown sugar or coconut blossom/nectar
    sugar

1 teaspoon orange juice

3 drops sweet orange essential oil

2 ounces ground almonds

2 ounces organic self-rising flour

Preheat the oven to 325°F. Separate the egg yolks and beat well. Place the grated carrots in a pan of boiling water and cook for 5 minutes; take off the heat and drain. Combine the carrot, egg yolks, and sugar, and mix well. Slowly add the orange juice and the sweet orange essential oil, then the almonds and flour. Beat the white of the eggs until stiff, and fold into the cake mix. Pour the mix into a greased cake pan and bake for about 40 minutes. Test with a skewer. The cake can be topped with orange butter frosting, or try cardamom or ylang ylang for something different. Alternatively, use the cream cheese frosting recipe below.

CREAM CHEESE FROSTING

6 ounces cream cheese (or substitute)

6 ounces sifted icing sugar

4 drops essential oil of your choice

Beat the cream cheese and sugar to a soft cream. Add the essential oil and beat well. The cream cheese frosting can be used for cake fillings, cupcake toppings, or as a topping for sweet pies.

Bread and Pastry

Essential oils can be added to pastry or bread dough just before baking. Small amounts are generally used depending upon taste. For example, add 1 drop per 8 oz. of dough. To make orange and cinnamon bread, add 4 drops of sweet orange and an extra 1 drop of cinnamon essential oil to 32 oz. of dough.

Included in a basic pastry mix, the essential oils add spice, citrus, or flower aroma as desired. Use 1 drop per 2 ounces of pastry.

Flower and Herb Syrups

These syrups are simply made and are reminiscent of sixteenth-century Elizabethan times. They can be used in desserts and drinks, as toppings, and as remedies. Rose syrup, for example, can ease a sore throat, and peppermint syrup helps indigestion. To make a true syrup, you need flowers as well as essential oils:

FLOWER OR HERB SYRUP

Fresh edible flowers or herbs, enough to fill
    a pint (475 mL) jar

2½ cups water

1 pound sugar or coconut blossom/nectar sugar

3 drops essential oil

Add the freshly picked and washed edible flowers or herbs to the water, and bring to a boil. Turn down the heat and simmer for 10 minutes. Leave to cool for 10 minutes, then strain to remove all the plant material. Now add water to the strained liquid so it again reaches 2½ cups. Heat this liquid along with the sugar on a low heat to prevent the sugar from burning, slowly stirring until the mixture thickens — the longer it cooks, the thicker the syrup. Add the essential oils to the syrup, pour into a jar or bottle, and store.

HONEY AND SUGAR

Fragrant honeys are useful in both the kitchen and the medicine chest. They can be used as drinks, spread on toast, or used in any recipe that calls for honey. For a 1-pound (454 g) jar of honey, stir in 1 or 2 drops of essential oil.

Sugar absorbs fragrance very well, but don't drop essential oils directly into the sugar. Instead place 2 drops on a piece of white paper towel and leave this in the sugar jar. Leave it for at least 24 hours before using the sugar. Try lavender, ylang ylang, rose, lemon, orange, or any essential oil you wish.

Aromatic Petals

Crystallized flower petals make wonderful decorations for cakes and desserts. Gum arabic is often used to make them, but I like to use egg white, although egg white petals can't be stored for as long as petals made using other methods. Whisk the egg white until stiff, pour into an egg cup, and add 1 drop of essential oil. Dip clean petals into the mixture, then place them on a wire tray to dry, sprinkling well with fragrant castor (finely granulated) sugar.

Fragrant Flower Jams

To make a flower jam, choose flowers or herbs with soft petals (lavender or rosemary, for example, will leave tough particles in the jam).

1 pound sugar
5 fl. oz. rose water or orange flower water
1 pound (454 g) fresh clean edible flowers or herbs
2 drops essential oil of choice
Heat the sugar and water until you have syrup, then add the edible petals or leaves. Simmer for 5 minutes, then add essential oil of your choice. Leave the mixture to simmer gently on a low heat for 45 minutes, stirring occasionally. Pour into small sterilized jars and store.

Jams made of fruit can also have essential oils incorporated into them. Some good combinations are strawberry and rose, raspberry and lemon, plum and sweet orange, sweet orange and neroli — the combinations are endless and need only a little imagination.

Jellies

Jellies make an interesting accompaniment to all manner of meat, fish, and vegetable dishes. Flower jellies can be used in pies and cakes, or melted to use as toppings, or incorporated into drinks. The following is a basic jelly that you can adapt as you please.

BASIC APPLE JELLY
1 pound apples
1 cup water
1 pound sugar
Edible flowers or herbs to fill a pint (475 mL) jar
3 drops essential oil of choice
Cut the apples, including the peel, into small pieces. Place in a pan with the water. Simmer gently until reduced to a pulp. Strain the pulp in a cook's jelly bag for as long as needed to extract (and reserve) the liquid from the pulp. Measure the liquid and top it up with water until it reaches 2½ cups. Add the sugar and stir over a low heat until the sugar melts, then add the flowers or herbs of your choice. Bring to a boil, stirring all the time — do not allow to burn. Continue boiling until the jelly starts to set, then add essential oil to complement the flowers or herbs used. Pour into sterilized jars and store.

Here are some suggestions for matching the essential oils used in your jellies with various accompanying dishes:

Basil: cold meat, tomato dishes, pasta, salads

Fennel: vegetables, fish, poultry

Lemongrass: vegetables, grains, poultry, red meat

Rosemary: lamb, poultry, vegetables, pulses

Lavender: meat, vegetables

Melissa: poultry, fish, vegetables

Geranium: meat, rice, curries

Rose: meat, poultry, vegetables, rice

Spearmint: meat, vegetables, grains

Bircher Muesli

Authentic muesli is not the dehydrated cereal and fruits you'll find in a package on a supermarket shelf, but a delicate mixture of cereals, oats, grated fresh apple, nuts, and fruits that's rich and creamy, with or without milk. The following recipe makes one serving:

MUESLI
1 tablespoon oats
3 tablespoons (45 mL) water or organic unfiltered
    apple juice
1 large apple, grated (with peel but not seeds)
1 tablespoon grated or flaked walnuts or almonds
    or a mixture of whole nuts
1 drop lemon essential oil (optional)
1 tablespoon organic cow's or goat's milk,
    almond or other nut milk, rice milk, or
    oat milk
Soak the oats overnight in the water or apple juice and store in the refrigerator. Before breakfast, grate the apple with the peel but not the seeds and add it, along with the rest of the ingredients, to the oats, sprinkling the nuts on top if you prefer. Although the base is always the same, any other fruits in season may be added, as well as yogurt, dried fruits such as goji berries and cherries, and seeds such as sesame, chia, and flax.

The combination of apples and oats can help to lower cholesterol, as well as assisting the body in the removal of heavy metals. As part of a whole-food diet, this recipe can be used by those with arthritis and rheumatism.

Nut Milks

Nut milks are delicious and nutritious. They can be used in cereals, in puddings, or as a base for drinks or sauces.

ALMOND MILK
2 tablespoons finely ground almonds
1 teaspoon fragrant or plain honey
5 fl. oz. water
Mix the almonds and honey in a blender. Add the water and leave to stand for one hour. If any residue remains after blending, strain it out. The same recipe can be used for milks of sesame seed, pistachio, or hazelnut.

Christmas

In England, Christmas isn't Christmas without meatless, spiced, and dried fruit mince pies, and even the most traditional recipe for the sweet, spiced mincemeat can be enhanced with a drop of essential oil of sweet orange or lemon. The combination of spices and fruit oils works deliciously, and as the pies cook the inviting aroma will fill the home.

The essential oils distilled from spices are excellent in various Christmas cakes and desserts. Ginger essential oil in the Christmas pudding or spice cake releases a heavenly aroma and does to the flavor what you would expect — spices it up! Try a few drops of any of the following in your seasonal dishes:

SPICE OILS FOR CHRISTMAS COOKING
Cinnamon (*Cinnamomum zeylanicum*)
Ginger (*Zingiber officinale*)
Mace (*Myristica fragrans*)
Nutmeg (*Myristica fragrans*)
Cardamom (*Elettaria cardamomum*)
Clove bud (*Syzygium aromaticum*)

The essential oils can be used in place of the spices in mulled wines too, and there is nothing more welcoming to a winter-chilled guest. Here is just one recipe; the amounts given are for 4 cups of red wine:

MULLED WINE
1 drop lemon essential oil
2 drops sweet orange essential oil
2 drops mandarin essential oil
2 tablespoons honey
4 cups red wine
1 clove bud
1 cinnamon stick (or pinch of cinnamon powder)
1 uncut orange
1 uncut lemon

Blend the essential oils together into the honey. In a nonmetallic pan, slowly heat the red wine with the clove bud, the cinnamon stick, and the orange and lemon. Add 1 teaspoon of the flavored honey, and stir well while still on the heat. More honey can be added if you prefer a sweeter wine; store the remainder for future use. When the wine starts to bubble, take it off the heat and serve. Alcohol evaporates with heating — the longer it's on the heat, the less alcohol it will contain. Merry Christmas!

Overeating

It often happens over the holidays: Each year we say to ourselves that we'll not overindulge and will ignore the table piled high with all manner of goodies. We'll give the boxes of chocolates to a local charity shop for the volunteer staff. We'll just keep it simple — no nuts or candied fruits, no mince pies or Christmas pudding and brandy butter. But really, this is all a waste of time because we'll do exactly what we did last year, which is overindulge, and then spend weeks feeling guilty and looking at the latest diet book!

The essential oils can't turn back the clock, yet alone forgive us our excesses. What they can do is help facilitate digestion, through the use of honey teas. This is a method for adults only. Mix 1 drop of any of the following essential oils into 1 tablespoon of honey and blend well. Add ¼ teaspoon of this honey mix to a large cupful of hot water with a squeeze of fresh lemon juice, and sip the drink slowly.

OVEREATING ESSENTIAL OILS
Lemon (*Citrus limon*)
Spearmint (*Mentha spicata*)
Ginger (*Zingiber officinale*)
Cardamom (*Elettaria cardamomum*)
Mandarin (*Citrus reticulata*)
Caraway seed (*Carum carvi*)
Coriander seed (*Coriandrum sativum*)

But why not be realistic and prepare the following blend so it's ready for the holiday season?

THE "WHY DID I DO IT?!" BLEND
Mandarin	8 drops
Spearmint	2 drops
Ginger	1 drop
Lemon	4 drops
Coriander seed	2 drops
Cardamom	2 drops

Blend together in these proportions and use ¼ drop in the honey-tea method described above.

Party Punches

Party punches can be hot or cold, alcoholic or nonalcoholic, and essential oils used for their flavoring and aroma make these easy-to-serve drinks very interesting. The oils we use fall into three groups:

SPICES
Cinnamon (*Cinnamomum zeylanicum*)
Coriander seed (*Coriandrum sativum*)
Cardamom (*Elettaria cardamomum*)
Nutmeg (*Myristica fragrans*)

CITRUS FRUITS
Lemon (*Citrus limon*)
Orange, sweet (*Citrus sinensis*)
Lime (*Citrus aurantifolia*)
Tangerine (*Citrus reticulata*)
Mandarin (*Citrus reticulata*)
Grapefruit (*Citrus paradisi*)

HERBS AND FLOWERS
Geranium (*Pelargonium graveolens*)
Rose otto (*Rosa damascena*)
Melissa (*Melissa officinalis*)
Neroli (*Citrus aurantium*)
Lemon verbena (*Lippia citriodora*)
Lavender (*Lavandula angustifolia*)

The recipes that follow are merely an indication of what can be done. Mix the essential oils into the alcohol before adding any other ingredients, as the alcohol will help disperse the essential oil throughout the mixture.

HOT OR COLD ORANGE WINE
1 drop sweet orange essential oil
1 drop geranium essential oil
1 bottle red wine
2 cups orange juice
Mix the essential oils into the red wine, then mix in the orange juice. If served hot, add sugar to taste. If served cold, add ice cubes in which marigold petals have been frozen.

MANDARIN GROG
In this variation of the traditional grog recipe, mandarin fruit and mandarin essential oil are substituted for oranges.

7 fl. oz. (207 mL) vodka, brandy, or orange juice
1 drop nutmeg essential oil
4 drops mandarin essential oil
1 drop lemon essential oil
7 fl. oz. (207 mL) water
2 mandarins or tangerines, washed
2 ounces (57 g) raisins
2 ounces (57 g) prunes
2 clove buds
1 cinnamon stick
2 ounces (57 g) raw cane sugar
2 bottles red wine or nonalcoholic alternative
2 ounces (57 g) blanched almonds, flaked
In a large, nonmetallic pan, mix the vodka (or alternative) and the essential oils together, then add the water, fruit (citrus, raisins, and prunes), clove, cinnamon, and sugar. Bring to a boil, then simmer on low heat for 30 minutes. Add the wine and bring back to a boil. Take the pan off the heat and allow to stand for at least eight hours. Cooking or boiling any alcohol will usually reduce the alcohol content. When ready to serve, reheat and add the almonds.

FRUIT PUNCH
4½ pounds sliced fruit
Small handful lemon balm and mint leaves, washed
6 bottles white wine or nonalcoholic alternative
2 drops melissa or lemon essential oil
4 teaspoons (20 mL) honey
Lemonade to taste
Put the fruit — peaches, apricots, oranges, apples, or the like — in a large bowl along with a few sprigs of lemon balm and mint. Add 1 bottle of the wine, the essential oil, and the honey, cover with a tight lid, and leave to stand for a couple of hours. When ready to serve, add the remaining bottles of wine, lemonade to taste, and ice cubes. Stir well.

Rose Cocktail

2 drops rose otto essential oil, or 1 drop of
   geranium oil
6 fl. oz. or 1½ wineglasses of brandy or
   nonalcoholic alternative
6 bottles rosé wine or nonalcoholic alternative
1 tablespoon (15 mL) grenadine syrup or
   pomegranate syrup
8 ounces (225 g) fresh or frozen strawberries
4 pints (1.9 liters) lemonade

Dissolve the essential oil in the brandy and mix with the wine and grenadine. Puree the strawberries, blend in with the lemonade, and add this to the wine mixture. Serve with ice cubes in which you have frozen clean rose petals, and decorate the whole beautiful creation by floating your best rose in the bowl.

Hangover Help

Good hospitality is all very well and good, but it can certainly take its toll. Too much alcohol leads to dehydration and results in the miserable sensations known collectively as a hangover — nausea, headache, dehydration, and loss of equilibrium. To a greater or lesser extent, the body is having to cope with a degree of toxic poisoning. Fortunately, there's quite a lot that can be done to lessen the effects and not feel so bad after a night of partying.

Wines and beers, alcoholic and nonalcoholic, vary enormously in their chemical content. Some are organic, in that their ingredients were not cultivated using chemicals and no preservatives or other harmful ingredients, such as sulfites, were added during their processing. Good-quality organic beverages will do far less damage — in terms of both your head the morning after and your liver over a longer period of time. You can buy organic wines and beers at most large chain food stores, but if you can't find them go for the more expensive bottles with less alcohol content and try to avoid those whose labels warn that they contain sulfites or that their ingredients are from more than one country. Where wine is concerned, you do usually get what you pay for. Studies have shown what the French have known for centuries: that one glass of red wine a day may help prevent heart disease. The theory is that antioxidants in red wine, particularly a polyphenol called *resveratrol*, may help prevent damage to the arteries, prevent blood clots, reduce the risk of inflammation, lower bad cholesterol (low-density lipoprotein), and raise good cholesterol (high-density lipoprotein). It all sounds too good to be true, yet scientific research is showing that a small glass of red wine could be good. On the other hand, we have to remember there are always other, not-so-good effects from alcohol consumption, including hangovers.

Other preventative measures against hangovers include drinking plenty of water before and after you drink alcohol, as this slows down the absorption rate and allows the body to cope better. Also, before going to sleep, take at least 1,000 mg of vitamin C, and do not drink black coffee, as this will make things worse.

Using essential oils has been known to assist the body return to its prealcoholic state:

The "Morning After" Essential Oils
Juniper berry (*Juniperus communis*)
Grapefruit (*Citrus paradisi*)
Cardamom (*Elettaria cardamomum*)
Rosemary (*Rosmarinus officinalis*)
Lavender (*Lavandula angustifolia*)
Lemon (*Citrus limon*)
Sandalwood (*Santalum album*)
Fennel, sweet (*Foeniculum vulgare var. dulce*)
Lavandin (*Lavandula x intermedia*)
Spearmint (*Mentha spicata*)
Peppermint (*Mentha piperita*)
Basil linalol (*Ocimum basilicum ct. linalool*)

Any of these essential oils can be used on their own or in a blend, using 3 drops in an inhalation. Use a total of 3–4 drops diluted in the same amount of carrier oil in a bath or shower, avoiding peppermint and spearmint as these may cause irritation on the skin.

Apart from helping to rid the body of the alcoholic residue by the usual elimination methods, sleep is the best remedy for a hangover. For those who can take it easy in the morning after the night before, a relaxing blend of essential oils will help your body deal with the onslaught that last night went by the name of "fun":

THE "PLEASE TREAD SOFTLY" BATH BLEND

Grapefruit	5 drops
Lavender	3 drops
Sandalwood	5 drops
Lemon	10 drops

Blend the essential oils together, then use 4 drops in a bath. If you bottle the blend beforehand, it'll be ready for this emergency, and the next.

You could also mix 2 drops of spearmint oil into a teaspoon of carrier oil and rub it over the back of the neck and shoulders. Drink plenty of water and eat fiber-loaded foods. For those who have to battle through the rush hour and get to work in the morning after a night of socializing, the following body and inhalation blend might give you the necessary enthusiasm:

THE "OH NO, I HAVE TO GET TO WORK" BLEND

Grapefruit	8 drops
Rosemary	7 drops
Peppermint	1 drop
Cardamom	2 drops
Geranium	2 drops
Juniper berry	3 drops

Blend the essential oils together, then dilute 2 drops in a teaspoon of carrier oil and rub over the back of the neck and the shoulders. Put 4 drops of the essential oil blend on a tissue and inhale when needed, throughout the day. If you get invited to lots of parties or late evenings out, it's worthwhile making up this blend for use when needed.

Natural Health for Animals

17

Animals generally get a rough deal in this world, with farming techniques that pump them full of chemicals and with food for herbivores sometimes containing animal matter. Even some pet foods have questionable sources, and caring for our pets as well as we would like can be difficult when veterinary fees are high.

Fortunately, natural treatments for animals are increasingly available, in stores and elsewhere. Professionals, including vets, breeders, trainers, and farmers, have come to appreciate that in some cases a natural option is the better way forward. Indeed, many commercial companies are now operating in this field. Some commentators have raised objection to this, using the same arguments of a few decades ago when the natural health movement for humans started. For example, those who held that homeopathy can't work in humans because the active ingredient is undetectable now question its use in animals. However, the argument that homeopathy's use in humans is due to the placebo effect — "It's all in the mind" — can't be applied to animals. The fact that animals respond so well to treatments like homeopathy and acupuncture argues in favor of the efficacy of these treatments, precisely because no psychological factors are involved.

Special consideration needs to be given when using essential oils on animals. First, they have a much more sensitive sense of smell than humans, and of course animals — especially dogs — come in very different sizes, so any essential oil or blend used should vary between, say, a dachshund and a Great Dane. Any aromatic or herbal product should be used with the same care on your pet as when administering pharmaceutical preparations.

Animals are very unlike human beings in the chemical compounds they are sensitive to, and different species of animals can have different tolerance levels to the various essential oils. So, when treating animals, don't simply apply essential oils appropriate to a condition that occurs in humans. Use small amounts in the first instance with animals, gradually increasing the amount in small incremental steps, and then only if necessary. Animals respond well to natural health methods and it would be a pity to deny animals access to them, especially as anecdotal evidence shows they respond so well, but do consult your veterinarian.

Methods of Use for Animals

Various application methods and techniques can be used on a variety of animals. Each method has its own advantages and is appropriate for a variety of purposes.

WATER-BASED SPRAYS

These can be used for pet body sprays and therapeutic skin applications. They can also be used on bedding areas, during travel, and as general air fresheners and room sprays. The sprays most often consist of an herbal or essential oil water-based mixture, or a pure plant hydrolat.

OILS/CARRIER OILS

Oils are mainly used for skin, coat, paw, or hoof applications of essential oils or to carry herbal concoctions. Essential oils are first diluted in carrier oils, and then this is added to gels, ointment, and balms. Some carrier oils, such as tamanu and neem oil, have excellent properties and can be used as treatments in their own right.

BALMS AND OINTMENTS

Used for specific skin areas and for paw and hoof applications, balms and ointments are made from carrier oils mixed with thicker natural agents, such as beeswax, shea butter, and cocoa butter.

GELS

Gels are very popular for most pet skin applications and can be used in place of ointments or balms. Generally, gels have a nonoily texture and include aloe vera gel and silica gel.

HYDROLATS AND ESSENTIAL OIL WATERS

A true hydrolat is created when plant material has been distilled purely to produce a product that contains traces of essential oils and the water-soluble properties of the plant material. For some smaller animals, hydrolats and essential oil waters are sometimes a better option than using essential oil in other methods.

First Aid Kit for Animals

NEEM OIL (*Azadirachta indica*)

Neem oil is useful for insect bites, cuts and minor wounds, skin irritations, and parasitic treatments. Neem oil is well known as a remedy for skin problems in humans and could be used in this way for animals too, having the additional advantage of deterring insects. Neem oil is a good addition in ointments and balms, although it's generally used undiluted. As neem is a cold-pressed vegetable oil, essential oils can be blended into it to create very effective treatments. Neem oil can sometimes become solid in cold temperatures, melting at room temperature or when blended with a carrier oil. Neem has a distinctive odor that some humans find unpleasant.

TAMANU OIL (*Calophyllum inophyllum*)

Tamanu oil is an analgesic, wound-healing oil that has antiseptic and antibiotic properties and is good for ulcerations, insect bites, and most all skin conditions. It can be used on its own or as a carrier oil blended with essential oils.

COLLOIDAL SILVER

A highly effective natural antiseptic, colloidal silver consists of minute particles of silver, invisible to the eye, suspended in water. It can be used almost anywhere that requires antiseptic or antibacterial treatment, including bites, cuts, and wounds. It can be used undiluted, and it is also useful in combination with hydrolats and essential oil waters. Essential oils can be used alongside colloidal silver.

CIDER VINEGAR

Cider vinegar is naturally astringent and antiseptic and can be incorporated into ointments and balms, combined with hydrolats and essential oil waters, and used to partially dilute essential oils before adding to other mediums. To use as a wash, dilute 1 teaspoon of cider vinegar in 1 fl. oz. (30 mL) of water. This solution can be used to ease sore skin and wash away dirt embedded in paws.

HYDROLATS

Hydrolats are useful in pet sprays and for topical application to the skin or fur of most animals. Hydrolats, unlike essential oils, can be used undiluted, blended with other hydrolats, or diluted with water.

Lavender Hydrolat

Lavender hydrolat is slightly antiseptic and has healing and calming properties. It can be used undiluted on the skin and can be added to water-based sprays. Its slight antiseptic and healing properties are useful for cleaning minor scratches and wounds, and it may help calm nervous and sensitive animals.

Thyme Hydrolat

This hydrolat has antiseptic and healing properties. Use undiluted when cleaning cuts, wounds, or bites. Can be combined with colloidal silver to boost its antibacterial effect.

Chamomile German or Chamomile Roman Hydrolat

These both have anti-inflammatory properties and are slightly antiseptic. Used as a spray, they are healing and calming. Both can be applied to the skin or fur of most animals.

SEAWEED POWDER OR SUPPLEMENTS

When added to food, seaweed powder may deter intestinal parasites. It is said to be good for tooth care by helping to remove plaque. It is useful when combined with gels and clays — use as directed by the manufacturer.

CLAY

Clay powders come in various forms. French green clay is used to make poultices.

OTHER USEFUL ADDITIONS TO THE FIRST AID KIT FOR ANIMALS

Lemongrass hydrolat or essential oil water
Geranium hydrolat or essential oil water
Eucalyptus lemon hydrolat or essential oil water
Peppermint or spearmint hydrolat or essential oil water

ANIMAL FIRST AID KIT ESSENTIAL OILS
Lavender (*Lavandula angustifolia*)
Chamomile german (*Matricaria recutita*)
Chamomile roman (*Anthemis nobilis*)
Lemongrass (*Cymbopogon citratus / flexuosus*)
Geranium (*Pelargonium graveolens*)
Manuka (*Leptospermum scoparium*)
Immortelle (*Helichrysum italicum*)
Spearmint (*Mentha spicata*)
Marjoram, sweet (*Origanum majorana*)
Bergamot (*Citrus bergamia*)
Frankincense (*Boswellia carterii*)

Sprays for Animals

In this section are a general calming spray and an antiseptic spray, both of which could be used on most animals. Because there's a huge difference in animal size and need, the blends should be diluted in water — to varying degrees — to allow for these variables.

CALMING SPRAY FOR ANIMALS

Animals can get anxious for a variety of routine reasons, such as taking a long journey or going to the veterinarian. But there are also many times when there are exceptional events and circumstances the animal can't understand, such as when the family is moving or even when the house is being renovated and there's general domestic upheaval. A pet may be upset when having to stay away from the family in a kennel or pet hotel. Family pets can also become anxious when there's been a bereavement in the family, including the death of other household pets. Most pets are very sensitive to their family's emotions and can feel the sad loss of a family member, be that human or animal. Like us, they feel as if their life has been turned upside down, and they may miss the love and security that family member gave them.

Different animal personalities show their anxiety and stress in very different ways. Some animals may become aggressive, others hide or refuse to eat, while others become clingy or just seem nervous. We know the personality of our individual pets and can judge for ourselves if they need a little help to alleviate anxiety and keep calm.

Because most animals have such a strong sense of smell, it's always best to use the least amount of essential oil, then progress to more only if and when it seems required.

General Calming Spray

Marjoram, sweet	5 drops
Clary sage	3 drops
Valerian	2 drops
Vetiver	3 drops
Lavender	4 drops

Organic cider vinegar	8 drops
Glycerin (vegetable)	1 teaspoon (5 mL)
Distilled water	2 fl. oz. (60 mL)

First, blend the essential oils and cider vinegar together. Add 2 drops of this blend into the water and glycerin, and shake really well. This is a starting dilution that can then be diluted further. The starting dilution can be added to a further 3½ fl. oz. (100 mL) of water or more, depending on the size of the animal and the situation — their emotional disposition and the degree of their stress or anxiety. Alternatively, blend all the essential oils and cider vinegar together, add to the glycerin and water, and shake well. Then add to 18 fl. oz. (510 mL) of warm water and shake well again. Leave for 24 hours in a lidded bottle and then filter the mixture through an unbleached paper coffee filter before using.

Use a new or unused plant mister or other clean sprayer. Spray around the animal and their living area, never directly on the animal. You could spray the bedding, for example, or where the animal is resting. If traveling, a good idea is to spray a small piece of fabric that can be placed in the traveling box. Avoid spraying near the animal's eyes and using the blend near valuable fabric materials or wooden objects that could be damaged by the water, vinegar, or essential oils.

GENERAL ANTISEPTIC SPRAY

The following blend of essential oils forms the basis of a general antiseptic spray. Three to 5 drops are diluted in an equal number of drops of cider vinegar, and then diluted again in a water and glycerin solution, and shaken well. The number of drops of essential oil used depends on the size of the animal and the conditions. As we can never be sure when we might need an antiseptic spray, either when out and about or at home, it's good to have a spray ready-made for any emergency.

This formula could also be incorporated into an essential oil water; see below.

GENERAL ANTISEPTIC SPRAY

Lavender	3 drops
Geranium	3 drops
Lemon	3 drops
Manuka	5 drops
Immortelle	4 drops
Lemongrass	3 drops
Cider vinegar	21 drops
Glycerin (vegetable)	1 teaspoon (5 mL)
Distilled water	2 fl. oz. (60 mL)

First, blend the essential oils and cider vinegar together, then dilute by adding 3–5 drops to the vegetable glycerin and distilled water and shake well. To make a larger amount, blend all the essential oils and cider vinegar together, add to the glycerin and 60 mL of water, and shake well. Then add this solution to 8 fl. oz. (240 mL) of warm water, shake well again, and leave for 24 hours in a lidded bottle. Then filter the mixture through an unbleached paper coffee filter before using. Avoid spraying near the animal's eyes or using the blend near valuable fabric materials or wooden objects that could be damaged by the water, vinegar, or essential oils.

MAKING AN ESSENTIAL OIL WATER

The essential oil blends above, used as the basis for the calming or antiseptic sprays, would also make an ideal basis for an essential oil water, although any essential oil or combination can be used in this method.

First, blend the essential oils together and mix as best you can with boiling water. Pour into a bottle, shake really well, and leave for 24 hours, shaking the bottle whenever you think about it or pass it on the kitchen counter. After the 24 hours are up, give the bottle another really good shake. As water and oil don't mix, pour the contents through an unbleached paper coffee filter

to help remove any essential oil globules. Bottle again, and store in the fridge. Colloidal silver can be added if you wish. The advantage of using this method is that you can make it fresh whenever you need it and use essential oils you may already have at hand.

Aromatherapy for Dogs

Dogs are the best companions — nonjudgmental, loving us just the way we are, always there when we need them, ready to comfort us when we're sad or distressed, and always pleased to see us. Dogs encourage humans to exercise — by getting the leash and taking us out in the fresh air for walks. They're an important part of the family and don't ask much in return — just a warm place to sleep, good food, water, a few words of praise, and lots of touch and love. Dogs who get massaged and pampered have landed in doggie heaven.

The first line of health for any dog is food. Dogs fed only on canned and dried foods are often sickly and can develop illness in later life, perhaps because of the ingredients and preservatives in processed foods. Like us, dogs need fresh food as often as possible, and because they are carnivores, that means fresh meat and occasional bones. The best way to provide this is to build up a good relationship with your local butcher.

When illness strikes a dog, it's more difficult to notice than in a human because our dog can't tell us what's wrong. We have to guess, and even the veterinarian relies on us to describe the symptoms causing concern. Dog owners know when their pooch is ill, just as parents know when their child is ill.

Because dogs have so many olfactory receptors, remember to avoid getting any type of aromatic or essential oil on their nose or too near their face. As far as animals in general, and dogs in particular, are concerned, less is always more.

When using this section please be aware that dogs vary hugely in size and weight — more than any other species. The great number of miniature dog breeds only illustrates how difficult it is to provide information that covers all types of dog. So please be aware of this and always keep in mind the size of your dog, in relation to the average-size dog, and use quantities of essential oil that are appropriate.

In pet shops there are shelves of beautifully packaged doggie products and all manner of dog clothing. Charming as all this attention is, clothing can rub on fur, and if the material is synthetic and there are metal fastenings, these could cause allergic reactions. This is just something to think about if your dog develops a skin problem.

FLEAS AND TICKS

Fleas can be as much of a problem for the rest of the household as for your dog, but thankfully certain essential oils are very effective at discouraging the fleas, ticks, and other minute skin parasites for which dogs seem inevitable homes. Neem oil from the neem tree is not only effective on humans but can be effective on animals too, with beneficial effects on skin disorders such as eczema, dermatitis, and itchy, dry, flaky skin. Unfortunately, neem oil does not have the most pleasant aroma for us humans. But dogs seem quite happy to have small amounts occasionally, well diluted, applied to their coats and skin. The following essential oils can be used in various methods to help discourage fleas and ticks:

Cedarwood atlas (*Cedrus atlantica*)
Eucalyptus lemon (*Eucalyptus citriodora*)
Geranium (*Pelargonium graveolens*)
Lavender (*Lavandula angustifolia*)
Lemongrass (*Cymbopogon citratus/flexuosus*)
Manuka (*Leptospermum scoparium*)
Neem (*Azadirachta indica*)
Spearmint (*Mentha spicata*)

Clary sage (*Salvia sclarea*)
Cypress (*Cupressus sempervirens*)
Thyme (*Thymus vulgaris*)
Vetiver (*Vetiveria zizanoides*)
Niaouli (*Melaleuca quinquenervia*)
Patchouli (*Pogostemon cablin*)
Peppermint (*Mentha piperita*)
Tea tree (*Melaleuca alternifolia*)

Shampooing

If you shampoo your dog, one of the easiest ways to deal with a flea situation is to add 1–3 drops of either cedarwood atlas, eucalyptus lemon, manuka, or neem oil to 3½ fl. oz. (100 mL) of their shampoo. Alternatively, use the blend below.

Special Care: Make sure you avoid getting the shampoo near or into the dog's eyes.

FLEA AND TICK BLEND FOR THE SHAMPOO
OR BRUSH METHODS

Manuka	5 drops
Patchouli	1 drop
Neem	2 drops
Cedarwood atlas	6 drops
Thyme linalol	2 drops
Eucalyptus lemon	4 drops

Blend the above amounts together and use 4 drops for 5 fl. oz. (150 mL) of shampoo for the shampoo method, or use 3 drops in a pint (475 mL) of warm water for the brushing method. Alternatively, use 8 drops of the blend to make an essential oil water using 8 fl. oz. (240 mL) of distilled water and 0.7 fl. oz. (20 mL) of colloidal silver; use as a deterrent spray.

Brushing

Take a brush that has strong steel or plastic bristles and a piece of material the same size as the face of the brush. The material needs to be quite thick, such as an old piece of toweling or washcloth. Pull the material down over the teeth of the brush, keeping the material as close to the tips of the brush as possible, away from the base. The more teeth the brush has, the better.

Prepare a bowl with a pint (475 mL) of warm water and mix in 4 drops of cedarwood atlas or lavender oil, or use 4 drops of the blend above, diluted in a teaspoon (5 mL) of castor oil or sesame oil, and soak the material of the prepared brush in this mixture before brushing your dog's coat. This treatment could condition the coat and will help collect the parasites and eggs on the brush — which should be rinsed out often during the brushing.

Combing

If your dog is suffering seriously from fleas or other parasites, mix 5 drops of the blend above, or cedarwood atlas or lavender oil, with 5 drops of vinegar, then add them directly onto a piece of material. Rub the cloth together to disperse the oil, and then place it over the teeth of a steel comb. Use this to comb your dog's hair, before shampooing.

MINOR CUTS AND GRAZES

Bathe the injured area with lavender or thyme hydrolat, or an essential oil water mix (see above). Alternatively, use 3 drops each of lavender and thyme linalol essential oil in 4 pints (2 liters) of water, swishing it around well to help disperse the essential oil. Remove any floating globules with a paper towel to avoid getting essential oil onto the wound. Also, use the antiseptic spray once a day above and around the bedding and rest areas, until the cuts have healed.

If your dog has an injury that has become ulcerous and weeps pus, follow your veterinarian's instructions. If you're unable to get veterinary help, wash the area thoroughly in a solution made up of 4 drops of lavender and 2 drops of thyme

linalol essential oil added to 2 fl. oz. (60 mL) of warm water, mixed together well, making sure no essential oil globules are applied directly to the wound.

The following essential oils can be used to treat cuts and grazes in dogs:

Chamomile german (*Matricaria recutita*)
Juniper berry (*Juniperus communis*)
Lavender (*Lavandula angustifolia*)
Manuka (*Leptospermum scoparium*)
Myrrh (*Commiphora myrrha*)
Tea tree (*Melaleuca alternifolia*)
Marjoram, sweet (*Origanum majorana*)
Thyme linalol (*Thymus vulgaris ct. linalool*)

COUGHS, COLDS, AND FLU

There are two methods to help dogs with coughs, colds, or flu — one oil based and the other water based. In either case, have respect for your dog's greater sense of smell and start with the minimum quantity of essential oil, increasing the dose slowly if necessary.

The following essential oils could be used for coughs, colds, and flu in dogs:

Niaouli (*Melaleuca quinquenervia*)
Ravensara (*Ravensara aromatica*)
Cajuput (*Melaleuca cajuputi*)

A tiny amount of the following rub can be applied over the dog's chest, around the rib cage, around the throat, and, most importantly, in a direct line from below the ears into the shoulders. For the oil-based treatment, add 1 drop each of any two essential oils listed above to 4 tablespoons (60 mL) of carrier oil. Some people don't like the idea of putting oil on a dog's coat, and with long-haired pets I can see their point. So for them, make a tincture by adding 2 drops of essential oil to 1 teaspoon (5 mL) of alcohol (vodka, for instance) and then adding this to 4 tablespoons

(60 mL) of water. Alternatively, dilute the essential oil into a little carrier oil and then add it to aloe vera gel. Whatever method you choose, apply once a day for three days only.

You could also spray the area where the dog sleeps. Blankets can be sprayed with a water-based essential oil spray and left to dry before using. Use 2 drops in 4 tablespoons (60 mL) of water. If you're washing the sleeping area, add 3 drops of essential oil to half a bucket of warm water; always avoid getting any spray or essential oil near the animal's face.

ARTHRITIS AND RHEUMATISM

Arthritis is as painful for dogs as it is for people, so be gentle when touching any painful area. Having said that, dogs generally love to be rubbed and stroked, and a dog with arthritis will both enjoy and benefit from gentle aromatherapy massage.

The following essential oils could be used to help ease arthritis and rheumatism:

Chamomile german (*Matricaria recutita*)
Chamomile roman (*Anthemis nobilis*)
Rosemary (*Rosmarinus officinalis*)
Immortelle (*Helichrysum italicum*)
Juniper berry (*Juniperus communis*)
Lavender (*Lavandula angustifolia*)
Marjoram, sweet (*Origanum majorana*)

PAINFUL JOINTS DOG BLEND 1

Rosemary	2 drops
Lavender	3 drops
Immortelle	3 drops
Chamomile roman	2 drops

Blend the essential oils together, and dilute in 2 tablespoons (30 mL) of carrier oil or in an oil and aloe vera gel mix. Jojoba is a nice oil to use, as it keeps the coat in good condition. Use a small amount, relative to the size of the dog, on your fingertips. Try to apply as close to the skin as

possible before gently massaging the affected area, and if the dog pulls away, stop. Avoid putting the oil near the dog's face.

PAINFUL JOINTS DOG BLEND 2

Marjoram, sweet	4 drops
Chamomile german	2 drops
Immortelle	2 drops

Blend the essential oils together, then dilute in 2 tablespoons (30 mL) of calendula or jojoba oil, or in an oil and aloe vera gel mix. Use a small amount, relative to the size of the dog, on your fingertips. Try to apply as close to the skin as possible before gently massaging the affected area, and if the dog pulls away, stop. Avoid putting the oil near the face.

If massaging your dog, don't rush into the massage, as the dog may feel it has to defend itself from potential further pain until it realizes the touch is going to be soothing. Starting on either side of the vertebrae, softly and gently massage the back and neck before moving on to the shoulders and haunches. Once the dog realizes the relief and attention it gets from massages, it will usually welcome them. Keep the dog warm, and ensure that he or she has a cozy sleeping area.

EARWAX

Dogs often suffer from a buildup of earwax, which can become smelly and offensive. This buildup may be the result of a plant seed or some other item having become lodged in the ear, and it's important not to remove anything that's not clearly visible — that is the veterinarian's job.

If there's no obstruction present, the wax buildup needs softening and removing, and the ear needs deodorizing and disinfecting, particularly if there are signs of redness or infection. The best essential oils to use for this are lavender and chamomile german. Dilute 1 drop of lavender or chamomile german in 2 teaspoons (10 mL) of olive oil and massage a small amount of this mixture around each ear and the pink underside of the ears. Gently massage the whole ear to soften the wax. If it's visible, gently remove as much wax as you can with cotton wool, without going into the ear canal itself.

DOGGIE BREATH

Dribbling and bad breath often indicate that a dog has dental problems. Gums should be pink, with no sign of bleeding. If the teeth are yellow or brownish, there could be a buildup of plaque, which inflames the gums. Dogs' teeth should be checked and cleaned regularly, ideally once a day. Use a specialist pet toothpaste, or try a small amount of the blend below — using only as much as your dog needs. Common baking soda (sodium bicarbonate) and essential oils provide a great way to keep teeth clean and fresh and help to remove plaque. If plaque is a problem, include dried food in your dog's diet.

Dog's Toothpaste and Breath Deodorizer

Baking soda	4 tablespoons (60 mL)
Almond oil, sweet	1 teaspoon (5 mL)
Cardamom	1 drop
Spearmint	1 drop

Make the toothpaste by mixing all the ingredients together, and store in a small pot in a cool place. Use a small amount when needed, applying with cotton wool or a very soft toothbrush to avoid damaging the gums. Dampen the cotton wool, dip it into the mixture, and use on the teeth.

Bad breath that's not caused by teeth or gums may indicate a stomach problem.

Doggie Breath Blend

Cardamom	2 drops
Coriander seed	2 drops
Spearmint	1 drop

Blend the essential oils together, then dilute in 1 tablespoon (15 mL) of sweet almond oil.

Apply a small amount of the diluted oil in a line from beneath the ears onto the shoulders, and over the stomach. Your dog may also benefit from canine probiotic supplements.

DIET

Dogs fed exclusively on canned food may not be hungry, but they could well be deficient in vitamins and minerals. Much food designed for the pet food trade contains meat considered unfit for human consumption, including perhaps meats full of antibiotics, metals, and other unnatural substances. We can help our pets nutritionally by giving them both raw and cooked fresh meats occasionally and by giving them supplements, such as small amounts of bonemeal for calcium, kelp and alfalfa for beneficial minerals, dolomite for nerves and fretfulness, and brewer's yeast for vitamin B and trace elements, as well as seaweed and dried liver tablets. Cod liver oil two or three times a week for its omega 3 fatty acids will give the coat a shining gleam and provide vitamins A and D, but be careful with the amount or you may have a pet with loose stools. Always start with low amounts; 1 drop initially should be sufficient and could gradually be increased to 2 or 3 drops, depending on the size of your dog.

Aromatherapy for Cats

Cats don't need daily walks, and they're independent and will hunt for both play and for food. Compared to dogs, cats are fairly easy to look after. They not only make good pets but cats can also help our health. It's known that stroking a cat has a calming effect on the nervous system and lowers blood pressure.

But no matter how much we love our cats,

they can be aggravating when they ruin the furniture by treating it as their favorite scratching board. As a preventative measure, make a scratching post from a smooth piece of wood and crush a piece of catnip (*Nepeta cataria*) over it. Cats adore catnip, and it's very easy to plant a patch of it in your garden, where cats will roll in it with great pleasure. It spreads quite rapidly, so one plant is usually quite sufficient to start with.

It's become quite popular to use hydrolats or floral waters with cats. Hydrolats by their very nature don't last too long and may develop what's known as a *bloom* — micro-organisms such as bacteria — at the bottom of the bottle. Although some herbalists may admire the bloom and say this shows the hydrolat is active, it's not something I'd want to be taking chances with. So always purchase the freshest you can find from reliable sources who sell true hydrolats or hydrosols.

TREATING CAT AILMENTS

A cat's body weight and size should be taken into consideration if using any product for external application, including natural medications such as plant remedies, herbs, hydrolats, essential oil waters, and essential oils. Cats are always cleaning and licking themselves, and if there's more than one cat in the house they may sleep entwined with each other, rubbing any external product onto the other cat.

There are many substances that cats come into contact with that could potentially cause them harm. Cats roam the streets and we often have no idea where they go. Yet many municipalities control weed growth with chemicals and our cats may be walking on this ground on a regular basis. Also, someone may be spraying weed killer in their backyard, or using substances to clean molds and fungi from paving stones, or laying rodent poison, and so on. And of course

when it rains, these substances will spread. Cleaning materials and artificial air sprays used in the home may even be responsible for a family cat's malaise.

There are a few herbs and aromatics that cats' digestive systems might find difficult to process, including chemical compounds that are both organic and inorganic. For example, salicin/salicylate compounds, such as those in aspirin, are unsuitable for cats. This compound is also found in wintergreen and birch essential oils. Although found in the plant material in very small amounts, it makes sense that any product containing birch or wintergreen should be avoided.

Cats can be treated quite successfully with a variety of nutritional supplements or with a change of diet, and often that's all that's required. Try feeding with raw fresh meats and fish instead of cooked meats. Cats often get dehydrated and may prefer drinking running water or rainwater to highly treated water from a tap that often contains chlorine, so filter your cat's drinking water or give them mineral or spring water. Adding to their food oils that contain essential fatty acids, such as flaxseed oil and safflower oil, can also enhance your cat's well-being.

If your cat has arthritis or rheumatism, supplements such as garlic, selenium, zinc, vitamin C, seaweed, and omega 3 fatty acids may help to alleviate stiff joints and pain. Homeopathic medicines are well tolerated by cats, and there are many good books on the subject. These are some of the remedies that could be used:

- Arnica 6c can be given after any injury or shock.
- Rhus Tox 6c can be used for arthritis.
- Hepar Sulph 6c can be given for infection.
- Chamomile granules can be given for gum inflammation and for inflammations in general.

SKIN CONDITIONS: PREVENTION AND CARE

Evening primrose seed (*Oenothera biennis*) oil can be added to food; selenium and zinc are also very helpful. Vitamin E, applied externally, can help to heal external wounds, and added to food it will often relieve dermatitis. Cod liver oil, which contains omega 3 fatty acids, helps the fur remain shiny and assists in maintaining good health in general.

ABSCESSES

Cats often get abscesses, usually as a result of a hectic night out on the prowl. To treat an abscess, it's your choice whether to use a veterinarian's preparation, head for your essential oil box, or both.

For Abscesses in Cats

Aloe vera gel	3 teaspoons (15 mL)
Chamomile german essential oil	1 drop

Clean the affected area with an equal mixture of water, lavender hydrolat, and colloidal silver. Then apply a small amount of the aloe vera blend above to the affected area only.

CANKER (OTITIS EXTERNA)

Canker of the ear, another problem that cats encounter, is caused by mites in the ear or bacterial or fungal infection. Canker can be contagious and should be seen by a veterinary practitioner before carrying out any home care methods. Always wear plastic gloves when touching or applying any product to an ear that has been diagnosed with canker, and follow your vet's advice.

Canker can cause soreness, inflammation, and infection. The ear will feel hot, and there could be a smelly discharge of wax. Try to clean the ear if possible with lavender or chamomile hydrolat. To prevent a sore from forming from the scratching, warm a teaspoon (5 mL) of olive oil to which 1 drop of neem oil has been added. Using a disposable cotton ball, wipe a small amount on the pink underside of the ear and around the opening of the ear canal, but not in the canal itself.

FLEAS

Fleas are one of the main causes of dermatitis in cats. The symptoms are intense itching and discomfort, sore or broken skin, and possibly loss of hair. These symptoms are caused by an allergic reaction to the bite. Often cats are also allergic to the preparations given to deter fleas and mites — which can just compound the problem. Lavender or chamomile hydrolat mixed with aloe vera gel could help soothe the skin. Tamanu oil applied to the sore area can often help cats afflicted with sore skin and dermatitis due to insect bites of all kinds and to other causes. However, because cats lick their fur and paws, care must be given to where the oil is used, and it should be applied in only very small amounts.

Brewer's yeast: A useful nutritional supplement for skin problems and flea infestation. A small amount of the powder can also be gently brushed into the fur at the back of the neck.

Odorless garlic capsules: The contents could be emptied out and added to food in small amounts to help deter fleas.

Cat's Herb Pillows

Herb pillows to deter fleas can be made very easily. Use the herbs of catnip, sage, mint, thyme, or lavender, or dried neem leaves, or a mixture. Place the pillow where the cat prefers to rest.

Rabbits

In the wild, rabbits run about in clean fields and woods, but in captivity they often have to put up with confined living quarters and urine-soaked straw under their feet. It really is only fair to ensure that their cages are kept clean and fresh. Dried herbs can be scattered among the straw on the floor of the cage, where they may help to prevent maggots from breeding and deter mites and other parasites. Many people want to avoid using disinfectants and other synthetically produced products in their rabbit's care and would prefer using herbal alternatives, which can include some essential oils, hydrolats, and products you can make yourself.

Sniffles and colds affect rabbits. While the rabbit is away in the rabbit run, wipe out the cage using a filtered, water-based essential oil solution you've made yourself using 2 drops of eucalyptus lemon to 2 pints (950 mL) of water. Allow the cage to dry and air before the rabbit goes back into the cage. Or use a freshly made essential oil water spray, using a clean or new plant mister. Use 4 drops of essential oil — a blend of eucalyptus radiata and niaouli — in 2 pints (950 mL) of water, following the instructions on page 481.

Canker is highly infectious and can easily spread between rabbits. Veterinary care should be sought and rubber gloves worn if carrying out any home treatment. Make up a bottle of oil using these proportions: blend together ½ teaspoon of warmed neem oil and 1 tablespoon of jojoba oil. Apply a small amount on cotton wool to the underside of the ear flap and around the ear canal but not inside it, once a day for three days. The area can also be washed in thyme hydrolat, lavender hydrolat, or an essential oil water made by using either lavender or thyme essential oil. You can also use a gel made by adding 1 drop of neem oil to a teaspoon of aloe vera gel. Use a small amount with each application.

Sore hocks can be eased by an application of $^1/_5$ teaspoon (1 mL) of tamanu oil combined with 4 teaspoons (20 mL) of jojoba oil and 1 drop of chamomile roman oil. Or add $^1/_5$ teaspoon (1 mL) of tamanu and 2 drops of chamomile roman to 1 ounce (30 g) of a natural balm, mixing well.

Hamsters

Hamsters should be kept clean and dry. A jam jar placed on its side will often be used by the hamsters as a toilet, and can be cleaned out quite easily. Use essential oil to wash the cage, just as for rabbits. Hamsters seem to like the smell of lavender, which is handy because it's antiseptic and antibiotic and will keep the hamsters healthy. Add 2 drops of lavender oil to 2 quarts (1.9 liters) of water and wipe a small amount around the whole of the cage after you've washed it in the usual way, letting it dry before putting the hamster back into the cage.

Hamsters store their food and this can rot, so to help prevent maggots use dried herbs such as thyme on the floor of the cage, or an antiseptic filtered essential oil water sprayed onto the floor. Only spray when the hamster is out of its cage and allow at least 30 minutes before putting the hamster back in.

Guinea Pigs

Guinea pigs seem to tolerate essential oils quite well, and many a breeder has used them successfully. There are several books that suggest using essential oils for a variety of problems. These are delicate animals, however, and need much care, and the dosage of any herb, vitamin, or essential oil should be very small, and then used only if required.

For coughs, bronchitis, or flu, some breeders use commercially prepared human decongestants and strong disinfectants in the cage. But why not try making the following remedy, which is gentler and very effective?

Eucalyptus radiata	1 drop
Niaouli	2 drops
Ravensara	2 drops

Blend the essential oils together, then add to 1 pint (475 mL) of water, mix well, and pour through an unbleached paper coffee filter to remove the globules before placing in a clean plant mister. Shake well. Alternatively, make a filtered essential oil water. Remove all the bedding from the guinea pig's cage, and clean as normal. Then spray the empty cage, and when dry, lay clean bedding.

To make your own decongestant, add 1 drop of the above essential oil blend to 1 dessertspoon of aloe vera gel. Alternatively, use an unscented natural ointment of your choice as a base. Dab a tiny smear of your preparation on the guinea pig's chest.

SKIN PROBLEMS

Skin infestations can be most distressing and are usually caused by parasites. Some essential oils do help when diluted and applied to the skin after shampooing. However, as most of the material to actually touch the animal's skin will be the base oil, it's preferable to use something that itself has anti-mite properties. Calendula macerated oil is effective at relieving skin disorders resulting from infestation. Also, tamanu oil (*Calophyllum inophyllum*) can be helpful for skin irritation: add 1 teaspoon (5 mL) of tamanu oil to 2 tablespoons (30 mL) of calendula macerated oil, and use a small amount for each application. This same oil may also help alleviate inflammation, sores, wounds, eczema, and dry cracks. For a deterrent, add 1 drop of neem oil to 1 fl. oz. (30 mL) of calendula macerated oil.

If you breed guinea pigs or have many of them, it may be worth making up the following blend:

SPECIAL SKIN BLEND FOR GUINEA PIGS

Neem oil	1 drop
Lemongrass	1 drop
Patchouli	1 drop
Manuka	1 drop
Lavender	2 drops
Chamomile roman	2 drops
Sweet almond oil	3 fl. oz. (90 mL)

Blend the essential oils together, add to the sweet almond oil, and bottle. After shampooing, smear a tiny amount on the affected areas of the skin. Leave it on, and repeat once a day for two days. Alternatively, the essential oil blend could be added to a balm.

Horses

Horses are by their very nature extremely sensitive creatures. They do seem to have an affinity with essential oils but, because of their sensitive nature, will turn away if a particular essential oil is not welcome. Essential oils have strong, intense aromas; you only have to sniff a bottle yourself to realize this. So it's unwise to put a bottle of essential oils underneath a horse's nose to test whether they like it or not. Instead, approach the horse with a diluted amount of the oil on your hand.

Horses like to be massaged, which is very useful when using herbal remedies and essential oil preparations, and many different equine massage techniques have evolved. However, you don't need to have equine massage skills to use essential oils, which can be a useful addition to your horse's stable.

MOVING HORSES

Moving a horse in any sort of trailer or box that's been used by other horses runs a slight risk of cross-infection, as well as a nervous reaction to the scent left behind by the previous occupant. If your horse is used to the aroma of essential oils and associates that with great massages, love, and healing, plus shows a good tolerance for and re-action to essential oils, then use the water spray method to help prevent stress. Make an essential oil water, and using a clean plant mister, spray the horse box or trailer with a mixture of viral-busting and bacteria-busting essential oils at least 30 min-utes before the horse is loaded, leaving the doors open. The following blend is aimed at reducing the stress and anxiety of travel, as well as having antibacterial and antimicrobial properties:

Ravensara	10 drops
Geranium	10 drops
Bergamot	10 drops
Lavender	10 drops
Thyme linalol	5 drops

From this blend, add 20 drops to 2 pints (950 mL) of water, and spray the walls and floor of the horse box, around 30 minutes before the horse en-ters, as described above.

The same mixture can be diluted in a carrier oil and brushed or wiped over the coat when groom-ing, when used in the following dilutions:

Oil Brush

To 1 pint (475 mL) of carrier oil add 15 drops of the above essential oil mixture. Blend together well. Dip a grooming brush into the mixture and brush over the coat, using a small amount each time.

Water Wipe

To 1 pint (475 mL) of plain water add 15 drops of the above essential oil mixture. Blend together well. Dip a cloth into the mixture and use to wipe over the horse's coat, using a small amount each time.

Moving a Nervous and Fretful Horse

The blend below can be used in a variety of ways, all aimed at making a horse's move less stressful. The goal is to bring a sense of familiarity and secu-rity to the horse. The blend can be diluted in a car-rier oil and brushed or wiped over the horse's coat when grooming — following the dilutions outlined in the Oil Brush and Water Wipe methods, above. When planning to move the horse, spray the walls and floor of the horse box before the horse enters, as described above, using 20 drops of the blend below diluted in 2 pints (950 mL) of water.

Juniper berry	10 drops
Orange, sweet	20 drops
Chamomile roman	10 drops
Lavender	20 drops

When loading and moving foals, only use laven-der hydrolat sprayed in the air when the foal is not in the vicinity. For older horses, hydrolats work really well and can be substituted for water in a water spray, not only when moving the horse but in other applications also. The same can be said for filtered essential oil waters.

WORMS

Horses get infested with several types of worm, including roundworms, tapeworms, and other in-testinal parasites, and need to be wormed regularly — especially if they don't have much freedom. To help prevent worm infestation, include in the feed a small handful of parsley leaves, rosemary, mint, mustard green, marigold petals, dande-lion leaves, or dried nettle tops — dried nettles contain no sting. Adding flaxseed oil to the diet helps keep the intestine healthy, while linseed oil added to the feed may help to expel worms. Seaweed powder is said to help in this regard too.

A simple way of keeping some species of worms at bay is to use garlic. Grate at least three cloves into each feed daily for a period of at least 14 days. Alternatively, use odorless garlic capsules or tablets, although fresh garlic does seem to be best. The added plus is that flies and fleas do not like the odor that comes through the skin and may stop biting and irritating garlic-fed horses.

FLIES

Flies are a problem in stables, and it's said that a walnut tree planted nearby will keep them away. But that isn't always possible! To stop horses from fretting with these annoying insects, put 3 neat drops of lemongrass or spearmint essential oil onto the brush you use to brush the horse down.

Spraying the stable with a mixture of water and essential oils does work for a while, but as essential oils evaporate very quickly the flies may then come back. Although it's wise to use a spray in the stable, the better idea is to try to stop the flies from biting the horse and, worse, trying to lay eggs in any wounds. The following is a list of essential oils that repel flies.

ESSENTIAL OILS TO DETER FLIES
Eucalyptus (*Eucalyptus dives, E. citriodora,*
      and *E. globulus*)
Basil (*Ocimum basilicum*)
Citronella (*Cymbopogon nardus*)
May chang (*Litsea cubeba*)
Garlic (*Allium sativum*)
Lavender (*Lavandula angustifolia*)
Lavandin (*Lavandula x intermedia*)
Lemongrass (*Cymbopogon citratus/flexuosus*)
Patchouli (*Pogostemon cablin*)
Peppermint (*Mentha avensis*)
Vetiver (*Vetiveria zizanoides*)
Neem (*Azadirachta indica*)

FLY WASH
The amount of fly wash needed will depend on the size of the horse. The following volumes will suffice for several washes of a large horse:

Vetiver	5 drops
Eucalyptus lemon	5 drops
Peppermint	15 drops
Patchouli	5 drops

Blend the essential oils together, then add to 4 pints (1.9 liters) of warm water. Oil and water don't mix, so you'll find that the oil does float on the surface of the water; try as best as you can to mix both together before dipping the cloth into the water. Wring out the cloth to remove excess water, then smooth it over your horse. This water blend can also be filtered through a paper coffee filter and used in a plant mister to spray the horse.

HOOF ROT

Hoof rot can affect all hoofed animals; the affected hooves should be treated with hot compresses. First, dilute the following essential oil blend in 3 fl. oz. (90 mL) of carrier oil, or in 3 fl. oz. (90 mL) of a gel such as aloe vera. From this, use 1 teaspoon (5 mL) for each compress, using any natural material, and hold it in place using horse socks.

Chamomile german	5 drops
Thyme	3 drops
Tea tree	3 drops
Manuka	5 drops
Chamomile roman	3 drops

STALL WASH

When washing down the stall, first dilute the essential oils listed below in 1 gallon (3.8 liters) of water, and from this mix take 4 cups, which is then added to another 1 gallon (3.8 liters) of water.

Oregano	10 drops
Thyme	10 drops
Lemongrass oil	20 drops

The stable needs to be kept clean and dry, but this environment also provides a perfect place for a family of mice to make their home. To help prevent this, wash the floor in the usual way and as a final rinse, wash down the whole stall with 1 gallon (3.8 liters) of water to which 15 drops of peppermint oil has been added. Dried peppermint herb can be added to the bedding as well.

LEG PROBLEMS

Horses are often struck down with leg problems. Fractures of the leg are about the worst thing that can happen to a horse, but healing may be helped by using essential oil compresses. All the following oils are helpful at this time:

Chamomile german (*Matricaria recutita*)
Chamomile roman (*Anthemis nobilis*)
Ginger (*Zingiber officinalis*)
Immortelle (*Helichrysum italicum*)
Hyssop decumbens (*Hyssopus officinalis var. decumbens*)
Lavender (*Lavandula angustifolia*)
Marjoram, sweet (*Origanum majorana*)
Peppermint (*Mentha piperita*)
Plai (*Zingiber cassumunar*)
Spikenard (*Nardostachys jatamansi*)

FRACTURED LEG BLEND
Ginger   10 drops
Immortelle   5 drops
Hyssop decumbens   5 drops

Blend the essential oils together and dilute in 2 fl. oz. (60 mL) of comfrey (*Symphytum officinale*) macerated oil. The comfrey oil can be substituted with arnica oil or gel, or calendula oil. Warm the mixture and add it to a material compress, which should be wrapped around the leg. Cabbage leaf compresses are also helpful (see page 304). Massaging the leg after the fracture has healed will strengthen the ligaments and help prevent calcification.

LEG MASSAGE OIL BLEND
Juniper berry   5 drops
Immortelle   5 drops
Plai   3 drops
Rosemary   3 drops

Blend the essential oils together, then dilute them in 5 fl. oz. (150 mL) of arnica oil, comfrey oil, or calendula macerated oil. Massage the oil over the whole leg and shoulder, or leg and flank, using a small amount each time.

NERVOUSNESS AND STRESS

Many horses have a very sensitive nature, and there are several essential oils that when used in massage may help reduce a nervous disposition, or stress. These include the following:

ESSENTIAL OILS FOR NERVOUS AND STRESSED HORSES
Chamomile roman (*Anthemis nobilis*)
Lavender (*Lavandula angustifolia*)
Clary sage (*Salvia sclarea*)
Sandalwood (*Santalum album*)
Valerian (*Valeriana officinalis*)
Vetiver (*Vetiveria zizanoides*)

Prepare a massage oil with one or several of the oils above — the choice will very much depend on your horse and the person who's carrying out the massage. Use no more than a total of 10 drops per 5 fl. oz. (150 mL) of oil. Often with nervousness, less is more. Homeopathic remedies are also very useful in treating nervous or high-strung horses, and in some cases it may be advisable to consult with a homeopathic veterinarian.

Small-Scale Farming

Many people like to keep what are thought of as traditional farm animals: the cow called Bluebell, to provide the family with fresh milk; or a goat called Barney, just for the fun of keeping a goat. Essential oils can be used to help deter flies and pests or to wash out animal pens, and they can be used in healing sprays and oils. With animals, always use small amounts, well diluted. Adjust the dilution according to the size of your animal, referring to other sections of this chapter.

Keeping Insects Away
The following essential oils can help in keeping unwanted insects away:

Patchouli (*Pogostemon cablin*)
Tea tree (*Melaleuca alternifolia*)
Lavender (*Lavandula angustifolia*)
Lemongrass (*Cymbopogon citratus/flexuosus*)
Eucalyptus peppermint (*Eucalyptus dives*)
Eucalyptus lemon (*Eucalyptus citriodora*)
Citronella (*Cymbopogon nardus*)
Garlic (*Allium sativum*)

Keeping Rodents Away
Peppermint (*Mentha piperita*)
Eucalyptus peppermint (*Eucalyptus dives*)
Patchouli (*Pogostemon cablin*)
Garlic (*Allium sativum*)
Oregano (*Origanum vulgare*)
Thyme (*Thymus vulgaris*)
Cinnamon leaf (*Cinnamomum zeylanicum*)

SHEEP

Mice are a problem in lambing sheds, so since mice dislike peppermint, grow some peppermint plants around the sheds as a border. Unfortunately, this doesn't seem to work with rats. When washing down the pens, use as a final rinse a gallon (3.8 liters) of water to which 5 drops of peppermint oil have been added. You can also drop neat peppermint oil around the outer edges of the shed. The peppermint seems to relax the mothers and makes a pen a pleasant place to be in.

COWS, BULLS, AND CALVES

Cows suffer a lot. They're fed antibiotics, growth hormones, drugs to increase their milk yield, and much more besides. The milk production of cows can be increased by adding to their feed the right herb instead of these worrying hormones that the unwitting consumer must drink along with the milk. Hazelnut leaves are said to increase the butterfat content of the milk, while also being very good for the cow's digestive system. The herb melissa (lemon balm) is thought to increase milk production. Use it dried in the feed, or make a melissa "herb tea" to spray onto the feed. The herb marjoram is also said to be useful for increased lactation: add dried marjoram to the feed or make a marjoram herb tea to spray on the feed.

Mastitis
The inflammation of mastitis may be painful to cows, and it causes a great deal of financial loss to the dairy farmer, in milk production and veterinary bills. One method to help reduce inflammation involves applying a diluted essential oil blend to the udders. This should be carried out at the first sign of problems.

Lavender	4 drops
Chamomile german	4 drops
Geranium	4 drops
Eucalyptus radiata	4 drops

Blend the essential oils together, then dilute in 4 fl. oz. (120 mL) of a carrier oil, such as safflower or rapeseed oil. From this dilution, use approximately ½ teaspoon for each application.

Another option is to blend the essential oils in a little calendula macerated oil and then dilute that in 4 fl. oz. (120 mL) of aloe vera gel. Adding 1 drop of peppermint oil to the essential oil blend above gives a slight cooling and anti-inflammatory effect. These methods of application can be used alongside any treatment recommended by your veterinarian, if they agree with their use.

Cow Tonics

Cows are sometimes fed tonics made from herbs and greens, especially in springtime, and all cows could benefit from a tonic. We're talking about old-fashioned tonics such as the following one:

Mix up a large handful of watercress, mint, dandelion leaves, nettle tops (wear gloves), sorrel leaves, and sage. Fresh leaves are best, but dried will do if fresh leaves aren't available. In a large pot, melt a teaspoonful of molasses in 5 pints (1.4 liters) of boiling water and put all the leaves in, plus 2 crushed garlic cloves. Leave to cool, stirring occasionally. Leave the pot standing for 24 hours, then strain off most of the liquid and add it to the drinking trough. The greenery left behind can be added to the feed.

BEES

Bees are extremely sensitive to aromas and are strongly attracted by them, as any aromatherapist using pure flower oils will confirm. To encourage bees to take to a new hive, try the following solution:

Geranium	1 drop
Chamomile roman	1 drop
Thyme	1 drop

Add the essential oils above to 1 tablespoon of water (15 mL), then soak a piece of material in the essential oil and water mix and use it to rub the inside walls of the hive.

All these essential oils could also be used on their own. Some organic beekeepers use a similar method — this time to deter mites. They wipe the inside of the hives using oregano and/or thyme essential oil.

The attraction of bees to the floral aromas can be a nuisance if you work with essential oils professionally, as I've found to my own cost. Once a year, I used to have swarms of bees trying to get into my clinic, crashing against the window, flying past clients as they went in and out of the door, crawling through the light fittings, blinds, and just about anywhere they could. The bees were manic in their attempts to get to what they thought was the most enormous field overflowing with delicious nectar-heavy blooms. I had to find an answer to this problem. I made a blend of essential oils derived from roots, not flowers — vetiver, valerian, and ginger — and smeared it all over the outside door frame and window frames, and the bees took a U-turn and left. Ever since then we've not had the problem of bees making a beeline — sorry for the pun — for the clinic. I tell you this story in case you too have had a similar experience.

18

Gardens for the Future

A garden is a community of plants, insects, birds, and small creatures. In a good community, everyone gets along, takes as much as they need to survive, and gives resources to their neighbors to help them thrive. In a dysfunctional community, bullies are allowed to take over, neighbors steal from each other, nobody helps anyone else, and eventually, the community disintegrates into chaos. A thriving garden is one in which the nutrients taken from the soil are replenished, the pests are under control, the weeds haven't taken over, neighboring plants give nutrients to each other, and everything grows healthy and strong.

Everything starts with the soil. Plants take their nutrients and moisture from the soil, and while we can expect rain to fall, it's up to us to think how the nutrients are going to get back into the soil for the next generation of plants. Worms are called "ecosystem engineers" because they dig tunnels that aerate the soil and provide easy channels for plant roots to expand into, and they eat plant debris that is turned into soil-enriching humus containing phosphorus, nitrogen, potassium, and other micronutrients. If there are no worms, the nutrients are going to get depleted.

So, it's up to us to make sure the worms are well fed and stay in our garden. A garden with no leaves or other organic matter doesn't offer the worms much incentive to stay around.

Fungi also take nutrients from dead matter and process it back into nutrient-rich humus. Without them, deadwood would never break down, so they're a vital element in the process of recycling nutrients. Indeed, half a million different types of microscopic creatures live in the soil, busily working away, keeping it rich and healthy. They're friends of the community, and their well-being has to be considered.

Drainage depends on the type of soil. Aside from the fertile humus created by our hardworking worms and fungi, soil is made up of sand, silt, and clay. Sand grains are the largest in size; silt, which is broken-down rock, is smaller; and then there's clay, which is extremely fine. If the soil's too sandy, when it rains the water just disappears below the level at which it's useful to most plants. Clay is so fine it becomes densely packed, and the rainwater can't get much below the surface. If a grain of sand were the size of a soccer ball, clay grains would be the size of a pinhead, and they're electro-charged, which attracts nutrients and water to them. The key with gardening is to try to ensure that the ground is not too sandy, nor too clay-heavy, so water can drain and yet there's enough for our plants. Achieving a good balance for plant growth means knowing the soil and feeding it so it's well balanced. It might need organic compost, and spending a few hours digging it in is going to pay big dividends in the long run.

Under normal weather conditions, the plants and soil generally get along, doing what they're supposed to do. But when there's a drought, or too much rain, catastrophe can occur. The Dust Bowl in the central United States and Canada in the 1930s was brought about by droughts, exacerbating farming practices that had left the soil vulnerable. The soil became dust and blew away. In many places soil erosion is caused by rain falling too heavily where not enough consideration has been given to how the crops are being grown. There are some easy measures that can be taken to hold on to the soil. The first is to allow grass to grow between rows of plants. This helps prevent excess rain from running off with the soil. Also, straw placed on unused areas of bare earth takes the brunt of the force when raindrops crash onto the soil, so the soil itself isn't so broken up and doesn't run off with the rainwater. On hillsides, rows of crops can be planted in directions that create barriers to prevent gushing rain from carrying the soil away.

Choosing a good community of plants involves knowing each plant's individual way of growing, the height it grows to, the depth of its roots, the type of soil it likes, the nutrients required, the insects that pollinate it, and the insects and microbes that could eat the plant, or bring disease to it. Choosing a good neighbor for each plant then depends on knowing which other plants can help in any of these regards.

Choosing a good community of insects means knowing which pollinate and which, on the other hand, use plants for food, as a home, or as a nursery for their eggs and growing young. Some insects are generally very good to have in the garden, as they prey on those that damage plants. For example, hoverflies lay their eggs in aphid colonies precisely so their young can eat them — and each hoverfly can munch through hundreds of aphids even before it pupates. You can attract hoverflies with nasturtiums, marigolds, and poppies.

Companion gardening is a term that describes good relationships between neighboring plants. At the simplest level, a good neighbor may be one that provides the shade and protection its neighbor needs. Or, if one plant has a deeper root system and takes nutrients from the lower levels of soil, that leaves nutrients in the upper levels for its shallow-rooted neighbor. Or one variety may excrete just the nutrients that its neighbor requires. One plant may emit an aroma that coincidentally deters insects that endanger its neighbor or an aroma that attracts insects that pollinate the neighbor. In some cases, the antibacterial or antiviral properties contained within the aroma emitted by one plant may protect the neighbors, as well as the plant itself.

The field of plant communication is now being seen as a way to manage crops on a large scale. Even plants we'd not consider aromatic emit volatile organic compounds (VOCs) that deter insect predators, and these VOCs can be detected not only by plants of their own kind but also by unrelated species. If one plant can pick up olfactory messages from another species, that opens up the possibility of surrounding a field of crops with a species that will warn the crop plant of predators in the neighborhood, so it too can protect itself. These crop-protective plants are being called *sentinels*, and they may play a part in the future of farming.

One problem facing farmers is insecticidal resistance, which leads to the practice of using even more insecticide, or stronger insecticides. Some essential oils and their compounds are seen as a solution to this situation because they can deter certain insects, are unlikely — because of their phytochemical diversity — to cause resistance over time, and, being natural, don't damage the environment. Research into this area is being carried out in the field of allelopathy, which is the broader study of how the biologically active compounds in plants — whether in their leaves or in their roots — interact with other plants and cause a reaction in them. There's a huge amount of information still to be gathered on each and every plant species, but it's quite likely that the future of farming will be based on a much deeper understanding of the ancient craft of companion gardening. Farmers may well put aside a portion of their land to grow their own insecticides and plants that could be used as antimicrobials to help control the bacteria, viruses, and fungi that affect crops.

Using Essential Oils in the Garden

Essential oils could play several roles in the garden. They can be used to attract pollinators and to deter unwanted pests — as well as dealing with the bacteria and viruses they carry. The antimicrobial properties of essential oils evolved over millions of years not to help us but to ensure the survival of the plants from which they came.

Strong, healthy plants are more disease resistant, and if we utilize the biochemical aspects of intercropping and use naturally derived plant food such as seaweeds, that strength can be built up. This gentle approach not only increases the yield but can improve the fragrance of flowers and the flavor of vegetables and fruit.

It's well known that tomato and basil make good companions in the cooking pot or salad bowl, but basil grown around the tomato plant can enhance the taste of tomatoes before they even leave the plant. Roses love to be in the company of garlic, basil, or thyme, and either these can be planted around the rosebush or trace amounts of essential oil can be incorporated into the watering can.

The secret of success in the battle with garden pests is to know your enemy — their likes and dislikes, their natural enemies and how to attract them, their life cycles, the parameters of their movements, and so forth. With that information it should be possible to construct a winning plan. When using essential oils in the garden use trace amounts in a watering can; that's all that's usually needed. The following list is a guide to which essential oils and plants may help deter insects and garden pests.

TABLE 18. THE NATURAL INSECT REPELLENTS

INSECT	REPELLENT PLANTS OR PLANT TEAS	ESSENTIAL OILS
Ant	Spearmint, tansy, pennyroyal, peppermint, rosemary, thyme Grow the plants near the doors of a house, either in the ground or in pots. Also put the essential oils on cotton balls and place by the doors. Spray the oils where the ants are seen, and on their nests.	Orange, rosemary, spearmint, peppermint, cinnamon, clove, thyme, pennyroyal, garlic, wintergreen
Aphid	Rosemary, marigold, nasturtium, spearmint, stinging nettle, southernwood, garlic, potatoes, parsley, basil, horseradish	Rosemary, tagetes, aniseed, spearmint, peppermint, cedarwood, hyssop, coriander, neem, wintergreen
Aphid (peas and legumes)	Savory, rosemary	Bay laurel, neem, coriander, savory, rosemary
Bean beetle	Potatoes, thyme, rosemary	Thyme, garlic, rosemary, peppermint
Blackfly	Stinging nettle, basil, lavender	Lavender, tagetes, peppermint, clove, rosemary
Cabbage root fly	Thyme, sage, rosemary	Thyme, sage, rosemary, peppermint
Cabbage white butterfly	Sage, rosemary, hyssop, thyme, peppermint, celery, mint, southernwood	Peppermint, sage, rosemary, hyssop, thyme
Carrot root fly	Rosemary, chives, sage, thyme, onions, leeks	Rosemary, oregano, tagetes, thyme
Caterpillar	Celery, celeriac family, tomatoes	Spearmint, sage, rosemary, geranium, peppermint, thyme, wintergreen
Cutworm	Oak leaf, oak bark	Thyme, sage, rosemary, clove, peppermint, wintergreen
Eelworm	Marigold	Tagetes, clove, rosemary
Flea	Lavender, peppermint	Lemongrass, citronella, pennyroyal, lavender, peppermint, thyme, rosemary, wintergreen

INSECT	REPELLENT PLANTS OR PLANT TEAS	ESSENTIAL OILS
Flea beetle (black)	Mint, lettuce	Lemongrass, pennyroyal, lavender, rosemary, clove, thyme, peppermint
Fly	Rue, peppermint, tansy, tomatoes Rue is very helpful grown around composts, manure piles, and barns.	Pennyroyal, clove, lemongrass, lavender, citronella, peppermint, rosemary, basil, spearmint, oregano, neem, vetiver, eucalyptus lemon, geranium, patchouli
Gnat	Pennyroyal	Spearmint, cinnamon, lemongrass, geranium, patchouli
Greenfly	Garlic Greenfly might be attracted by basil and grapefruit oils. Don't use grapefruit skins to catch slugs in the greenhouse.	Lavender, manuka, tea tree, oregano, thyme, rosemary, peppermint, neem
Lice	Spearmint, pennyroyal, peppermint, nettle, basil	Spearmint, peppermint, cedarwood, neem, pennyroyal, basil
Mite	Peppermint, southernwood	Eucalyptus, lemongrass, bergamot, peppermint
Mosquito	Sassafras, pennyroyal, southernwood, rosemary, sage, santolina, lavender, mint, basil Castor oil plants may help.	Catnip, ajowan, basil, rosemary, eucalyptus lemon, lavender, oregano, thyme, pennyroyal, geranium, clove, patchouli, vetiver, citronella, lemongrass
Moth	Southernwood, rosemary, sage, santolina, lavender, peppermint, tansy	Cedarwood, pine, spearmint, lavender, hyssop, pennyroyal, citronella, peppermint, vetiver, lemongrass
Plant lice	Stinging nettles	Spearmint, pennyroyal, peppermint
Slug	Garlic, chives Crush eggshells, and add a drop of rosemary to them before scattering around the vegetable patch. Slugs don't like any intense aroma or too rough a surface. Cut coarse sandpaper into strips to create a barrier.	Garlic, cedarwood, hyssop, pine, peppermint, clove, rosemary

INSECT	REPELLENT PLANTS OR PLANT TEAS	ESSENTIAL OILS
Snail	Garlic, peppermint, spearmint Snails dislike many essential oils.	Lemongrass, clove, spearmint, cinnamon, peppermint, cedarwood, pine, garlic, patchouli
Tick	Rue, pennyroyal, sage, peppermint	Citronella, lemongrass, thyme, sage, rue, rosemary, clove, peppermint
Weevil	Garlic	Cedarwood, rue, sandalwood, patchouli
White fly	Marigolds, tomatoes, tagetes	Tagetes, lavender, sage, neem, rosemary, peppermint, wintergreen
Woolly aphid	Nasturtium	Neem, pine

Essential oils will be affected by light and rain, so using 1 drop of an ecofriendly dish soap or castile soap in the watering can may help the aroma of the essential oil last a little longer.

GENERAL INSECT DETERRENT SPRAY BLEND

Cinnamon	1 drop
Rosemary	4 drops
Clove	2 drops
Thyme	1 drop
Eucalyptus lemon (or lemongrass)	3 drops

Use 2 drops of the blend per 1 pint (475 mL) of water. Pour the mixture through an unbleached paper coffee filter, then add 1 tablespoon (15 mL) of this liquid to each pint (475 mL) of water. It may take several days before the insects give up and decide to go elsewhere.

You'll see in table 18 (on page 498) that ants can be deterred by orange and peppermint and will go to great lengths to avoid it. To clear an ant nest, put 2 neat drops of peppermint oil directly onto the nest and wait for the exodus. An orange and peppermint tea can be used for both the home and garden. Collect orange peels and add 1 drop of peppermint oil to the pithy part of the peel, leave for a couple of days, then add to 3 pints (1.5 liters) of boiling water. Leave it to steep for at least 24 hours before removing the peel. Use this liquid as an ant deterrent spray. If you don't have any orange peel, use a drop of orange oil instead, and filter before using.

If ants are coming into your home, put 1 or 2 drops of peppermint, spearmint, or clove oil on the threshold, or wherever they enter, but avoid using neat essential oil on any carpeted, wooden, or laminate floors, as it may cause damage. You can create a mobile barrier with a peppermint plant in a pot that can be placed at the back door and moved as the ants get smart and try to find another entrance point. Alternatively, chop the leaves of a peppermint plant, add peppermint essential oil, and scatter them to create a barrier. As mice try to avoid peppermint too, these same methods can be used to discourage them.

Peppermint is a useful plant or oil to have for deterring all sorts of insects, including the cabbage white butterfly. Again, scatter the dried leaves or use a trace amount of essential oil in the watering can. Refer to the various methods of use that follow; 1 drop of essential oil is enough for a large watering can — less is always more when using essential oils in the garden.

Insects are essential for pollination, including bees, wasps, and butterflies. Bees can be encouraged to visit your garden by using essential oils from flowering herbs — 1 drop on a dish of water — as they're attracted by the smell of what they think are real flowers. If you have fruit trees that need pollinating, this trick is something to consider! If you have a hive of bees, thyme and oregano essential oil are useful antimicrobials (see "Bees" in chapter 17, "Natural Health for Animals"). Essential oils extracted from roots do not attract bees.

There are many tribes of mosquito — yes, *tribes* is what they're called — and many species within each tribe. Each will have different aroma preferences and dislikes, and varying strengths of essential oils will be required to deter them. In all this, there will have to be a degree of experimentation to discover the perfect solution to the particular mosquito that's bothering you. The essential oil of catnip is a really good deterrent used in the garden — use as you would citronella or combine it with other essential oils from the lists above. Bear in mind, though, that if you use catnip it may attract all the local cats. The aroma of lemongrass, citronella, neem, or lavender oil, among others, can take the sting out of hot summer nights.

All flying insects are a nuisance in the garden, especially if you're having a barbecue. Ribbons hung from trees are an attractive way to deter flying insects such as midges, gnats, or mosquitoes, and this method is easy to prepare and refresh. Add 5 drops of your chosen essential oil(s) to a small bowl of water and soak some colorfast ribbons in this mixture before attaching them to the underside of the garden parasol or to branches of trees, garden fences, or whatever border you have, to deter insects from entering your airspace.

Refresh with additional neat essential oil as needed. If any water has accumulated in garden pots or buckets, pour it away as it just encourages insects into the area.

Avoid getting essential oil into pond or lake water. Insects hovering over a pond can be deterred by putting neat essential oil on ribbons on a long pole and sticking that in the ground near the water. If your summer evenings are being spoiled by moths, use the same methods described above, but use lavender or cedarwood oil, which moths try to avoid. For insect deterrents, you can use essential oils that are past their therapeutic-use expiration date as it's the aroma that's needed to deter insects.

Methods of Using Essential Oils in the Garden

When using essential oils in the garden, less is best. Essential oils are highly concentrated, and although we may not detect an aroma, insects and animals will. It only takes a trace of essential oil aroma to confuse an insect that's generally attracted to a particular plant because of the aroma it emits. There are many methods of using essential oils in the garden, so decide which method to use depending on the type of insect and the kind of plant you want to protect, its proximity to other plants, and what plants they are.

SPRAYS

Sprays can be used as insect deterrents or to help banish mold and mildew. Add 3 drops of essential oil to 3½ fl. oz. (100 mL) of water, shake well, and leave to stand for 24 hours. Finally, filter the liquid by pouring it through an unbleached paper coffee filter. Use 1 tablespoon (15 mL) of this mixture to each 2 pints (950 mL) of water.

When spraying onto flowers, fruit, or vegetables make sure the mixture has been well shaken

— as oil and water don't mix — and shake again each time before you spray. If you can see essential oil globules floating on the top of the water, simply remove them by dipping the corner of an absorbent paper towel into the globules.

ESSENTIAL OIL TEAS

Add 8 drops of essential oil to 2½ pints (1.2 liters) of water. Boil and leave to cool before pouring through a paper coffee filter to remove any essential oil globules. Dilute 2 tablespoons of this in each 4 pints (1.9 liters) of water, and use in the usual watering methods.

STRING

String soaked in a solution of water and essential oil could be strung between rows of vegetables to confuse the sense of smell of flying insects, such as cabbage white butterflies or carrot root flies. Use appropriate essential oils from table 18.

HANGING STRIPS

Place 1 drop of neat essential oil on a strip of material and hang it from a stick or a branch of a tree. This method saves you from the arduous task of spraying a large area. Renew as needed.

COTTON BALLS

This method can be used to deter insects or help deter burrowing animals such as moles. Place 3 drops of essential oil on a cotton ball and place it in the burrow or on the nest and repeat as needed. Try to use essential oils that are very pungent.

CARTONS

The carton method is useful for deterring slugs, snails, mice, cats, dogs, and all ground-moving insects. Bury an old plastic food carton such as a yogurt container so that the open top rim is level with the surface of the ground. Pour a little water or vegetable oil into the container, and add 2 drops of essential oil. This method can also be helpful in discouraging cats and dogs from urinating in the area. Cover the carton when it rains.

Plant Teas

Herbal, floral, and other plant teas use plant material to gently transport the active principle of an herb or flower to another plant. The plant material used could be dried, although fresh is always better. Pick the plant early in the morning, preferably when the dew is still on the leaves. Use young plant material that may have more growth constituents in the stem and leaves.

Use 1 cup of fresh or dried plant material to 2 cups of water. Pour boiling water over the plant material, cover, and leave it to stand for at least four hours. Strain off the liquid and store it in the fridge. Further dilute the tea by using 2 tablespoons (30 mL) of this liquid to each 8 pints (3.8 liters) of water in a watering can or garden spray.

For a more concentrated plant tea for the garden, fill a lidded jar with the plant material, cover with boiling water, and leave it to stand overnight. Strain off, and repeat the process but instead of using boiling water, use the already prepared plant tea — which should be boiled. The process can be repeated several times. Then, use 1–2 teaspoons of this concentrated tea in 1 pint (475 mL) of water in a plant mister. For ideas about which herbs and flowers to use, refer to the good companions lists that follow.

Slugs and Birds

Slugs have obviously made a lot of enemies over the years, because so many methods of dealing with them have been devised. The best option is to try to deter them from eating your plants in the first place. Slugs have an acute sense of smell and hate garlic in any shape or form. The essential oil of garlic is so aromatically powerful that it's rather unpleasant to handle, so another option is to break a garlic bulb into its cloves and place these in the ground, especially along the edges of the garden where slugs may be laying their eggs. Look under stones or clumps of earth for the little telltale white pearls. Alternatively, use nondeodorized garlic capsules: pierce a couple of holes in them with a pin and dig them in around the vegetable patch or garden's borders. Another method is to add 1 table-spoon of crushed garlic to a watering can of water, mix well, and water the areas where the slugs are causing damage, but not on the plant itself.

The plants that attract the slugs — usually the thickest and most succulent plants in the garden — might be protected by laying a physical barrier around them. Dried pine needles or dried holly work well, but any prickly material is an option, such as crushed eggshells, coarse sandpaper, or copper wire. Another approach is to put some-thing on the surface that sticks to the slugs' un-dersides and dries them out, such as raw oat bran.

Unless there are fruits in the garden that you want to keep birds away from, in general birds are good to have around because they feed on aphids, caterpillars, and slugs. Invite them into the garden with bird feeders and baths. String or cotton strung across flower or vegetable beds and between fruit trees will deter birds, but these should be brightly colored so the birds can see them clearly, and strung tightly so their legs don't get entangled in them.

Mold and Mildew

Mold and mildew are often the result of overwa-tering, or watering the leaves of plants rather than the roots. An occasional light sprinkle is fine, but leaving large spots of water on leaves can encour-age mildew and mold, especially when the sum-mer weather becomes cooler. Treat with the tea or spray methods; choosing from the list below, use 1 or 2 drops of essential oil to every 4 pints (1.9 liters) of water in your usual gardening spray.

Elderflower plant tea discourages most molds, while chive plant tea is particularly good with the gray, dusty mold that blights the delicate rose. Nettle tea treats mildew on cucumbers, while horsetail tea helps to protect plants against many types of vegetable-loving mold due to its high sil-ica content.

ANTI–MOLD AND MILDEW ESSENTIAL OILS
Patchouli (*Pogostemon cablin*)
Cinnamon leaf (*Cinnamomum zeylanicum*)
Tea tree (*Melaleuca alternifolia*)
Clove bud (*Syzygium aromaticum*)
Oregano (*Origanum vulgare*)
Geranium (*Pelargonium graveolens*)
Manuka (*Leptospermum scoparium*)

Gardeners and farmers alike are plagued by tomato and potato blight, caused by a fungus-like organism. The plants can be sprayed with a com-bination of essential oils and aspirin or, alterna-tively, with willow tea or other products from the willow tree bark (*Salix alba*) from which the sal-icylic acid in aspirin is derived. Part of the prob-lem with this organism is that it can genetically mutate and outrun chemical treatments. Essential oils, on the other hand, can keep pace with the genetic mutations because not only are there sev-eral essential oils that can help, but when they are combined together, and in a changing variety of proportions, new solutions are made. When using aspirin tablets, ensure they are water soluble. Use around 500 mg to each quart of water (950 mL) and spray the foliage, including under the leaves.

TOMATO AND POTATO BLIGHT SOLUTION

Water-soluble aspirin, crushed	500 mg
Water	2 pints (950 mL)
*Essential oil	1 drop

Choose from the anti–mold and mildew essential oil list on page 503.

Crush the aspirin tablets, or use herbal willow tablets or powder. (Alternatives to the aspirin and water combination could be willow water, or an infused willow solution made by soaking *Salix alba* bark or twigs in water for a couple of weeks.) Put the aspirin in a plant mister, along with the water and essential oil. Shake the mister well, before spraying, to thoroughly dissolve the aspirin. An alternative method is to use 1 tablespoon of baking soda (sodium bicarbonate) instead of the aspirin.

The Friendly Bunch

Certain aromatic plants have a beneficial effect on most flowers and vegetables when grown among them. Marigolds were considered sacred by the Aztecs and associated with their god of agriculture — no doubt because when grown next to many plants, the marigolds increased their crop. Sage is beneficial to many vegetables, as are lavender, rosemary, and thyme. Plant lavender and rosemary along the borders of vegetable patches, rather than between them, simply because they're so permanent, and prune them to prevent them from becoming too tall.

The herb tarragon can be grown most everywhere because it doesn't leech the soil of nutrients, as many other plants do. Yarrow is said to increase the aromatic quality of most herbs and could make a good companion for medicinal plants and herbs. Valerian contains phosphorus and might attract beneficial earthworms. Foxglove has a good effect on most plants when grown in a border at the back of the flower beds. Avoid planting fennel near vegetables — most just aren't comfortable with it growing close by.

Strawberries planted next to the following vegetables are said to improve their growth: dwarf green beans, leeks, lettuce, onions, and spinach. On the other hand, they're not good neighbors to cabbage, red cabbage, or potatoes.

TABLE 19. VEGETABLES' GOOD COMPANIONS

VEGETABLES AND PLANTS	HERBS	FLOWERS	OTHER VEGETABLE PLANTS	ESSENTIAL OILS
Asparagus	Parsley, dill, basil, comfrey	Marigold	Tomatoes, carrots	Basil, dill, parsley
Beans, broad	Savory, basil		Potatoes, sweet corn	Lavender, basil, savory (summer)
Beans: green, dwarf/bush	Savory		Carrots, peas, potatoes, radishes, sweet corn, squash, cucumbers, eggplant, lettuce	Lavender, basil, savory (summer)

VEGETABLES AND PLANTS	HERBS	FLOWERS	OTHER VEGETABLE PLANTS	ESSENTIAL OILS
Beans, runner	Savory		Potatoes, sweet corn, radishes, pumpkin, squash	Lavender, basil, savory (summer)
Beetroots	Marjoram, sage		Onions, cabbage, leeks, sweet corn	Marjoram, sage
Broccoli	Valerian, dill, rosemary, sage, thyme, peppermint, chamomile	Nasturtium	Cabbage, peas, tomatoes, celery, cucumbers, onions, lettuce, potatoes	Basil, thyme, rosemary, peppermint, sage
Cabbage	Peppermint, sage, dill, rosemary, feverfew, thyme, peppermint, chamomile	Marigold	Cucumbers, celery, beetroot, onions, lettuce	Peppermint, sage, thyme, clary sage, chamomile, rosemary
Carrots	Chives, rosemary, sage		Peas, beans, leeks, lettuce, onions	Sage, rosemary
Cauliflower	Thyme, sage, rosemary, chives		Runner beans, celery, cucumbers, lettuce, brassicas, beetroot, carrots	Thyme, sage, peppermint, rosemary, chamomile
Celery	Yarrow	Daisies	Cabbage, leeks, dwarf beans, celeriac, tomatoes, cauliflower	Geranium, yarrow
Cucumbers	Chives	Sunflowers	Peas, cabbage, brassicas, sweet corn, carrots, spinach	Sage, yarrow
Eggplant/aubergine	Tarragon, thyme, dill	Marigold	Peas, spinach, radishes, beans	Catnip, thyme
Leeks	Valerian		Celery, carrots	Celery, hyssop
Lettuce	Basil	Tagetes	Carrots, radishes, beans, cucumbers, beetroot	Carrot seed, tagetes, basil

VEGETABLES AND PLANTS	HERBS	FLOWERS	OTHER VEGETABLE PLANTS	ESSENTIAL OILS
Onions	Chamomile, savory (summer)	Roses	Beetroot, tomatoes, cabbage, carrots, lettuce	Chamomile, savory (summer)
Peas	Caraway	Nasturtium	Brassicas, sweet corn, celery, lettuce, carrots, broccoli, radishes, cucumbers	Geranium, carrot seed, caraway, coriander
Peppers	Basil, marjoram	Sunflowers	Beans, tomatoes	Basil, marjoram
Potatoes	Horseradish, borage	Foxgloves	Beans (all), sweet corn, cabbage, peas	Basil, sage
Pumpkins	Borage, oregano	Nasturtium	Sweet corn, beans, radishes, cucumbers, onions	Oregano
Radishes	Chervil, parsley		Carrots, peas, lettuce	Parsley seed, savory (summer)
Spinach	Borage, chives		Carrots, onions, lettuce, cauliflower, runner beans	Thyme, lavender
Squash	Borage	Nasturtium, marigolds	Radishes, cucumbers, onions, sweet corn, beans	Oregano
Sweet corn	Borage, savory, dill, chamomile	Marigolds	Cucumbers, broad beans, runner beans, peas, potatoes, squash, eggplant, pumpkin, marrow	Savory (summer), tagetes
Tomatoes	Basil, chives, parsley, peppermint	Marigolds, tagetes, foxgloves	Asparagus, celery, carrots, onions, celeriac, eggplant	Tagetes, basil
Zucchini/courgette	Borage	Nasturtium, marigold	Radishes, cucumbers, sweet corn, beans	Oregano

TABLE 20. FRUITS' GOOD COMPANIONS

FRUIT	HERBS	FLOWERS	VEGETABLE PLANTS	ESSENTIAL OILS
Apples	Southernwood, chives	Nasturtium, wallflowers, fox-gloves, lavender	Legumes, climbing beans	Lavender
Grapes	Hyssop	Clematis		Hyssop, lavender
Strawberries	Borage, nettles, sage, rosemary, mint, thyme		Leeks, onions, peas, beans, spinach, lettuce	Sage, rosemary, thyme

NATURE'S NURSEMAIDS

When hyssop is grown among other plants, it's said to prevent bacterial invasion. Chamomile is another plant that appears to have a protective nature when grown next to ailing plants — either move your chamomile plants next to the ailing patient, make a plant tea spray with chamomile flowers, or follow the instructions for making an essential oil spray or tea. Once the plant is recovering, leave it to Mother Nature to do her work.

Stinging nettles are one of the great unappreciated nurses of the plant world. Whenever you find nettles growing somewhere inconvenient or unwelcome, cut them down and make a plant tea; it can become the standby emergency "medicine" for all your plants. Nettles also make good fertilizing material. When cooked, the sting goes out of nettles and they can be used in teas to drink, or included in soups.

Just as there are plants that find each other's company mutually beneficial, there are those that do *not* thrive close to each other. Sometimes we can explain why — because they're competing for resources, for example, or they attract insects and micro-organisms that harm each other — but sometimes the reasons as yet are unclear. Certain planting arrangements just don't work well. Growing any type of bean near onions, garlic, and shallots, for example, is a grouping in which none will do well, whatever the soil and weather conditions. Perhaps you can find in the list below the answer to one of your most mystifying gardening failures. Fennel and rue are generally bad for all plants — they should be grown on their own or in pots, so I suppose in gardening terms they're the outcasts.

TABLE 21. THE UNFRIENDLY NEIGHBORS

VEGETABLE PLANT	HERBS	FLOWERS	OTHER VEGETABLE PLANTS
Beans, green (all)	Fennel	Gladioli, sunflowers	Beetroot, kohlrabi, onions, shallots, garlic
Beetroot	Fennel, mustard	Marigolds	Beans (all)
Cabbage	Fennel, parsley		Onions, beans, tomatoes
Cabbage, red	Fennel		Tomatoes, beans
Carrots	Fennel, dill		Radishes, parsnips
Cucumbers	Fennel, thyme, peppermint		Potatoes
Lettuce	Fennel, parsley		Cress, cabbage, celery
Peas	Fennel	Gladioli	Onions, garlic
Potatoes	Fennel	Sunflowers	Pumpkin, tomatoes, squash, cucumbers
Tomatoes	Fennel		Kohlrabi, cabbage, sweet corn, chili peppers

Weed Control

Weeds take resources from the ground, making those resources unavailable to other plants. If allowed to grow tall they may restrict sunlight reaching other plants, and they can also harbor pests.

GENERAL WEED CONTROL SPRAY

Clove bud	2 drops
Peppermint	2 drops
Thyme	2 drops

Blend the essential oils together in these proportions. Add 1 drop of the blend to 1 teaspoon (5 mL) of vinegar, then dilute again into 1 pint (475 mL) of water.

Vinegar does not discriminate and will attack your precious plants as well as the weeds, so ensure the direction of the spray is on the weeds only. On really tough weeds, such as those growing in your pathway or those that have invaded the sides of the house with long roots, spray as usual or try brushing the tops with the mixture every day for a few days. This is only really suitable in dry, hot weather, as any rainfall will, of course, dilute and disperse the mixture.

Trees and Fruits

In companion gardening terms, trees have their friends too. All the following plants help trees to flourish if grown nearby: chamomile, chives, garlic, feverfew, tansy, southernwood, nasturtium, and stinging nettle. Nasturtiums planted around the base of a tree or encouraged to grow up its trunk will protect it from aphids, and will also have a discouraging effect on scab and molds on apple trees. The aphids love nasturtiums so much they will be attracted to them, leaving most everything else in peace. However, aphids do need some controlling, and clumps of chives or southernwood planted nearby will help keep their numbers under control. Wallflowers, either grown around apple trees or made into a plant tea and sprayed onto trees, might have a similarly protective action. Legumes in general may help most trees and could be encouraged to grow up their trunks. Beans are said to aid the growth of apricot trees.

Southernwood planted around trees may repel fruit tree moths, while tansy keeps away flying insects in general. On the other hand, bees are vital for pollination, and they can be encouraged by planting coriander or flowers that bees love between the trees. To try and deter insects from eating fruit, use lavender, rosemary, or clove bud essential oil, placed on cotton balls and put in small plastic bags. Then pierce the bags with a pin a few times so the odor can escape but not evaporate completely, and hang them on branch tips, away from the fruit. Fresh or dried plant material such as lavender could also be used, tied into little gauze bags. Confusing insects' sense

of smell is best carried out in the morning and at night.

It's a great shame to go to all the trouble of protecting your trees and bringing in a terrific crop if the whole effect is ruined by bad storage. Flowers and fruit do not generally store well together. Apples don't do well if stored near potatoes, and they don't like growing near each other, either, while carrots stored by apples lose their sweetness.

Brown rot is the scourge of fruit farmers, but they have four very good friends in horseradish, garlic, onion, and chive. These can either be grown between the trees or made into a plant tea and used to water or spray the fruit plants. Stinging nettles are a very useful plant because they contain nitrogen, magnesium, iron, phosphates, mineral salt, and trace elements, and when grown between any type of currant, whether black, red, or white, they may bring in a bigger and tastier crop. Alternatively, use a stinging nettle plant tea.

Strawberries do very well grown beside dwarf beans, spinach, lettuce, and borage. Borage flowers also encourage the bees needed for pollination. Lettuces and strawberries both can endure slugs if the conditions are right and if pine needles are used for bedding. The sharpness and dryness of the needles discourage slugs from traveling over them, and the needles can sometimes give strawberries a hint of wild strawberry flavor — a trick not entirely unknown to certain catering suppliers.

Flowers and Indoor Plants

Flowers have pests, just as vegetables do. Roses have problems with blackflies, for example, and can develop mildew and black spot. As a general rule the essential oils used against mold and mildew may work well with flowers, and geranium and lemongrass oil seem to reduce mildew on roses. There's only one important point to remember — a particular flower will loathe being sprayed with the essential oil tea of its relatives, so don't use rose oil to spray your roses unless you want a flower strike on your hands!

Bicarbonate of soda used in the watering can have a beneficial effect on sweet peas and other flowers, increasing the number and size of blooms. You only need to give the flowering plants this treatment once a month or less: use ¼ teaspoon of bicarbonate of soda to 1 gallon (3.8 liters) of water, and water the roots. Try not to get the mixture on the leaves or flowers. Always underuse rather than overuse. This same dilution can also be used in cut flower water.

The vase life of any flower is easy to prolong with any number of effective methods. One of the simplest is to add white or brown sugar to the water, but don't use more than a pinch of sugar to 4 pints of water. Flowers of the daffodil family, such as narcissus and jonquil, last longer if a pinch of salt is added to the water. Tea brewed in a teapot need never go to waste. Any leftover tea can be added to water in china vases — not glass for obvious reasons — while the tea leaves make an excellent mulching material for any plant in the garden.

Houseplants and plants in window boxes could be watered with dilutions of milk, so when you've finished with a carton fill it with water and use a little of this to water the plants. It's thought the plants benefit from the proteins in the milk.

Essential oils that are too old to use for therapeutic purposes can be added to the water used to wash out plant pots before being stored. Use 2–3 drops per bucket of water This will help reduce any remaining plant bacteria and viruses.

Herbs

Herbs are very useful as an intercrop between vegetables and flowers. Good companions of the herb variety are rosemary and sage, and anise and coriander; while all herbs benefit from having yarrow or stinging nettles nearby. Generally speaking, herbs like sunny, well-drained conditions, although this can be difficult to arrange when intercropping. Try the following among your vegetables and flowers: borage, lavender, sage, basil, thyme, marjoram, chamomile, hyssop, chervil, and tarragon. Cabbage, broccoli, brussels sprouts, and kale are just some of the vegetables that produce large, good-quality produce when scattered among the herbs and flowers. Sweet corn does particularly well near dill.

Getting the Best from the Soil

Fertile soil is the key to good gardening, and if you feed the soil rather than the plants, your plants can take care of themselves. Nitrogen helps promote growth and strength. Lupins produce a lot of nitrogen and are often the first plants to grow on barren waste — for example, after a volcanic eruption. Legumes have bacterial nodules on their roots that bring nitrogenous compounds into the soil. Beans, peas, clover, alfalfa, lentils, peanuts, and soy fall into this group. Some legumes are cultivated expressly so they can be dug back into the ground as "green manure," and moving the position in which legumes are grown each year as part of crop rotation will bring their benefits to soil in other parts of the garden. Mustard is a fast-growing plant that adds nitrogen to the soil, and if sown where there's spare land it'll be ready to dig in within four to six weeks. If you wait longer, the flowers will pod and create seeds that can overrun the garden, so harvest early if using for green manure.

Moving vegetables around in the garden each growing season allows each plant to use the nutrients it needs without depleting the soil, while also releasing nutrients that can be used by the next occupant of the space. There is a science to crop rotation too complex to go into here, but it's worth exploring if you're growing vegetables on a regular basis.

Green manure need not be green at all. Banana skins make excellent fertilizer for roses and peonies, among other plants — just dig them in around the base. Roses can be given a stronger perfume by digging in garlic and onion leftovers. Melon leaves and stems contain calcium and could make a good mulching material.

For shrubs or vegetables that need lots of water but have deep roots and tend to get over-thirsty in dry weather, sink into the ground an old pipe or length of hose, alongside the plant. This can be used to water the plant in a way that ensures it reaches the roots.

A method thought to be centuries old involves planting seeds according to the phases of the moon, and a number of high-tech farmers throughout the world take the principle seriously enough to apply it to large-scale farming. The planets exert silent influences on us all, and although the agreed beneficial effect of planting according to the moon has been put down to the simple fact that there tends to be heavy rain after the new and full moons and the first and third quarters, and thus seeds germinate more quickly, there's probably more to it than this. There is only one way to decide whether moon planting works or not, and that's to do it yourself. There are also those who maintain that growing north-south gives different results than planting east-west. This is thought to be due to electromagnetic forces and their pull on living organisms.

In gardening there's so much to consider, and it's all a delicate balancing act. Gardeners spend an entire lifetime building up a fund of knowledge, and they know there is always so much more to learn. Yet a child can plant a simple seed, watch a whole plant grow from it, and learn that all life begins with the seed. Gardening can be as complicated, or as simple, as you like. Essential oils have played their part in gardening and will continue to do so even more in the future, and they're a valuable tool to put in the gardening kit. It's good to remember, as we do so, that the evolved wisdom of nature herself gave us essential oils.

19

Carrier Oils and Hydrolats

In the world of aromatherapy, carrier oils and hydrolats play a large part: carrier oils because they are used to dilute essential oil, and water-based hydrolats because they provide a range of products containing water-soluble or hydrophilic plant molecules that are not normally present within an essential oil. Both offer methods by which the use of nature's fragrant pharmacy can be expanded.

Carrier Oils

Essential oils are rarely used undiluted at present, and throughout this book you'll find references to diluting agents that could be used for specific conditions. In diluted form essential oils have far more potential, as the various ways of using them become more easily available. And one of the easiest ways of diluting essential oils is to use a carrier oil.

The most suitable carrier oil for all the blends in this book, unless another carrier has been specifically mentioned, is sweet almond oil. Sweet almond is suitable for all ages and skin types — it's gentle on the skin, nourishing, easily absorbed, and generally nonirritating to the skin.

This section outlines profiles for a wide range

of carrier oils, some of which can be combined with a base carrier oil to maximize the healing potential of the whole blend. Essential oils are always diluted in a carrier oil for any type of body rub or massage treatment; the dilution enables an equal amount of essential oil to be spread over the whole body or particular part of the body.

VEGETABLE, CARRIER, AND BASE OILS — WHAT'S THE DIFFERENCE? AND WHY DO I NEED THEM?

A huge number of people around the world use aromatherapy, and there's no hard and fast rules as to what the oil the essential oils are diluted in is called. People use the word *vegetable* just to distinguish between an oil that derives from a plant (such as a nut, kernel, seed, or flower) and one that derives from petrochemicals. Essential oils should not be diluted in mineral oils, nor should they be diluted in other nonplant oils, such as those derived from fish or from animal fats.

The terms *carrier oil* and *base oil* are often used interchangeably. I use *carrier oil* to describe any oil (vegetable of course) that acts as a means to carry the essential oil molecules; and sometimes I use *base oil* to describe a base carrier oil to which other carrier oils, or plant additions, are added, in differing quantities, for specific applications.

Each oil has its own characteristics and therapeutic properties — some are profiled individually below. They've been divided into four categories: main carrier oils, oils that could comprise a certain proportion of the main carrier oil, specialist oils, and infused/macerated oils; and two butters. It's not only essential oils that make wonderful therapeutic blends. Combinations of carrier oils can have therapeutic healing potential that, when combined with essential oils, adds to the overall potency. However, so long as you have a bottle of good-quality sweet almond oil, you can cover most eventualities.

The physical absorption rate of a diluted essential oil will depend on how thick or light the carrier oil is, and whether during and after skin application the area has been covered to prevent evaporation. Because essential oils, whether diluted or undiluted, start evaporating as soon as they're applied to the skin, the carrier oil could help prevent too many of the lighter aromatic molecules from evaporating. These volatile molecules won't be entirely lost because they'll be inhaled through the nose in the process of olfaction. The fact that you can smell an essential oil when it's being applied tells you there's the possibility that healing is taking place on two levels — through olfaction as well as through skin absorption.

BLENDING CARRIER OILS

When blending carrier oils, the basic rule is to put the larger amounts into the bottle first, adding the other ingredients in order of next greatest volume. Then, put the top on the bottle and roll it vigorously between the palms of your hands, allowing all the parts to become well blended. The following suggestions are for professional-style body and facial carrier oil blends that can be used with any essential oil formula:

BODY CARRIER OIL BLEND

Almond oil, sweet	2 teaspoons (10 mL)
Apricot kernel oil	2 teaspoons (10 mL)
Macadamia oil	1 teaspoon (5 mL)
Grapeseed oil	1 teaspoon (5 mL)
Carrot oil	4 drops
Jojoba oil	4 drops

FACIAL CARRIER OIL FOR MOST SKIN TYPES

Camellia seed oil	1 tablespoon (15 mL)
Almond oil, sweet	2 teaspoons (10 mL)
Rosehip seed oil	1 teaspoon (5 mL)
Avocado oil	$1/5$ teaspoon (1 mL)
Borage seed oil	5 drops

THE IMPORTANCE OF QUALITY

The vegetable oils we see in supermarkets are primarily a food source. As such, they each have their own nutrient and energy capacities. The industrial production of food-grade vegetable oils often involves processes to remove traces of pesticides, herbicides, fungicides, and chemical fertilizers. Commercial consideration has also to be given to the need for a long shelf life. And there's the perception that customers want a product that's colorless and odorless. All these things add up to a situation in which vegetable oils are subjected to many chemical and heat processes during the journey from plant growth, through extraction and storage, to store shelf. The processes used to obtain vegetable oils can diminish the natural nutrients and health-giving properties of the oil, and to distinguish them from natural oils, they're here called *processed oils*.

Processed oils are put through a lengthy series of procedures involving the use of chemical solvents and clay-based earths to remove waxes, gums, lecithin, free fatty acids, monoacylglycerols, diacylglycerols, colored compounds, odors (volatile compounds), pesticides, and so on. The solvents and earths themselves have to be removed by further procedures. Using processed oils on the skin can cause irritation and sensitivity if they still have residues of biocides or chemical solvents used in their production. All this is important when thinking about which carrier oils to purchase. Some of the processes involved could have been chemical washing due to long storage, solvent extraction, degumming (or filtration), neutralization, bleaching, and deodorization.

THE IMPORTANCE OF USING PURE, ORGANIC, NATURAL PLANT OILS

By comparison to the processed oils discussed above, pure, organic oils are produced with different customer requirements and don't need to be subjected to the processes involved in extracting remaining traces of the chemicals used in the cultivation of the plant material. When buying vegetable oils for use with essential oils, look for the following words: *pure, organic, first-pressing, cold-pressed,* and *virgin.*

Pure: The word *pure* indicates the oil has not been mixed with any other oil species or put through processes that leech from it the vitamins, minerals, and other positive elements that exist in natural vegetable oils.

Organic: Organic oils are those extracted from plants that have not been grown with the use of pesticides, herbicides, or fungicides (known collectively as *biocides*), or with chemical fertilizers or growth enhancers. Also, organically cultivated vegetable oils should not be genetically modified (GM).

Natural: Natural oils are those that contain only natural substances. A surprising number of cosmetic oils and products contain ingredients that are synthetic — which means they've been manufactured to fulfill certain commercial objectives.

Carrier Oil Profiles

The following carrier oil profiles represent only a few of the many oils that are available. The countries where they are produced change over time, so the entries under "Source" are by no means set in stone.

MAIN CARRIER OILS

Almond Oil (Sweet), *Prunus amygdalus var. dulcis* (Plant Family: Rosaceae)

- General-purpose oil; can be used up to 100% in body and facial oils, or could be included in carrier oil blends
- Can be used as a carrier oil for all blends in this book unless otherwise stated

Qualities: emollient — softening, moisturizing, nourishing, restructuring, conditioning, soothing
Skin types: all face and body skin types, including sensitive, inflamed, psoriasis, and eczema
Uses: multiple uses, including dryness, itchiness, inflammation, and irritation
Used in: body oils, face oils, creams, lotions, balms, ointments
Source: seeds/nuts; produced in many countries
Color: pale yellow
Contains: vitamins E and K, omegas 9 and 6 fatty acids
Note: For those with nut sensitivity — take a skin test prior to use.

Apricot Kernel Oil, *Prunus armeniaca* (Plant Family: Rosaceae)

- General-purpose oil; can be used up to 100% in body and facial oils, or could be included in carrier oil blends
- Can be used as a carrier oil for all blends in this book unless otherwise stated

Qualities: emollient — softening, moisturizing, soothing, nourishing, anti-aging

Skin types: all skin types, including dry, sensitive, inflamed, mature, and prematurely aged skin
Uses: multiple uses, including dryness, inflammation, irritation; improving skin elasticity; rejuvenation
Used in: body oils, face oils, creams, lotions, balms, ointments
Source: kernel; produced in several countries
Color: pale yellow to yellow
Contains: vitamin E, omegas 9 and 6 fatty acids
Note: For those with nut sensitivity — take a skin test prior to use.

Argan Oil, *Argania spinosa* (Plant Family: Sapotaceae)

- Can be used up to 100% in facial or body oil or in a carrier oil blend for body or face, at 15%–50%

Qualities: antioxidant, reconstructing, softening, toning, regenerative, protective
Skin types: all skin types including mature and prematurely aging
Uses: dryness and flaking skin, scarring, sun damage, damaged skin; improving skin elasticity; hair care
Used in: body oils, face oils, creams, lotions, balms, ointments
Source: kernels; produced in Morocco
Color: yellow
Contains: vitamin E, omegas 9 and 6 fatty acids

Camelina, *Camelina sativa* (Gold of Pleasure) (Plant Family: Brassicaceae)

- Can be used up to 100% in body and facial oils, or could be included in carrier oil blends at 20%–60%

Qualities: antioxidant, emollient, anti-inflammatory, moisturizing, regenerating, improving skin elasticity, conditioning

Skin types: dry skin, mature skin, oily skin, combination skin, acne, problem skin
Uses: psoriasis, eczema, dryness, inflammation, damaged skin; anti-aging
Used in: body oils, face oils, creams, lotions, balms, hair care
Source: seeds; produced in northern Europe and the United Kingdom
Color: golden
Contains: remarkably high vitamin E content; omegas 3, 6, 7, and 9 fatty acids
Note: Also known as *Gold of Pleasure*; possible skin irritant on sensitive skins; purchase cold-pressed

Camellia Seed Oil, *Camellia japonica* (Plant Family: Theaceae)

- Can be used up to 100% in body and facial oils, or could be included in carrier oil blends at between 30% and 70%

Qualities: antioxidant, moisturizing, nourishing, regenerative, anti-aging, conditioning, restructuring
Skin types: all skin types including dry skin, mature skin, and sensitive skin
Uses: aging skin, scarring, dry flaky skin, eczema, psoriasis, sun damage
Used in: body oils, face oils, creams, lotions, balms, ointments, hair care
Source: seeds; produced mainly in Japan
Color: very pale yellow
Contains: omegas 9 and 6 fatty acids

Coconut Oil, *Cocos nucifera* (Plant Family: Palmaceae)

- Can be used up to 100% in body oils or included in carrier oil blends at 30%–50%

Qualities: nourishing, emollient, protective
Skin types: dry and dehydrated skin, mature skin

Uses: irritation, itching, sun damage; softening and smoothing; hair care
Used in: body oils, balms, ointments
Source: virgin coconut oil obtained from fresh mature coconut kernels; mainly produced in the Asia-Pacific region
Color: colorless; white when cold and solid
Contains: lauric acid (saturated fatty acid)
Note: In its natural state: a pure, white, semisolid oil when cold; melts in the warmth of the hand. Avoid use on oily, pimpled, or acne-prone skins. Can cause irritation on sensitive skins. For those with nut sensitivity — take a skin test prior to use.

Grapeseed Oil, *Vitis vinifera* (Plant Family: Vitaceae)

- Can be used up to 100% in body oils
- Can be used as a carrier oil for all adult body blends in this book, unless otherwise stated

Qualities: restorative, smoothing, antioxidant, restructuring
Skin types: all skin types including combination skin, oily skin, and those prone to pimples
Uses: massage; dehydration; moisturizing and soothing
Used in: body oils, face oils, creams, lotions, balms
Source: seed; produced in many countries
Color: light green
Contains: vitamin E, omegas 6 and 9 fatty acids
Note: Purchase only organically grown, cold-pressed oil. New oils are available from specific wine grapes, such as chardonnay.

Hazelnut Oil, *Corylus avellana* (Plant Family: Betulaceae)

- Can be used up to 100% in body and facial oils, or could be included in carrier oil blends at 30%–70%

Qualities: emollient, moisturizing, nourishing, revitalizing, regenerative, toning
Skin types: all skin types including dry, mature, combination, stressed, damaged, and sensitive
Uses: anti-aging; scarring, dryness, sun damage; has a slight astringent action
Used in: body oils, face oils, creams, lotions, balms
Source: nuts; produced mainly in the United States, Europe, and Turkey
Color: yellow
Contains: vitamin E, omegas 9 and 6 fatty acids
Note: For those with nut sensitivity — take a skin test prior to use.

Hemp Seed Oil, *Cannabis sativa* (Plant Family: Cannabaceae)

- Can be used up to 100% in body oils, or included in body or facial oil carrier blends at 10%–20%

Qualities: firming, moisturizing, soothing, nourishing, anti-inflammatory
Skin types: mature skin, combination skin, dry skin, damaged skin, psoriasis
Uses: inflammation and dryness; toning and balancing
Used in: body oils, face oils, balms, ointments, gels, hair care
Source: seeds; produced in China, France, the United States, Canada, and Germany
Color: green, light to dark
Contains: omegas 3, 6, and 9 fatty acids; gamma linolenic acid (GLA)
Note: Has a nutty odor.

Jojoba Oil, *Simmondsia chinensis* (Plant Family: Buxaceae)

- Can be used up to 100% in body and facial oils, or could be included in carrier oil blends at 30%–80%

Qualities: protective, moisturizing, anti-inflammatory, anti-infectious, nourishing, balancing

Skin types: all skin types including mature skin, prematurely aged skin, sensitive skin, oily skin, acne, and problem skin

Uses: skin infections, dryness, rashes, inflammation, rosacea, eczema, psoriasis; soothing, cleansing, and conditioning

Used in: body oils, face oils, creams, lotions, balms, ointments, gels

Source: beans; produced in the United States, Egypt, and Argentina

Color: pale yellow

Contains: vitamin E; omegas 3, 6, and 9 fatty acids

Note: Classified as a liquid wax due to wax particles in the oil; used as a diluent in natural perfumery. Closely resembles human sebum.

Kukui, *Aleurites moluccana* (Plant Family: Euphoreaceae)

- Can be used as a carrier oil for all blends in this book unless otherwise stated

Qualities: emollient, moisturizing, nourishing, regenerative, restorative, protective

Skin types: all skin types including sensitive skin and mature skin

Uses: dryness, irritation, eczema, psoriasis, acne, soreness, sun damage

Used in: body oils, base oils, creams, lotions, balms

Source: nuts; Hawaii, Southeast Asia

Color: light yellow

Contains: vitamins A and E; omegas 6, 3, and 9 fatty acids

Note: For those with nut sensitivity — take a skin test prior to use.

Macadamia Nut Oil, *Macadamia ternifolia* (Plant Family: Proteaceae)

- Can be used up to 100% in body and facial oils, or could be included in carrier oil blends at 30%–70%

Qualities: antioxidant, nourishing, moisturizing, restructuring, regenerative, promotes skin elasticity

Skin types: good for all skin types particularly prematurely aged, mature, combination, or sensitive

Uses: anti-aging; dryness, redness, eczema, psoriasis

Used in: body oils, face oils, creams, lotions, balms, ointments

Source: nuts; produced in Australia, Hawaii, Kenya, and South America

Color: yellow

Contains: omegas 9 and 7 fatty acids

Note: For those with nut sensitivity — take a skin test prior to use. Macadamia has a fatty acids profile similar to human sebum.

Meadowfoam Seed Oil, *Limnanthes alba* (Plant Family: Limnanthaceae)

- Can be used up to 100% in body and facial oils, or could be included in carrier oil blends at 20%–70%

Qualities: antioxidant, emollient, moisturizing, smoothing, nourishing, protective

Skin types: all skin types, including mature skin and dry skin

Uses: dryness, roughly textured skin; hair care

Used in: body oils, lotions, balms, gels, hair care

Source: seeds/nutlets; produced in the United States

Color: light golden

Contains: unique structure — exceptionally long-chain fatty acids

Note: Extremely stable oil, excellent oxidative stability — does not deteriorate quickly.

Moringa Oil, *Moringa oleifera* (Plant Family: Moringaceae)

- Can be used up to 100% in body and facial oils, or could be included in carrier oil blends at 30%–60%

Qualities: emollient, antioxidant, regenerating, nourishing, balancing, protective
Skin types: all skin types, including mature skin, prematurely aged skin, acne, problem skin
Uses: anti-aging; dryness, damaged skin, infected skin, premature aging
Used in: body oils, face oils, creams, lotions, balms, ointments, hair care
Source: seeds; produced in India, Senegal, Rwanda, and South Africa
Color: pale to golden yellow
Contains: vitamins A, C, and E; omegas 9 and 3 fatty acids
Note: Also known as *ben oil*.

Peach Kernel Oil, *Prunus persica* (Plant Family: Rosaceae)

- Can be used up to 100% in body and facial oils, or could be included in carrier oil blends at 30%–70%
- Can be used as a carrier oil for all blends in this book, unless otherwise stated

Qualities: moisturizing, revitalizing, regenerative, nourishing, protective
Skin types: all skin types, including mature skin, dehydrated skin, and sensitive skin
Uses: dryness, itching, irritation, inflammation, eczema, psoriasis; improving skin elasticity
Used in: body oils, face oils, creams, lotions, balms, ointments, hair care
Source: kernels; produced in several countries, including China
Color: pale golden yellow
Contains: vitamins A and E, omegas 9 and 6 fatty acids

Rice Bran Oil, *Oryza sativa* (Plant Family: Poaceae/Gramineae)

- Can be used up to 100% in body and facial oils, or could be included in carrier oil blends at 30%–70%
- Can be used as a carrier oil for all adult blends in this book, unless otherwise stated

Qualities: antioxidant, protective, nourishing, soothing, moisturizing, reconstructing
Skin types: all skin types including mature skin, prematurely aged skin, dry skin, sensitive skin
Uses: anti-aging, softening; sun damage, irritations, itching
Used in: body oils, face oils, creams, lotions, hair care
Source: germ and inner husk of rice; produced in Japan, United States, Italy, Vietnam, and China
Color: pale to golden yellow
Contains: vitamin E, omegas 9 and 6 fatty acids

Safflower Oil, *Carthamus tinctorius* (Plant Family: Cynareae)

- Can be used up to 100% in body and facial oils, or could be included in carrier oil blends at 30%–50%
- Can be used as a carrier oil for all adult body blends, unless otherwise stated

Qualities: nourishing, moisturizing, balancing
Skin types: all skin types, including dry skin, oily skin, mature skin, acne-prone skin
Uses: sore or flaky skin, dryness, itchiness, dehydrated skin
Used in: body oils, face oils, creams, lotions, balms, ointments
Source: seeds; produced in the United States, Mexico, India, Germany, and China
Color: golden yellow
Contains: vitamin E, omegas 6 and 9 fatty acids

Sunflower Oil, *Helianthus annuus* (Plant Family: Asteraceae/Compositae)

- Can be used up to 100% in body and facial oils, or could be included in carrier oil blends at 30%–70%
- Can be used for all adult body blends in this book, unless otherwise stated

Qualities: softening, moisturizing, regenerative, conditioning, protective
Skin types: all skin types including sensitive skin, combination skin, acne, and oily skin
Uses: dryness, irritation, rashes, redness, dehydrated skin
Used in: body oils, face oils, creams, lotions, balms, ointments
Source: seeds; produced in Europe, Ukraine, Russia, and Argentina
Color: pale yellow
Contains: vitamin E, omega 9 and 6 fatty acids
Note: Use only cold-pressed organic sunflower oil, not culinary. Sunflower oil has a fatty acid profile similar to human sebum.

Walnut Oil, *Juglans regia* (Plant Family: Juglandaceae)

- Can be used up to 100% in body and facial oils, or could be included in carrier oil blends at 30%–70%

Qualities: regenerative, moisturizing, toning, nourishing
Skin types: all skin types, including dry skin, mature skin, sun-damaged skin, and oily skin
Uses: anti-aging; itchiness, damaged skin, dryness and dry patches
Used in: body oils, face oils, creams, lotions, balms, ointments
Source: nuts; produced in the United States, Australia, and France
Color: yellow
Contains: omegas 6, 9, and 3 fatty acids

Note: For those with nut sensitivity — take a skin test prior to use.

OILS THAT COULD BE USED AS A PERCENTAGE OF THE MAIN CARRIER

Avocado Oil, *Persea americana/gratissima* (Plant Family: Lauraceae)

- Could be used at 100%, although generally used as an addition in body and facial oils, at 10% and 40%

Qualities: emollient — soothing, softening, regenerative, protective, nourishing, toning, moisturizing, restorative
Skin types: suits all skin types, including dry skin, mature skin, and prematurely aged skin
Uses: dehydration, inflammation, scarring, rashes, eczema; anti-aging
Used in: body oils, face oils, creams, lotions, balms, hair care
Source: flesh of the fruit; produced in the United States, Italy, and South Africa
Color: light to rich dark green; refined oil is yellow
Contains: vitamins A, B, D, and E; omegas 6, 9, and 3 fatty acids
Note: Unrefined oil can solidify in very low temperatures.

Borage Seed Oil, *Borago officinalis* (Plant Family: Boraginaceae)

- Generally used as an addition in body and facial oils, at 10% and 30%

Qualities: emollient, moisturizing, regenerating, revitalizing, nourishing, soothing
Skin types: all skin types, including dry skin, mature skin, prematurely aged skin, and sensitive skin
Uses: psoriasis, eczema, scarring; anti-aging; improving skin elasticity
Used in: body oils, face oils, creams, lotions

Source: seeds; produced in the United Kingdom, China, and Kenya

Color: light yellow to pale golden yellow

Contains: extremely high in fatty acids; omegas 3, 6, and 9 fatty acids; gamma linolenic acid (GLA)

Evening Primrose Seed Oil, *Oenothera biennis* (Plant Family: Onagraceae)

- Generally used as an addition in body and facial oils, at 10% and 30%

Qualities: nourishing, moisturizing, regenerating, soothing, conditioning

Skin types: all skin types, including mature skin, dry skin, and combination skin

Uses: anti-aging; eczema, psoriasis, dryness, inflammation, damaged skin, scarring

Used in: body oils, face oils, creams, lotions

Source: seeds; produced in the United Kingdom and China

Color: pale yellow

Contains: omega 6, 3, and 9 fatty acids; gamma linolenic acid (GLA)

Neem Oil, *Azadirachta indica* (Plant Family: Meliaceae)

- Not a carrier oil as such; can be used neat for skin infections or as insect repellent; could be included in carrier oil blends at 10%–20%

Qualities: antibacterial, antifungal, antimicrobial, antiseptic, antiparasitic

Skin types: most skin types for therapeutic application, although use with care on sensitive skin

Uses: cuts, stings, wounds, fungal infections, infected skin, dandruff, scalp conditions

Used in: oils, lotions, balms, ointments, gels

Source: kernel; produced in India

Color: highly varied: light brown, yellow, reddish brown, greenish brown, red

Contains: omegas 9 and 6 fatty acids, palmitic acid, azadirachtin

Note: Has a strong odor; generally a semisolid oil that needs heat to transform into a usable liquid

Olive Oil, *Olea europaea* (Plant Family: Oleaceae)

- Could be included in carrier oil blends at 30%–50%

Qualities: nourishing, regenerating, moisturizing, protective, anti-inflammatory

Skin types: all skin types, including mature skin and dry skin

Uses: dryness, itching, chapped skin, damaged skin, bruising, sun damage; soothing

Used in: body oils, lotions, ointments, hair conditioners, hair care

Source: olives; produced in Europe and North Africa

Color: light to medium green

Contains: vitamins E and K, omegas 9 and 6 fatty acids

Note: Use only cold-pressed virgin organic olive oil, not culinary oil.

Olive Squalane, *Olea europaea* (Plant Family: Oleaceae)

- Could be included in body carrier oil blends at 10%–50%
- Could be used up to 100% in facial oils

Qualities: emollient, moisturizing, nourishing, protective, regenerative

Skin types: all skin types, including mature skin, combination skin, damaged skin, and prematurely aged skin

Uses: smoothing, soothing, anti-aging; for dehydration

Used in: body oils, face oils, creams, lotions, balms

Source: olive pits; produced mainly in France

Color: clear
Note: An organically composed lipid extracted from olives; molecular structure similar to the hydrolipidic film and sebum in humans.

Sesame Seed Oil, *Sesamum indicum* (Plant Family: Pedaliaceae)

- Generally used on specific areas for therapeutic reasons, could be included in carrier oil blends at 30%–50%

Qualities: emollient, antioxidant, moisturizing, nourishing, conditioning, antibacterial, antifungal
Skin types: combination skin, dry skin, mature skin, damaged skin, problematic skin
Uses: psoriasis, eczema, dryness, sun damage, skin infections
Used in: body oils, balms, ointments, gels
Source: seeds; produced in many countries
Color: dark yellow/light golden yellow
Contains: vitamins E and K, omegas 6 and 9 fatty acids
Note: Can cause allergic reactions; for those with any sensitivity — take a skin test prior to use

Wheatgerm Oil, *Triticum vulgare* (Plant Family: Poaceae/Gramineae)

- Generally used on specific areas for therapeutic reasons, could be included in carrier oil blends at 10%–30%

Qualities: emollient, nourishing, moisturizing, antioxidant, regenerative, revitalizing, soothing
Skin types: all skin types, including mature skin, dry skin, and dehydrated skin
Uses: dryness, irritation, itchiness, damaged skin, sun-damaged skin, scarring, inflammation
Used in: body oils, face oils, balms, ointments
Source: germ of wheat kernel; produced in Canada and Germany
Color: yellow

Contains: very high in vitamin E, omegas 6 and 3 fatty acids
Note: May cause irritation and sensitivity in those with wheat allergies.

SPECIALIST OILS

Blackcurrant Seed Oil, *Ribes nigrum* (Plant Family: Grossulariaceae)

- Generally used in facial skin care preparations at 0.5%–5%

Qualities: revitalizing, regenerative, protective, moisturizing, anti-inflammatory
Skin types: all skin types including mature, prematurely aged
Uses: anti-aging; skin elasticity; dry skin, damaged skin; revitalizing
Used in: body oils, face oils, creams, lotions
Source: seeds; produced in Germany, Finland, and China
Color: light yellow to honey colored
Contains: vitamin E, omegas 6 and 3 fatty acids, gamma linolenic acid (GLA)

Passion Flower Seed Oil, *Passifloria incarnata* (Plant Family: Passifloraceae)

- Can be used at 100% in body and facial oils; generally used as an ingredient in body and facial carrier oil blends at 10%–30%

Qualities: emollient, nourishing, anti-inflammatory, revitalizing
Skin types: all skin types, including mature skin, prematurely aged skin, and sensitive skin
Uses: dryness; conditioning, toning; skin elasticity
Used in: body oils, face oils, creams, lotions
Source: seeds; produced in Brazil and Peru
Color: golden yellow
Contains: vitamins A and E, omegas 6 and 9 fatty acids
Note: also called *maracuja oil.*

Rosehip Seed Oil, *Rosa rubiginosa* (Plant Family: Rosaceae)

- Can be used up to 100% in facial oils, or could be included in carrier oil blends at 20%–30%

Qualities: antioxidant, cell and tissue regenerating, stimulating, moisturizing, conditioning, rebalancing, restructuring, toning, anti-inflammatory, regenerative
Skin types: all skin types, especially mature skin, prematurely aged skin, acne, and sensitive skin
Uses: anti-aging; scarring, eczema, damaged skin, sun damage; skin elasticity, revitalization
Used in: body oils, face oils, creams, lotions
Source: seeds; produced in Chile
Color: orange/reddish gold
Contains: omega 3, 6, and 9 fatty acids; trans-retinoic acid
Note: Can have a strong smell; some rosehip seed oils may stain skin or clothes.

Sea Buckthorn Oil, *Hippophae rhamnoides* (Plant family: Elaeagnaceae)

- In some circumstances, can be applied in facial oils up to 10%, or could be included in a carrier oil blend at 1%–5%

Qualities: antioxidant, anti-inflammatory, cellular regeneration, conditioning, nourishing, rebalancing, toning, cell and tissue revitalizing, restorative
Skin types: all skin types, including mature skin, prematurely aged skin, acne
Uses: anti-aging; skin elasticity; sun damage; tissue damage, wounds, sores, irritation, eczema, rosacea
Used in: body oils, face oils, creams, lotions, balms, ointments
Source: oils extracted from pulp and/or seeds of berry; produced in Russia, Germany, and Finland
Color: deep orange-red
Contains: vitamins A, C, E, and K; carotenoids;

very high in omegas 3, 6, 7, and 9 fatty acids — seed oil higher in omega 6, pulp oil higher in omega 7
Note: If used undiluted, the orange-red color may temporarily stain skin and clothing.

Tamanu, *Calophyllum inophyllum* (Plant Family: Guttiferae)

- In some circumstances can be applied in body or facial oils up to 100%, or could be included in a carrier oil blend at 30%–50%.

Qualities: emollient, tissue regenerative, anti-inflammatory, antiseptic, antimicrobial, antioxidant, analgesic
Skin types: all skin types including mature skin and sensitive skin
Uses: damaged skin, acne, infections, wounds, cuts, grazes, ulcers, dermatitis, eczema, scarring; anti-aging
Used in: body oils, lotions, balms, ointments, hair care
Source: fruit kernel; produced in Polynesia, Melanesia, and Madagascar
Color: dark green
Contains: vitamins E and A; omegas 9, 6, and 3 fatty acids
Note: For those with skin sensitivity — take a skin test prior to use; could have irritant effect on sensitive skins when applied undiluted; also called *foraha*.

MACERATED/INFUSED OILS

The term *macerated oils* refers to those oils produced by traditional methods, which involves infusing the plant material in a suitable vegetable oil over an extended period of time. Repeated maceration is when the plant material is removed, the macerated oil is infused with fresh plant material, and the process repeated. This is carried out to increase the concentration of active constituents in the oil. Sometimes plant material is extracted, by CO_2 extraction, for example, and then diluted in a vegetable carrier oil. This is not the traditional meaning of the word *maceration* — please inquire of your supplier the specific production methods being used.

Arnica Macerated Oil, *Arnica montana* (Plant Family: Asteraceae/Compositae)

- Can be used in specific-area body oils up to 20% for short-term therapeutic purposes, or included in carrier oil blends at 2%–5%

Qualities: analgesic, anti-inflammatory, tissue conditioning
Skin types: all skin types when used in therapeutic applications
Uses: bruises, skin tissue trauma, bumps and knocks, aching, rheumatism, overstretched limbs, stiff muscles, repetitive strain
Used in: body oils, ointments, gels
Source: macerated oil of fresh flowers; produced in Germany, Switzerland, Holland, and France
Color: greenish yellow
Contains: Carotenoids, inulin, selenium, manganese
Note: Not to be applied on broken skin. Unsuitable for facial skin care; can cause skin sensitivity in some people. Not to be confused with the essential oil of arnica.

Calendula (Marigold), *Calendula officinalis* (Plant Family: Asteraceae)

- Can be used up to 100% for specific body applications, or could be included in carrier oil blends at 30%–70%

Qualities: emollient, soothing, anti-inflammatory, tissue regeneration, astringent
Skin types: all skin types, including sensitive skin
Uses: skin tissue repair; bruising, irritation,

itchiness, eczema, psoriasis, soreness, sun damage, chapped skin, rough skin
Used in: body oils, creams, lotions, ointments
Source: flower petals; produced in many countries including the United States, the United Kingdom, and Germany
Color: yellow to orange
Contains: carotenoids — beta-carotene; saponins; vitamins A, B, D, and E
Note: The percentages and uses suggested above relate to traditionally macerated oils only and not to CO_2 extracted calendula oil, to which none of the uses or percentage dilutions above refer.

Carrot Root Oil, *Daucus carota* (Plant Family: Apiaceae/Umbelliferae)

- Generally used in carrier oil blends at 5%–20%

Qualities: antioxidant, soothing, calming, regenerative, revitalizing, nourishing
Skin types: all skin types, including dry skin, dehydrated skin, mature skin, acned and pimple-prone skin
Uses: anti-aging, soothing; itchiness, dryness, soreness, sun-damaged skin, psoriasis, scarring
Used in: body oils, face oils, creams, lotions, balms, ointments, gels
Source: tissue/root; Canada and Europe
Color: light to dark orange
Contains: vitamins A and E, carotenoids — beta-carotene
Note: Use macerated oil from carrot tissue; not to be confused with carrot seed oil. Highly colored and can stain the body and clothes.

Monoi Oil, *Gardenia taitensis* + *Cocos nucifera* (Plant Families: Rubiaceae + Arecaceae)

- Can be used up to 100% for body care, or could be included in carrier oil blends at 30%–60%
- Most suitable for body and hair care

Qualities: emollient — softening, soothing, moisturizing, regenerating, protective
Skin types: all skin types, including dry skin, dehydrated skin, and mature skin
Uses: smoothing, anti-aging; dryness, sun damage
Used in: body oils, lotions, balms, hair care
Source: flowers macerated in copra/coconut oil; produced in Polynesia
Color: light cream
Contains: oleic acid, linoleic acid, potassium, magnesium, vitamins B and C
Note: Monoi oil is a maceration of the tiare flower in virgin copra/coconut oil that can solidify when cold and melt in warmth, such as on contact with hands. Has a sweet floral fragrance.

St. John's Wort Oil, *Hypericum perforatum* (Plant Family: Hypericaceae)

• Can be used in specific-area body oils up to 100% for short-term therapeutic purposes, or included in carrier oil blends at 30%–50%

Qualities: analgesic, anti-inflammatory, soothing, antiseptic
Skin types: all skin types in therapeutic applications only
Uses: injuries, bruises, skin tissue trauma, bumps and knocks, wounds, sun damage, aching, rheumatism, overstretched limbs, stiff muscles
Used in: body oils, ointments, gels
Source: stems, leaves, flowers; produced in France and the United Kingdom
Color: reddish brown
Contains: hypericin, hyperforin, tannins, flavonoids
Note: Avoid sun exposure after application because of its photosensitizing effect. The percentages and uses suggested above relate to traditionally macerated oils only and not to CO_2 extracted St. John's Wort oil.

BUTTERS

A few butters can be used on their own for specific applications, but they are more likely to be incorporated into carrier oils and products such as balms. The traditional way of producing butters is to roast and/or crush the plant material to extract the fat components. Some products that are called butters are actually a combination of oils and minute wax particles. Waxes are used as thickening agents in creams and to give structure to ointments and balms. Waxes maintain solidity at room temperature and require heating before being incorporated into products. The best-known wax is beeswax, but many plant waxes are available that have no animal content, including laurel, candelilla, and carnauba.

Cocoa Butter, *Theobroma cacao* (Plant Family: Malvaceae)

• Solid; has to be melted with heat before it can be included in any body product such as a balm, lotion, cream or oil; usually no more than 10% in a carrier oil

Qualities: emollient, moisturizing, softening, smoothing, soothing, antioxidant
Skin types: all skin types
Uses: dryness, itchiness, flaky skin; skin elasticity
Used in: balms, lotions, creams, oils
Source: cacao beans or cocoa liquor; produced in Uganda, Kenya, and central and southern South America
Color: pale cream
Contains: vitamin E, omega 6 fatty acid, theobromine
Note: Also known as *theobroma oil*. Sometimes has a faint chocolate aroma.

Shea Butter, *Vitellaria paradoxa/Butyrospermum parkii* (Plant Family: Sapotaceae)

- Semisolid; needs to be melted before it can be included in any product, melts on contact with warmth

Qualities: moisturizing/emollient, soothing, softening, anti-inflammatory, protective

Skin types: all skin types

Uses: dryness, irritation, flaky skin, soreness, sun damage, rashes; smoothing

Used in: creams, lotions, balms, soaps, hair care

Source: nuts; produced in West Africa

Color: white to cream

Contains: vitamins A, E, and F, omega 9 fatty acids

Note: For those with nut sensitivity — take a skin test prior to use. Also known as *African karite butter.*

Hydrolats

Hydrolats were in regular use in my childhood home — peppermint for stomachache, dill for indigestion, and rose for skin care. During my time traveling and studying phytotherapy in Europe, I learned how valuable hydrolats can be, not only as a therapeutic tool but also when used in cooking and in many more applications. Being invited to visit the renowned French artisan *distillateur* Henri Viaud at his home in the south of France many years ago gave me further opportunity to explore hydrolats from a distiller's perspective. He picked wild thyme from the slopes around his house, which was built into the side of a mountain, and distilled it into the most wonderful essential oil and hydrolat. He told me about the value of the therapeutic marriage that can be accomplished when distilling two different plant materials together at the same time. This practice of double-distillation was commonplace

at the time among the artisan distillers of the region, who took great pride and joy in being able to create a variety of active plant products. Over the years I've enjoyed experimenting and making my own hydrolats, and this option is explained in chapter 15, "Fragrant Care for Your Home," in the section "Making Your Own Essential Oil Waters and Hydrolats" (see page 456).

I use the word *hydrolat* throughout this book to describe a product that's produced during the distillation of essential oils, or to describe a product distilled for the sole purpose of producing a hydrolat. When essential oils are stream distilled, a large volume of water in the form of condensed steam is used to release the volatile fragrant compounds from the plant material, producing essential oil. This liquid is siphoned off, leaving behind a watery distillate that contains traces of essential oil along with water-soluble (hydrophilic) molecules of the plant material that are not normally present in an essential oil. The name given to this water is *hydrola* (*hydrolat*). Although both hydrolats and essential oils come from the same plant material, they each contain components not present in the other. Hydrolats are therefore a different tool than essential oils, with different properties and uses.

In Europe, where aromatherapy originated, the term used was *hydrolated* followed by the name of the plant — for example, *hydrolated lavender.* Hydrolats are distinguished from a whole range of other water-based products — some of which have valuable therapeutic properties and some that do not (a fact established not by the name but by the method of production) — called *hydrosols, herbal distillates, floral waters, aromatic distillates, aromatic waters, aqueous extracts, plant water essences,* and *essential oil waters,* to name a few. In other words, there are many processes that involve the manufacture of a water (*hydro*)-and-plant product that are not hydrolats. As the benefits of hydrolats are increasingly recognized, the tendency has arisen for all these terms to be used interchangeably.

To try to make sense of all this, let's begin at the beginning. References dating back hundreds of years show that throughout time people have been boiling up plant material and producing waters from them. Some might have been intended for medicinal use, some for cooking, and some for beauty. Some, no doubt, were used for all three. In a sense, this history is part of the herbal tradition, yet it's also a tradition that any household could be part of.

These products, made in ways specific to a locality, were most probably used quite quickly, according to the season of the plant's growth. Bacteria thrive in water, and expecting a long life of these products was probably not wise, given the unhygienic circumstances most people lived in.

In some countries steam distillation was traditionally used to produce fragrant waters, such as rose and orange blossom, which became part of the culture. Rose water, for example, has been used in cooking in Turkey, Lebanon, and Iran for centuries, where it's still added to rice puddings, yogurt, pastry, and the aromatic candy Turkish delight. In India, rose water is used in a dessert called *gulab jamun*. Orange blossom was and is still used in much the same way as rose water.

So, to summarize, making water-and-plant products has a long tradition, and over the years people have made the waters for their own intrinsic values. This brings us to the present time. The herbal tradition continues, and those waters are still as valuable as they have always been. In some parts of the world oregano and thyme water are commonly found in grocery stores and are used medicinally and in cooking. And peppermint water, for example, has been in the official pharmacopeias of many countries for as long as anyone can remember.

However, these products are not always hydrolats, which are specifically a by-product of essential oil production. The water by-product of essential oil distillation contains traces of the essential oil — more of those chemical constituents that are slightly more soluble in water, such as the alcohol group, and fewer of the elements that do not disperse so easily in water, such as the ketones. In addition, they contain hydrophilic molecules of the plant material not normally present in an essential oil, which are themselves valuable. This makes an essential oil and a hydrolat from the same plant material quite different from each other in terms of their components, properties, and uses. Sometimes a hydrolat smells like the essential oil, sometimes it doesn't. In terms of aroma, there's a huge variation in the degree of similarity between particular plants and hydrolats. Much depends on the distillation process, particularly the degree of heat and the length of time involved. A hydrolat may be reused for a second or even third distillation, making it stronger each time.

Two things are happening with the availability of hydrolats. First, there's increasing recognition of the value of those hydrolats that remain after essential oil distillation. Second, the herbal tradition of immersing plant material in water to produce an herbal infusion is being revived. Both have their value, but they're being conflated, so it's wise to know whether one is being sold a hydrolat or an herbal distillate. It matters because of the range of quality: if there can be a variation between a good and a bad essential oil on a scale of 1 to 10, when it comes to a water-based product the scale goes from 1 to 100. Being informed helps us avoid products that may not be what they purport to be.

Many methods are being used to create products advertised as hydrolats, hydrosols, or floral waters. One method involves adding a fragrance to water. It might smell like a rose water, but it has absolutely nothing whatsoever to do with natural rose. Basic plant material is boiled like a tea and filtered, rather than going through a distillation process. In another method, essential oil is added to water along with a surfactant that emulsifies the essential oil and allows it to be dissolved in the water.

You can begin to see the problem. As always, ensuring quality is about having confidence in the integrity of your suppliers. Ideally, a hydrolat will come from organically grown plant material, use only pure water, contain no preservatives or alcohol, and be hygienically prepared and bottled to avoid the risk of microbial contamination. A good supplier will tell you if anything has been added to increase the shelf life and advise you if a bloom has developed — a misty, milky look at the bottom of the container. If you intend to use the hydrolat for medicinal purposes or in cooking or food, ask the supplier if the hydrolat being purchased is food grade and suitable for ingestion. Without any form of preservative, hydrolats may deteriorate, so store them in a cool place away from light and heat.

HYDROLAT METHODS OF USE

Humidifiers: hung over radiators — used as a room freshener
House sprays: used as a room freshener
Compresses: health care or skin care
Face wipes: health care or skin care
Body wipes: health care, skin care, or baby care
Baths or foot baths: health care or well-being
Sitz baths: health care or well-being
In teas/drinks: health care or well-being
Food: cooking flavor and well-being
Skin care: problem skin; facial tonic
Baby care: sore bottom or well-being

For more information on the use of hydrolats in beauty preparations, please see chapter 13, "The Fragrant Way to Beauty," pages 382–384.

EXAMPLES OF SOME HYDROLATS AND THEIR GENERAL APPLICATIONS

Aniseed Hydrolat (*Pimpinella anisum*)
Health and well-being: halitosis, poor digestion, digestive problems, appetite
Skin care/body care: none
Food: flavoring soups, seasonings, fish, baking
Home: room sprays, radiators, diffusers, surfaces

Basil Hydrolat (*Ocimum basilicum*)
Health and well-being: general tonic, invigorating; for digestion when taken as a hydrolat tea
Skin care/body care: stimulating, invigorating, tonic, refreshing; combination skin, tired lifeless skin
Use in: toners, lotions, creams, gels, hair conditioners, shampoo; added to baths
Food: flavoring sauces, seasoning, meats, vegetables, preserves, baking, sorbets, desserts
Home: room spray, diffusers, radiators

Calendula Hydrolat (*Calendula officinalis*)
Health and well-being: anti-inflammatory, soothing; various skin conditions such as rashes and grazes when combined with lavender and chamomile
Skin care/body care: soothing, calming; dryness, flaky skin, sluggish skin, oily skin, acne, pimples; added to baths for inflamed or irritated skin
Use in: sprays, skin tonics, creams, lotions, gels, hair products
Food: none
Home: none

Chamomile German Hydrolat
(*Matricaria recutita*)
Health and well-being: calming, soothing; rashes, inflammation, eczema, psoriasis, antiseptic; sore eyes — apply on cotton pads over closed eyelids

Skin care/body care: most skin types: normal skin, acne, pimples, sensitive skin, dry skin, fragile skin, aging skin; regenerative, balancing, softening, soothing

Use in: sprays, tonics, creams, lotions, gels, compresses, poultices

Food: calming teas

Home: bedrooms, diffusers, radiators

Chamomile Roman Hydrolat
(*Anthemis nobilis*)
Health and well-being: nervousness, anxiety, insomnia, rashes, skin disorders, eczema, psoriasis, inflammation, itchiness; use combined with lavender hydrolat; sore eyes — apply on eye pads over closed eyelids

Skin care/body care: most skin types: normal skin, sensitive skin, delicate skin, dry skin, aging skin; moisturizing, regenerative, balancing, soothing; for acne, pimples, redness, scarring

Use in: sprays, skin tonics, creams, lotions, gels, compresses, poultices, hair products; added to baths

Food: calming teas

Home: room sprays, radiators, diffusers

Cornflower Hydrolat (*Centaurea cyanus*)
Health and well-being: soothing and cooling; for tired eyes or irritated eyes from pollution or computer strain — apply on cotton pads over closed eyelids

Skin care/body care: moisturizing, soothing, calming

Use in: sprays, skin tonics, creams, lotions, gels

Food: none

Home: none

Eucalyptus Radiata Hydrolat
(*Eucalyptus radiata*)
Health and well-being: coughs, colds, respiratory conditions, inflammation; deodorizing, cooling, soothing

Skin care/body care: oily skin, sluggish skin, acne, pimples; astringent, refreshing, invigorating; tonic

Use in: sprays, skin tonics, gels, compresses, poultices, hair products; added to baths

Food: teas for respiratory conditions mixed with honey and lemon

Home: room sprays, radiators, diffusers

Fennel (Sweet) Hydrolat
(*Foeniculum vulgare var. dulce*)
Health and well-being: swollen eyes — apply on cotton pads over closed eyelids; fatigue, exhaustion, digestion

Skin care/body care: normal skin, dry skin, aging skin; tonic, refreshing, softening, toning; cellulite

Use in: lotions, gels, compresses, poultices; added to baths

Food: vegetables, soups, broths, fish, baking, desserts

Home: radiators, diffusers; better in combinations for use as room sprays

Geranium Hydrolat
(*Pelargonium graveolens*)
Health and well-being: circulatory conditions, infections, swelling; balancing, refreshing

Skin care/body care: all skin types; anti-aging, regenerative, balancing, toning; cellulite

Use in: sprays, tonics, lotions, gels, creams, compresses

Food: baking, fruit dishes, desserts, drinks, sorbets

Home: room sprays, diffusers, radiators

Ginger Hydrolat (*Zingiber officinale*)

<u>Health and well-being:</u> digestion, digestive problems, stomach cramps, nausea, travel sickness, nervousness

<u>Body care:</u> stimulating, balancing, toning; cellulite

<u>Use in:</u> body spritzes, body tonics, gels, compresses, poultices

<u>Food:</u> teas, sauces, soups, meat dishes, baking — pie fillings — preserves, sorbets, vegetables

<u>Home:</u> room sprays, radiators, diffusers

Juniper Berry Hydrolat (*Juniperus communis*)

<u>Health and well-being:</u> deodorant; general fatigue, nervousness, swelling, and aching legs and feet

<u>Skin care/body care:</u> cleansing, toning; stimulates skin; oily skin, acne, pimples, swelling, bruising

<u>Use in:</u> skin sprays, tonics, gels, compresses, poultices; added to baths

<u>Food:</u> tea, meat, fish, drinks, soups

<u>Home:</u> atmospheric cleansing, energy clearing; use in sprays and diffusers

Lavender Hydrolat (*Lavandula angustifolia*)

<u>Health and well-being:</u> gentle tonic for the nervous system; soothing, calming, antiseptic; cuts, grazes, rashes, stings, soreness, inflammation, eczema, psoriasis, sore eyes — apply on cotton pad over closed eyelids

<u>Skin care/body care:</u> all skin types: normal skin, sensitive skin, dry skin, oily skin, combination skin, aging skin; acne, pimples, redness; refreshing, regenerative, soothing, anti-inflammatory; tones and brightens

<u>Use in:</u> sprays, skin tonics, creams, lotions, gels, compresses, poultices, hair products; added to baths

<u>Food:</u> baking, desserts, sorbets, fish, meats, preserves

<u>Home:</u> room sprays, radiators, diffusers, laundry

Lemon Balm (Melissa) Hydrolat (*Melissa officinalis*)

<u>Health and well-being:</u> calming, uplifting; insomnia, nervousness, anxiety, exhaustion, infections; convalescence

<u>Skin care/body care:</u> oily skin, itchy skin, sensitive skin, dry skin, sluggish skin, pimples; refreshing, regenerative, softening, astringent, tonic

<u>Use in:</u> sprays, tonics, creams, lotions, gels, added to baths, compresses, poultices

<u>Food:</u> drinks, baking, desserts, sauces, soups, fish, meats, vegetables, preserves, fruit dishes, sorbets

<u>Home:</u> room sprays, radiators, diffusers

Lemon Verbena Hydrolat (*Lippia citriodora*)

<u>Health and well-being:</u> inflammation; calming, soothing, balancing, uplifting

<u>Skin care/body care:</u> most skin types; astringent effect, decongestive, soothing, calming

<u>Use in:</u> sprays, skin tonics, creams, lotions, gels

<u>Food:</u> baking, desserts, sauces, soups, fish, meats, vegetables, preserves, fruit dishes

<u>Home:</u> room sprays, radiators, diffusers

Linden Blossom (Lime Tree Flowers) Hydrolat (*Tilia vulgaris/cordata*)

<u>Health and well-being:</u> insomnia; relaxing, calming

<u>Skin care/body care:</u> dry skin, flaky skin, sensitive skin; moisturizing, soothing, toning

<u>Use in:</u> sprays, tonics, creams, lotions, gels

<u>Food:</u> teas, desserts

<u>Home:</u> room sprays, radiators, diffusers

Marjoram (Sweet) Hydrolat (*Origanum majorana*)

Health and well-being: calming; nervousness, tiredness; general tonic

Skin care / body care: problem skin, skin prone to acne and discoloration, oily skin, blotchy, uneven skin tone

Use in: sprays, skin tonics, creams, lotions, gels, compresses, poultices; added to baths

Food: sauces, soups, vegetables, meat, fish

Home: room sprays, radiators, diffusers

Orange Blossom (Neroli) Hydrolat (*Citrus aurantium*)

Health and well-being: calming, soothing; insomnia, general fatigue, nervousness, digestive upsets

Skin care / body care: most skin types: sensitive skin, aging skin, sluggish skin; irritation, scarring; astringent, refreshing, regenerative, balancing, soothing; rebalances sensitized skin

Use in: sprays, tonics, creams, lotions, gels, compresses, poultices

Food: desserts, baking, preserves, drinks, sorbets, fruit dishes

Home: room sprays, radiators, diffusers

Oregano Hydrolat (*Origanum vulgare*)

Health and well-being: infections, cuts, grazes, wounds, coughs, colds, respiratory conditions, sore throats, gum infection, aches

Body care: skin infections, rashes, cellulite; stimulating

Use in: sprays, gels, compresses, poultices

Food: sauces, meat, vegetables

Home: sprays, diffuser, radiators, surfaces

Peppermint Hydrolat (*Mentha piperita*)

Health and well-being: digestive problems, bloating, intestinal gas, inflammation, tiredness; general tonic; calming

Skin care / body care: problem skin, skin prone to acne, oily skin; cooling

Use in: sprays, skin tonics, gels, compresses, poultices; added to baths

Food: teas, sauces, meat, fish, preserves, desserts, sorbets, fruit dishes

Home: room sprays, radiators, diffusers

Pine Hydrolat (*Pinus sylvestris*)

Health and well-being: deodorant; fatigue, exhaustion, infections; vitality

Skin care / body care: toning, vitality

Use in: sprays, tonics, lotions, gels, shampoos, conditioners

Food: none

Home: room sprays, radiators, diffusers, surfaces

Rose Hydrolat (*Rosa damascena / centifolia*)

Health and well-being: coughs, sore throats, sore eyes — apply on cotton pads over closed eyelids; gargles, mouthwashes; nervousness, anxiety; uplifting, general tonic

Skin care / body care: most skin types: normal skin, combination skin, dry skin, aging skin, sensitive skin; soothing, refreshing, firming, regenerative, balancing, softening; scarring

Use in: sprays, tonics, creams, lotions, gels, compresses, poultices; added to baths

Food: baking, pastries, drinks, preserves, juices, sorbets, desserts

Home: room sprays, radiators, diffusers

Rosemary Hydrolat (*Rosmarinus officinalis*)

Health and well-being: headaches, respiratory conditions, soreness; tonic

Skin care / body care: skin infections, oily skin, acne, pimples, sluggish skin; decongestive, stimulating, refreshing, regenerative

Use in: sprays, tonics, creams, lotions, gels, poultices, compresses

Food: sauces, soups, meat, fish, vegetables, sorbets

Home: room sprays, radiators, diffusers, surfaces

Sage Hydrolat (*Salvia officinalis*)

Health and well-being: mouthwashes, gargles; sore throats

Skin care / body care: mature skin, dull skin, scarring; regenerative, balancing, softening

Use in: sprays, tonics, lotions, gels, compresses, poultices, hair products

Food: vegetables, soups, sauces, meat, fish

Home: atmospheric cleansing, energy clearing; use in sprays and diffusers; generally mixed with other hydrolats

Spearmint Hydrolat (*Mentha spicata*)

Health and well-being: deodorant, tonics, mouthwashes; cooling, refreshing

Skin care / body care: oily skin, pimples, stretch marks; toning

Use in: sprays, tonics, creams, lotions, gels, compresses, poultices; added to baths

Food: baking, desserts, sauces, soups, fish, meats, vegetables, fruit dishes, sorbets

Home: room sprays, radiators, diffusers

Thyme Hydrolat (*Thymus vulgaris*)

Health and well-being: antiseptic; infections, respiratory conditions, coughs, colds, fatigue

Skin care / body care: skin infections, acne, sluggish skin, tired and lifeless skin; balancing, cleansing

Use in: sprays, tonics, lotions, gels, compresses, poultices, hair products

Food: sauces, soups, meat, fish, vegetables

Home: room sprays, radiators, diffusers, surfaces

Witch Hazel Hydrolat (*Hamamelis virginiana*)

Health and well-being: bumps, bruising, aches, scrapes, swelling, sore eyes — apply on cotton pads over closed eyelids; astringent, soothing

Skin care / body care: astringent, purifying, toning

Use in: sprays, tonics, gels, compresses, poultices

Food: none

Home: none

The Essential Oils and Absolutes

This chapter contains a quick and easy chart for immediate reference, plus 125 comprehensive profiles of individual essential oils and absolutes. The chart provides information on therapeutic uses, therapeutic properties, and precautionary advice for each essential oil. To find out more about a particular essential oil or absolute, refer to the full individual essential oil profiles that follow the chart.

The information listed under "Therapeutic Uses" in this chapter is not a definitive list of all the conditions that a particular essential oil could be used for. When deciding which essential oils to use for a specific condition, first look under "Therapeutic Uses" to see if the condition is listed there, and if it's not, refer to the "Therapeutic Properties" entry. That may provide a more comprehensive picture of the potential healing spectrum of a particular essential oil. For example, if the symptoms of the condition involve painful muscular spasms, look for an essential oil that has analgesic, antispasmodic, or spasmolytic therapeutic properties.

An explanation of the terms used can be found in appendix 2, "Glossary of Therapeutic Properties."

A few essential oils in the following profiles are defined as absolutes. Absolute oils are usually produced from flowers or plant material not generally suitable for extraction by the usual methods of steam distillation or hydrodistillation. For the most part absolutes are obtained by solvent extraction, after which the solvent is removed, or by CO_2 extraction, which uses carbon dioxide to obtain the oil.

For advice on which essential oils can be used on children, please refer to chapter 7, "The Gentle Touch for Babies, Children, and Teenagers."

For advice on which essential oils to use during pregnancy, please refer to chapter 8, "A Woman's Natural Choice."

For dilution ratios and blending advice, please refer to the section "Quantities to Use and Blending" in chapter 1 (pages 10–13).

TABLE 22. QUICK REFERENCE CHART

COMMON NAME(S) (*Botanical Name*)	THERAPEUTIC USES	THERAPEUTIC PROPERTIES	PRECAUTIONARY ADVICE
AMYRIS (*Amyris balsamifera*)	Coughs, chest congestion, restlessness, stress, tension, a generally relaxing tonic, skin care	Antiseptic, antispasmodic, balsamic, emollient, expectorant, regenerative, sedative, slight anti-inflammatory	No contraindications known
ANGELICA ROOT (*Angelica archangelica*)	Coughs, sinus infection, viral infection, rheumatism, arthritis, gout, physical fatigue, fortifying and strengthening, stress-related conditions	Anti-infectious, antispasmodic, antitussive, diuretic, mucolytic, stomachic	Has photosensitization potential; avoid sunlight exposure after application. Best avoided during pregnancy.
ANGELICA SEED (*Angelica archangelica*)	Menstrual problems, coughs, colds, fevers, digestive problems, indigestion, flatulence, stress, anxiety, nervousness; calming	Antiseptic, carminative, cholagogue, depurative, digestive, expectorant, stomachic, tonic	No contraindications known
ANISEED (*Pimpinella anisum*)	Coughs, bronchitis, catarrh, flatulence, intestinal spasm, indigestion, digestive-linked migraines and headaches; calms nervous digestive tract conditions	Antiseptic, antispasmodic, carminative, expectorant, stomachic	May cause irritation on highly sensitive skins; a skin patch test is advisable. Best avoided during pregnancy and while breast-feeding.
BALSAM DE PERU (*Myroxylon balsamum*)	Skin conditions, rashes, wounds, pruritus, scabies, ringworm, bedsores, cuts, ulcers, hemorrhoids, coughs, bronchitis, head lice, dandruff, coughs, respiratory conditions	Anthelmintic, antibacterial, antifungal, anti-inflammatory, antiseptic, antitussive, balsamic, calmative, cicatrizing, expectorant	May cause irritation on highly sensitive skins; a skin patch test is advisable.

COMMON NAME(S) (Botanical Name)	THERAPEUTIC USES	THERAPEUTIC PROPERTIES	PRECAUTIONARY ADVICE
BASIL, SWEET (Ocimum basilicum)	Muscular spasm and contraction, rheumatism, digestive problems, nausea, flatulence, menstrual cramps, dysmenorrhea, headache, migraines, tension, stress, physical and mental exhaustion	Antibacterial, anti-infectious, antiseptic, antispasmodic, carminative, digestive, restorative, stomachic, tonic	May cause irritation on highly sensitive skins; a skin patch test is advisable. Avoid use in baths and showers. Always dilute before use. Avoid during pregnancy and while breast-feeding.
BASIL LINALOL (Ocimum basilicum ct. linalool)	Muscular spasm and contraction, rheumatism, respiratory conditions, menstrual cramps, menstrual problems, headache, migraines, intestinal cramps, nausea, cystitis, mental and physical fatigue, stress, tension	Antibacterial, antidepressant, anti-infectious, antiseptic, antispasmodic, calmative, carminative, nervine, restorative, tonic	Best avoided during pregnancy
BASIL TULSI / HOLY BASIL / TULSI (Ocimum tenuiflorum/ O. sanctum)	Muscular spasm and contraction, respiratory conditions, cystitis, intestinal spasm, parasitic infections, cramp, menstrual cramp, menstrual problems, headache, migraine, mental and physical fatigue	Antibacterial, anti-infectious, antiseptic, antispasmodic, calmative, carminative, pectoral, restorative	May cause irritation on highly sensitive skins; a skin patch test is advisable. Avoid use in baths and showers. Always dilute before use. Avoid during pregnancy and while breast-feeding.
BAY, WEST INDIAN (Pimenta racemosa)	Muscular aches and pains, neuralgia, arthritis, circulatory conditions, bronchial infections, digestive problems	Analgesic, anti-infectious, anti-neuralgic, anti-rheumatic, antiseptic, antispasmodic, circulatory, nervine, tonic	Can be a skin irritant; carry out a skin patch test. Best used for acute conditions. Best avoided during pregnancy.

COMMON NAME(S) (Botanical Name)	THERAPEUTIC USES	THERAPEUTIC PROPERTIES	PRECAUTIONARY ADVICE
BAY LAUREL (Laurus nobilis)	Influenza, rheumatism, muscular aches and pains, neuralgia, arthritis, circulatory conditions, candida, respiratory and bronchial infections, digestive problems, flatulence, colds, flu, skin rashes, spots, sores, dental infection, fungal foot conditions, nervousness, general fatigue	Analgesic, antibacterial, antifungal, anti-infectious, antimicrobial, antineuralgic, antiviral, circulatory, expectorant, pectoral	Those prone to allergic skin reactions are advised to carry out a skin patch test. Avoid during pregnancy.
BENZOIN (Styrax benzoin)	Catarrh, bronchitis, coughs, colds, scar tissue, nervous tension, stress, emotional crisis	Antidepressant, anti-inflammatory, antiseptic, carminative, expectorant, pectoral, vulnerary	Those with highly sensitive skin or those prone to allergic skin reactions are advised to carry out a skin patch test.
BERGAMOT (Citrus bergamia)	Infections, fevers, indigestion, cystitis, wounds, acne, herpes sores, depression, stress, tension, insomnia, fear, emotional crisis, emotional strengthening, convalescence	Antibacterial, antidepressant, antiseptic, antispasmodic, calmative, carminative, febrifuge, sedative, stomachic, vulnerary	Photosensitizer; do not apply to the skin prior to sun exposure. Rectified bergamot FCF is a nonphotosensitizer.
BIRCH, SWEET (Betula lenta)	Muscular aches and pains, rheumatism, arthritis, muscular injury, skeletal inflammation, lumbago, neuralgia, circulatory conditions, detoxifying, edema, heavy limbs	Analgesic, anti-inflammatory, antispasmodic, circulatory, diuretic, stimulant	To be avoided by those on multiple medications or anticoagulants. Not recommended for nonprofessional users. Not to be used during pregnancy and while breast-feeding.

COMMON NAME(S) (Botanical Name)	THERAPEUTIC USES	THERAPEUTIC PROPERTIES	PRECAUTIONARY ADVICE
BLACK PEPPER (Piper nigrum)	General aches and pains, stomach cramp, digestive problems, rheumatism, circulatory conditions, cold limbs, chills, exhaustion, convalescence; a general nerve tonic	Analgesic, anti-catarrhal, anti-infectious, anti-microbial, anti-septic, circulatory, diuretic, febrifuge, general tonic, immunostimulant, nervine, restor-ative, tonic	May cause irritation on highly sensitive skins
CAJUPUT (Melaleuca cajuputi)	Arthritis, rheumatism, neural-gia, muscular spasms and con-tractions, sciatica, sore throats, sinusitis, bronchitis, coughs, colds, parasite-induced skin problems, skin infections, head lice, insect bites, fatigue	Analgesic, anti-bacterial, anti-infectious, anti-microbial, anti-spasmodic, decon-gestant, expecto-rant, febrifuge, insect deterrent, pectoral, stimulant, tonic	No contraindications known
CAMPHOR, WHITE (Cinnamomum camphora)	Muscular aches and pains, rheumatism, muscular injuries, chesty coughs, bronchitis, colds, sinus problems, acne, rashes, parasitic skin infection, contusions, bruises; stimulat-ing, insect repellent	Anthelmintic, antibacterial, anti-infectious, anti-inflammatory, antiseptic, expecto-rant, stimulant	Best avoided during pregnancy and while breast-feeding. White camphor should not be confused with brown or yellow cam-phors, both of which should not be used.
CANANGA (Cananga odorata ct. macrophylla)	Circulatory conditions, inflamed skin, physical exhaustion, stress, tension, ner-vousness, anxiety; perfumery, skin care	Antidepressant, anti-inflammatory, antiseptic, antispas-modic, calmative, hypotensive, sedative	No contraindications known

COMMON NAME(S) (Botanical Name)	THERAPEUTIC USES	THERAPEUTIC PROPERTIES	PRECAUTIONARY ADVICE
CARAWAY SEED (*Carum carvi*)	Gastrointestinal conditions, dyspepsia, abdominal spasm, colic, flatulence, intestinal cramps and spasms, IBS, colitis, diverticulitis, gastric ulceration, allergic rhinitis, bronchitis, coughs, nervousness	Antibacterial, antihistaminic, anti-inflammatory, antimicrobial, antiseptic, antispasmodic, calmative, carminative, digestive, expectorant, nervine, pectoral, stomachic	No contraindications known
CARDAMOM (*Elettaria cardamomum*)	Indigestion, intestinal cramp, flatulence, dyspepsia, nausea, gastric migraine, constipation, IBS, colitis, Crohn's disease, muscular cramps and strains, muscular spasm, bronchial congestion, exhaustion and mental fatigue; strengthening, fortifying	Analgesic, anti-inflammatory, antispasmodic, calmative, carminative, nervine, pectoral, stomachic	No contraindications known
CARNATION ABSOLUTE (*Dianthus caryophyllus*)	Stress, insomnia, overactive mind, workaholism, insecurity, inability to communicate feelings, feeling detached from reality, sense of aloneness; relaxation	Calmative, relaxant, tonic	No contraindications known
CARROT SEED (*Daucus carota*)	Arthritis, rheumatism, indigestion, water retention, genito-urinary infections, urinary tract infections, detoxifying, eczema, ulcers, psoriasis, acne, pimples	Calmative, cytophylactic, depurative, diuretic, hepatic, regenerative, vasodilatory	Best avoided during pregnancy and while breast-feeding

COMMON NAME(S) (*Botanical Name*)	THERAPEUTIC USES	THERAPEUTIC PROPERTIES	PRECAUTIONARY ADVICE
CEDARWOOD, VIRGINIA (*Juniperus virginiana*)	Respiratory infections, catarrh, bronchitis, coughs, urinary tract infections, cellulite	Antiseptic, astringent, balsamic, decongestant, depurative, diuretic, expectorant, insect deterrent, pectoral	May cause irritation on sensitive skins; a skin patch test is advisable. Avoid during pregnancy.
CEDARWOOD ATLAS (*Cedrus atlantica*)	Chest infections, catarrh, detoxifying, cellulite, anxiety, stress, tension, physical exhaustion, acne, scalp disorders	Anti-inflammatory, antiseborrheic, antiseptic, depurative, pectoral, regenerative, restorative, tonic	No contraindications known
CELERY SEED (*Apium graveolens*)	Varicose veins, heavy legs, congestion, constipation, hemorrhoids, detoxifying, stress-related digestive conditions, nervousness, depression	Antiseptic, calmative, circulatory, depurative, digestive, sedative	No contraindications known
CHAMOMILE GERMAN (*Matricaria recutita*)	Pain relief, inflammation, fever, rheumatism, arthritis, muscular spasm, neuralgia, endometriosis, menstrual cramp, detoxification, abdominal cramp, stomachache, inflamed skin conditions, infected skin conditions, wounds, rashes, psoriasis, eczema, acne, spots, chilblains	Analgesic, anti-bacterial, anti-inflammatory, anti-phlogistic, antiseptic, antispasmodic, calmative, cicatrizing, emmenagogue, febrifuge, hepatic, immunostimulant, stomachic, vulnerary	No contraindications known
CHAMOMILE MAROC (*Ormenis multicaulis*)	Muscular spasm, menstrual cramp, intestinal cramp, stomachache, migraine, headaches, nervousness, irritability, anxiety	Anthelmintic, anti-infectious, antiseptic, antispasmodic, calmative, carminative, relaxant, sedative	No contraindications known

COMMON NAME(S) (*Botanical Name*)	THERAPEUTIC USES	THERAPEUTIC PROPERTIES	PRECAUTIONARY ADVICE
CHAMOMILE ROMAN (*Anthemis nobilis*)	Muscular spasm and contraction, rheumatism, menstrual cramp, rashes, acne, eczema, psoriasis, skin irritation, inflammatory skin infections, sunburn, dental and teething problems, insomnia, anxiety, nervousness, depression, stress-related conditions, insect bites and stings	Analgesic, antibacterial, anti-infectious, anti-inflammatory, antineuralgic, antispasmodic, calmative, cicatrizing, immunostimulant, nervine, sedative, vulnerary	No contraindications known
CINNAMON LEAF (*Cinnamomum zeylanicum*)	Bacterial and viral infections, parasitic infection, intestinal infection, fungal infection, respiratory infection, fevers, coughs, flu, muscular injury, aches and pains, rheumatism, arthritis, cold limbs, general physical debility, exhaustion, fatigue, tired all the time	Analgesic, anthelmintic, antibacterial, antifungal, antimicrobial, antiputrescent, antiseptic, antispasmodic, antiviral, carminative, circulatory, depurative, immunostimulant, stimulant, tonic	Best avoided if using multiple medications or anticoagulants. Those with hypersensitive skin are advised to carry out a skin patch test.
CISTUS/ LABDANUM/ ROCKROSE (*Cistus ladaniferus*)	Viral infection, influenza, bronchial conditions, joint aches and pains, muscular pain, arthritis, cuts, wounds, spots, acne, stems bleeding, scarring, nervousness, tension, stress	Analgesic, antibacterial, antiseptic, antispasmodic, antiviral, calmative, cicatrizing, immunostimulant	Best avoided during pregnancy
CITRONELLA (*Cymbopogon nardus*)	Muscular aches and pains, infectious skin conditions, fevers, heat rash, excessive perspiration, fungal infection, fungal foot infection, fatigue, insect deterrent, insect bites	Antibacterial, antifungal, anti-inflammatory, antiphlogistic, antiseptic, febrifuge, insect repellent	May cause irritation on highly sensitive skin; a patch test is advisable. Skin applications are best avoided during pregnancy.

COMMON NAME(S) (Botanical Name)	THERAPEUTIC USES	THERAPEUTIC PROPERTIES	PRECAUTIONARY ADVICE
CLARY SAGE (*Salvia sclarea*)	Menstrual problems, menstrual cramps, endometriosis, PMS, menopausal problems, hot flashes, muscular aches and pains, muscular fatigue, muscular spasm, excessive perspiration, headache, loss of concentration, memory, insomnia, nervousness, depression, anxiety, physical stress, psychological stress	Analgesic, antibacterial, antidepressant, antiseptic, antisudorific, calmative, emmenagogue, nervine, restorative, soporific, spasmolytic, tonic	Best avoided during pregnancy
CLOVE BUD (*Syzygium aromaticum*)	Pain relief, bacterial infection, fungal infection, viral skin infections, warts, verrucas, toothache, gum disease, muscle pain, rheumatism, flu, bronchitis, tired limbs, nausea, flatulence, stomach cramps, abdominal spasm, parasitic infection, scabies, ringworm	Analgesic, anthelmintic, antibacterial, antifungal, anti-infectious, antineuralgic, antiseptic, carminative, spasmolytic, stomachic	Avoid prolonged use. Avoid using undiluted on skin; apply a skin patch test for highly sensitive skins. Avoid during pregnancy.
COPAIBA (*Copaifera officinalis*)	Bronchitis, sore throats, tonsillitis, varicose conditions, varicose veins, hemorrhoids, urinary tract infection, cystitis, intestinal cramp and spasm, stomachache, stomach discomfort, *Helicobacter pylori*, muscular pain, bacterial and inflammatory skin conditions, fungal skin infection, onychomycosis, nail infection, athlete's foot	Analgesic, antifungal, anti-inflammatory, antimicrobial, antiseptic, astringent, cicatrizing, circulatory, diuretic, expectorant, stimulant	No contraindications known

COMMON NAME(S) (*Botanical Name*)	THERAPEUTIC USES	THERAPEUTIC PROPERTIES	PRECAUTIONARY ADVICE
CORIANDER SEED (*Coriandrum sativum*)	Digestive problems, flatulence, dyspepsia, bloating, indigestion, abdominal spasm, abdominal discomfort, IBS, detoxifying, nervous tension, muscular fatigue, muscular aches and pains, mental fatigue, tired all the time, emotional exhaustion	Analgesic, antibacterial, antispasmodic, carminative, depurative, regenerative, sedative, stimulant, stomachic	No contraindications known
CYPRESS (*Cupressus sempervirens*)	Varicose veins, fluid retention, hemorrhoids, congestive conditions, heavy and tired legs, edema, rheumatism, menstrual cramp, menopausal fatigue, hot flashes, cellulite, dry cough, bronchial spasm, asthma, respiratory conditions	Antispasmodic, antisudorific, antitussive, astringent, circulatory, diuretic, hepatic, restorative, vasoconstrictor, venous decongestant.	Avoid prolonged use. Best avoided in pregnancy and while breast-feeding.
DAMIANA (*Turnera diffusa*)	Catarrh, respiratory tract irritation, menstrual cramp, menopausal symptoms, headache, migraine, impotency, lack of sexual desire, nervous tension, nervous exhaustion	Antidepressant, antiseptic, aphrodisiac, astringent, cholagogue, diuretic, expectorant, nervine, stimulant, stomachic, tonic	Best avoided during pregnancy and while breast-feeding
DAVANA (*Artemisia pallens*)	Bacterial infections, bronchial congestion, coughs, colds, influenza, nervous stomach, indigestion, nausea, menstrual cramp, menopausal symptoms, general debility, anxiety, stress, irritability, tension	Antidepressant, anti-infectious, antimicrobial, antiseptic, calmative, decongestive, mucolytic, nervine, restorative, stomachic	Best avoided during pregnancy

COMMON NAME(S) (Botanical Name)	THERAPEUTIC USES	THERAPEUTIC PROPERTIES	PRECAUTIONARY ADVICE
DILL SEED (Anethum graveolens)	Colic, indigestion, dyspepsia, flatulence, gastrointestinal spasm, intestinal cramp, gastric spasm, IBS, diverticulosis, constipation, detoxifying, headache, nervous stomach, menstrual pain, digestive stimulant, nervousness	Antiputrescent, antiseptic, antispasmodic, calmative, carminative, cholagogue, decongestive, depurative, digestive, hepatic, sedative	Best avoided if using multiple medications
ELEMI (Canarium luzonicum)	Respiratory tract infections, chronic coughs, catarrh, stress-related bronchial conditions, muscular fatigue, overworked muscles, infectious skin conditions, wounds, cuts and grazes, tiredness; soothing and calming	Analgesic, anti-infectious, antiseptic, antispasmodic, cicatrizing, expectorant, pectoral, stimulant, stomachic, tonic	No contraindications known
EUCALYPTUS GLOBULUS (Eucalyptus globulus)	Respiratory infections, bronchitis, fever, catarrh, sinusitis, fever, muscular aches and pains, rheumatism, arthritis, urinary infection, cystitis, parasitic infection	Analgesic, anthelmintic, antibacterial, antifungal, anti-infectious, anti-inflammatory, antimicrobial, antiputrescent, antirheumatic, antiseptic, antiviral, expectorant, febrifuge, pectoral	Eucalyptus radiata is preferable for use with seniors and those convalescing. Best avoided during pregnancy and while breast-feeding.
EUCALYPTUS LEMON (Eucalyptus citriodora/ Corymbia citriodora)	Muscular injuries, fungal skin infection, bacterial skin infection, sores, wounds, respiratory tract conditions, asthma, fever, candida, insect bites; insect repellent	Analgesic, antibacterial, antifungal, anti-infectious, anti-inflammatory, antiseptic, antispasmodic, calmative, insect deterrent, vulnerary	No contraindications known

COMMON NAME(S) (Botanical Name)	THERAPEUTIC USES	THERAPEUTIC PROPERTIES	PRECAUTIONARY ADVICE
EUCALYPTUS PEPPERMINT (Eucalyptus dives)	Respiratory infections, sinusitis, sinus headaches, influenza, fever, headache, migraine, rheumatism, arthritis, muscular aches and pains, leg cramps, abdominal cramp, menstrual cramp, neuralgia, inflammatory conditions, candida, cellulite, parasitic infections, head lice, fatigue, exhaustion, acne, pimples	Analgesic, anti-bacterial, anti-inflammatory, antineuralgic, antiseptic, expectorant, mucolytic, pectoral, spasmolytic, stimulant, vasodilatory	Those prone to allergic skin reactions are advised to carry out a skin patch test. Best avoided during pregnancy and while breast-feeding.
EUCALYPTUS RADIATA (Eucalyptus radiata)	Respiratory tract infection, bronchitis, catarrh, sinusitis, rhinitis, colds, influenza, fever, asthma, rheumatism, muscular aches and pains, neuralgia, abdominal cramp, menstrual cramp, headache, mental exhaustion, fatigue, general stimulant and tonic, insect stings and bites	Analgesic, antibacterial, anti-infectious, anti-inflammatory, antiphlogistic, antirheumatic, antiseptic, antispasmodic, antitussive, antiviral, expectorant, febrifuge, immunostimulant, pectoral, tonic, vulnerary	No contraindications known
FENNEL, SWEET (Foeniculum vulgare var. dulce)	Digestive disorders, colic, dyspepsia, gastrointestinal spasm, flatulence, nausea, constipation, IBS, abdominal spasm, menstrual problems, menstrual cramp, premenstrual syndrome, infertility, endometriosis, menopausal symptoms, detoxifying, cellulite, fluid retention, heavy legs, bronchitis, respiratory conditions, parasitic infection	Anti-inflammatory, antiseptic, antispasmodic, carminative, depurative, diuretic, emmenagogue, expectorant, spasmolytic, stomachic, vermifuge	Avoid if using multiple medications. Avoid during pregnancy and while breast-feeding.

COMMON NAME(S) (*Botanical Name*)	THERAPEUTIC USES	THERAPEUTIC PROPERTIES	PRECAUTIONARY ADVICE
FIR, SILVER (*Abies alba*)	Catarrh, sinusitis, bronchitis, bronchial tract discomfort, dry cough, rheumatism, muscular aches and pains, feverishness, anxiety, tension; general tonic	Analgesic, antiseptic, antitussive, expectorant, pectoral, tonic	Best avoided by those with respiratory problems
FRAGONIA (*Agonis fragrans*)	Respiratory conditions, bronchitis, catarrh, sinus congestion, colds, bacterial and fungal infections, skin infection, pains, acne, pimples, inflammatory muscular conditions, muscular aches and pains	Analgesic, anti-infectious, anti-inflammatory, antimicrobial, antiputrescent, immunostimulant, mucolytic, pectoral, restorative, spasmolytic, vulnerary	No contraindications known
FRANKIN-CENSE (*Boswellia carterii*)	Coughs, colds, bronchitis, nervous asthma, skin infections, scars, wounds, urinary tract infection, mental fatigue, depression, nervousness, stress, tension, inability to communicate	Antibacterial, antidepressant, antimicrobial, antiseptic, calmative, cicatrizing, cytophylactic, expectorant, nervine, restorative, tonic	No contraindications known
GALBANUM (*Ferula galbaniflua*)	Skin infections, inflammatory skin disorders, acne, pimples, cuts and grazes, wounds, scarring, bronchitis, coughs, respiratory difficulties, inflammatory muscular aches and pains, rheumatoid arthritis, indigestion, stress and nerve-related conditions	Anti-inflammatory, antimicrobial, antiseptic, calmative, carminative, cicatrizing, digestive, nervine, spasmolytic, tonic	No contraindications known

COMMON NAME(S) (*Botanical Name*)	THERAPEUTIC USES	THERAPEUTIC PROPERTIES	PRECAUTIONARY ADVICE
GERANIUM (*Pelargonium graveolens/ Pelargonium x asperum*)	Female reproductive disorders, menstrual cramp, infertility, endometriosis, PMS, menopausal symptoms, circulatory disorders, Raynaud's disease, varicose veins, hemorrhoids, neuralgia, nervous skin disorders, depression, fatigue, emotional crisis, stress-related conditions	Analgesic, antibacterial, antidepressant, anti-infectious, anti-inflammatory, antiseptic, astringent, circulatory, hemostatic, nervine, restorative, spasmolytic, stimulant, tonic, vulnerary	No contraindications known
GERANIUM, BULGARIAN/ ZDRAVETZ (*Geranium macrorrhizum*)	Menstrual problems, menopausal symptoms, infertility, insomnia, nervous depression, fatigue, skin conditions — irritation, soreness, problematic skin	Antidepressant, anti-infectious, antispasmodic, carminative, diaphoretic, febrifuge, hypertensive, nervine, sedative, stimulating	No contraindications known
GINGER (*Zingiber officinale*)	Fractures, rheumatism, arthritis, muscle fatigue, muscular weakness, numbness, menstrual cramp, gastrointestinal spasm, digestive problems, flatulence, diverticulosis, IBS, constipation, nausea, sea and travel sickness, colds, chills, influenza, sinus congestion, chronic catarrh, circulatory tonic, Raynaud's disease, cold limbs, nervousness, mental exhaustion, general debility	Analgesic, antiseptic, antispasmodic, antitussive, carminative, circulatory, expectorant, febrifuge, fortifying, pectoral, stimulant, stomachic, thermogenic	No contraindications known

COMMON NAME(S) (Botanical Name)	THERAPEUTIC USES	THERAPEUTIC PROPERTIES	PRECAUTIONARY ADVICE
GINGER LILY ROOT (*Hedychium spicatum*)	Cuts, scratches, wounds, respiratory conditions, insomnia, nausea, coughs, chest infection, mental fatigue, anxiety, chronic fatigue, anxiety, stress, nervousness	Antibacterial, anti-inflammatory, antiseptic, carminative, digestive, expectorant, stimulant, tonic	Those with highly sensitive skin or prone to allergic skin reaction are advised to carry out a skin patch test.
GRAPEFRUIT (*Citrus paradisi*)	Muscle fatigue, muscular weakness, cellulite, migraine, headache, fluid retention, IBS, detoxifying, physical exhaustion, mental exhaustion, depression, stress	Anti-infectious, antiseptic, cholagogue, depurative, digestive, diuretic, hepatic, immunostimulant, tonic	Avoid if using multiple medications. Is a low-risk photosensitizer; do not apply to the skin prior to sun exposure.
GREENLAND MOSS/ LABRADOR TEA (*Ledum groenlandicum*)	Circulatory dysfunction, internal and soft tissue inflammation, liver conditions, detoxifying, water retention, edema, swellings, injuries, muscular aches and pains, stress-related conditions, anxiety, tension	Analgesic, antibacterial, antidepressant, anti-inflammatory, antiseptic, antispasmodic, circulatory, depurative, diuretic, hepatic, immunostimulant, spasmolytic, tonic	Avoid prolonged use. May cause irritation on highly sensitive skins; a patch test is advisable. Best avoided during pregnancy and while breast-feeding.
HOP (*Humulus lupulus*)	Neuralgia, bruising, analgesic, menstrual problems, menopausal symptoms, insomnia, coughs, stress-related asthma, stress-related digestive conditions, nervousness, stress, tension	Antimicrobial, astringent, calmative, carminative, emollient, estrogenic, nervine, soporific, spasmolytic	Best avoided during pregnancy and while breast-feeding

COMMON NAME(S) (*Botanical Name*)	THERAPEUTIC USES	THERAPEUTIC PROPERTIES	PRECAUTIONARY ADVICE
HO WOOD (*Cinnamomum camphora ct. linalool*)	Influenza, colds, chills, bacterial and viral respiratory infections, menstrual cramp, vaginal infections, parasitic skin infection, wounds, cuts, grazes, eczema, acne, stress and stress-related conditions, anxiety, tension	Analgesic, anthelmintic, antibacterial, antidepressant, antifungal, anti-infectious, antiseptic, antiviral, cytophylactic, immunostimulant, restorative, tonic	No contraindications known
HYSSOP DECUMBENS (*Hyssopus officinalis var. decumbens*)	Coughs, colds, influenza, bronchitis, catarrh, asthma, bronchial infections, contusions, bruising, wounds, arthritis, rheumatism, muscular aches and pains, digestive problems	Antibacterial, antiviral, astringent, carminative, cicatrizing, circulatory, digestive, diuretic, expectorant, pectoral, spasmolytic	Avoid during pregnancy and while breast-feeding
IMMORTELLE/ ITALIAN EVERLASTING/ HELICHRYSUM (*Helichrysum italicum*)	Pain relief, bruising, wounds, contusions, coughs, bronchial congestion, rhinitis, abdominal cramp, muscular spasm, rheumatism, arthritis, carpel tunnel, tendonitis, edema, varicose veins, hemorrhoids, circulatory conditions, ulceration, acne, pimples, eczema, psoriasis	Analgesic, anticholagogue, anticoagulant, anti-inflammatory, cicatrizing, circulatory, diuretic, expectorant, hepatic, mucolytic, spasmodic, stimulant, vulnerary	Avoid prolonged use. Best avoided during pregnancy.
JASMINE ABSOLUTE (*Jasminum grandiflorum/ officinale*)	Fertility, menstrual cramp, abdominal spasm, nervous tension, nervousness, stress-related conditions, lethargy, apathy, fatigue, insecurity, low esteem, anxiety, depression	Antidepressant, antiseptic, antispasmodic, calmative, cicatrizing, nervine, sedative, stimulant	No contraindications known

COMMON NAME(S) (Botanical Name)	THERAPEUTIC USES	THERAPEUTIC PROPERTIES	PRECAUTIONARY ADVICE
JUNIPER BERRY (Juniperus communis)	Fluid retention, cystitis, urinary tract infections, abdominal bloating, menstrual cramp, heavy legs, detoxifying, cellulite, gout, rheumatism, arthritis, acne, ulceration, eczema, mental exhaustion, chronic fatigue, anxiety, tension	Analgesic, anthelmintic, anti-inflammatory, antiseptic, carminative, depurative, diuretic, emmenagogue, nervine, spasmolytic, tonic	Best avoided by those with kidney disorders. Best avoided during pregnancy.
LAVANDIN (Lavandula x intermedia)	Skin infections, wounds, menstrual cramp, muscular cramp and contractions, muscular spasm, muscular injuries, migraine, stress, tension, respiratory tract infections, rashes, pimples, acne, nervous tension, pain relief	Analgesic, antibacterial, anti-infectious, anti-inflammatory, antiseptic, antispasmodic, nervine, sedative, vulnerary	No contraindications known
LAVENDER (Lavandula angustifolia)	Inflammatory conditions, skin infections, wounds, cuts, grazes, rashes, itching, stress-related eczema, nervous psoriasis, sunburn, burns, muscular spasm, muscular contraction, abdominal cramp, headache, migraine, insomnia, nervousness and related conditions, acne, pimples, insect bites, stress, tension, anxiety, tension, panic; insect deterrent	Analgesic, anthelmintic, antibacterial, antidepressant, anti-infectious, anti-inflammatory, antimicrobial, antiseptic, antivenomous, calmative, cicatrizing, cytophylactic, sedative, soporific, spasmolytic, vulnerary	No contraindications known

COMMON NAME(S) (*Botanical Name*)	THERAPEUTIC USES	THERAPEUTIC PROPERTIES	PRECAUTIONARY ADVICE
LAVENDER, SPIKE (*Lavandula latifolia*)	Muscular aches and pains, muscular spasm, muscular injuries, migraine, catarrh, bronchial congestion, headaches, pimples, rashes, nervous tension, insect bites	Analgesic, antibacterial, antifungal, antiseptic, antitoxic, antiviral, cicatrizing, decongestant, expectorant, immunostimulant, insect repellent, spasmolytic	No contraindications known
LEMON (*Citrus limon*)	Digestive problems, loss of appetite, detoxifying, cellulite, bronchial conditions, influenza, sore throat, laryngitis, varicose veins, hemorrhoids, acne, skin infections, herpes, abscesses, physical exhaustion, fatigue, debilitation, anxious depression, nervous tension, inability to concentrate or focus	Anti-infectious, antimicrobial, antiseptic, antispasmodic, antiviral, astringent, calmative, carminative, cicatrizing, circulatory, depurative, digestive, diuretic, hemostatic, stimulant, tonic, vermifuge	Expressed lemon oil is a photosensitizer; do not apply to the skin prior to sun exposure. Distilled lemon oil is a nonphotosensitizer. May cause irritation on highly sensitive skin; skin patch test is advisable.
LEMONGRASS (*Cymbopogon citratus/flexuosus*)	Muscular aches and pains, muscular ligament and tendon injury, gastrointestinal disorders, indigestion, colitis, diuretic, detoxifying, cellulite, fever, nonspecific infections, physical and mental exhaustion, acne, pimples, insect bites	Analgesic, anthelmintic, antifungal, anti-infectious, antimicrobial, antiseptic, astringent, depurative, digestive, diuretic, febrifuge, insect deterrent, tonic	May cause irritation on highly sensitive skins; a patch test is advisable. Best avoided during pregnancy. Avoid if using multiple medications.

COMMON NAME(S) (Botanical Name)	THERAPEUTIC USES	THERAPEUTIC PROPERTIES	PRECAUTIONARY ADVICE
LEMON VERBENA (*Lippia citriodora*)	Nervous indigestion, abdominal cramp, muscular spasm, gastrointestinal problems, diverticulosis, IBS, insomnia, stress, depression, nervous asthma, anxiety, restlessness	Anthelmintic, anti-inflammatory, antiseptic, antispasmodic, carminative, digestive, sedative, stimulant	Photosensitizer; do not apply to the skin prior to sun exposure. May cause irritation on highly sensitive skins; a patch test is advisable.
LIME (*Citrus aurantifolia*)	Digestive problems, loss of appetite, detoxifying, cellulite, heavy and sore legs, throat infections, tonsillitis, sore throats, bronchial conditions, influenza, lethargy, chronic fatigue, mental exhaustion, intestinal parasites	Anthelmintic, antimicrobial, antiseptic, antiviral, astringent, cholagogue, depurative, digestive, restorative	Expressed lime oil is a photosensitizer; do not apply to the skin prior to sun exposure. Distilled lime oil is a nonphotosensitizer.
LINDEN BLOSSOM ABSOLUTE (*Tilia vulgaris/ cordata*)	Nervous tension, nervous spasm, muscular spasm, insomnia, soothing, calming, emotional crisis, stress- and anxiety-related conditions	Antidepressant, antiseptic, antispasmodic, astringent, calmative, emollient, expectorant, nervine, sedative	Avoid during pregnancy
MAGNOLIA FLOWER (*Michelia alba*)	Scars, wounds, muscular aches, abdominal cramp, intestinal spasm, fear-induced anxiety, insomnia, inability to communicate, stress-related tension, depression	Analgesic, antidepressive, antiseptic, antispasmodic, calmative, cytophylactic, nervine, restorative, sedative	No contraindications known
MANDARIN (*Citrus reticulata/ C. nobilis*)	Digestive conditions, nervous spasm, intestinal spasm, IBS, stomachache, constipation, cellulite, insomnia, sleeping disorders, nervous tension, irritability, stress, convalescence, problem skin	Antiseptic, antispasmodic, calmative, digestive, sedative, stomachic, tonic	No contraindications known

COMMON NAME(S) (*Botanical Name*)	THERAPEUTIC USES	THERAPEUTIC PROPERTIES	PRECAUTIONARY ADVICE
MANUKA (*Leptospermum scoparium*)	Bronchial infections, bronchitis, catarrh, coughs, influenza, skin infections, wounds, cuts, grazes, contusions, ulceration, *Helicobacter pylori*, fungal skin infection, athlete's foot, parasitic infection, ringworm, mites, head lice, scabies	Analgesic, antibacterial, antifungal, anti-infectious, anti-inflammatory, antimicrobial, antiseptic, cytophylactic, expectorant, immunostimulant, spasmolytic, vulnerary	No contraindications known
MARJORAM, SWEET (*Origanum majorana*)	Muscle relaxant, muscular spasm, muscular pain, general aches, numbness, bodily stiffness, abdominal pain, menstrual cramp, menstrual problems, menopausal symptoms, contusion, bruises, head pain, gastrointestinal disorders, abdominal spasm, indigestion, intestinal spasm, constipation, IBS, diverticulosis, insomnia, stress-related conditions, anxiety	Analgesic, antibacterial, antiseptic, antispasmodic, calmative, circulatory, digestive, nervine, sedative, vasodilatory	No contraindications known
MASTIC (*Pistacia lentiscus*)	Bronchial disorders, coughs, colds, arthritis, rheumatism, varicose veins, circulatory conditions, *Helicobacter pylori*, ulceration, wounds, cuts and grazes, hemorrhoids, aching and heavy legs, cold lower limbs and numbness, dental hygiene	Analgesic, anti-inflammatory, antimicrobial, antiseptic, antispasmodic, antitussive, circulatory, decongestant, expectorant, pectoral, vasoconstrictor, vulnerary	No contraindications known

COMMON NAME(S) (Botanical Name)	THERAPEUTIC USES	THERAPEUTIC PROPERTIES	PRECAUTIONARY ADVICE
MAY CHANG (Litsea cubeba)	Cellulite, stomachache, abdominal cramp, indigestion, muscular aches and pains, tendonitis, arthritis, rheumatism, problematic skin conditions — acne, pimples, boils — circulation conditions, nervous tension, anxiety, stress	Anthelmintic, antidepressant, antifungal, anti-infectious, anti-inflammatory, antiseptic, astringent, carminative, circulatory, insect deterrent, sedative, stimulant	May cause irritation on highly sensitive skins; a patch test is advisable. Best avoided during pregnancy.
MELISSA (Melissa officinalis)	Insomnia, sleep disorders, indigestion, nausea, fungal infection, candida, viral skin infection, herpes, menopausal symptoms, detoxifying, nervousness, stress- and anxiety-related symptoms, depression	Antibacterial, antidepressant, antifungal, antiseptic, antiviral, calmative, circulatory, depurative, insect repellent, nervine, soporific, spasmolytic, stomachic	Avoid if using multiple medications. May cause irritation on highly sensitive skins; a patch test is advisable. Best avoided during pregnancy and while breast-feeding.
MIMOSA ABSOLUTE (Acacia decurrens/ A. farnesiana)	Nervous tension, nerve-related conditions, stress-related fatigue, stress, depression, intestinal infection, diarrhea, upset stomach	Antiseptic, astringent, calmative, emollient	Best avoided during pregnancy and while breast-feeding
MYRRH (Commiphora myrrha)	Coughs, catarrh, bronchitis, bronchial congestion, wounds, sores, ulceration, eczema, skin infections, ringworm, scabies, insect bites, parasitic bites, excess mucus, gum disease, mouth ulcers, fungal nail infection	Antifungal, anti-inflammatory, antimicrobial, antiseptic, astringent, balsamic, carminative, cicatrizing, expectorant, pectoral, vulnerary	Avoid during pregnancy and while breast-feeding

COMMON NAME(S) (*Botanical Name*)	THERAPEUTIC USES	THERAPEUTIC PROPERTIES	PRECAUTIONARY ADVICE
MYRTLE (*Myrtus communis*)	Bronchitis, sinus infection, laryngitis, bronchial infections, coughs, colds, cystitis, urinary tract infection, heavy legs, insomnia, tired all the time, skin disorders, psoriasis, acne, pimples, boils, parasitic infection, head lice, mite bites, emotional, mental, and physical exhaustion	Antibacterial, anti-catarrhal, antiviral, astringent, expectorant, pectoral, regenerative, restorative, soporific, stimulant, tonic	Best avoided during pregnancy and while breast-feeding. Avoid if using multiple medications.
NARCISSUS ABSOLUTE (*Narcissus poeticus*)	Stress, tension, anxiety, insomnia, muscular spasm, aches and pains, nervousness, inability to relax, troubled minds	Antispasmodic, hypnotic, nervine, sedative, soporific	May cause headaches in susceptible people. Best avoided during pregnancy.
NEEM/ MARGOSA (*Azadirachta indica*)	Psoriasis, eczema, parasitic skin infection, ringworm, scabies, ulceration, bacterial skin infection, scalp infection, dandruff, head lice, acne, sores, pimples, insect bites, insect stings	Analgesic, anthelmintic, antibacterial, antifungal, anti-inflammatory, antiviral, insecticide, pesticide, sedative	May cause irritation on sensitive skin. Best avoided during pregnancy.
NEROLI/ ORANGE BLOSSOM (*Citrus aurantium*)	Insomnia, convalescence, indigestion, abdominal spasm, intestinal cramp, stress and related conditions, scar tissue, scarring, skin regenerating, acne, problematic skins, stretch marks, menopausal anxieties, insomnia, sleep disorders, nervousness, depression, tension, emotional exhaustion	Antidepressant, anti-infectious, antimicrobial, antiseptic, calmative, carminative, cicatrizing, circulatory, cytophylactic, regenerative, restorative, sedative, spasmolytic, tonic	No contraindications known

COMMON NAME(S) (Botanical Name)	THERAPEUTIC USES	THERAPEUTIC PROPERTIES	PRECAUTIONARY ADVICE
NIAOULI (Melaleuca quinquenervia)	Bronchitis, respiratory tract disorders, influenza, sinus congestion, sore throats, catarrh, coughs, colds, uterine infection, rheumatism, muscular injuries, rashes, pimples, acne, herpes, wounds, cuts and grazes	Analgesic, antibacterial, anticatarrhal, antifungal, antiseptic, antiviral, balsamic, decongestant, expectorant, insect deterrent, pectoral, tonic, vulnerary	No contraindications known
NUTMEG (Myristica fragrans)	Gastrointestinal spasm, nausea, upset stomach, rheumatism, arthritis, muscular aches and pains, muscular injuries, menstrual cramp, insomnia, restlessness, nervousness, tension	Analgesic, antiinfectious, antiseptic, calmative, carminative, digestive, nervine, sedative, spasmolytic	Avoid if using multiple medications. Best avoided during pregnancy and while breast-feeding.
ORANGE, SWEET (Citrus sinensis)	Nervous anxiety, constipation, intestinal spasm, fluid retention, detoxifying, heavy legs, cellulite, insomnia, depression, anxiety- and stress-related conditions, tension, convalescence	Antibacterial, antiseptic, calmative, cholagogue, depurative, diuretic, sedative, stimulant, stomachic, tonic	No contraindications known
OREGANO (Origanum vulgare)	Viral infection, bacterial infection, respiratory tract infection, muscular pain	Analgesic, anthelmintic, antibacterial, antifungal, antiseptic, antiviral, expectorant, rubefacient, stimulant	May cause skin sensitivity; a skin patch test is advisable. Avoid during pregnancy and while breast-feeding. Avoid if using multiple medications.
OREGANO, GREEK (Origanum heracleoticum)	Viral infection, bacterial infection, parasitic infection, respiratory tract infection, gastrointestinal infection, bronchitis, catarrh, colds, influenza, rheumatism, muscular pain, acne, abscesses	Analgesic, anthelmintic, antibacterial, antifungal, anti-infectious, antiseptic, antiviral, immunostimulant, stimulant	May cause irritation on highly sensitive skins; a patch test is advisable. Best avoided during pregnancy and while breast-feeding.

COMMON NAME(S) (Botanical Name)	THERAPEUTIC USES	THERAPEUTIC PROPERTIES	PRECAUTIONARY ADVICE
PALMAROSA (*Cymbopogon martinii*)	Sinusitis, excess mucus, cystitis, urinary tract infection, bacterial infection, gastrointestinal disorders, scarring, wounds, acne, pimples, boils, fungal infection, general fatigue, muscular aches, overexercised muscles, stress, irritability, restlessness, insect bites and stings	Antibacterial, antifungal, anti-infectious, antiseptic, antiviral, cicatrizing, cytophylactic, digestive, immunostimulant, insect deterrent, vulnerary	Best avoided during pregnancy
PATCHOULI (*Pogostemon cablin*)	Fungal infection, parasitic skin infection, ringworm, scabies, mites, scalp infection, problematic skin conditions, sores, abscess, cuts, grazes, insect repellent, insect bites and stings, PMS, depression, moodiness, irritability	Antidepressant, antifungal, anti-infectious, anti-inflammatory, antimicrobial, antiseptic, astringent, calmative, cicatrizing, cytophylactic, insect deterrent, nervine	No contraindications known
PEPPERMINT (*Mentha piperita*)	Headache, migraine, digestive problems, nausea, colic, gastrointestinal disorders, flatulence, colitis, diverticulitis, Crohn's disease, IBS, sinus congestion, sinusitis, muscular aches and pains, muscular injuries, muscular spasm, sciatica, sprains, rheumatism, menstrual cramp, neuralgia, mental exhaustion, tension, physical exhaustion, fatigue, apathy	Analgesic, antibacterial, anti-infectious, anti-inflammatory, antiseptic, antispasmodic, antiviral, carminative, cholagogue, circulatory, decongestant, digestive, emmenagogue, stimulant, stomachic, tonic	Avoided during pregnancy and while breast-feeding. Avoid using undiluted in baths and showers.

COMMON NAME(S) (Botanical Name)	THERAPEUTIC USES	THERAPEUTIC PROPERTIES	PRECAUTIONARY ADVICE
PETITGRAIN (Citrus aurantium)	Stress-related conditions, nervous spasm, muscular spasm, general aches, hypertension, nervous asthma, insomnia, depression, general debility, stress, tension, irritability	Antidepressant, anti-inflammatory, antiseptic, antispasmodic, calmative, cicatrizing, cytophylactic, nervine, relaxant, sedative, tonic	No contraindications known
PINE (Pinus sylvestris)	Rheumatism, muscular pain, muscular injury, muscular fatigue, fatigued and heavy legs, gout, bronchial infection, sinus congestion, general debility, fatigue, mental and nervous exhaustion	Anti-infectious, antimicrobial, antiseptic, balsamic, decongestant, diuretic, expectorant, pectoral, tonic	May cause irritation on highly sensitive skin or skin prone to allergic reaction; a patch test is advisable. Best avoided by those with respiratory problems.
PLAI (Zingiber cassumunar)	Arthritis, joint pains, muscle pain, muscular injuries, torn ligaments, muscular spasm, tendonitis, menstrual cramp, abdominal spasm, colitis, diverticulosis	Analgesic, anti-inflammatory, anti-neuralgic, antispasmodic, calmative, carminative,	No contraindications known
RAVENSARA (Ravensara aromatica)	Colds, influenza, bacterial infection, viral infection, herpes, shingles, bronchial infection, bronchitis, respiratory tract infection, rhinitis, sinusitis, muscular pain	Antibacterial, anti-infectious, antiseptic, antiviral, expectorant, immunostimulant, stimulant	Best avoided during pregnancy
RAVINTSARA (Cinnamomum camphora ct. cineole)	Bronchitis, bronchial congestion, colds, sinusitis, rhinitis, excess mucus, laryngitis, respiratory infection, viral infection	Anthelmintic, antibacterial, anticatarrhal, antifungal, anti-infectious, antiseptic, antiviral, expectorant, immunostimulant, mucolytic	Best avoided during pregnancy

COMMON NAME(S) (Botanical Name)	THERAPEUTIC USES	THERAPEUTIC PROPERTIES	PRECAUTIONARY ADVICE
ROSALINA/ SWAMP PAPERBARK (*Melaleuca ericifolia*)	Respiratory tract infections, sinusitis, sinus headache, coughs, colds, restlessness, nervousness, irritability, acne, pimples, insect bites	Analgesic, antibacterial, anti-infectious, antimicrobial, antiseptic, antispasmodic, antiviral, calmative, expectorant, immunostimulant, nervine, pectoral	No contraindications known
ROSE ABSOLUTE (*Rosa centifolia*)	Infertility, menstrual problems, endometriosis, dysmenorrhea, menstrual cramp, abdominal cramp, circulatory problems, depression, anxiety, tension, phobias, nervous tension, stress-related conditions, scarring	Antidepressant, antiseptic, antispasmodic, astringent, calmative, cicatrizing, cytophylactic, hypnotic, nervine, sedative, tonic	No contraindications known
ROSEMARY (*Rosmarinus officinalis*)	Muscular aches and pains, rheumatism, arthritis, muscular weakness, muscular injuries, headache, migraine, gastric upset, abdominal spasm, respiratory conditions, sinus congestion, fluid retention, heavy legs, edema, cellulite, detoxifying, memory enhancement, general debility, acne, pimples, boils, abscesses, dandruff, hair loss	Analgesic, antimicrobial, antiseptic, antispasmodic, carminative, cicatrizing, decongestant, depurative, diuretic, immunostimulant, insect deterrent, restorative, spasmolytic, stomachic, stimulant	Best avoided during pregnancy

COMMON NAME(S) (*Botanical Name*)	THERAPEUTIC USES	THERAPEUTIC PROPERTIES	PRECAUTIONARY ADVICE
ROSE OTTO/ BULGARIAN ROSE/TURKISH ROSE (*Rosa damascena*)	Female reproductive problems, infertility, menstrual irregularity, endometriosis, dysmenorrhea, menstrual cramp, abdominal cramp, circulatory conditions, acne, skin dehydration, scarring, premature aging, depression, anxiety, emotional anxiety, nervous tension, stress-related conditions	Antidepressant, anti-infectious, antiseptic, astringent, calmative, cicatrizing, circulatory, cytophylactic, emmenagogue, emollient, sedative, spasmolytic, tonic	No contraindications known
ROSEWOOD/ BOIS DE ROSE (*Aniba rosaeodora*)	Bronchial infections, tonsillitis, coughs, stress headache, convalescence, acne, eczema, psoriasis, scarring, insect bites and stings, nervousness, depression, anxiety, stress-related conditions; tonic	Analgesic, anthelmintic, antifungal, antimicrobial, antiseptic, antiviral, calmative, cytophylactic, spasmolytic, tonic	No contraindications known
SAGE (*Salvia officinalis*)	Arthritis, rheumatism, muscular aches and pains, muscular injury, tendonitis, painful joints, menstrual pain, menstrual cramp, menopausal symptoms, hot flashes, excess perspiration, varicose congestion, heavy and tired legs	Antibacterial, antifungal, anti-inflammatory, antiseptic, antispasmodic, antiviral, astringent, cholagogue, cicatrizing, expectorant, digestive, diuretic, emmenagogue, mucolytic, stomachic, tonic	Use with care and avoid prolonged use. Use well diluted. Do not use if subject to seizures, epilepsy, or high blood pressure. Avoid all use during pregnancy and while breast-feeding.

COMMON NAME(S) (Botanical Name)	THERAPEUTIC USES	THERAPEUTIC PROPERTIES	PRECAUTIONARY ADVICE
SAGE, GREEK (Salvia fruticosa/ tribola)	Muscular aches and pains, muscular injury, painful joints, headache, stomachache, sore throat, menstrual cramp, acne, pimples	Anti-inflammatory, antimicrobial, antiseptic, antispasmodic, astringent, stomachic, tonic	Use with care for a short length of time, in low dosage. Avoid during pregnancy and while breast-feeding.
SANDALWOOD (Santalum album)	Coughs, sore throats, urinary infection, cystitis, vaginal infections, heavy legs, scarring, insomnia, anxiety, nervous tension, nervous exhaustion, depression	Antidepressant, anti-inflammatory, antiseptic, antispasmodic, astringent, calmative, cicatrizing, diuretic, emollient, nervine, pectoral, restorative, sedative, tonic	No contraindications known
SANDALWOOD, PACIFIC (Santalum austrocaledonicum)	Insomnia, stress, uterine spasms, depression, nervous anxiety	Antiseptic, antispasmodic, calmative, emollient, expectorant, sedative	No contraindications known
SARO/ MANDRAV-ASAROTRA (Cinnamosma fragrans)	Bronchitis, catarrh, coughs, colds, influenza, sinusitis, muscular pain, muscular injuries, cellulite, physical exhaustion	Analgesic, antifungal, antimicrobial, antiparasitic, antiseptic, antispasmodic, expectorant, mucolytic	Best avoided during pregnancy
SAVORY, SUMMER (Satureja hortensis)	Bronchial infections, catarrh, influenza, muscular aches and pains, fungal infection, insect bites	Anthelmintic, antifungal, anti-infectious, antimicrobial, astringent, carminative, immunostimulant	Can cause skin irritation; a patch test is advisable. Avoid during pregnancy and while breast-feeding. Avoid if using multiple medications.

COMMON NAME(S) (Botanical Name)	THERAPEUTIC USES	THERAPEUTIC PROPERTIES	PRECAUTIONARY ADVICE
SAVORY, WINTER/ MOUNTAIN (Satureja montana)	Viral infection, bacterial infection, respiratory infection, bronchitis, fungal infection, muscular aches and pains, skeletal aches and pains, digestive problems, wounds, abscesses	Anthelmintic, antibacterial, antifungal, anti-infectious, antiparasitic, antiviral, immuno-stimulant, tonic	Can cause skin irritation; a patch test is advisable. Avoid during pregnancy and while breast-feeding. Avoid if using multiple medications.
SPEARMINT (Mentha spicata)	Colic, dyspepsia, nausea, flatulence, digestive upsets, stomachache, neuralgia, lumbago, muscular aches, nervous migraine, nervous fatigue	Antiseptic, calmative, decongestant, digestive, nervine, restorative, spasmolytic, stimulant, stomachic	No contraindications known
SPIKENARD (Nardostachys jatamansi)	Insomnia, menstrual problems, muscular spasm, muscular contraction, neuralgia, sciatica, bodily congestion, aging skin, rashes, urticaria, physical tension, stress-related conditions, anxiety, nervous tension; calming	Analgesic, antibacterial, anti-infectious, anti-inflammatory, antiseptic, calmative, nervine, regenerative, restorative, sedative, soporific, spasmolytic	No contraindications known
SPRUCE (Picea abies)	Bronchitis, respiratory problems, physical fatigue, mental exhaustion, rheumatism, general aches and pains, acne, anxiety, stress	Antibacterial, antifungal, anti-inflammatory, antispasmodic, antitussive, expectorant, tonic	May cause irritation on sensitive skins; a patch test is advisable. Best avoided during pregnancy.
SPRUCE, BLACK (Picea mariana)	Bronchial infections, catarrh, sinus congestion, arthritis, rheumatism, gout, over-exercised muscles, stiff joints, muscular strains, tendonitis, cellulite	Analgesic, anthelmintic, antibacterial, antifungal, anti-inflammatory, antispasmodic, diuretic, expectorant, insect deterrent, pectoral	May cause irritation on highly sensitive skins; a patch test is advisable. Best avoided during pregnancy.

COMMON NAME(S) (*Botanical Name*)	THERAPEUTIC USES	THERAPEUTIC PROPERTIES	PRECAUTIONARY ADVICE
TAGETES (*Tagetes minuta*)	Athlete's foot, corns, calluses, bunions, parasitic infestations, resistant fungal infections	Antifungal, anti-microbial, anti-septic, insect deterrent, parasitic	Photosensitizer; do not apply to the skin prior to sun exposure. May cause irritation on sensitive skin; a skin patch test is advisable. Best avoided during pregnancy and while breast-feeding.
TANGERINE (*Citrus reticulata/ C. nobilis*)	Stress-induced insomnia, nervous exhaustion, mild muscular spasm, cellulite, digestive problems, detoxifying, flatulence, constipation, bodily congestion, tired all the time, irritability, generally dispirited, overly anxious	Antiseptic, antispasmodic, cytophylactic, depurative, digestive, sedative, stomachic, tonic	No contraindications known
TARRAGON (*Artemisia dracunculus*)	Dyspepsia, flatulence, indigestion, intestinal spasm, gastrointestinal problems, constipation, nausea, muscular cramp, muscular spasm, rheumatism, abdominal congestion and swelling	Anti-inflammatory, antispasmodic, antiviral, carminative, diuretic, stomachic, tonic	Avoid if using multiple medications. Avoid prolonged use. May cause irritation on highly sensitive skins; a skin patch test is advisable. Avoid during pregnancy and while breast-feeding.
TEA TREE (*Melaleuca alternifolia*)	Bacterial skin infections, parasitic skin infection, respiratory tract infection, sinusitis, rhinitis, wounds, ulceration, pimples, acne, abscesses, head and body lice, athlete's foot, fungal foot infection, warts, verrucas	Anthelmintic, antibacterial, antifungal, antiseptic, antiviral, decongestant, immunostimulant, vulnerary	May cause irritation on sensitive skins; a patch test is advisable.

COMMON NAME(S) (*Botanical Name*)	THERAPEUTIC USES	THERAPEUTIC PROPERTIES	PRECAUTIONARY ADVICE
THYME (*Thymus vulgaris*)	Bacterial and viral skin infections, respiratory tract infection, catarrh, bronchitis, muscular spasm, infected and weeping wounds, herpes, chronic fatigue, mental fatigue	Analgesic, anthelmintic, antifungal, anti-infectious, antimicrobial, antiputrescent, antiseptic, antispasmodic, antiviral, immunostimulant, stimulant, tonic, vermifuge	Avoid prolonged use. May cause irritation; a patch test is advisable. Best avoided during pregnancy.
THYME LINALOL (*Thymus vulgaris ct. linalool*)	Influenza, coughs, colds, bronchitis, sinusitis, rhinitis, laryngitis, sore throat, mucus congestion, viral and bacterial skin infection, circulatory problems, cold limbs, numbness, muscular pain, tendonitis, arthritis, rheumatism, acne, warts, verrucas, lethargy, inability to concentrate	Analgesic, antibacterial, antifungal, anti-infectious, antiputrescent, antiseptic, antispasmodic, antiviral, expectorant, immunostimulant, pectoral, restorative, stimulant, tonic, vermifuge	No contraindications known
TUBEROSE ABSOLUTE (*Polianthes tuberosa*)	Muscular spasm, stress-induced conditions, physical tension, insomnia, nervousness, restlessness, irritability, anxiety, depression	Antidepressant, calmative, carminative, hypnotic, relaxant, sedative, spasmodic, stimulant	May cause irritation on sensitive skins; a patch test is advisable. Best avoided during pregnancy and while breast-feeding.
TURMERIC (*Curcuma longa*)	Gastrointestinal conditions, indigestion, dyspepsia, stomach cramp, general aches and pains, rheumatism, rheumatoid arthritis	Analgesic, anti-inflammatory, antimicrobial, antispasmodic, cholagogue, digestive, diuretic, restorative, stimulant, stomachic, tonic	Avoid prolonged use. May cause irritation on sensitive skins; a patch test is advisable. Best avoided during pregnancy. Avoid if using multiple medications.

COMMON NAME(S) (*Botanical Name*)	THERAPEUTIC USES	THERAPEUTIC PROPERTIES	PRECAUTIONARY ADVICE
VALERIAN (*Valeriana officinalis*)	Insomnia, nervousness, stress, tension, tension headache, stress-induced migraine, muscular spasm, cramp, restlessness, inability to relax, restless leg, trembling disorders	Antimicrobial, antispasmodic, calmative, depurative, diuretic, hypnotic, nervine, sedative, soporific, stomachic	Avoid if taking sedatives or antidepressant medication. Best avoided during pregnancy and while breast-feeding.
VANILLA ABSOLUTE (*Vanilla plantifolia*)	Stress-induced conditions, nervous anxiety, nervousness, insomnia and restlessness, nervous stomach, inability to relax	Antidepressant, balsamic, calmative, sedative, stimulant	May cause irritation on highly sensitive skins; a patch test is advisable.
VETIVER (*Vetiveria zizanoides*)	Stress-induced conditions, nervous tension, muscular spasm, muscular pain, menstrual cramping, premenstrual syndrome, restlessness, restless legs, workaholism, physical exhaustion, irritability, depression	Antimicrobial, antiseptic, antispasmodic, depurative, nervine, restorative, sedative, tonic	No contraindications known
VIOLET LEAF ABSOLUTE (*Viola odorata*)	Fluid retention, edema, cellulite, stress-induced acne, prematurely aged skin, bruising, sore skin, nervous exhaustion	Analgesic, antibacterial, antiseptic, astringent, cytophylactic, diuretic, emollient, soporific, stimulant	No contraindications known
YARROW (*Achillea millefolium*)	Rheumatism, arthritis, inflammation, muscular injury, menstrual cramp, wounds, scarring	Anti-inflammatory, antiseptic, antispasmodic, astringent, carminative, cicatrizing, circulatory, expectorant	Avoid if using multiple medications. May cause irritation on highly sensitive skins; a patch test is advisable.

COMMON NAME(S) (Botanical Name)	THERAPEUTIC USES	THERAPEUTIC PROPERTIES	PRECAUTIONARY ADVICE
YLANG YLANG (Cananga odorata)	Hypertension, circulation, muscular cramp, menstrual cramp, intestinal spasm, insomnia, nervous tension, stress, nervousness, depression, physical exhaustion	Antidepressant, antiphlogistic, antiseptic, antispasmodic, calmative, nervine, sedative, tonic	May cause irritation on highly sensitive skin; a skin patch test is advisable.
YUZU (Citrus junos)	General tonic, nervous stomach cramp, cellulite, neuralgia, influenza, colds, postviral convalescence, stress-induced skin conditions, nervous tension, anxiety, nervous exhaustion	Analgesic, antibacterial, antiinfectious, antiseptic, antiviral, calmative, diuretic, nervine, sedative, stimulant, tonic	May cause irritation. With highly sensitive skin, a skin patch test is advisable.
ZDRAVETZ	See Geranium, Bulgarian		

The Essential Oil Profiles

The essential oil listings under the headings "Blends well with" in the profiles below are not exhaustive lists of the essential oils that complement or blend well with the profiled oil. These lists merely provide suggestions; there are no hard and fast rules about which essential oil complements another. The following lists are a general guide as to which essential oils complement the profiled essential oil when it is being used as a major component in a therapeutic healing blend. Ultimately, complementarity depends upon the intended use of the blend.

Under the "Precautionary advice" sections, some essential oils are described as "GRAS status," which means "generally recognized as safe for their intended use." This is a designation allocated by the United States Food and Drug Administration to describe substances that have been identified as safe to use in food, provided they are solvent-free and used in the way generally intended.

AMYRIS, Amyris balsamifera
(Plant Family: Rutaceae)

Type of plant: A small, flowering evergreen tree with glossy green leaves and clusters of small white flowers
Part used: Wood
Method of extraction: Steam distillation
Data: It takes years to produce this oil, as the wood has to dry for up to three years before

distillation and then rest for up to a year afterward so the aroma can fully develop. The tree grows wild in Haiti, where it's traditionally called candlewood, as the resin is highly flammable and the wood was traditionally made into torches. The wood is used to make furniture, while the oil is used in perfumery.

Principal places of production: Haiti, Jamaica, Cuba, Dominican Republic

When buying look for: Pale-yellow liquid, slightly viscous, with a sweet, slightly woody aroma, similar to sandalwood. This essential oil is sometimes mis-sold as sandalwood — which is more expensive and increasingly difficult to obtain. Although amyris oil is substituted for sandalwood in the perfumery trade, it cannot be substituted in aromatherapy.

Therapeutic properties: Antiseptic, antispasmodic, balsamic, emollient, expectorant, regenerative, sedative, slight anti-inflammatory

Therapeutic uses: Coughs, chest congestion, restlessness, stress, tension; a generally relaxing tonic, skin care

Blends well with: Bay (West Indian), bergamot, cananga, cardamom, carnation, cedarwood, frankincense, geranium, grapefruit, ho wood, hyacinth, lavender, lemon, lime, magnolia, nutmeg, orange (sweet), palmarosa, petitgrain, rose absolute, rosewood, sandalwood, spikenard, tangerine, tuberose, valerian, vetiver, ylang ylang

Precautionary advice: No contraindications known

ANGELICA ROOT, *Angelica archangelica* (Plant Family: Apiaceae/Umbelliferae)

Type of plant: Tall herb with large flower heads carrying clusters of small, ball-like, green-white flowers

Part used: Roots

Method of extraction: Steam distillation

Data: Not to be confused with angelica seed oil.

The stems, leaves, roots, and seeds of this plant are all aromatic. Angelica has been used in many countries' systems of medicine throughout history. See **Angelica Seed** below.

Principal places of production: Belgium, France, China, Spain, Russia, Egypt, India, Hungary, Holland, Germany

When buying look for: From colorless through pale yellow, darkening to light amber with age, with a musky, spicy, rooty aroma

Therapeutic properties: Anti-infectious, antispasmodic, antitussive, diuretic, mucolytic, stomachic

Therapeutic uses: Coughs, sinus infection, viral infection, rheumatism, arthritis, gout, physical fatigue, stress-related conditions; fortifying and strengthening

Blends well with: Black pepper, cajuput, cardamom, cedarwood, chamomile german, cypress, elemi, geranium, ginger, grapefruit, juniper berry, lemon, manuka, marjoram (sweet), niaouli, orange (sweet), palmarosa, ravensara, rosalina, tea tree, turmeric, vetiver, yarrow

Precautionary advice: Has photosensitization potential; avoid sunlight exposure after application. Best avoided during pregnancy and while breast-feeding. GRAS status.

ANGELICA SEED, *Angelica archangelica* (Plant Family: Apiaceae/Umbelliferae)

Type of plant: Tall herb with large flower heads carrying clusters of small, ball-like, green-white flowers

Part used: Seeds

Method of extraction: Steam distillation

Data: Not to be confused with angelica root oil (see above). There are over 30 types of angelica in the world. Its name comes from the fact that its floral top evokes thoughts of angel's wings. The plant was used by the ancient Romans and medieval Europeans, and it continues to be used in traditional European, Chinese, and American First Nations medicine. The stems are often candied/crystallized and used as cake decoration.

Principal places of production: Belgium, Hungary, Russia, Germany

When buying look for: A colorless to pale-yellow liquid with a fresh, musky, green peppery aroma

Therapeutic properties: Antiseptic, carminative, cholagogue, depurative, digestive, expectorant, stomachic, tonic

Therapeutic uses: Menstrual problems, coughs, colds, fevers, digestive problems, indigestion, flatulence, stress, anxiety, nervousness; calming

Blends well with: Basil, bergamot, black pepper, cardamom, chamomile roman, clary sage, coriander seed, dill seed, fennel (sweet), ginger, grapefruit, juniper berry, lavender, lemon, lime, marjoram (sweet), melissa, orange (sweet), petitgrain, rose, tangerine, valerian

Precautionary advice: No contraindications known. GRAS status.

ANISEED, *Pimpinella anisum*
(Plant Family: Apiaceae/Umbelliferae)

Type of plant: Flowering herb growing 2–3 feet high with white flowers and fern-like leaves

Part used: Seeds

Method of extraction: Steam distillation

Data: Aniseed is also known as *anis* or *anise* (not to be confused with star anise, which is a different essential oil). Aniseed is widely used as a flavoring in food and drink, as well as by the pharmaceutical and dentistry industries. Widely used in historical times, including by the Greeks and Romans, particularly for disorders of the digestive system.

Principal places of production: Spain, Egypt, Central and South America, Indonesia, India, China

When buying look for: A colorless to pale-yellow liquid with a spicy-sweet aroma, typical of aniseed

Therapeutic properties: Antiseptic, antispasmodic, carminative, expectorant, stomachic

Therapeutic uses: Coughs, bronchitis, catarrh, flatulence, intestinal spasm, indigestion, and digestive-linked migraines and headaches; calms nervous digestive tract conditions

Blends well with: Angelica seed, bay laurel, black pepper, caraway seed, cardamom, cinnamon leaf, clove bud, eucalyptus peppermint, fennel (sweet), geranium, ginger, grapefruit, lemon, orange (sweet), peppermint, spearmint, tangerine

Precautionary advice: May cause irritation on highly sensitive skins; a skin patch test is advisable. Best avoided during pregnancy and while breast-feeding. GRAS status.

BALSAM DE PERU, *Myroxylon balsamum*
(Plant Family: Fabaceae/Leguminosae)

Type of plant: Evergreen tree growing to 140 feet with large leaves; flowers each produce a single seed that's 3–4 inches (7–10 cm) long.

Part used: Oleoresin

Method of extraction: Solvent extraction/vacuum distillation

Data: The huge size of the seed makes it very hardy, and when introduced into foreign territory with no natural predators the tree can proliferate easily and cause environmental havoc among indigenous plants. Despite its name, this tree does not grow in Peru — it's indigenous to El Salvador, Honduras, and Guatemala. The essential oil is extracted from the oleoresin, which is tempted out of the tree in different ways. The bark can be cut to make the resin exude; when dry it is collected. Or a portion of the bark is burned to stimulate exudation of the resin, then wrapped in cloths to absorb the resin for some weeks, before pressing the cloth to extract the resin.

Principal places of production: El Salvador, Paraguay, Venezuela, Colombia

When buying look for: Pale- to medium-amber viscous liquid with a unique, warm, sweet balsamic aroma. Also called *Peru balsam*.

Therapeutic properties: Anthelmintic, antibacterial, antifungal, anti-inflammatory, antiseptic, antitussive, balsamic, calmative, cicatrizing, expectorant

Therapeutic uses: Skin conditions, rashes, wounds, pruritus, scabies, ringworm, bedsores, cuts, ulcers, hemorrhoids, coughs, bronchitis, head lice, dandruff, coughs, respiratory conditions

Blends well with: Benzoin, cajuput, chamomile german, cinnamon leaf, clove bud, copaiba, cypress, elemi, frankincense, geranium, ho wood, lavandin, lavender, lemongrass, manuka, myrrh, orange (sweet), palmarosa, rosewood, valerian, vanilla

Precautionary advice: May cause irritation on highly sensitive skins; a skin patch test is advisable. GRAS status.

BASIL, SWEET, *Ocimum basilicum*
(Plant Family: Lamiaceae/Labiatae)

Type of plant: Bushy annual herb growing up to 2 feet high, with white, pink, or purple flowers

Part used: Leaves and flowering tops

Method of extraction: Steam distillation

Data: The plant is cut when flowering and distilled immediately, as it loses aroma when dried. Basil is a sacred plant in many countries, including India. In the Mediterranean area it's grown around the house to confer protection and keep away flies. In Greece, a pot of basil is often found outside houses and shops. There are several types of basil; please see below.

Principal places of production: Vietnam, India, United States, Réunion (France), Comoro

Islands, Madagascar, Seychelles, Thailand, France, South Africa, Egypt

When buying look for: A colorless to pale-yellow liquid with a warm, slightly peppery, aniseed-like aroma

Therapeutic properties: Antibacterial, anti-infectious, antiseptic, antispasmodic, carminative, digestive, restorative, stomachic, tonic

Therapeutic uses: Muscular spasm and contraction, rheumatism, digestive problems, nausea, flatulence, menstrual cramp, dysmenorrhea, headache, migraines, tension, stress, physical and mental exhaustion

Blends well with: Bay laurel, bergamot, black pepper, cedarwood, chamomile roman, clary sage, coriander seed, cypress, eucalyptus radiata, fennel (sweet), fragonia, geranium, ginger, grapefruit, juniper berry, lavender, lemon, lemongrass, manuka, marjoram (sweet), mastic, may chang, niaouli, orange (sweet), oregano, palmarosa, peppermint, petitgrain, rosemary, spearmint, tea tree, thyme linalol, ylang ylang

Precautionary advice: May cause irritation on highly sensitive skins; a skin patch test is advisable. Avoid use in baths and showers. Always dilute before use. Avoid during pregnancy and while breast-feeding. GRAS status.

BASIL LINALOL, *Ocimum basilicum ct. linalool* (Plant Family: Lamiaceae/Labiatae)

Type of plant: Bushy annual herb growing up to 2 feet high, with white, pink, or purple flowers

Part used: Leaves and flowering tops

Method of extraction: Steam distillation

Data: The oil called *Ocimum basilicum* chemotype (ct.) *linalool* has similar therapeutic properties to basil, *Ocimum basilicum*. There are at least 35 different species of basil grown around the world, and many cultures have attributed spiritual as well as healing properties to it. Basil linalol is a species of basil grown for its linalol content.

Principal places of production: Egypt, Nepal, Italy, France

When buying look for: Colorless to pale-yellow liquid with a soft, warm, peppery aroma

Therapeutic properties: Antibacterial, antidepressant, anti-infectious, antiseptic, antispasmodic, calmative, carminative, nervine, restorative, tonic

Therapeutic uses: Muscular spasm and contraction, rheumatism, respiratory conditions, menstrual cramp, menstrual problems, headache, migraines, intestinal cramp, nausea, cystitis, mental and physical fatigue, stress, tension

Blends well with: Bay (West Indian), bergamot, cardamom, cedarwood, chamomile roman, cistus, clary sage, coriander seed, cypress, eucalyptus radiata, fragonia, geranium, grapefruit, immortelle, juniper berry, lavender, lemon, manuka, marjoram (sweet), mastic, niaouli, orange (sweet), oregano, palmarosa, peppermint, petitgrain, plai, rosemary, sandalwood, spearmint, thyme linalol, ylang ylang

Precautionary advice: Best avoided during pregnancy.

BASIL TULSI, *Ocimum tenuiflorum*, *O. sanctum* (Plant Family: Lamiaceae)

Type of plant: Shrub growing up to 2 feet with green or purple aromatic leaves and small purple flowers

Part used: Leaves and flowering tops

Method of extraction: Steam distillation

Data: Also known as *holy basil* and *tulasi*, basil tulsi originated in north India and is now widespread throughout southern Asia. It is used in Ayurvedic medicine and medicinal teas. Basil tulsi is so valued that it has acquired the moniker "the elixir of life." The plant is considered sacred in Hinduism and offered to the god Vishnu in his many forms. The leaves are seen as representative of Lakshmi, consort of Krishna. The plant is often found outside Hindu homes.

Principal place of production: India

When buying look for: Colorless to pale-yellow liquid, with a warm, green, spicy aroma

Therapeutic properties: Antibacterial, anti-infectious, antiseptic, antispasmodic, calmative, carminative, pectoral, restorative

Therapeutic uses: Muscular spasm and contraction, respiratory conditions, cystitis, intestinal spasm, parasitic infections, cramps, menstrual cramps, menstrual problems, headache, migraines, mental and physical fatigue

Blends well with: Bay laurel, bergamot, black pepper, cardamom, cedarwood, clary sage, coriander seed, frankincense, geranium, ginger, immortelle, lemon, lemongrass, mandarin, marjoram (sweet), myrtle, niaouli, orange (sweet), oregano, peppermint, plai, rosemary, sandalwood, spearmint, spikenard, thyme linalol, turmeric

Precautionary advice: May cause irritation on highly sensitive skins; a skin patch test is advisable. Avoid use in baths and showers, and always dilute before use. Avoid during pregnancy and while breast-feeding.

BAY, WEST INDIAN, *Pimenta racemosa* (Plant Family: Myrtaceae)

Type of plant: Evergreen tree growing over 30 feet high with small, highly fragrant leaves, small white flowers, and black berries

Part used: Leaves

Method of extraction: Steam distillation

Data: Distilled from the dried leaves. The *Pimenta racemosa* tree is very common in the Caribbean and Central America, where the leaves have long been distilled with alcohol to produce bay rum — a tonic used for colds, muscle pains, and hair treatments. Used in many male fragrances.

Principal places of production: Dominica, Jamaica, Virgin Islands
When buying look for: A deep amber to light-brown liquid with a spicy, sweet, clove-like aroma. Should not be confused with bay laurel (*Laurus nobilis*) oil.
Therapeutic properties: Analgesic, anti-infectious, antineuralgic, antirheumatic, antiseptic, antispasmodic, circulatory, nervine, tonic
Therapeutic uses: Muscular aches and pains, neuralgia, arthritis, circulatory conditions, bronchial infection, digestive problems
Blends well with: Bergamot, black pepper, cardamom, cinnamon leaf, clove bud, coriander seed, frankincense, geranium, ginger, grapefruit, hyssop decumbens, lavender (spike), lemon, mandarin, marjoram (sweet), mastic, nutmeg, orange (sweet), palmarosa, petitgrain, rosemary, sandalwood, ylang ylang
Precautionary advice: Avoid prolonged use. Can be a skin irritant. Those prone to allergic skin reactions are advised to carry out a skin patch test. Best avoided during pregnancy. GRAS status.

BAY LAUREL, *Laurus nobilis*
(Plant Family: Lauraceae)

Type of plant: Evergreen tree growing to 60 feet in height with glossy leaves, creamy-green flowers, and small black berries
Part used: Leaves
Method of extraction: Steam distillation
Data: Native to the Mediterranean and to the Near East, where from ancient times the leaves took on special significance. Ancient Greeks made headdresses of laurel leaves to crown winning sportsmen, warriors, and scholars. The name "Poet Laureate," given to the official national poet of the United Kingdom, derives from this tradition, as does the French word *baccalauréat*, which describes the multisubject exam taken at the end of secondary schooling. The leaves are widely used as flavoring in cooking.

Principal places of production: Croatia, Turkey, Crete (Greece), Bosnia and Herzegovina
When buying look for: Pale-yellow to pale-green liquid with a sweet, herbaceous, yet camphorous aroma
Therapeutic properties: Analgesic, antibacterial, antifungal, anti-infectious, antimicrobial, antineuralgic, antiviral, circulatory, expectorant, pectoral
Therapeutic uses: Influenza, rheumatism, muscular aches and pains, neuralgia, arthritis, circulatory conditions, candida, respiratory and bronchial infections, digestive problems, flatulence, colds, flu, skin rash, spots, sores, dental infections, fungal foot conditions, nervousness, general fatigue
Blends well with: Basil linalol, benzoin, bergamot, black pepper, chamomile roman, clove bud, cypress, eucalyptus lemon, eucalyptus radiata, frankincense, geranium, ho wood, immortelle, lavender, lavender (spike), lemon, manuka, marjoram (sweet), myrtle, oregano, palmarosa, peppermint, saro, tea tree, thyme linalol, yarrow
Precautionary advice: Those prone to allergic skin reactions are advised to carry out a skin patch test. Avoid during pregnancy. GRAS status.

BENZOIN, *Styrax benzoin, S. tonkinensis*
(Plant Family: Styracaceae)

Type of plant: Tree growing up over 80 feet high with green-yellow flowers
Part used: Resin
Method of extraction: Solvent extraction
Data: Benzoin is a resin from the tree trunk that is a yellowish color when it initially exudes and darkens as it dries. Benzoin has been valued for millennia, especially in the Middle East and Asia. Sometimes called *benjamin gum*. There are four varieties of benzoin tree and oil, although *Styrax benzoin dryander* is mostly used medicinally, with all types being used in perfumery.

Principal places of production: Laos, Indonesia, Thailand, Cambodia, Vietnam, China
When buying look for: An amber-colored, honey-like liquid with a warm, balsamic, vanilla-like aroma. Benzoin is sometimes labeled in grades.
Therapeutic properties: Antidepressant, anti-inflammatory, antiseptic, carminative, expectorant, pectoral, vulnerary
Therapeutic uses: Catarrh, bronchitis, coughs, colds, scar tissue, nervous tension, stress, emotional crisis
Blends well with: Bay laurel, bergamot, black pepper, cardamom, chamomile german, coriander seed, frankincense, geranium, ginger, grapefruit, jasmine, lavender, lemon, mastic, may chang, myrrh, myrtle, niaouli, nutmeg, orange (sweet), palmarosa, patchouli, petitgrain, rose absolute, sandalwood, tuberose, vanilla, ylang ylang
Precautionary advice: Those with highly sensitive skin and those prone to allergic skin reactions are advised to carry out a skin patch test.

BERGAMOT, *Citrus bergamia*, *Citrus aurantium ssp. bergamia*
(Plant Family: Rutaceae)

Type of plant: Small tree growing to 15 feet, with white star-shaped flowers and small yellow-green citrus fruits
Part used: Rind of fruit
Method of extraction: Cold expression then distillation
Data: Bergamot is the main flavoring in Earl Grey tea. It's also widely used in eau de cologne. It was named after the north Italian town of Bergamo but is mainly produced in southern Italy. There is an annual herb that is also called bergamot (*Monarda didyma*) but is unrelated to bergamot essential oil. "FCF" indicates the oil is bergapten- or furocoumarin-free.

Principal places of production: Ninety percent of the world's crop is produced in the Reggio di Calabria region of Italy or on the nearby island of Sicily.
When buying look for: A green liquid with a fruity, fresh citrus aroma, with spicy floral undertones
Therapeutic properties: Antibacterial, antidepressant, antiseptic, antispasmodic, calmative, carminative, febrifuge, sedative, stomachic, vulnerary
Therapeutic uses: Infections, fevers, indigestion, cystitis, wounds, acne, herpes sores, depression, stress, tension, insomnia, fear, emotional crisis, convalescence, emotional strengthening
Blends well with: Bay (West Indian), black pepper, cananga, chamomile maroc, clary sage, cypress, frankincense, geranium, ginger, immortelle, jasmine, lavender, lavender (spike), magnolia flower, mandarin, myrtle, neroli, nutmeg, orange (sweet), rose absolute, rosemary, rose otto, sandalwood, spikenard, tea tree, thyme linalol, vetiver, ylang ylang
Precautionary advice: Photosensitizer; do not apply to the skin prior to sun exposure. Rectified bergamot FCF is a nonphotosensitizer. GRAS status.

BIRCH, SWEET, *Betula lenta*
(Plant Family: Betulaceae)

Type of plant: Tall deciduous leafy tree that produces male pendulant seed flowers called catkins that hang down from the branches while the female catkins are upright.
Part used: Bark
Method of extraction: Steam distillation
Data: Native to the east coast of the United States and southern Canada and to parts of Russia. The *sweet* in the name derives from the sugar syrup made from the boiled sap of the tree, traditionally gathered by American First

Nations peoples. Sweet birch oil was formerly used as a substitute for wintergreen oil (*Gaultheria procumbens*).

Principal places of production: United States, Canada, Russia

When buying look for: Colorless to pale-yellow liquid with a strong, sweet, wintergreen-like aroma. Not to be confused with white birch essential oil (*Betula alba*).

Therapeutic properties: Analgesic, anti-inflammatory, antispasmodic, circulatory, diuretic, stimulant

Therapeutic uses: Muscular aches and pains, rheumatism, arthritis, muscular injury, skeletal inflammation, lumbago, neuralgia, circulatory conditions, edema, heavy limbs

Blends well with: Basil linalol, cedarwood, chamomile roman, clary sage, eucalyptus radiata, frankincense, geranium, juniper berry, lavandin, lavender, lemon, marjoram (sweet), peppermint, plai, rosalina, sage (Greek), saro.

Precautionary advice: To be avoided by those on multiple medications or anticoagulants. Not recommended for nonprofessional users. Not to be used during pregnancy or while breast-feeding.

BLACK PEPPER, *Piper nigrum* (Plant Family: Piperaceae)

Type of plant: Climbing, woody vine with dark-green leaves, small white flowers, and when mature, drupes of dark-red berries. The vine clings to trees and can live for 20 years.

Part used: Berries

Method of extraction: Steam distillation

Data: The peppercorns are picked when green and unripe, and they are usually slightly boiled before being left to dry in the sun for a few days, which turns them dark brown and ready for distillation. Black pepper has been used continuously in Indian Ayurvedic medicine for thousands of years. Its value as a spice fueled wars between the Portuguese, British, Dutch, and French colonialists, vying to gain access to it. In the eighteenth century a Frenchman called Pierre Poivre managed to take the plant to the French colony of Madagascar, breaking the Portuguese monopoly. This was such a crucial move for the French that his name is immortalized in the French word for pepper — *poivre*. Black pepper became an alternative form of currency known as *black gold*, and its value led to the expression "peppercorn rent."

Principal places of production: India, Sri Lanka, Madagascar, Malaysia, China, Indonesia

When buying look for: Colorless to pale-yellow liquid with a strong, warm, peppery aroma

Therapeutic properties: Analgesic, anticatarrhal, anti-infectious, antimicrobial, antiseptic, circulatory, diuretic, febrifuge, general tonic, immunostimulant, nervine, restorative, tonic

Therapeutic uses: General aches and pains, stomach cramp, digestive problems, rheumatism, circulatory conditions, cold limbs, chills, exhaustion, convalescence; general nerve tonic

Blends well with: Bay (West Indian), bergamot, cardamom, cinnamon leaf, clary sage, clove bud, fennel (sweet), fragonia, geranium, ginger, grapefruit, juniper berry, lavender, lavender (spike), lemon, lemongrass, lime, mandarin, marjoram (sweet), nutmeg, orange (sweet), palmarosa, patchouli, plai, rose absolute, rosemary, sage, sandalwood, tangerine, tea tree, ylang ylang

Precautionary advice: May cause irritation on highly sensitive skins. GRAS status.

CAJUPUT, *Melaleuca cajuputi, M. leucadendron* (Plant Family: Myrtaceae)

Type of plant: Tall evergreen flowering tree with gray, papery bark and white or green flower spikes

Part used: Leaves and twigs

Method of extraction: Steam distillation

Data: Also known as *cajeput*. This is the original species from which all the melaleuca species evolved. It's sometimes called *white tree*, due to its light-colored bark. The tree bark has been used as roofing and flooring material, and in Australia the plant was traditionally used by Aboriginal people for aches, pains, and headaches. In an herbal dated 1876, cajuput is mentioned as useful in treating intestinal problems.

Principal places of production: Indonesia, Vietnam, Malaysia, India, Australia

When buying look for: A colorless to pale-yellow liquid with a strong, fruity, camphor-like aroma

Therapeutic properties: Analgesic, antibacterial, anti-infectious, antimicrobial, antispasmodic, decongestant, expectorant, febrifuge, insect deterrent, pectoral, stimulant, tonic

Therapeutic uses: Arthritis, rheumatism, neuralgia, muscular spasm and contractions, sciatica, sore throat, sinusitis, bronchitis, coughs, colds, parasite-induced skin problems, skin infection, head lice, insect bites, fatigue

Blends well with: Bay laurel, bergamot, camphor (white), cardamom, cinnamon leaf, clove bud, eucalyptus lemon, eucalyptus radiata, geranium, ginger, hyssop decumbens, juniper berry, lavandin, lemon, myrtle, niaouli, nutmeg, orange (sweet), oregano, peppermint, pine, rosemary, sage (Greek), sandalwood, spruce, tea tree, thyme linalol

Precautionary advice: No contraindications known

CAMPHOR, WHITE, *Cinnamomum camphora* (Plant Family: Lauraceae)

Type of plant: Evergreen broadleaf tree growing to 100 feet with rough bark, glossy fragrant leaves, a profusion of white flowers, and black berries

Part used: Chipped wood and roots

Method of extraction: Steam distillation

Data: This plant is sometimes called *camphor laurel*. Camphor has been in use for many centuries in Asian medicinal systems, especially in China. In India and elsewhere, lumps of crude camphor used to be worn around the neck to ward off infection and parasites.

Principal places of production: China, Indonesia, Japan

When buying look for: A colorless liquid with a characteristic camphor aroma. Only the white camphor essential oil is used in aromatherapy; yellow camphor or brown camphor should never be used.

Therapeutic properties: Anthelmintic, antibacterial, anti-infectious, anti-inflammatory, antiseptic, expectorant, stimulant

Therapeutic uses: Muscular aches and pains, rheumatism, muscular injury, chesty cough, bronchitis, colds, sinus problems, acne, rashes, parasitic skin infections, contusions, bruises; stimulating insect repellent

Blends well with: Basil linalol, birch (silver), black pepper, cedarwood, chamomile german, cinnamon leaf, clove bud, elemi, eucalyptus radiata, frankincense, ginger, immortelle, lavender, manuka, marjoram (sweet), niaouli, peppermint, pine, ravensara, rosemary, tea tree, thyme linalol, yarrow

Precautionary advice: Avoid during pregnancy and while breast-feeding. White camphor should not be confused with brown or yellow camphors, both of which are toxic.

CANANGA, *Cananga odorata* ct. *macrophylla* (Plant Family: Annonaceae)

Type of plant: Flowering tree growing to 50 feet with glossy leaves and large, fragrant yellow flowers

Part used: Flowers

Method of extraction: Hydro or steam distillation

Data: The tree grows in tropical areas of Indonesia, Malaysia, the Philippines, and other Asian countries, where the flowers are used in

decoration and ceremony. It is sometimes used as a substitute for ylang ylang, as the aroma of cananga is similar, although less intensely floral.
Principal places of production: Indonesia, Thailand, Malaysia
When buying look for: A colorless to pale-yellow liquid with a floral-type aroma
Therapeutic properties: Antidepressant, anti-inflammatory, antiseptic, antispasmodic, calmative, hypotensive, sedative
Therapeutic uses: Inflamed skin, physical exhaustion, stress, tension, nervousness, anxiety; perfumery, skin care
Blends well with: Bergamot, carnation, cinnamon leaf, clary sage, clove bud, eucalyptus lemon, frankincense, geranium, ginger, grapefruit, jasmine, lavandin, lemon, linden blossom, magnolia leaf, mandarin, may chang, neroli, orange (sweet), palmarosa, patchouli, petitgrain, rose absolute, sandalwood, vetiver
Precautionary advice: No contraindications. GRAS status.

CARAWAY SEED, *Carum carvi*
(Plant Family: Apiaceae/Umbelliferae)

Type of plant: Flowering plant growing up to 2 feet in height, with feathery leaves and umbels of small white or pink flowers
Part used: Seeds
Method of extraction: Steam distillation
Data: The seeds are sickle-shaped and striped. As the plant easily self-seeds, it can be found in many parts of Asia, Europe, and the United States. Caraway seeds have been found fossilized in ancient European sites, so we know they were being consumed at least 8,000 years ago. Caraway was known to the ancient Egyptians and the Romans, and indeed, caraway is still used across a huge geographical area, including all of Europe and India.

Principal places of production: Finland, Egypt, Poland, Holland, Denmark, Hungary, Germany, Austria, India, Spain, Russia, Tunisia, Pakistan, England
When buying look for: Colorless to pale-yellow liquid that darkens with age, with a fresh, fruity, spicy aroma
Therapeutic properties: Antibacterial, antihistaminic, anti-inflammatory, antimicrobial, antiseptic, antispasmodic, calmative, carminative, digestive, expectorant, nervine, pectoral, stomachic
Therapeutic uses: Gastrointestinal conditions, dyspepsia, abdominal spasm, colic, flatulence, intestinal cramp and spasms, irritable bowel syndrome, colitis, diverticulitis, gastric ulceration, allergic rhinitis, bronchitis, coughs, nervousness
Blends well with: Angelica seed, aniseed, bergamot, cardamom, carrot seed, chamomile roman, clary sage, copaiba, coriander seed, dill seed, eucalyptus peppermint, fennel (sweet), galbanum, geranium, grapefruit, mandarin, marjoram (sweet), palmarosa, petitgrain, spearmint
Precautionary advice: No contraindications known. GRAS status.

CARDAMOM, *Elettaria cardamomum*
(Plant Family: Zingiberaceae)

Type of plant: Perennial herb of the rush type, with blade-type leaves, small yellow flowers with violet tips, and capsules containing reddish brown seeds
Part used: Seed pods
Method of extraction: Steam distillation
Data: Originating in Asia, cardamom was used by ancient cultures as both a medicine and a spice for at least 2,000 years before first being distilled in Europe in the sixteenth century. The seeds are dried before distillation. Cardamom remains an important component of traditional medicine in India and China and in some Middle

Eastern countries. It is used as a digestive aid, for flavoring, and as an aphrodisiac.

Principal places of production: Guatemala, India, Sri Lanka

When buying look for: A colorless to pale-yellow liquid with a warm, soft, spicy aroma with subtle citrus notes

Therapeutic properties: Analgesic, anti-inflammatory, antispasmodic, calmative, carminative, nervine, pectoral, stomachic

Therapeutic uses: Indigestion, intestinal cramp, flatulence, dyspepsia, nausea, gastric migraine, constipation, irritable bowel syndrome, colitis, Crohn's disease, muscular cramp and strains, muscular spasm, bronchial congestion, exhaustion and mental fatigue; strengthening, fortifying

Blends well with: Bay (West Indian), benzoin, bergamot, black pepper, cedarwood, cinnamon leaf, clove bud, coriander seed, fennel (sweet), geranium, ginger, grapefruit, ho wood, jasmine, lavandin, lemon, mandarin, marjoram (sweet), may chang, nutmeg, orange (sweet), palmarosa, petitgrain, pimento berry, rosewood, sandalwood, turmeric, valerian, ylang ylang

Precautionary advice: No contraindications known. GRAS status.

CARNATION (ABSOLUTE), *Dianthus caryophyllus* (Plant Family: Caryophyllaceae)

Type of plant: Perennial plant with long, thin, silver-gray leaves and pink flowers of various shades with ragged-edged petals

Part used: Flower heads

Method of extraction: Solvent extraction, then alcohol extraction, which produces an absolute

Data: This flower is commonly grown as an ornamental garden plant, known as *clove pink*, as the aroma is reminiscent of clove. Carnations were often sent to signify love. The name is derived from the word *coronation*, as the flowers were once formed into garlands and crowns.

Principal places of production: France, Egypt

When buying look for: A greenish-brown tinged to dark-amber-brown slightly viscous liquid with a rich, floral, spicy aroma

Therapeutic properties: Calmative, relaxant, tonic

Therapeutic uses: Stress, insomnia, overactive mind, workaholism, insecurity, inability to communicate feelings, feeling detached from reality, sense of aloneness; relaxant

Blends well with: Bay (West Indian), benzoin, bergamot, black pepper, cananga, cardamom, chamomile maroc, clove bud, coriander seed, hyacinth, immortelle, jasmine, lemon, linden blossom, magnolia leaf, narcissus, orange (sweet), rose absolute, sandalwood, tuberose, ylang ylang, yuzu

Precautionary advice: No contraindications known

CARROT SEED, *Daucus carota* (Plant Family: Apiaceae/Umbelliferae)

Type of plant: A wild-growing herbal plant with large, feathery leaves and tiny white flowers

Part used: Seeds

Method of extraction: Steam distillation

Data: The flowers grow in dense umbels that gather into nest-like clumps to protect the seeds, which are dried and crushed before distillation. There's a long history of medicinal use of carrot seeds in Europe and Asia. Not to be confused with the culinary carrot seed that produces the orange carrot root vegetable.

Principal places of production: France, Hungary

When buying look for: A light-yellow to dark-yellow liquid with a warm, fruity, earthy odor

Therapeutic properties: Calmative, cytophylactic, depurative, diuretic, hepatic, regenerative, vasodilatory

Therapeutic uses: Detoxifying, arthritis, rheumatism, indigestion, water retention, genitourinary infection, urinary tract infection, eczema, ulcers, psoriasis, acne, pimples

Blends well with: Basil linalol, bergamot, black pepper, cananga, cedarwood, chamomile german, chamomile roman, cinnamon leaf, cistus, clove bud, cypress, fennel (sweet), frankincense, geranium, grapefruit, greenland moss, immortelle, juniper berry, lavender, lemon, mandarin, petitgrain, rose otto, rosewood, sandalwood, yarrow

Precautionary advice: Best avoided during pregnancy and while breast-feeding. GRAS status.

CEDARWOOD, VIRGINIA, *Juniperus virginiana* (Plant Family: Cupressaceae)

Type of plant: Evergreen tree growing up to over 100 feet high, with needles and berries

Part used: Wood shavings and sawdust

Method of extraction: Steam distillation

Data: Native to the eastern slopes of the Rocky Mountains in the United States. The redness of the wood earned the tree the name *red cedar*, but despite this name, this tree is in the family of juniper, and related to cypress. The purple-brown berries, leaves, and bark have long been used by American First Nations people for medicinal purposes.

Principal place of production: United States

When buying look for: A colorless to yellowish-orange, slightly viscous liquid with a clean, woody, balsamic odor

Therapeutic properties: Antiseptic, astringent, balsamic, depurative, diuretic, expectorant, insect deterrent, pectoral

Therapeutic uses: Respiratory infections, decongestant, catarrh, bronchitis, coughs, urinary tract infections, cellulite

Blends well with: Basil linalol, bergamot, black pepper, clary sage, cypress, frankincense,

geranium, grapefruit, juniper berry, lavender, lemon, marjoram (sweet), myrrh, niaouli, patchouli, petitgrain, ravintsara, rosemary, rosewood, sandalwood, thyme linalol, ylang ylang

Precautionary advice: May cause irritation on highly sensitive skins; a skin patch test is advisable. Avoid during pregnancy.

CEDARWOOD ATLAS, *Cedrus atlantica* (Plant Family: Pinaceae)

Type of plant: An evergreen tree growing to over 100 feet, with wide-spreading branches, needles, and cones

Part used: Wood chips and shavings

Method of extraction: Steam distillation

Data: The cedar species *Cedrus atlantica* is native to the Atlas Mountains of North Africa. Cedars have been recorded to live for up to 2,000 years. The majestic cedarwood atlas has associations with Judaism, Christianity, and Islam. As the tree is a protected species, the essential oil is distilled from the chips and shavings from certified sawmills.

Principal places of production: Morocco, France, Algeria

When buying look for: A slightly viscous, pale-yellow to dark-yellow liquid with a balsamic, soft, woody, sweet, warm aroma. There are other species of so-called cedarwood, but these are junipers from the *Cupressaceae* family and do not have the same properties.

Therapeutic properties: Anti-inflammatory, antiseborrheic, antiseptic, depurative, pectoral, regenerative, restorative, tonic

Therapeutic uses: Chest infection, catarrh, congestion, acne, scalp disorders, cellulite, anxiety, stress, tension, physical exhaustion; detoxifying

Blends well with: Basil linalol, bay (West Indian), bergamot, cardamom, chamomile roman, clary sage, cypress, frankincense, geranium, grapefruit, ho wood, juniper berry, lavender (spike), lemon, lemongrass, marjoram (sweet), orange (sweet), petitgrain, ravintsara, rose absolute, rosemary, rosewood, sandalwood, thyme linalol, ylang ylang

Precautionary advice: No contraindications known

CELERY SEED, *Apium graveolens* (Plant Family: Apiaceae/Umbelliferae)

Type of plant: A wild celery with upright rosettes of green leaves on a tall flowering stem, producing small greenish-white flowers and tiny seeds

Part used: Seeds

Method of extraction: Steam distillation

Data: Thought to originate in Europe, the plant naturally prefers growing in salt marshes or near coastlines. Widely cultivated as a vegetable, it's now found growing throughout the world. It appears in many countries' traditional herbals. The essential oil is distilled from wild celery. After harvest the plant needs threshing to release the seeds, which are crushed before distillation.

Principal places of production: India, France, United States, Hungary, Holland

When buying look for: A colorless to pale-yellow liquid with a deep aroma of celery. Not to be confused with celery leaf. If celery seed oil is not stored well it becomes oxidized and shouldn't be used for therapeutic purposes.

Therapeutic properties: Antiseptic, calmative, circulatory, depurative, digestive, sedative

Therapeutic uses: Varicose veins, heavy legs, congestion, constipation, hemorrhoids, stress-related digestive conditions, nervousness, depression; detoxifying

Blends well with: Amyris, angelica root, basil tulsi, cedarwood, clove bud, coriander seed, cypress, fennel (sweet), geranium, ginger, grapefruit, greenland moss, ho wood, immortelle,

juniper berry, lemon, lemongrass, myrtle, orange (sweet), petitgrain, rosemary, sage

Precautionary advice: No contraindications known. GRAS status.

CHAMOMILE GERMAN, *Matricaria recutita* (Plant Family: Asteraceae/Compositae)

Type of plant: Plant with feathery leaves and white daisy-like flowers with yellow centers

Part used: Flowering tops

Method of extraction: Steam distillation

Data: Sometimes known as *Chamomilla recutita* or *Matricaria chamomilla*, the herb is dried before distillation, and the blue color is due to chamazulene being produced during the distillation process. The name *matricaria* comes from the Latin *matrix*, meaning "womb," because of the plant's widespread use by women for gynecological conditions and during childbirth. The herb is an ingredient in some French liqueurs.

Principal places of production: Germany, Hungary, Morocco, Egypt, Chile, England, France, South America, South Africa

When buying look for: A dark-blue liquid with a sweet, straw-like, herbaceous aroma

Therapeutic properties: Analgesic, antibacterial, anti-inflammatory, antiphlogistic, antiseptic, antispasmodic, calmative, cicatrizing, depurative, emmenagogue, febrifuge, hepatic, immunostimulant, stomachic, vulnerary

Therapeutic uses: Pain relief, inflammation, fever, rheumatism, arthritis, muscular spasm, neuralgia, endometriosis, menstrual cramp, detoxifying, abdominal cramp, stomachache, inflamed skin conditions, infected skin conditions, wounds, rashes, psoriasis, eczema, acne, pimples, chilblains

Blends well with: Bergamot, cedarwood atlas, chamomile roman, clary sage, cypress, eucalyptus radiata, frankincense, geranium, grapefruit, immortelle, juniper berry, lavandin, lavender,

lemon, marjoram (sweet), niaouli, plai, ravensara, rose absolute, rosemary, spikenard, tea tree, vetiver, yarrow
Precautionary advice: No contraindications known. GRAS status.

CHAMOMILE MAROC (ORMENIS FLOWER), *Ormenis multicaulis, O. mixta* (Plant Family: Asteraceae/Compositae)

Type of plant: Perennial herb with daisy-like yellow flowers and hairy leaves
Part used: Flowering tops
Method of extraction: Steam distillation
Data: Although the flower of *Ormenis* looks like a typical chamomile, it's a different species and has quite different therapeutic qualities. When buying any chamomile, it's important to look at the botanical name and ensure it is the chamomile you seek. This chamomile is sometimes referred to as *chamomile mixta* or *wild chamomile*. There is also a tansy (*Tanacetum annuum*) that's sometimes called Moroccan chamomile, but this isn't a chamomile at all.
Principal place of production: Morocco
When buying look for: A greenish-yellow to amber liquid with a balsamic, herbaceous, sweet aroma. See Data above regarding the name.
Therapeutic properties: Anthelmintic, anti-infectious, antiseptic, antispasmodic, calmative, carminative, relaxant, sedative
Therapeutic uses: Muscular spasm, menstrual cramp, intestinal cramp, stomachache, migraine, headache, nervousness, irritability, anxiety
Blends well with: Bay laurel, bergamot, black pepper, cardamom, cistus, clary sage, coriander seed, frankincense, geranium, grapefruit, jasmine, lavender, lemon, lemongrass, mandarin, marjoram (sweet), melissa, orange (sweet), patchouli, petitgrain, rose absolute, sandalwood, ylang ylang

Precautionary advice: No contraindications known

CHAMOMILE ROMAN, *Anthemis nobilis* (Plant Family: Asteraceae/Compositae)

Type of plant: Small plant with feathery leaves and small white daisy-like flowers
Part used: Flowers and stems
Method of extraction: Steam distillation
Data: For at least 2,000 years chamomile has been used extensively as a medicine. The botanical name derives from the Greek *anthemis*, meaning "little flower." One variety of *anthemis* has been found at ancient Egyptian sites dating from the predynastic period. In early Scandinavian culture, chamomile was associated with the sun god, and chamomile appeared in all the European herbals.
Principal places of production: France, England, Bulgaria, Hungary, Chile
When buying look for: A pale-blue to slightly blue-green tinged liquid with a fruity, sweet, fresh, herby apple-like aroma
Therapeutic properties: Analgesic, antibacterial, anti-infectious, anti-inflammatory, antineuralgic, antispasmodic, calmative, cicatrizing, immunostimulant, nervine, sedative, vulnerary
Therapeutic uses: Muscular spasm and contractions, rheumatism, menstrual cramp, rashes, acne, eczema, psoriasis, skin irritation, inflammatory skin infection, sunburn, dental and teething problems, insect bites and stings, insomnia, anxiety, nervousness, depression, stress-related conditions
Blends well with: Bergamot, cedarwood atlas, chamomile german, clary sage, cypress, eucalyptus lemon, eucalyptus radiata, fennel (sweet), frankincense, geranium, grapefruit, immortelle, juniper berry, lavender, lemon, mandarin, marjoram (sweet), melissa, neroli, nutmeg, orange

*ayurveda meds —
headache*

(sweet), palmarosa, ravintsara, rosemary, rose otto, sandalwood, spikenard, valerian, vetiver
Precautionary advice: No contraindications known. GRAS status.

CINNAMON LEAF, *Cinnamomum zeylanicum, C. verum*
(Plant Family: Lauraceae)

Type of plant: Evergreen tree that can grow to 20–30 feet but is cultivated as a bush, with thick bark, greenish-orange speckled shoots, small white flowers, and fruit that when ripe, becomes bluish with white spots
Part used: Leaves and twigs
Method of extraction: Steam distillation
Data: Sri Lanka, the jewel-shaped island country off the south coast of India, has been fought over many times because of its valuable cinnamon crop — first by the Portuguese in 1505, then the Dutch, then the English. Valued for its medicinal as well as its spice and fragrance uses, cinnamon has been traded around the world for many centuries. The name comes from the ancient Greek *kinnamon*, meaning "tube" — the classic rolled bark of cinnamon.
Principal places of production: Sri Lanka, India, Madagascar, Comoro Islands, Seychelles
When buying look for: The leaf oil, which is used in aromatherapy, is a darkish yellow. The viscosity can vary from medium to thin, and the aroma is warm, earthy, and spicy. Essential oils are also produced from the bark, stems, and roots, but these have different properties and are not recommended for home use.
Therapeutic properties: Analgesic, anthelmintic, antibacterial, antifungal, antimicrobial, antiputrescent, antiseptic, antispasmodic, antiviral, carminative, circulatory, depurative, immunostimulant, stimulant, tonic
Therapeutic uses: Bacterial and viral infection, parasitic infection, intestinal infection, fungal infection, respiratory infection, fevers, coughs, flu, muscular injury, aches and pains, rheumatism, arthritis, cold limbs, general physical debility, exhaustion, fatigue, tired all the time
Blends well with: Bay laurel, benzoin, bergamot, cardamom, carnation, carrot seed, clove bud, coriander seed, eucalyptus lemon, eucalyptus radiata, frankincense, geranium, ginger, grapefruit, lavandin, lavender, lavender (spike), lemon, lemongrass, mandarin, may chang, myrtle, nutmeg, orange (sweet), oregano, palmarosa, petitgrain, pimento berry, rose absolute, tangerine, tarragon, ylang ylang, yuzu
Precautionary advice: Best avoided if using multiple medications or anticoagulants. Those with hypersensitive skin are advised to carry out a skin patch test. Best avoided during pregnancy and while breast-feeding. GRAS status.

CISTUS (LABDANUM/ROCKROSE), *Cistus ladaniferus* (Plant Family: Cistaceae)

Type of plant: Bush growing to 10 feet in height and having large, fragrant, white flowers
Part used: Fresh flowering plant, flowers, young branches, and leaves/gum
Method of extraction: Steam distillation
Data: There is a great deal of confusion regarding this essential oil because the plant it comes from (often called rockrose) is processed in so many ways — each producing a different essential oil. The essential oil referred to here is produced by steam distillation from the fresh fragrant flowers and leafy branches. This is an entirely different oil from one made in the following ways: (a) The leaves and twigs are boiled in water, producing a gum on the surface; this is skimmed off and dried; the result is the crude gum, which is steam distilled. (b) Oil is steam distilled directly from the leaves and twigs and smells of pine. (c) A concrete, or absolute, is processed differently, again from the leaves and

twigs, using a solvent. All these oils will have *Cistus ladaniferus* as their botanical source, but will be entirely different essential oils. To confuse things further, there is a flower essence called rockrose, which is actually from the plant *Helianthemum canadense*. When purchasing the essential oil of cistus, check that it's produced by steam distillation.

Principal places of production: France, Spain, Cyprus, Morocco, Greece, Portugal

When buying look for: Liquid ranging from dark yellow through amber to brown with a rich, resinous, warm, amber, herbaceous aroma

Therapeutic properties: Analgesic, antibacterial, antiseptic, antispasmodic, antiviral, calmative, cicatrizing, immunostimulant

Therapeutic uses: Viral infection, influenza, bronchial conditions, joint aches and pains, muscular pain, arthritis, cuts, wounds, pimples, acne, scarring, nervousness, tension, stress

Blends well with: Bay laurel, cananga, carrot seed, cedarwood atlas, chamomile roman, clary sage, cypress, elemi, eucalyptus lemon, frankincense, geranium, grapefruit, immortelle, lavandin, lavender, lemon, myrrh, orange (sweet), palmarosa, pine, ravintsara, rosewood, sage (Greek), sandalwood, tangerine, ylang ylang, yuzu

Precautionary advice: Best avoided during pregnancy.

CITRONELLA, *Cymbopogon nardus*
(Plant Family: Poaceae)

Type of plant: Tall perennial grass with tufts of narrow fragrant leaves

Part used: Leaves

Method of extraction: Steam distillation

Data: Citronella comes from the grass colloquially known as *mana grass* in Sri Lanka. It's an important export for several Asian countries, where it's used in cooking as well as to deter

moths, fleas, spiders, ticks, mosquitoes, and other insects. In Chinese medicine, it's used as a remedy for rheumatic pain.

Principal places of production: Sri Lanka, China, Taiwan, Indonesia, Brazil, Madagascar

When buying look for: A thin, yellow to light brown liquid with a fresh, citrus/lemony aroma

Therapeutic properties: Antibacterial, antifungal, anti-inflammatory, antiphlogistic, antiseptic, febrifuge; insect repellent

Therapeutic uses: Muscular aches and pains, infectious skin conditions, fevers, heat rash, excessive perspiration, fungal infections, fungal foot infections, fatigue, insect bites; insect deterrent

Blends well with: Bay (West Indian), cedarwood, cinnamon leaf, clove bud, cypress, eucalyptus radiata, geranium, ginger, juniper berry, lemon, lemongrass, lime, may chang, myrtle, orange (sweet), palmarosa, patchouli, pine, rosemary, spearmint, spruce, tangerine, vetiver, ylang ylang

Precautionary advice: May cause irritation on highly sensitive or damaged skins; a skin patch test is advisable. Skin applications are best avoided during pregnancy. GRAS status.

CLARY SAGE, *Salvia sclarea*
(Plant Family: Lamiaceae/Labiatae)

Type of plant: Biennial herb growing to 3 feet high with hairy stems, large, fragrant, velvety leaves, and lilac-pink flower spikes

Part used: Flowering tops

Method of extraction: Steam distillation

Data: The plant material is distilled either dried, when it is known as traditional clary sage, or fresh, when it is known as green crushed clary sage. The whole plant has glandular hairs containing essential oil. Native to southern and central Europe and to western Asia, clary sage was known to many ancient cultures. Indian sages said it gave illumination, while the Romans attributed to it the ability to confer good health. In Germany, it was used along with elderflowers as an additive to cheap wine to make it taste like muscatel.

Principal places of production: France, Bulgaria, Russia, Hungary, England, Germany, Spain, China

When buying look for: A colorless to pale-yellow liquid with a nutty, warm, light, musky, herbaceous aroma

Therapeutic properties: Analgesic, antibacterial, antidepressant, antiseptic, antisudorific, calmative, emmenagogue, nervine, restorative, soporific, spasmolytic, tonic

Therapeutic uses: Menstrual problems, menstrual cramp, endometriosis, premenstrual syndrome, menopausal problems, hot flashes, muscular aches and pains, muscular fatigue, muscular spasm, excessive perspiration, headaches, loss of concentration, memory, insomnia, nervousness, depression, anxiety, stress, psychological stress

Blends well with: Amyris, bergamot, black pepper, cananga, cardamom, chamomile maroc, chamomile roman, coriander seed, cypress, damiana, geranium, grapefruit, ho wood, jasmine, lavender, lemon, lime, mandarin, patchouli, rose absolute, rose otto, sandalwood, tangerine, valerian

Precautionary advice: Avoid during pregnancy and while breast-feeding. GRAS status.

CLOVE BUD, *Syzygium aromaticum*
(Plant Family: Myrtaceae)

Type of plant: All parts of this 40-foot evergreen tree are fragrant: the wood, flowers, and leaves.
Part used: Buds
Method of extraction: Steam distillation
Data: Clove buds are harvested then sun-dried until they turn to the characteristic deep red-brown color before being distilled. Clove was in use in the Levant from 1700 BCE, mentioned in Indian Ayurvedic medicine from 1500 BCE, and known from at least the third century BCE in China, where it continues to be part of Chinese medicine. Clove's value as a medicine and spice led to it being the cause of spice wars from Asia to the Caribbean, with European nations fighting over access to it. Clove continues to be an important component in cooking and perfumery.

Principal places of production: Madagascar, Indonesia, Sri Lanka, Tanzania, Caribbean, Philippines

When buying look for: A pale-yellow to pale-brown liquid with a rich, warm, sweet spice aroma. There are also essential oils of clove leaf and of clove stems, and these are avoided because they're strong skin irritants. Only clove oil distilled from the buds is used in aromatherapy.

Therapeutic properties: Analgesic, anthelmintic, antibacterial, antifungal, anti-infectious, antineuralgic, antiseptic, carminative, spasmolytic, stomachic

Therapeutic uses: Pain relief, bacterial infection, fungal infection, viral skin infection, warts, verrucas, toothache, gum disease, muscle pain, rheumatism, flu, bronchitis, tired limbs, nausea, flatulence, stomach cramp, abdominal spasm, parasitic infection, scabies, ringworm

Blends well with: Bay (West Indian), benzoin, bergamot, black pepper, cardamom, chamomile maroc, chamomile roman, cinnamon leaf, cistus, elemi, fennel (sweet), geranium, ginger, grapefruit, jasmine, lavender (spike), lemon, lemongrass, linden blossom, mandarin, marjoram (sweet), may chang, myrtle, orange (sweet), oregano, palmarosa, peppermint, ravensara, rose maroc, tangerine, thyme linalol, ylang ylang

Precautionary advice: Avoid prolonged use. Avoid using undiluted on skin; apply a patch test for highly sensitive skins. Avoid during pregnancy and while breast-feeding.

COPAIBA, *Copaifera officinalis*
(Plant Family: Fabaceae)

Type of plant: Copaiba is a rain forest tree growing to between 50 and 90 feet in height with long, flowering panicles and small white flowers

Part used: Oleoresin

Method of extraction: Steam distillation

Data: This species of copaiba tree is found throughout South America and the Amazon region. The resin is extracted by tapping or drilling holes into the tree, which then exudes resin from the holes. No trees are destroyed using this process of extraction. The oleoresin is then distilled to make the essential oil. The resin was first mentioned in Europe in the early 1600s. It's been used by indigenous people of the Amazon for a multitude of medicinal purposes and is part of the traditional healer's pharmacopeia; much ongoing scientific research is being carried out into its medical properties.

Principal place of production: Brazil

When buying look for: A colorless to light-brown viscous liquid with a soft, sweet, earthy, resinous aroma

Therapeutic properties: Analgesic, antifungal, anti-inflammatory, antimicrobial, antiseptic, astringent, cicatrizing, circulatory, diuretic, expectorant, stimulant

Therapeutic uses: Bronchitis, sore throats, tonsillitis, varicose conditions, varicose veins, hemorrhoids, urinary tract infections, cystitis, intestinal cramps and spasms, stomachache, stomach discomfort, *Helicobacter pylori*, muscular pain, bacterial and inflammatory skin conditions, fungal skin infections, onychomycosis, foot candida nail infections, athlete's foot

Blends well with: Benzoin, black pepper, cajuput, cardamom, chamomile german, chamomile roman, coriander seed, elemi, eucalyptus radiata, geranium, ginger, greenland moss, hyssop decumbens, juniper berry, lavender, lemon,

manuka, mastic, may chang, myrtle, niaouli, ravensara, thyme linalol, turmeric

Precautionary advice: No contraindications known

CORIANDER SEED, *Coriandrum sativum*
(Plant Family: Apiaceae/Umbelliferae)

Type of plant: Annual or biennial plant, with small, delicate shapely leaves. The whitish-pink flowers give way to green seeds.

Part used: Seeds

Method of extraction: Steam distillation of crushed ripe seeds

Data: This oil is produced from the seeds of the cilantro plant — widely used in cooking worldwide. The seeds were found in Tutankhamen's tomb. Fourteenth-century nuns used the seeds to produce the famous Carmelite water, used for rejuvenation, while French monks continue the long tradition of using them to produce Chatreuse and Benedictine liqueurs. The seeds are widely used in cooking all around the world.

Principal places of production: Hungary, Russia, Ukraine, India, Egypt, Tunisia, Morocco, United States, Italy

When buying look for: A colorless to pale-yellow liquid with a sweet, warm, fresh, spicy, slightly woody aroma

Therapeutic properties: Analgesic, antibacterial, antispasmodic, carminative, depurative, regenerative, sedative, stimulant, stomachic

Therapeutic uses: Digestive problems, flatulence, dyspepsia, bloating, indigestion, abdominal spasm, abdominal discomfort, irritable bowel syndrome, detoxifying, nervous tension, muscular fatigue, muscular aches and pains, mental fatigue, tired all the time, emotional exhaustion

Blends well with: Bergamot, black pepper, cajuput, cardamom, cinnamon leaf, clary sage, frankincense, geranium, ginger, grapefruit, jasmine, juniper berry, lemon, manuka, melissa, neroli,

nutmeg, orange (sweet), palmarosa, patchouli, petitgrain, sandalwood, spearmint, tarragon, vetiver, ylang ylang
Precautionary advice: No contraindications known. GRAS status.

CYPRESS, *Cupressus sempervirens*
(Plant Family: Cupressaceae)

Type of plant: Coniferous evergreen tree that can grow to over 100 feet high with tiny dark-green leaves on small branchlets, and both female and male flowers
Part used: Foliage and twigs
Method of extraction: Steam distillation
Data: Known as the Mediterranean cypress, this is a long-living tree with a symbolic history of use in mourning and in cemeteries. A cypress tree in Iran is estimated to be over 4,000 years old. The tree gave its name to the island of Cyprus. Due to the essential oil content, the wood is impervious to woodworm — making it useful for works of art and furniture. Cypress essential oil is a common ingredient in men's colognes.
Principal places of production: France, Morocco, Spain
When buying look for: A colorless to pale-yellow liquid with a warm, green, slightly spicy, woody aroma. Not to be confused with blue cypress essential oil.
Therapeutic properties: Antispasmodic, anti-sudorific, antitussive, astringent, circulatory, diuretic, hepatic; restorative, venous decongestant
Therapeutic uses: Varicose veins, fluid retention, hemorrhoids, congestive conditions, heavy and tired legs, edema, rheumatism, menstrual cramp, menopausal fatigue, hot flashes, cellulite, dry coughs, bronchial spasm, asthma, respiratory conditions
Blends well with: Bergamot, cedarwood atlas, chamomile roman, clary sage, frankincense, geranium, ginger, grapefruit, immortelle, juniper berry, lavandin, lavender, lemon, mandarin, manuka, marjoram (sweet), orange (sweet), petitgrain, pine, ravensara, ravintsara, rosemary
Precautionary advice: Avoid prolonged use. Best avoided during pregnancy and while breast-feeding.

DAMIANA, *Turnera diffusa*
(Plant Family: Passifloraceae)

Type of plant: A small aromatic shrub with dark-green leaves and small, fragrant, bright-yellow flowers and small, sweet-smelling fruits
Part used: Leaves
Method of extraction: Steam distillation
Data: Damiana leaves have a long history of medicinal use, and it is also used to flavor beverages. The reputation of damiana as an aphrodisiac derives from various indigenous people's traditional use of the shrub, and now several patents have been awarded for its use in medications to enhance the sexual experience.
Principal places of production: Caribbean, Mexico
When buying look for: A deep greenish-yellow to light-brown liquid with a slightly spicy, green aroma
Therapeutic properties: Antidepressant, antiseptic, aphrodisiac, astringent, cholagogue, diuretic, expectorant, nervine, stimulant, stomachic, tonic
Therapeutic uses: Catarrh, respiratory tract irritation, menstrual cramp, menopausal symptoms, headaches, migraine, impotency, lack of sexual desire, nervous tension, nervous exhaustion
Blends well with: Basil tulsi, cananga, cardamom, cajuput, clary sage, cedarwood, fennel (sweet), geranium, ginger lily root, jasmine, lavandin, lemon, magnolia leaf, neroli, orange (sweet), patchouli, petitgrain, pimento berry, ravensara, ravintsara, rose absolute, sandalwood, tuberose, vanilla, vetiver, ylang ylang

Precautionary advice: Best avoided during pregnancy and while breast-feeding.

DAVANA, *Artemisia pallens*
(Plant Family: Asteraceae)

Type of plant: Small herbaceous plant that grows to around 2 feet in height, with downy silvery-white leaves, small yellow flowers, and tiny seeds

Part used: Leaves and flowering tops

Method of extraction: Steam distillation

Data: In India the flowers are cultivated for garlands to be used in ceremonies and for essential oil production. The plant has a spiritual association with the Hindu god Shiva, and the blossoms are offered as decorations for the altars and are used in traditional Indian Ayurvedic medicine. The essential oil is used in perfumes and fragrances, due to its unique fruity odor. In some parts of the world davana is used as a flavoring ingredient in beverages and baking.

Principal place of production: India

When buying look for: A dark-yellow to amber liquid with a complex aroma of sweet fruit with a slightly warm, citrus, herbaceous, aroma

Therapeutic properties: Antidepressant, anti-infectious, antimicrobial, antiseptic, calmative, decongestant, mucolytic, nervine, restorative, stomachic

Therapeutic uses: Bacterial infection, bronchial congestion, coughs, colds, influenza, nervous stomach, indigestion, nausea, menstrual cramp, menopausal symptoms, general debility, anxiety, stress, irritability, tension

Blends well with: Basil linalol, basil tulsi, cardamom, clary sage, frankincense, galbanum, geranium, ginger, grapefruit, lavender (spike), lemon, lime, manuka, mastic, may chang, rosemary, rosewood, spikenard, vetiver, ylang ylang

Precautionary advice: Best avoided during pregnancy and while breast-feeding.

DILL SEED, *Anethum graveolens*
(Plant Family: Apiaceae/Umbelliferae)

Type of plant: Tall herb with green feathery leaves and a large flower head with many small yellow flowers and small seeds

Part used: Seeds

Method of extraction: Steam distillation

Data: Dill has been used for thousands of years in cooking and in medicine and has been an integral part of herb gardens since the Middle Ages. Dill is still a part of many European pharmacopeias. The main ingredient of babies' gripe water for colic is dill. The recipe for cucumbers pickled in dill was first made for King Charles I in 1640.

Principal places of production: England, Hungary, France, Spain, Germany

When buying look for: A colorless to yellow liquid with a fresh, grassy, sweet, slightly spicy aroma. Not to be confused with Indian dill (*Anethum sowa*).

Therapeutic properties: Antiputrescent, antiseptic, antispasmodic, calmative, carminative, cholagogue, decongestive, depurative, digestive, hepatic, sedative

Therapeutic uses: Colic, indigestion, dyspepsia, flatulence, gastrointestinal spasm, intestinal cramp, gastric spasm, irritable bowel syndrome, diverticulosis, constipation, detoxifying, headaches, nervous stomach, menstrual pain, digestive stimulant, nervousness

Blends well with: Angelica seed, aniseed, bergamot, caraway seed, cardamom, cinnamon leaf, coriander seed, fennel (sweet), grapefruit, juniper berry, lemon, mandarin, may chang, nutmeg, orange (sweet), petitgrain, spearmint

Precautionary advice: Best avoided if using multiple medications.

ELEMI, *Canarium luzonicum*
(Plant Family: Burseraceae)

Type of plant: Tall evergreen tree with glossy, dark-green leaves, yellow flowers and olive-like fruits

Part used: Gum resin

Method of extraction: Steam distillation

Data: The tree trunk is cut in long horizontal lines, from which the white gum resin exudes profusely and is collected daily or weekly, depending on the age of the tree. Most often the gum is exported to Europe, where it is distilled. The tree, known as the *canary tree*, is native to the Philippines. Also known as *Manila elemi*. Long used as an ingredient in incense and for its medicinal uses, elemi was introduced into the European pharmacopeias in the sixteenth century and was said to heal wounds and broken bones. Elemi was once added to artists' lacquers and varnish.

Principal places of production: Moluccas Islands (Philippines), Indonesia

When buying look for: A colorless to pale-yellow liquid with a fresh, citrus, slightly peppery, balsamic aroma

Therapeutic properties: Analgesic, anti-infectious, antiseptic, antispasmodic, cicatrizing, expectorant, pectoral, stimulant, stomachic, tonic

Therapeutic uses: Respiratory tract infection, chronic cough, catarrh, stress-related bronchial conditions, muscular fatigue, overworked muscles, infectious skin conditions, wounds, cuts and grazes, tiredness; soothing and calming

Blends well with: Benzoin, bergamot, chamomile maroc, cinnamon leaf, citronella, clove bud, eucalyptus lemon, eucalyptus radiata, frankincense, grapefruit, lavender, lemon, lemongrass, manuka, marjoram (sweet), myrrh, myrtle, palmarosa, pimento berry, ravensara, rosemary, sage (Greek), tea tree, thyme linalol

Precautionary advice: No contraindications known

EUCALYPTUS GLOBULUS (BLUE GUM),
Eucalyptus globulus (Plant Family: Myrtaceae)

Type of plant: Fast-growing tree that can grow to over 300 feet with a smooth, whitish-blue bark, long, silver-green, sickle-shaped leaves, and large white or cream-colored flowers

Part used: Leaves and twigs

Method of extraction: Steam distillation

Data: Native to Tasmania and New South Wales in Australia, the tree was first recorded in Tasmania in 1792 and the oil was first distilled in Australia in the 1850s. By the turn of the twentieth century the Tasmanian Eucalyptus Oil Company, with its platypus logo, was the most highly respected supplier. The medicinal properties of eucalyptus were quickly recognized, while the tree itself was appreciated because it uses large amounts of water and can turn swamp into usable land while at the same time eliminating the standing water in which mosquitoes thrive. The tree has been exported to many areas north and south of the Mediterranean and elsewhere in the world. In the late nineteenth century it was exported to South Africa, where the wood was used for mine building.

Principal places of production: Tasmania, Australia, China, Portugal, Spain, United States, Brazil, Nepal

When buying look for: A thin, colorless to pale-yellow liquid with an intense, fresh, green, camphorous, woody aroma

Therapeutic properties: Analgesic, anthelmintic, antibacterial, antifungal, anti-infectious, anti-inflammatory, antimicrobial, antiputrescent, antirheumatic, antiseptic, antiviral, expectorant, febrifuge, pectoral

Therapeutic uses: Respiratory infection, bronchitis, infectious disease, fever, catarrh, sinusitis,

586   *The* Complete Book *of* Essential Oils *and* Aromatherapy

fever, muscular aches and pains, rheumatism, arthritis, urinary infection, cystitis, parasitic infection

Blends well with: Basil linalol, black pepper, cedarwood, chamomile german, cypress, elemi, fragonia, frankincense, geranium, ginger, immortelle, juniper berry, lavandin, lemon, manuka, peppermint, rosemary, tangerine, thyme linalol

Precautionary advice: Eucalyptus radiata is preferable for use with seniors and those convalescing. Avoid during pregnancy and while breast-feeding.

EUCALYPTUS LEMON, *Eucalyptus citriodora, Corymbia citriodora* (Plant Family: Myrtaceae)

Type of plant: Evergreen tree growing over 100 feet in height with a smooth, blotchy, white, pink, or copper-colored trunk, slim leaves, fluffy, white flowers, and reddish-black glossy seeds

Part used: Leaves and twigs

Method of extraction: Steam distillation

Data: Also known as lemon-scented gum, or spotted gum, the tree is native to Queensland in northeastern Australia, although it has been extensively exported over the years. In oil production, the tree is sometimes cut back to encourage new growth because most oil is concentrated in the new leaves. The wood is used in situations requiring strength and flexibility, such as in ship building, bridge construction, flooring, handles of shovels and picks, and so on. The tree is also valued because it attracts bees and facilitates honey production.

Principal places of production: Australia, Tasmania, Brazil, China, India, Paraguay, Madagascar

When buying look for: A colorless to light-yellow liquid with an intense citrus, balsamic aroma.

Therapeutic properties: Analgesic, antibacterial, antifungal, anti-infectious, anti-inflammatory, antiseptic, antispasmodic, calmative, insect deterrent, vulnerary

Therapeutic uses: Muscular injury, fungal skin infection, bacterial skin infection, sores, wounds, respiratory tract conditions, asthma, fever, candida, insect bites, insect repellent

Blends well with: Basil linalol, black pepper, cedarwood, cypress, elemi, eucalyptus peppermint, eucalyptus radiata, fragonia, geranium, ginger, immortelle, juniper berry, lavandin, lavender, manuka, marjoram (sweet), peppermint, pine, ravensara, ravintsara, rosemary, tangerine, tea tree, thyme linalol, vetiver

Precautionary advice: No contraindications known

EUCALYPTUS PEPPERMINT, *Eucalyptus dives* (Plant Family: Myrtaceae)

Type of plant: Tree growing to 60 feet in height with a furrowed gray bark and broader leaves than other eucalyptus varieties, with small fluffy flowers

Part used: Leaves and twigs

Method of extraction: Steam distillation

Data: Two species of Australian eucalyptus are known as eucalyptus peppermint, and the oil most commonly used in aromatherapy is *Eucalyptus dives*. The other, *Eucalyptus piperita*, was known as the Sydney Peppermint and is native to New South Wales. In 1790 the British "Surgeon to the First Fleet," Dr. John White, published his *Journal of a Voyage to New South Wales*, in which he states that he personally distilled essential oil from *Eucalyptus piperita* in 1788, making it the earliest known eucalyptus distillation. *Eucalyptus dives* is native to the coastal regions of New

South Wales and Victoria and can flower and fruit when only six feet in height. Known as broad-leafed peppermint, this species was used by native Aborigines as a medicine, especially in cases of fever, when the smoke is wafted over the person. It's in some pharmaceutical preparations, mouthwashes, and veterinary medicines.

Principal places of production: Australia, Tasmania

When buying look for: A thin, pale-yellow liquid with a woody, balsamic aroma and a characteristic peppermint note

Therapeutic properties: Analgesic, antibacterial, anti-inflammatory, antineuralgic, antiseptic, expectorant, mucolytic, pectoral, spasmolytic, stimulant, vasodilatory

Therapeutic uses: Respiratory infection, sinusitis, sinus headache, influenza, fever, headache, migraine, rheumatism, arthritis, muscular aches and pains, leg cramp, abdominal cramp, menstrual cramp, neuralgia, inflammatory conditions, candida, cellulite, parasitic infections, head lice, fatigue, exhaustion, acne, pimples

Blends well with: Bay laurel, bergamot, black pepper, chamomile german, cypress, elemi, fennel (sweet), frankincense, geranium, immortelle, lavandin, lavender, lemon, manuka, myrtle, ravintsara, tangerine, thyme linalol, yuzu

Precautionary advice: Those prone to allergic skin reactions are advised to carry out a skin patch test. Best avoided during pregnancy and while breast-feeding.

EUCALYPTUS RADIATA, *Eucalyptus radiata* (Plant Family: Myrtaceae)

Type of plant: Tree growing to 100 feet with black bark at the lower level and smooth bark at the top, with thin, lance-shaped leaves and numerous flowers

Part used: Leaves and twigs

Method of extraction: Steam distillation

Data: The natural habitat of this tree is along banks of creeks or rivers and coastal mountain ranges in New South Wales, Australia. The tree is known as river white gum and has more oil glands in its leaves than other eucalyptus species. The first known record of *Eucalyptus radiata* distillation dates to 1898, although a Melbourne pharmacist was apparently using it decades before this. Today *Eucalyptus radiata* is considered the most appropriate eucalyptus oil for general aromatherapy use.

Principal places of production: Australia, Tasmania, South Africa, Russia

When buying look for: A thin, colorless to yellow-tinged liquid with a softer eucalyptus aroma and a slightly woody note. Also known as *Eucalyptus australiana.*

Therapeutic properties: Analgesic, antibacterial, anti-infectious, anti-inflammatory, antiphlogistic, antirheumatic, antiseptic, antispasmodic, antitussive, antiviral, expectorant, febrifuge, immunostimulant, pectoral, tonic, vulnerary

Therapeutic uses: Respiratory tract infection, bronchitis, catarrh, sinusitis, rhinitis, colds, influenza, fever, asthma, rheumatism, muscular aches and pains, neuralgia, abdominal cramp, menstrual cramp, headaches, mental exhaustion, fatigue, insect stings and bites; general stimulant and tonic

Blends well with: Basil linalol, black pepper, cedarwood, chamomile german, chamomile roman, elemi, eucalyptus peppermint, eucalyptus radiata, fragonia, geranium, grapefruit, immortelle, juniper berry, lavandin, lavender, lemon, manuka, niaouli, pine, ravensara, ravintsara, rosemary, tangerine, tea tree, thyme linalol

Precautionary advice: No contraindications known

FENNEL, SWEET, *Foeniculum vulgare var. dulce* (Plant Family: Apiaceae/Umbelliferae)

Type of plant: Tall herb growing up to 5 feet tall with delicate, feathery, lace-like leaves and small yellow flowers on a flowering head

Part used: Seeds

Method of extraction: Steam distillation

Data: The seeds are dried before distillation. Fennel was a favorite with the ancient Greeks and Romans, who used it extensively in medicine and cooking. They believed it gave strength and long life, helped the eyesight, aided lactation, and eased menstrual problems, as well as being able to stave off hunger. The plant originated in the Mediterranean area but is now grown all over the world.

Principal places of production: Hungary, France, Germany, Italy, India, Japan, Bulgaria, Russia, Moldova, Romania

When buying look for: A thin, colorless to pale yellow liquid with a warm, sweet, aniseed-like, peppery aroma. Not to be confused with bitter fennel (*Foeniculum vulgare var. amara*).

Therapeutic properties: Anti-inflammatory, antiseptic, antispasmodic, carminative, depurative, diuretic, emmenagogue, expectorant, spasmolytic, stomachic, vermifuge

Therapeutic uses: Digestive disorders, colic, dyspepsia, gastrointestinal spasm, flatulence, nausea, constipation, irritable bowel syndrome, abdominal spasm, menstrual problems, menstrual cramp, premenstrual syndrome, fertility, endometriosis, menopausal symptoms, detoxifying, cellulite, fluid retention, heavy legs, bronchitis, respiratory conditions, parasitic infection

Blends well with: Bergamot, black pepper, cananga, caraway seed, cardamom, chamomile german, chamomile roman, geranium, ginger, grapefruit, ho wood, juniper berry, lavandin, lavender, lemon, mandarin, orange (sweet)

Precautionary advice: Best avoided if using multiple medications. Avoid during pregnancy and while breast-feeding. GRAS status.

FIR, SILVER, *Abies alba* (Plant Family: Pinaceae)

Type of plant: Coniferous tree growing to over 150 feet high with flattened needle foliage and long cones

Part used: Needles and twigs

Method of extraction: Steam distillation

Data: Native to central Europe, the silver fir tree grows at altitudes between 1,000 and 6,000 feet. Sometimes known as *silver* or *white spruce*. Fir is used as an ingredient in cough preparations and, in combination with camphor, for rheumatic treatments. Often used in aftershaves and deodorants. The needles are put on the heat source in saunas. Often grown as Christmas trees.

Principal places of production: Austria, Poland, Germany, Croatia, Russia

When buying look for: A colorless to pale-yellow-tinged liquid with a soft balsamic, fresh fir aroma

Therapeutic properties: Analgesic, antiseptic, antitussive, expectorant, pectoral, tonic

Therapeutic uses: Catarrh, sinusitis, bronchitis, bronchial tract discomfort, dry cough, rheumatism, muscular aches and pains, feverishness, anxiety, tension; general tonic

Blends well with: Black pepper, cedarwood, chamomile german, chamomile maroc, cypress, eucalyptus radiata, frankincense, geranium, lavandin, lavender (spike), lemon, orange (sweet)

Precautionary advice: Best avoided by those with respiratory problems

FRAGONIA, *Agonis fragrans* (Plant Family: Myrtaceae)

Type of plant: Flowering shrub growing up to 7 or 8 feet high with small clusters of white flowers with pink centers

Part used: Leaves and twigs

Method of extraction: Steam distillation

Data: Grows wild along the southern coast

of Western Australia and was only recently identified as an essential oil–bearing plant with therapeutic properties. For this reason there has been little scientific research into the various chemotypes of oil that could be produced. However, what research has been done has shown that fragonia is antibacterial, antifungal, and anti-inflammatory. It is distilled when the leaves are fresh. This is a well-balanced, powerfully medicinal essential oil, gentle on the skin, with a pleasant aroma. It has therapeutic similarities to tea tree oil, but its aroma is far more appealing. Sometimes called *coarse tea tree*.

Principal place of production: Australia

When buying look for: Thin, colorless to yellow liquid with a fresh, green, slightly spicy, balsamic, fruity aroma

Therapeutic properties: Analgesic, antibacterial, antifungal, anti-infectious, anti-inflammatory, antimicrobial, antiputrescent, immunostimulant, mucolytic, pectoral, restorative, spasmolytic, vulnerary

Therapeutic uses: Respiratory conditions, bronchitis, catarrh, sinus congestion, colds, bacterial and fungal infection, skin infection, pain, acne, pimples, inflammatory muscular conditions, muscular aches and pain

Blends well with: Basil linalol, bay laurel, bergamot, chamomile german, chamomile roman, elemi, eucalyptus lemon, eucalyptus peppermint, frankincense, geranium, ho wood, lemon, lemongrass, manuka, mastic, orange (sweet), oregano, palmarosa, ravensara, ravintsara, spearmint, tea tree, thyme linalol

Precautionary advice: No contraindications known

FRANKINCENSE, *Boswellia carterii*
(Plant Family: Burseraceae)

Type of plant: Small, woody tree that grows to around 25 feet high with sparse, small green leaves and small, waxy, white flowers with yellow and orange centers

Part used: Oleoresin

Method of extraction: Steam distillation

Data: Frankincense has always been prized as an incense material. It was one of the three gifts brought to the baby Jesus and is used around the world in religious practice and ceremony. It is also used as incense to clear negative energy and bring good fortune to both business and home life. To obtain the resin, the tree is slashed to make an incision, causing the tree to exude an opaque, whitish-yellowish resin that forms into pear-shaped tears that, when hardened, can be collected. The tears are graded, with the whitest being the most prized. The essential oil is distilled from the crude gum. Several varieties of frankincense are used for essential oil production, but the properties usually attributed to frankincense in aromatherapy are from the species *Boswellia carterii* and *Boswellia sacra*. Other varieties used to produce essential oil include Indian frankincense (*Boswellia serrata*).

Principal places of production: Oman (Plain of Dhofar), Somalia, Ethiopia

When buying look for: Thin, colorless to pale-yellow liquid with a warm, sweet, balsamic, spicy, incense-like aroma

Therapeutic properties: Antibacterial, antidepressant, antimicrobial, antiseptic, calmative, cicatrizing, cytophylactic, expectorant, nervine, restorative, tonic

Therapeutic uses: Coughs, colds, bronchitis, nervous asthma, skin infection, scars, wounds, urinary tract infection, mental fatigue, depression, nervousness, stress, tension, inability to communicate

Blends well with: Angelica root, bergamot, carnation, chamomile maroc, chamomile roman, cistus, clary sage, coriander seed, cypress, geranium, ginger, grapefruit, immortelle, juniper berry, lavender, lemon, linden blossom,

mandarin, mastic, myrrh, neroli, orange (sweet), patchouli, rose absolute, rose otto, sandalwood, spikenard, valerian, ylang ylang
Precautionary advice: No contraindications known

GALBANUM, *Ferula galbaniflua, F. gummosa* (Plant Family: Apiaceae/Umbelliferae)

Type of plant: Tall plant that can grow up to 6 feet high with thick stalks and large flower heads covered in small, yellow, seed-bearing flowers, reminiscent of fennel
Part used: Gum resin
Method of extraction: Steam distillation
Data: The gum is harvested from an outgrowth on the root collar of the plant, which has to be deliberately exposed before scoring, allowing the gum resin to exude. It hardens into brownish tears over a couple of days and is then collected. Further cuts at the site release more gum resin, and the process is repeated. Galbanum is one of the ingredients in the anointing oil instructions given to Moses on Mount Sinai. Hippocrates is known to have used it as a medicine, while Pliny ascribed magical powers to it. In the Middle East, galbanum is still used in medicine, perfumery, incense, and purification ceremonies.
Principal places of production: Iran, Lebanon
When buying look for: A colorless to pale-yellow or slightly green liquid with an intense, green, earthy, peppery aroma
Therapeutic properties: Anti-inflammatory, antimicrobial, antiseptic, calmative, carminative, cicatrizing, digestive, nervine, spasmolytic, tonic
Therapeutic uses: Skin infection, inflammatory skin disorders, acne, pimples, cuts and grazes, wounds, scarring, bronchitis, coughs, respiratory difficulties, inflammatory muscular aches and pains, rheumatoid arthritis, indigestion, stress- and nerve-related conditions

Blends well with: Bergamot, cardamom, cedarwood, chamomile german, chamomile roman, cinnamon leaf, clove bud, frankincense, geranium, juniper berry, lavender, lemon, lemongrass, manuka, melissa, myrtle, narcissus, niaouli, nutmeg, orange (sweet), patchouli, ravensara, rose maroc, spikenard, valerian, violet leaf, yarrow
Precautionary advice: No contraindications known

GERANIUM, *Pelargonium graveolens, P. roseum, P. asperum* (Plant Family: Geraniaceae)

Type of plant: Plant with shapely, finely divided, deeply cut leaves with clusters of small pink flowers
Part used: Leaves and stalks
Method of extraction: Steam distillation
Data: The essential oil is distilled from the aromatic, freshly cut young plant tops. The plant material can be left in the field to partially dry before distillation so the fragrance is more intense. The final aroma can depend on the variety being distilled, as well as the age of the leaves and stems being distilled. The essential oil is concentrated in the young growth and will turn from a lemony-rose to a rose-type aroma when crushed. Omitting the older stems during distillation produces a more rose-like aroma. The essential oil is native to southern Africa, although the most prized oil for perfumery comes from an island off Madagascar, Réunion, formerly known as Ile de Bourbon, hence the name *geranium bourbon*. Several varieties of geranium are distilled for their oil: *Pelargonium graveolens, P. roseum, P. asperum, P. radens*, and *P. capitatum*.
Principal places of production: Réunion, Madagascar, South Africa, Egypt, China
When buying look for: A pale-yellow to pale-

Beware

green liquid with a sweet, soft, flowery-rose, green aroma
Therapeutic properties: Analgesic, antibacterial, antidepressant, anti-infectious, anti-inflammatory, antiseptic, astringent, circulatory, hemostatic, nervine, restorative, spasmolytic, stimulant, tonic, vulnerary
Therapeutic uses: Female reproductive disorders, menstrual cramp, infertility, endometriosis, premenstrual syndrome, menopausal symptoms, circulatory disorders, Reynaud's disease, varicose veins, hemorrhoids, neuralgia, nervous skin disorders, depression, fatigue, emotional crisis, stress-related conditions
Blends well with: Basil linalol, bay (West Indian), benzoin, bergamot, black pepper, cajuput, cananga, cardamom, carnation, chamomile german, chamomile maroc, chamomile roman, cistus, clary sage, cypress, fennel (sweet), frankincense, ginger, grapefruit, hyssop decumbens, immortelle, jasmine, juniper berry, lavender, lemon, mandarin, myrtle, neroli, orange (sweet), peppermint, patchouli, rose absolute, rosemary, rose otto, sandalwood, spearmint, vetiver, ylang ylang
Precautionary advice: No contraindications known. GRAS status.

GERANIUM, BULGARIAN (ZDRAVETZ), *Geranium macrorrhizum*
(Plant Family: Geraniaceae)

Type of plant: Fast-growing, self-rooting perennial plant growing to 2 feet high with pink flowers
Part used: Leaves and stems
Method of extraction: Steam distillation
Data: Often called Bulgarian geranium or geranium Robert because the plant is in the *Robertium* subgenus of the genus *Geranium*. The plant is also called *bigroot geranium* or *rock cranesbill*, as it grows in rocky, shaded areas and is found on almost all of Bulgaria's mountain ranges. Zdravetz is known as a health bringer in Bulgaria, where it has long been part of the traditional herbal healing system.
Principal place of production: Bulgaria
When buying look for: A crystalline consistency of light-green to dark-green color with a warm, green, spicy, herbaceous, floral aroma. Crystallizes when cold and becomes liquid when warm.
Therapeutic properties: Antidepressant, anti-infectious, antispasmodic, carminative, diaphoretic, febrifuge, hypertensive, nervine, sedative, stimulating
Therapeutic uses: Menstrual problems, menopausal symptoms, infertility, insomnia, nervous depression, fatigue, skin conditions — irritation, soreness, problematic skin
Blends well with: Basil linalol, basil tulsi, bay laurel, carrot seed, chamomile german, clary sage, cypress, hyssop decumbens, juniper berry, lavandin, lavender, lavender (spike), marjoram (sweet), myrtle, oregano, rosemary, sage (Greek), thyme linalol, valerian, yarrow
Precautionary advice: No contraindications known

GINGER, *Zingiber officinale*
(Plant Family: Zingiberaceae)

Type of plant: Perennial herb grown from a rhizome with downward extending roots. Long, thin leaves grow from the central stalk, to a height of around 4 feet.
Part used: Rhizomes
Method of extraction: Steam and CO_2 distillation
Data: The rhizomes are dried for a couple of weeks after harvesting, then crushed, dried again, sieved, then distilled. Ginger is native to China and spread throughout Asia, where it was and is still considered highly medicinal. It also has a reputation for being an aphrodisiac. Ginger was

brought to Europe by Arab traders in the Middle Ages. Aside from its medicinal uses, the essential oil is also an ingredient in exotic, oriental-type perfumes. In the food industry, ginger is valuable in both sweet and savory dishes and for making ginger beer and wine.

Principal places of production: China, India, Sri Lanka, Caribbean

When buying look for: A pale-yellow to dark-yellow liquid with the warm, earthy, and spicy aroma typical of ginger

Therapeutic properties: Analgesic, antiseptic, antispasmodic, antitussive, carminative, circulatory, expectorant, febrifuge, fortifying, pectoral, stimulant, stomachic, thermogenic

Therapeutic uses: Fractures, rheumatism, arthritis, muscle fatigue, muscular weakness, numbness, menstrual cramp, gastrointestinal spasm, digestive problems, flatulence, diverticulosis, irritable bowel syndrome, constipation, nausea, sea and travel sickness, colds, chills, influenza, sinus congestion, chronic catarrh, circulatory tonic, Raynaud's disease, cold limbs, nervousness, mental exhaustion, general debility

Blends well with: Bay (West Indian), bergamot, black pepper, cardamom, cistus, clove bud, coriander seed, cypress, frankincense, geranium, grapefruit, immortelle, jasmine, juniper berry, lemon, lime, mandarin, marjoram (sweet), niaouli, orange (sweet), palmarosa, patchouli, petitgrain, plai, rosalina, rose maroc, rosemary, rose otto, sandalwood, spearmint, turmeric, vanilla, vetiver, ylang ylang

Precautionary advice: No contraindications known. GRAS status.

GINGER LILY ROOT (ABSOLUTE),
Hedychium spicatum
(Plant Family: Zingiberaceae)

Type of plant: Hardy perennial with horizontal root stock and large glossy leaves, growing to

3 feet high with a single stalk atop, which is a dense spike of fragrant white flowers with long, thin petals

Part used: Rhizome

Method of extraction: Steam extraction

Data: Native to China, Nepal, Bhutan, northern India, Thailand, and Myanmar. Grows at altitudes between 3,500 and 9,000 feet. Used in Ayurvedic medicine for multiple purposes. The dried and powdered rhizomes are used in incense production, and also in cooking.

Principal places of production: Nepal, India, China

When buying look for: Pale-yellow to dark-yellow liquid with a musky, green, woody, balsamic, peppery aroma

Therapeutic properties: Antibacterial, anti-inflammatory, antiseptic, carminative, digestive, expectorant, stimulant, tonic

Therapeutic uses: Cuts, scratches, wounds, respiratory conditions, insomnia, nausea, cough, chest infection, mental fatigue, anxiety, chronic fatigue, anxiety, stress, nervousness

Blends well with: Bay (West Indian), bergamot, black pepper, cardamom, coriander seed, frankincense, geranium, immortelle, jasmine, juniper berry, lemon, lime, mandarin, marjoram (sweet), niaouli, orange (sweet), palmarosa, patchouli, petitgrain, plai, rosalina, sandalwood, spearmint, turmeric, vanilla, vetiver, ylang ylang

Precautionary advice: Those with highly sensitive skin or prone to allergic skin reaction are advised to carry out a skin patch test.

GRAPEFRUIT, *Citrus paradisi*
(Plant Family: Rutaceae)

Type of plant: Subtropical evergreen tree with fragrant white flowers and large yellow fruit

Part used: Fruit rind

Method of extraction: Cold expression

Data: The origin of the plant is uncertain, being a hybrid. Some say it was introduced into the

Caribbean from China by a Captain Shaddock, leading to the fruit being known as Shaddock fruit; others say it was crossbred by the botanist Griffith Hughes in Barbados in 1750, leading to the name Barbados fruit. Either way, in 1809 the seeds traveled with Spanish settlers to the United States, where from 1880 on it began to be commercially grown. Today, Florida is the source of most grapefruit essential oil. Grapefruit seed has been found to be a natural preservative.

Principal places of production: United States, Mexico, Israel, Argentina, South Africa, Turkey

When buying look for: A pale-yellow liquid with a sweet, fresh, fruity, citrus aroma

Therapeutic properties: Anti-infectious, antiseptic, cholagogue, depurative, digestive, diuretic, hepatic, immunostimulant, tonic

Therapeutic uses: Muscle fatigue, muscular weakness, cellulite, obesity, migraine, headaches, fluid retention, irritable bowel syndrome, detoxifying, physical exhaustion, mental exhaustion, depression, stress

Blends well with: Angelica root, basil linalol, bergamot, black pepper, cananga, caraway seed, cardamom, clary sage, clove bud, cypress, fennel (sweet), frankincense, geranium, ginger, jasmine, juniper berry, lavandin, lavender, mandarin, myrtle, neroli, orange (sweet), patchouli, peppermint, pimento berry, rosemary, spearmint, thyme linalol, ylang ylang

Precautionary advice: Best avoided if using multiple medications. Is a low-risk photosensitizer; do not apply to the skin prior to sun exposure. GRAS status.

GREENLAND MOSS (LABRADOR TEA),
Ledum groenlandicum
(Plant Family: Ericaceae)

Type of plant: Woody, perennial evergreen shrub growing to 1 meter high, with leathery, underfolding leaves, hairy on the underside, and a single stalk atop with clusters of white flowers

Part used: Leaves

Method of extraction: Steam distillation

Data: Often wild-crafted. Although called moss, the plant is not at all moss-like. It grows well in moist soil such as peatland and is also found in coniferous forests with open canopy. A tea is made from the leaves, hence the name *Labrador tea*. The leaves are also placed in closets to deter insects and among grain to deter animal and insect pests. Canadian First Nations people have used the plant for a wide variety of medicinal purposes.

Principal place of production: Canada

When buying look for: Pale-yellow liquid with an herbaceous, balsamic, woody aroma

Therapeutic properties: Analgesic, antibacterial, antidepressant, anti-inflammatory, antiseptic, antispasmodic, circulatory, depurative, diuretic, hepatic, immunostimulant, spasmolytic, tonic

Therapeutic uses: Circulatory dysfunction, internal and soft tissue inflammation, liver conditions, detoxifying, obesity, water retention, edema, swellings, injuries, muscular aches and pains, stress-related conditions, anxiety, tension

Blends well with: Angelica root, bay laurel, cajuput, cardamom, chamomile german, chamomile roman, clary sage, cypress, geranium, ginger, hyssop decumbens, immortelle, juniper berry, lavender, lemongrass, marjoram (sweet), may chang, niaouli, ravintsara, rosemary, spearmint

Precautionary advice: Avoid prolonged use. May cause irritation on highly sensitive skins; a skin patch test is advisable. Best avoided during pregnancy and while breast-feeding.

HOP, *Humulus lupulus*
(Plant Family: Moraceae)

Type of plant: Perennial climbing plant with male and female cone-shaped strobiles, made up of imbricated scales

Part used: Female strobiles

Method of extraction: Steam distillation; solvent extraction

Data: The best known use for hops is as an ingredient in beer. It has phytoestrogenic properties, which account for its traditional use as an aid to encourage breast milk and, some say, is the cause of the "beer belly" effect. Hops have been known as a sedative for hundreds of years, and hop pillows to aid sleep are still sold the world over.

Principal places of production: England, Hungary, Croatia, Germany, France

When buying look for: A pale-yellow to dark-yellow liquid with a green, herbaceous aroma

Therapeutic properties: Antimicrobial, astringent, calmative, carminative, emollient, estrogenic, nervine, soporific, spasmolytic

Therapeutic uses: Neuralgia, bruising, analgesic, menstrual problems, menopausal symptoms, insomnia, coughs, stress-related asthma, stress-related digestive conditions, nervousness, stress, tension

Blends well with: Amyris, cananga, carnation, cedarwood, chamomile maroc, chamomile roman, clary sage, geranium, lemon, mandarin, marjoram (sweet), nutmeg, orange (sweet), spikenard, spruce, valerian, vetiver

Precautionary advice: Best avoided during pregnancy and while breast-feeding. GRAS status.

HO WOOD (LINALOOL), *Cinnamomum camphora ct. linalool* (Plant Family: Lauracea)

Type of plant: Evergreen broadleaf tree growing to 100 feet high with rough bark, glossy fragrant leaves, a profusion of white flowers, and black berries

Part used: Bark, leaves, and twigs

Method of extraction: Steam distillation

Data: Widely used in perfumery as an alternative for rosewood essential oil since rosewood became an endangered tree. Native to China,

Taiwan, Vietnam, and Japan. There are different species of this tree and they're structurally very similar, so differentiation is established by analyzing the essential oil chemotype produced by the leaves. These fall into five groups: linalool, 1,8-cineole, camphor, borneol, and nerolidol. The camphor subtype has long been an important commercial source of natural camphor. The 1,8-cineole subtype produces ravintsara essential oil. Ensure that the chemotype linalool is purchased when looking for ho wood.

Principal places of production: China, Taiwan, Vietnam

When buying look for: A colorless to pale-yellow liquid with a warm, woody, herbaceous, sweet floral aroma. Also known as *Ho-Sho* oil.

Therapeutic properties: Analgesic, anthelmintic, antibacterial, antidepressant, antifungal, anti-infectious, antiseptic, antiviral, cytophylactic, immunostimulant, restorative, tonic

Therapeutic uses: Influenza, colds, chills, bacterial and viral respiratory infection, menstrual cramp, vaginal infection, parasitic skin infection, wounds, cuts, grazes, eczema, acne, stress and stress-related conditions, anxiety, tension

Blends well with: Amyris, angelica seed, basil linalol, bay (West Indian), benzoin, black pepper, caraway seed, cedarwood, chamomile roman, clary sage, copaiba, cypress, elemi, frankincense, geranium, lemon, lemongrass, marjoram (sweet), myrtle, lavandin, lavender, ravensara, rosalina, sandalwood, tangerine

Precautionary advice: No contraindications known

HYSSOP DECUMBENS, *Hyssopus officinalis var. decumbens* (Plant Family: Lamiaceae/Labiatae)

Type of plant: Herbaceous plant growing to 2 feet high with leafy stems and spikes of purplish-blue flowers

Part used: Leaves and flowering tops
Method of extraction: Steam distillation
Data: The essential oil is distilled from fresh plant material in late summer. Hyssop was sacred to the ancient Hebrews, who used it to purify temples, and it's still used at Passover as one of the "bitter herbs." Hyssop's medicinal properties were recognized also by the ancient Greeks, who used it for chest complaints and to increase blood circulation. Also used by the Romans and throughout the Middle Ages in Europe, where it was a common sight in herb gardens.
Principal places of production: France, Spain, Slovenia, Croatia, Brazil, Palestine
When buying look for: A colorless or yellow-tinged, pale-yellow through pale-brown liquid with a fresh, intense, spicy, camphor-like, herbaceous aroma. The type referred to in this book is *Hyssop officinalis var. decumbens.*
Therapeutic properties: Antibacterial, antiviral, astringent, carminative, cicatrizing, circulatory digestive, diuretic, expectorant, pectoral, spasmolytic
Therapeutic uses: Coughs, colds, influenza, bronchitis, catarrh, asthma, bronchial infection, contusions, bruising, wounds, arthritis, rheumatism, muscular aches and pains, digestive problems
Blends well with: Bergamot, camphor (white), clary sage, eucalyptus radiata, fragonia, frankincense, geranium, immortelle, juniper berry, lavandin, lavender, lemon, mandarin, manuka, marjoram (sweet), myrtle, orange (sweet), palmarosa, ravintsara, rosemary, sage (Greek), tea tree
Precautionary advice: Avoid during pregnancy and while breast-feeding. GRAS status.

IMMORTELLE (ITALIAN EVERLASTING/ HELICHRYSUM), *Helichrysum italicum* (Plant Family: Asteraceae/Compositae)

Type of plant: Bushy herb with very small, velvety leaves off long stems, each with a cluster of small yellow flowers

Part used: Flowering-head clusters
Method of extraction: Steam distillation
Data: The flowers are comprised of dry bracts rather than petals and last a very long time — hence the name *everlasting*. Listed as a medicinal herb in many Greek, Roman, and medieval European texts. There are hundreds of helichrysum/ immortelle varieties, but few produce essential oil.
Principal places of production: France (Corsica), Spain, Italy, Hungary, Bulgaria, Croatia
When buying look for: A pale-yellow liquid with a warm, earthy, herbaceous, slightly floral and hay-like aroma
Therapeutic properties: Analgesic, anticholagogue, anticoagulant, anti-inflammatory, cicatrizing, circulatory diuretic, expectorant, hepatic, mucolytic, spasmodic, stimulant, vulnerary
Therapeutic uses: Pain, bruising, wounds, contusions, coughs, bronchial congestion, rhinitis, abdominal cramp, muscular spasm, rheumatism, arthritis, carpel tunnel, tendonitis, edema, varicose veins, hemorrhoids, circulatory conditions, ulceration, acne, pimples, eczema, psoriasis
Blends well with: Basil linalol, bay laurel, bergamot, chamomile roman, clary sage, cypress, fragonia, frankincense, geranium, grapefruit, juniper berry, lavender, lavender (spike), lemon, marjoram (sweet), niaouli, orange (sweet), palmarosa, pine, plai, ravensara, rosemary, tea tree, thyme linalol, vetiver, ylang ylang
Precautionary advice: Avoid prolonged use. Best avoided during pregnancy and while breast-feeding.

JASMINE (ABSOLUTE), *Jasminum grandiflorum, J. officinale* (Plant Family: Oleaceae)

Type of plant: Climbing shrub with dark-green leaves and small, star-shaped, highly fragrant, white flowers
Part used: Flowers

Method of extraction: CO_2 or solvent extraction

Data: The delicate flowers are hand-picked before dawn, when their aroma is most intense, then they're processed to produce a concrete from which the absolute is obtained. Over a ton of flowers are required to produce 4 pounds of absolute. This is a very labor-intensive process, which accounts for the high price of jasmine. Native to the valleys of the Himalayas in northeast India, the highly fragrant jasmine was brought to Europe by Spanish seafarers in the sixteenth century. When perfumery became an important industry in Grasse, France, jasmine was at its core. The medicinal qualities of jasmine have been utilized for centuries in India, China, and Arabia — the native source of a jasmine variety with fleshier petals, *Jasminum sambac.* Today, jasmine tea is valued in China, and jasmine flower garlands are offered to guests in India.

Principal places of production: France, India, Egypt, China

When buying look for: Viscous, golden amber to orange-brown liquid with a sweet, rich, intensely, floral aroma

Therapeutic properties: Antidepressant, antiseptic, antispasmodic, calmative, cicatrizing, nervine, sedative, stimulant

Therapeutic uses: Infertility, menstrual cramp, abdominal spasm, nervous tension, nervousness, stress-related conditions, lethargy, apathy, fatigue, insecurity, low self-esteem, anxiety, depression

Blends well with: Amyris, bergamot, black pepper, cardamom, chamomile roman, cistus, clary sage, coriander seed, frankincense, geranium, ginger, grapefruit, lemon, linden blossom, mandarin, melissa, neroli, orange (sweet), petitgrain, rose maroc, sandalwood, ylang ylang, yuzu

Precautionary advice: No contraindications known. GRAS status.

JUNIPER BERRY, *Juniperus communis*
(Plant Family: Cupressaceae)

Type of plant: Low-growing woody shrub or tree growing to 30 feet high, with short green needles and dark-blue, berry-like seed cones

Part used: Berries

Method of extraction: Steam distillation

Data: A wide-ranging plant covering all areas of the northern hemisphere. Juniper branches are still used in spiritual ceremonies in Tibet and by First Nations peoples in America. Juniper berries were used in many medicinal systems, including in China and in ancient Egypt from the predynastic period. Juniper was burned in Paleolithic times in Europe, and in historic times was used to ward off disease. Juniper berries are best known as the raw material of gin.

Principal places of production: Italy, France, Spain, Hungary, Croatia, United States

When buying look for: A colorless to pale-yellow liquid with a fresh, green, fruity, slightly woody aroma, reminiscent of gin

Therapeutic properties: Analgesic, anthelmintic, anti-inflammatory, antiseptic, carminative, depurative, diuretic, emmenagogue, nervine, spasmolytic, tonic

Therapeutic uses: Fluid retention, cystitis, urinary tract infection, abdominal bloating, menstrual cramp, heavy legs, detoxifying, cellulite, obesity, gout, rheumatism, arthritis, acne, ulceration, eczema, mental exhaustion, chronic fatigue, anxiety, tension

Blends well with: Basil linalol, basil tulsi, bay laurel, bergamot, caraway seed, cardamom, carrot seed, cedarwood, celery seed, chamomile german, chamomile roman, cistus, citronella, clary sage, copaiba, cypress, fennel (sweet), frankincense, geranium, grapefruit, greenland moss, immortelle, lavandin, lavender, lavender (spike), lemon, mandarin, marjoram (sweet), myrtle, orange (sweet), oregano, peppermint, pine, plai, rose absolute, rosemary, rose otto, sage (Greek), sandalwood, saro, tarragon, thyme linalol, turmeric, violet leaf, yarrow

Precautionary advice: Best avoided by those with kidney disorders. Best avoided during pregnancy. GRAS status.

LAVANDIN, *Lavandula x intermedia* (Plant Family: Lamiaceae/Labiatae)

Type of plant: Shrub-like bush that grows taller than lavender, with three flowering heads on each stem, ranging from grayish-blue to intense purple

Part used: Flowering tops

Method of extraction: Steam distillation

Data: Also known as *Lavandula hybrida, L. hybrida grosso,* or *L. abrialis,* lavandin is a spontaneous hybrid between true lavender and spike lavender. It developed due to insect pollination in the area crossed by the two parent varieties, which is above 500 meters in altitude but below 700 meters. The essential oil has been produced for over 100 years. It should not be confused with lavender, which has therapeutic properties not matched by lavandin.

Principal places of production: France, Spain, Hungary, Bulgaria

When buying look for: Colorless to pale-yellow liquid with an herbaceous, floral, camphor-like aroma

Therapeutic properties: Analgesic, antibacterial, anti-infectious, anti-inflammatory, antiseptic, antispasmodic, nervine, sedative, vulnerary

Therapeutic uses: Skin infection, wounds, menstrual cramp, muscular cramp and contraction, muscular spasm, muscular injury, migraine, stress, tension, respiratory tract infection, pimples, acne, pain relief

Blends well with: Basil linalol, bergamot, black pepper, cedarwood, chamomile german, chamomile roman, clary sage, cypress, elemi, eucalyptus lemon, eucalyptus radiata, frankincense, geranium, ginger, greenland moss, immortelle, juniper berry, lemon, mandarin, manuka, marjoram (sweet), myrtle, niaouli, orange (sweet), oregano, palmarosa, plai, ravensara, spearmint, tangerine, tarragon, tea tree, thyme linalol, vetiver, yarrow, ylang ylang

Precautionary advice: No contraindications known

LAVENDER, *Lavandula angustifolia* (Plant Family: Lamiaceae/Labiatae)

Type of plant: A shrubby evergreen bush with silver, spike-shaped, grayish-green leaves and flowers in various shades of lavender to purple on top of tall, stiff stems

Part used: Flowering tops

Method of extraction: Steam and CO_2 distillation

Data: The plant is harvested in midsummer, left to dry for a couple of days to maximize the aroma, then distilled. Wild French lavender, grown at high altitude — over 2,800 feet — is categorized as "true" French lavender, particularly when grown in the Alpes de Haute region of Provence. Generally in France, lavender grows above 1,650 feet. Today lavender is grown in many countries, each version having somewhat different properties. The ancient Greeks, Persians, and Romans burned lavender in rooms where people were sick. The word *lavender* is derived from the Latin word *lavera,* "to wash," because the Romans used the flowers in their baths.

Principal places of production: France, United Kingdom, Bulgaria, Hungary, Croatia, China, Russia, Tasmania

When buying look for: Colorless to yellow-tinged liquid with a fresh, soft, floral, herbaceous aroma

Therapeutic properties: Analgesic, anthelmintic, antibacterial, antidepressant, anti-infectious, anti-inflammatory, antimicrobial, antiseptic, antivenomous, calmative, cicatrizing, cytophylactic, sedative, soporific, spasmolytic, vulnerary

Therapeutic uses: Inflammatory conditions, skin infection, wounds, cuts, grazes, rashes, itching, stress-related eczema, nervous psoriasis, sunburn, burns, muscular spasm, muscular contraction, abdominal cramp, headache, migraine, insomnia, nervousness and related conditions, acne, pimples, insect bites, stress, tension, anxiety, tension, panic; insect deterrent

Blends well with: Basil linalol, bergamot, black pepper, cedarwood, chamomile german, chamomile roman, clary sage, cypress, elemi, eucalyptus lemon, eucalyptus radiata, frankincense, geranium, ginger, ginger lily root, grapefruit, greenland moss, immortelle, juniper berry, lemon, lemongrass, mandarin, manuka, marjoram (sweet), melissa, myrtle, niaouli, orange (sweet), oregano, palmarosa, petitgrain, pine, plai, ravensara, ravintsara, rose maroc, rosemary, rose otto, spearmint, spikenard, spruce, tangerine, tea tree, thyme linalol, valerian, vetiver, yarrow

Precautionary advice: No contraindications known. GRAS status.

LAVENDER, SPIKE, *Lavandula latifolia*, *L. spica* (Plant Family: Lamiaceae/Labiatae)

Type of plant: A bushy, herbaceous plant with spike-shaped, silver leaves and purple flowers on top of tall stiff stems

Part used: Flowering tops

Method of extraction: Steam distillation

Data: During distillation, spike lavender produces three times as much essential oil as true lavender and is sometimes used as an adulterant. Being lower-priced, spike was once very popular with the perfume industry and was used in "lavender" soaps and fragrances. Wild spike lavender grows at much lower altitudes than true

lavender, and today it is mostly gathered from wild locations in Spain. It's known in France as broadleaf lavender, as its leaves are wider.

Principal places of production: Spain, France, Croatia, Hungary

When buying look for: A colorless to yellow-tinged liquid with a fresh, herbaceous, floral aroma and a camphorous note

Therapeutic properties: Analgesic, antibacterial, antifungal, antiseptic, decongestant, expectorant, spasmolytic, insect repellent

Therapeutic uses: Skin infection, wounds, cuts, grazes, muscular spasm, muscular contraction, abdominal cramp, headache, migraine, acne, pimples, insect bites; insect deterrent

Blends well with: Basil linalol, bay laurel, cajuput, camphor (white), cinnamon leaf, clary sage, clove bud, cypress, eucalyptus radiata, fir (silver), geranium, grapefruit, ho wood, hyssop decumbens, juniper berry, lemon, lemongrass, manuka, marjoram (sweet), myrtle, palmarosa, peppermint, pine, plai, sage (Greek), spruce, ravensara, rosemary, tea tree, vetiver, ylang ylang

Precautionary advice: No contraindications known. GRAS status.

LEMON, *Citrus limon* (Plant Family: Rutaceae)

Type of plant: A small evergreen tree with glossy leaves, highly fragrant white flowers, and yellow fruit

Part used: Fresh fruit rind

Method of extraction: Cold expression / steam distillation

Data: The lemon tree produces fruit all year, so fruits are harvested when ripe, all year round. In cold expression, the lemon is pressed to release the essential oil, and then centrifugation separates any water from the essential oil. The lemon was unknown in Europe until Alexander the Great brought it back from Asia. India is thought to be its country of origin. The essential oil contains vitamins and minerals, and the juice is a source of citric acid. Lemon essential oil is effective in removing stains and polishing metal and is used as a solvent.

Principal places of production: Argentina, United States, Italy, Spain, Brazil, Greece, South Africa, China

When buying look for: A pale-yellow to faintly greenish liquid with a sweet, light, fruity, fresh citrus aroma

Therapeutic properties: Anti-infectious, antimicrobial, antiseptic, antispasmodic, antiviral, astringent, calmative, carminative, cicatrizing, circulatory, depurative, digestive, diuretic, hemostatic, stimulant, tonic, vermifuge

Therapeutic uses: Digestive problems, loss of appetite, detoxifying, cellulite, bronchial conditions, influenza, sore throats, laryngitis, acne, skin infections, herpes, abscesses, physical exhaustion, fatigue, debilitation, insect bites, anxious depression, nervous tension, inability to concentrate or focus

Blends well with: Most other essential oils: bay (West Indian), bay laurel, black pepper, cananga, cedarwood, chamomile maroc, chamomile roman, cinnamon leaf, cistus, clary sage, coriander seed, cypress, eucalyptus lemon, eucalyptus peppermint, eucalyptus radiata, fennel (sweet), fragonia, frankincense, galbanum, geranium, ginger, grapefruit, immortelle, jasmine, juniper berry, lavandin, lavender, linden blossom, manuka, myrtle, orange (sweet), oregano, peppermint, pimento berry, ravintsara, rose absolute, rosemary, rose otto, sage, spearmint, tarragon, tea tree, thyme linalol, vetiver, ylang ylang

Precautionary advice: Expressed lemon oil is a photosensitizer; do not apply to the skin prior to sun exposure. Distilled lemon oil is a nonphotosensitizer. May cause irritation on highly sensitive skin; skin patch test is advisable. GRAS status.

LEMONGRASS, *Cymbopogon flexuosus, C. citratus* (Plant Family: Poaceae)

Type of plant: Perennial grass with long thin leaves, usually growing to around 3 feet high

Part used: Leaves

Method of extraction: Steam distillation

Data: Either fresh or partly dried leaves are distilled. Lemongrass is best known as an important component of Indian and other Asian cooking, where the bulb is also utilized, and it is also used in traditional Indian Ayurvedic medicine. Widely used as an insect deterrent.

Principal places of production: Nepal, India, Sri Lanka, Madagascar, Guatemala, Brazil

When buying look for: A pale-yellow to golden-yellow liquid with an herbaceous, earthy, citrus aroma

Therapeutic properties: Analgesic, anthelmintic, antifungal, anti-infectious, antimicrobial, antiseptic, astringent, depurative, digestive, diuretic, tonic

Therapeutic uses: Muscular aches and pains, gastrointestinal disorders, indigestion, colitis, diuretic, detoxifying, cellulite, fever, nonspecific infection, physical and mental exhaustion, acne, pimples, insect bites, insect repellent

Blends well with: Basil, black pepper, caraway seed, cedarwood, clary sage, coriander seed, cypress, eucalyptus peppermint, eucalyptus radiata, fennel (sweet), fragonia, geranium, ginger, immortelle, juniper berry, lavender (spike), manuka, orange (sweet), oregano, palmarosa, patchouli, peppermint, pimento berry, plai, ravintsara, rosemary, spearmint, tea tree, thyme linalol, vetiver, ylang ylang

Precautionary advice: May cause irritation on highly sensitive skins; a skin patch test is advisable. Best avoided during pregnancy. Best avoided if using multiple medications. GRAS status.

LEMON VERBENA, *Lippia citriodora, Aloysia triphylla* (Plant Family: Verbenaceae)

Type of plant: Bushy perennial shrub growing to around 6 feet high, with slim lemon-scented leaves and stems carrying spikes of tiny white to light-pink or lilac flowers

Part used: Flowering tops

Method of extraction: Steam distillation

Data: The leaves are harvested along with the flowers and distilled straight away. Originally from South America, lemon verbena was introduced into Europe by the Spanish in the seventeenth century and now grows widely throughout the world. It's a popular scented garden shrub, and the leaves are often used in potpourris and herbal pillows.

Principal places of production: France, Spain, Morocco, Algeria, Réunion

When buying look for: A yellow to golden yellow liquid with a fresh, sweet, soft, herbaceous, citrus aroma. Not to be confused with vervain (*Verbena officinalis*) or Spanish verbena oil.

Therapeutic properties: Anthelmintic, antiinflammatory, antiseptic, antispasmodic, carminative, digestive, sedative

Therapeutic uses: Nervous indigestion, abdominal cramp, muscular spasm, gastrointestinal problems, diverticulosis, irritable bowel syndrome, insomnia, stress, depression, nervous asthma, anxiety, restlessness

Blends well with: Black pepper, cananga, cardamom, clove bud, coriander seed, cypress, elemi, fennel (sweet), ginger, jasmine, juniper berry, mandarin, marjoram (sweet), myrtle, orange (sweet), peppermint, petitgrain, rosemary, spearmint, valerian, vetiver, ylang ylang

Precautionary advice: Photosensitizer; do not apply to the skin prior to sun exposure. May cause irritation on highly sensitive skins; a skin patch test is advisable.

LIME, *Citrus aurantifolia* (Plant Family: Rutaceae)

Type of plant: Thorned evergreen tree growing to around 15 feet high with dark glossy leaves, cream-colored flowers, and small green fruits

Part used: Fruit rind

Method of extraction: Steam distillation / cold expression

Data: Essential oil of lime is produced in two ways: steam distillation and cold expression. All parts of the lime are widely used throughout the world in cooking. Lime is utilized in the soft drinks and food industry and in perfumes, aftershaves, and deodorants. Lime is indigenous to Asia and was introduced into Europe by Arabian traders, and then into the Americas by the Spanish, probably earlier than the sixteenth century.

Principal places of production: Mexico, Peru, India, Brazil

When buying look for: A colorless to greenish-yellow liquid with a typically fresh, fruity, tangy, citrus aroma

Therapeutic properties: Anthelmintic, antimicrobial, antiseptic, antiviral, astringent, cholagogue, depurative, digestive, restorative

Therapeutic uses: Digestive problems, loss of appetite, detoxifying, cellulite, throat infection, tonsillitis, sore throat, influenza, lethargy, chronic fatigue, mental exhaustion, intestinal parasites

Blends well with: Bay (West Indian), benzoin, black pepper, cardamom, citronella, clary sage, cypress, elemi, eucalyptus peppermint, geranium, fragonia, frankincense, ginger, juniper berry, lavandin, lemon, manuka, myrtle, nutmeg, orange (sweet), pimento berry, rose absolute, rosemary, sage (Greek), tangerine, tuberose, turmeric, vanilla, vetiver, ylang ylang

Precautionary advice: Expressed lime oil is a photosensitizer; do not apply to the skin prior to sun exposure. Distilled lime oil is a nonphotosensitizer. GRAS status.

LINDEN BLOSSOM (ABSOLUTE), *Tilia vulgaris/cordata, T. europaea, T. platyphyllos* (Plant Family: Tiliaceae)

Type of plant: Tall deciduous tree growing to 80 feet high with heart-shaped leaves and clusters of small, fragrant, creamy-colored flowers

Part used: Flowers

Method of extraction: Solvent and CO_2 extraction; maceration

Data: Commonly known as the *lime tree*. The flowers are made into a tea, which calms, aids sleep, and helps in cases of nervousness. The honey produced by bees attracted to the flowers is valued for its sedative properties. The tree can live for 800 years, and in Europe avenues of the trees are often found in municipal parks and in the grounds of stately homes.

Principal place of production: France

When buying look for: Slightly viscous, greenish-yellow to dark-yellow-brown liquid with a light, warm, sweet, floral aroma

Therapeutic properties: Antidepressant, antiseptic, antispasmodic, astringent, calmative, emollient, expectorant, nervine, sedative

Therapeutic uses: Nervous tension, nervous spasm, muscular spasm, insomnia, emotional crisis, stress- and anxiety-related conditions; soothing, calming

Blends well with: Balsam de Peru, benzoin, bergamot, black pepper, cananga, cinnamon leaf, coriander seed, geranium, grapefruit, jasmine, lemon, lime, mandarin, may chang, neroli, orange (sweet), petitgrain, rose absolute, rose otto, sandalwood, spikenard, valerian, ylang ylang, yuzu

Precautionary advice: Avoid during pregnancy. GRAS status.

MAGNOLIA FLOWER, *Michelia alba* (Plant Family: Magnoliaceae)

Type of plant: Tree growing to over 50 feet high with large glossy leaves and delicate, highly fragrant white flowers with 12 long, slim petals

Part used: Flowers

Method of extraction: Steam distillation

Data: The tree is a hybrid and is not found in the wild. In Asia it's often cultivated as a decorative tree. In China magnolia flowers are used in traditional Chinese medicine and to fragrance tea. Throughout Asia magnolia flowers are offered in temples to mark births and other celebrations. Magnolias in general are some of the oldest plants known, developing before winged insects and so pollinated by the more ancient beetles. Fossils of magnolia date to over 100 million years ago and show it was once growing in Europe, as well as in America and Asia, now its native habitat.

Principal place of production: China

When buying look for: A greenish-yellow to brown liquid with a fresh, sweet, floral aroma. Not to be confused with magnolia leaf essential oil.

Therapeutic properties: Analgesic, antidepressive, antiseptic, antispasmodic, calmative, cytophylactic, nervine, restorative, sedative

Therapeutic uses: Scars, wounds, muscular aches, abdominal cramp, intestinal spasm, fear-induced anxiety, insomnia, inability to communicate, stress-related tension, depression

Blends well with: Amyris, benzoin, bergamot, cananga, cedarwood, chamomile maroc, cistus, frankincense, geranium, immortelle, jasmine, lavender, mandarin, marjoram (sweet), neroli, orange (sweet), petitgrain, rose, rosewood, ylang ylang

Precautionary advice: No contraindications known

MANDARIN, *Citrus reticulata*
(Plant Family: Rutaceae)

Type of plant: Small evergreen tree with small leaves, fragrant white flowers, and orange-colored fruits

Part used: Fruit rind

Method of extraction: Cold expression

Data: It's said that the name *mandarin* comes from the color of the clothing worn by the officials of the old Chinese empire, the mandarins. The dried rind of the fruit is used in cooking and in traditional Chinese medicine to regulate chi. Mandarin originated in China and Vietnam and spread through Asia, only coming to Europe in the nineteenth century, particularly to the southern tip of Italy. The fruit is pressed to extract the essential oil before being fully ripe. This is a very gentle oil, good for blending and excellent for the more delicate among us, including children and those convalescing.

Principal places of production: Italy, Spain, Argentina, Egypt, Brazil, China, United States

When buying look for: A yellowish-green through orangey-gold liquid with a sweet, light, floral, fruity-citrus aroma. Mandarin essential oil is available in three different stages — green, yellow, and red — all with slightly differing fragrance notes. Not to be confused with the essential oil of tangerine, which has different properties.

Therapeutic properties: Antiseptic, antispasmodic, calmative, digestive, sedative, stomachic, tonic

Therapeutic uses: Digestive conditions, nervous spasm, intestinal spasm, irritable bowel syndrome, stomachache, constipation, cellulite, insomnia, sleeping disorders, nervous tension, irritability, stress, convalescence

Blends well with: Basil linalol, bay (West Indian), bay laurel, bergamot, black pepper, cananga, cardamom, chamomile german, chamomile maroc, chamomile roman, clary sage, clove bud, coriander seed, cypress, fennel (sweet), frankincense, geranium, ginger, grapefruit, jasmine, juniper berry, lavandin, lavender, lemon, lime, linden blossom, marjoram (sweet), neroli, nutmeg, orange (sweet), patchouli, petitgrain, pine, ravensara, rosalina, rose absolute, rosemary, rose otto, rosewood, sandalwood, spearmint, spikenard, thyme linalol, valerian, ylang ylang

Precautionary advice: No contraindications known. GRAS status.

MANUKA, *Leptospermum scoparium*
(Plant Family: Myrtaceae)

Type of plant: Hardy, fast-growing shrub growing to 12 feet high with prickly leaves and small, whitish-pink flowers with a deep pinkish-red center.

Part used: Leaves and end branches

Method of extraction: Steam distillation

Data: Manuka, a plant native to New Zealand, is becoming known internationally as a very useful essential oil. It's distilled from both wild and cultivated bushes. In the wild it often grows alongside kanuka, and the plant materials should be separated before distillation into the two essential oils. All parts of the bush have been used by the Maori people as an important part of their indigenous medicinal system. Manuka is said to be the original tea tree; Captain James Cook wrote that it "has a very agreeable bitter taste and flavor when [the leaves] are recent, but loses some of both when they are dried."

Principal places of production: New Zealand, Australia

When buying look for: A clear to pale-yellow liquid with an earthy, slightly sweet, balsamic, camphorous aroma

Therapeutic properties: Analgesic, antibacterial, antifungal, anti-infectious, anti-inflammatory, antimicrobial, antiseptic, cytophylactic, expectorant, immunostimulant, spasmolytic, vulnerary

Therapeutic uses: Bronchial infection, bronchitis, catarrh, coughs, influenza, skin infection, wounds, cuts, grazes, contusions, ulceration, *Helicobacter pylori*, fungal skin infection, athlete's foot, parasitic infection, ringworm, mites, head lice, scabies

Blends well with: Basil, bergamot, cedarwood, chamomile german, chamomile roman, cypress, eucalyptus peppermint, eucalyptus radiata, fragonia, lavender, lavender (spike), lemon, mastic, niaouli, oregano, peppermint, pine, rosemary, spruce, tea tree, thyme linalol

Precautionary advice: No contraindications known

MARJORAM, SWEET, *Origanum majorana, Majorana hortensis*
(Plant Family: Lamiaceae/Labiatae)

Type of plant: Bushy, low-growing perennial herb with grayish-green leaves and terminal clusters of tiny white or purple flowers

Part used: Fresh flowering tops, leaves, and stems

Method of extraction: Steam distillation

Data: The plant material is harvested when flowering, and distilled while still fresh. Marjoram leaves and branches have been found in burial sites dating from the Roman period of ancient Egypt. Marjoram has been incorporated since that time in ointments and used in spiritual cleansing. Known to the ancient Greeks, the plant spread through Europe from Turkey and Cyprus and is now on the coat of arms of the town of Marjora in Sicily. Valued throughout history in Europe, it was once one of the most commonly found herbs.

Principal places of production: Egypt, Spain, France, Morocco, Tunisia, Bulgaria, Hungary, Germany, Portugal

When buying look for: A clear, slightly yellow-tinged to pale-yellow liquid with a warm, green, spicy, herbaceous aroma

Therapeutic properties: Analgesic, antibacterial, antiseptic, antispasmodic, calmative, circulatory, digestive, nervine, sedative, vasodilatory

Therapeutic uses: Muscle relaxant, muscular spasm, muscular pain, general aches, numbness, bodily stiffness, abdominal pain, menstrual cramp, menstrual problems, menopausal symptoms, contusion, bruises, headache, gastrointestinal disorders, abdominal spasm, indigestion, intestinal spasm, constipation, irritable bowel syndrome, diverticulosis, insomnia, stress-related conditions, anxiety

Blends well with: Basil linalol, bergamot, black pepper, cardamom, cedarwood, chamomile german, chamomile roman, clary sage, cypress, frankincense, geranium, grapefruit, juniper berry, lavandin, lavender, lemon, lime, orange (sweet), peppermint, petitgrain, pine, ravensara, rosalina, rosemary, rosewood, sandalwood, spearmint, spikenard, thyme linalol, valerian, vetiver

Precautionary advice: No contraindications known. GRAS status.

MASTIC, *Pistacia lentiscus*
(Plant Family: Anacardiaceae)

Type of plant: Hardy, shrub-like evergreen tree growing to around 15 feet high with small red fruits

Part used: Resin

Method of extraction: Steam distillation

Data: Although native to the Mediterranean area and the Near East, the mastic tree is processed for essential oil on the Greek island of Chios, particularly in seven villages in the southwest collectively known as the Mastichochoria. The tree variety there is *Pistacia lentiscus var. chia*. The trunk is cut, allowing sap to drop to the ground. This dries and hardens into a translucent form and will return to liquid if allowed to become too warm. Raw mastic is an extremely versatile substance and has been used for thousands of years as a medicine, cosmetic, perfume, and incense, and for food flavoring. It was the world's first recorded chewing gum, deriving its name perhaps from the Spanish word for "chew" — *masticar.* The Greeks call the resin *mastiha* and value it as an addition, when ground, to both sweet and savory dishes. An essential oil is also made from the leaves and twigs.

Principal places of production: Greece, Morocco

When buying look for: A colorless to pale-yellow liquid with a green, balsamic, resinous aroma

Therapeutic properties: Analgesic, anti-inflammatory, antimicrobial, antiseptic, anti-spasmodic, antitussive, circulatory, decongestant, expectorant, pectoral, vasoconstrictor, vulnerary

Therapeutic uses: Bronchial disorders, coughs, colds, arthritis, rheumatism, *Helicobacter pylori*, ulceration, wounds, cuts and grazes, hemorrhoids, cold lower limbs and numbness, dental hygiene

Blends well with: Amyris, angelica seed, balsam de Peru, bay laurel, benzoin, bergamot, black pepper, cedarwood, chamomile german, chamomile roman, cistus, copaiba, cypress, eucalyptus radiata, frankincense, galbanum, geranium, ho wood, juniper berry, pimento berry, sage (Greek), sandalwood, spikenard

Precautionary advice: No contraindications known

MAY CHANG, *Litsea cubeba*
(Plant Family: Lauraceae)

Type of plant: Shrubby tree growing to 35 feet high, with slender bright-green leaves and fluffy white or pale-yellow lemon-scented flowers and small pepper-like fruits

Part used: Ripe berries and leaves

Method of extraction: Steam distillation

Data: Native mostly to mountainous areas of China, Taiwan, and Indonesia but now grown commercially elsewhere. All parts of this tree are used. The fruits are green when unripe, turning red then dark brown when ripe. They're made into a hot spice in Asia; the flowers are used as flavoring for medicinal tea; while the branches and roots are valued in traditional Chinese medicine. The essential oil is a popular component of citrus-type perfumes. It's also processed commercially to obtain pure citral.

Principal places of production: China, Taiwan, Indonesia

When buying look for: A pale-yellow to yellow liquid with a sweet, herbaceous, intensely fruity, citrus aroma

Therapeutic properties: Anthelmintic, anti-depressant, antifungal, anti-infectious, anti-inflammatory, antiseptic, astringent, carminative, circulatory, insect deterrent, sedative, stimulant

Therapeutic uses: Cellulite, stomachache, abdominal cramp, indigestion, muscular aches and pain, tendonitis, arthritis, rheumatism, problematic skin conditions — acne, pimples, boils — circulation conditions, nervous tension, anxiety, stress

Blends well with: Basil linalol, black pepper, cananga, cedarwood, chamomile german, chamomile maroc, coriander seed, cypress, eucalyptus radiata, frankincense, geranium, ginger, marjoram (sweet), orange (sweet), palmarosa, peppermint, petitgrain, rosemary, thyme linalol, vetiver, ylang ylang

Precautionary advice: May cause irritation on highly sensitive skins; a patch test is advisable. Best avoided during pregnancy.

MELISSA, *Melissa officinalis*
(Plant Family: Lamiaceae/Labiatae)

Type of plant: Bushy perennial herb growing to 3 feet high with lemon-scented serrated leaves and small white flowers

Part used: Flowering tops, leaves, and stems

Method of extraction: Steam distillation

Data: Melissa is also known as *lemon balm, lemon melissa,* or *sweet balm.* It acquired the name *bee balm* because beekeepers once used it to attract bees to their hives. Valued by European herbalists since the Middle Ages, it's mentioned in many old pharmacopeias and was the key ingredient in Carmelite water. Although the fragrance is easily released by crushing a leaf, a very large amount of plant material is required to produce a small volume of essential oil, a fact reflected in its price.

Principal places of production: France, Hungary, Germany, Ireland, United Kingdom, South Africa

When buying look for: A pale-yellow to yellowish-green liquid with a slightly floral, green, herbaceous, citrus aroma. Melissa is sometimes adulterated with other, cheaper citrus-type essential oils.

Therapeutic properties: Antibacterial, antidepressant, antifungal, antiseptic, antiviral, calmative, circulatory, depurative, insect repellent, nervine, soporific, spasmolytic, stomachic

Therapeutic uses: Insomnia, sleep disorders, indigestion, nausea, fungal infections, candida, viral skin infections, herpes, menopausal symptoms, detoxifying, nervousness, stress and anxiety-related symptoms, depression

Blends well with: Bergamot, cananga, carnation, chamomile roman, clary sage, frankincense, geranium, myrtle, neroli, orange (sweet), petitgrain, rose absolute, rose otto, rosewood, sandalwood, spikenard, tangerine, tuberose, valerian, vanilla, ylang ylang

Precautionary advice: Best avoided if using multiple medications. May cause irritation on highly sensitive skins; a skin patch test is advisable. Best avoided during pregnancy and while breastfeeding. GRAS status.

MIMOSA (ABSOLUTE), *Acacia dealbata, A. decurrens* (Plant Family: Mimosaceae)

Type of plant: Tall shrubby tree with bipinnate leaves and a profusion of bright-yellow pom-pom shaped flowers and black seed pods

Part used: Flowers, leaves, and twigs

Method of extraction: Solvent extraction

Data: The mimosa shrub, which can grow over 10 feet high, has long been used in the traditional Aboriginal medicine of Australia, where its common name is *wattle.* In the south of France and Italy, where mimosa thrives well in the wild due to the high temperatures, it's said to herald the start of spring. The bark was used in the tanning industry for its astringent effects. The flowers and leaves produce this highly perfumed absolute, which is utilized in perfumes and aftershaves. Mimosa is a close relative of cassie.

Principal places of production: France, India, Italy, Morocco

When buying look for: Viscous, golden yellow through greenish-brown liquid with a soft, green, warm, sweet, floral aroma and an almond note. This absolute is extremely sticky and sometimes has a solid appearance.

Therapeutic properties: Antiseptic, astringent, calmative, emollient

Therapeutic uses: Nervous tension, nerve-related conditions, stress-related fatigue, stress, depression, intestinal infection, diarrhea, upset stomach

Blends well with: Bergamot, carnation, cinnamon leaf, cistus, clove bud, geranium, ginger, grapefruit, ho wood, immortelle, jasmine, lavandin, lavender, lemon, mandarin, may chang, nutmeg, orange (sweet), palmarosa, petitgrain, rose maroc, spearmint, tuberose, vanilla, violet leaf, ylang ylang, yuzu

Precautionary advice: Best avoided during pregnancy and while breast-feeding.

MYRRH, *Commiphora myrrha*
(Plant Family: Burseraceae)

Type of plant: Small thorny tree growing up to 9 feet high, with small oval leaves and white flowers. On old trees the bark is white.

Part used: Oleoresin gum

Method of extraction: Steam distillation

Data: Native to northeast Africa and areas of Arabia adjacent to the Red Sea. The tree produces a pale-yellow liquid from cuts in its bark, which on contact with air becomes a hard, brittle reddish-brown. The resin is often exported, then distilled in Europe. Myrrh was used by the ancient Egyptians, for embalming and as a medicine and an incense ingredient; the resin has been found in pots placed in burials and tombs. Known as a wound healer for millennia. Famously given as a gift to baby Jesus. Myrrh has been in use as a spiritual fumigant for thousands of years and remains today in the British Pharmacopoeia.

Principal places of production: Somalia, Ethiopia, Sudan

When buying look for: A viscous, dark greenish-yellow through amber-brown liquid with a warm, slightly musty, earthy, balsamic aroma. The term *sweet myrrh* usually refers to the essential oil of opoponax, which is generally not used in aromatherapy.

Therapeutic properties: Antifungal, anti-inflammatory, antimicrobial, antiseptic, astringent, balsamic, carminative, cicatrizing, expectorant, pectoral, vulnerary

Therapeutic uses: Coughs, catarrh, bronchitis, bronchial congestion, wounds, sores, ulcerations,

eczema, skin infection, ringworm, scabies, insect bites, parasitic bites, intestinal disorders, excess mucus, gum disease, mouth ulcers, fungal nail infection

Blends well with: Benzoin, black pepper, cajuput, cardamom, cedarwood, chamomile german, chamomile roman, elemi, frankincense, geranium, ginger, greenland moss, hyssop decumbens, lavandin, lavender, lemon, mastic, may chang, myrtle, niaouli, turmeric

Precautionary advice: Avoid during pregnancy and while breast-feeding.

MYRTLE, *Myrtus communis*
(Plant Family: Myrtaceae)

Type of plant: Bushy evergreen shrub-like tree growing to 15 feet high with fragrant leathery leaves, white flowers with tufts of white stamens, and bluish-black berries

Part used: Leaves, twigs, and flowers

Method of extraction: Steam distillation

Data: The myrtle grown in the French island of Corsica is known as *green myrtle*. A favorite garden plant due to its aromatic leaves. The essential oil is used in medicines, skin preparations, perfumes, aftershaves, and as food flavoring. Myrtle has long had a reputation as an aphrodisiac, being variously associated with weddings, sexual potency, and marital happiness from Roman times to the present day, from the Levant to Scandinavia.

Principal places of production: France, Tunisia, Morocco, Spain

When buying look for: A pale-yellow to golden-amber liquid with a fresh, sweet, peppery, herbaceous, camphorous aroma

Therapeutic properties: Antibacterial, anticatarrhal, antiviral, astringent, expectorant, pectoral, regenerative, restorative, soporific, stimulant, tonic

Therapeutic uses: Bronchitis, sinus infection,

laryngitis, bronchial infection, coughs, colds, cystitis, urinary tract infection, heavy legs, insomnia, tired all the time, skin disorders, psoriasis, acne, pimples, boils, parasitic infection, head lice, mite bites, emotional, mental, and physical exhaustion
Blends well with: Basil linalol, bergamot, black pepper, chamomile roman, cistus, eucalyptus lemon, eucalyptus radiata, frankincense, geranium, ginger, hyssop decumbens, immortelle, lavandin, lavender, lemon, lemongrass, mandarin, niaouli, orange (sweet), petitgrain, rosemary, spruce, thyme linalol
Precautionary advice: Best avoided during pregnancy and while breast-feeding. Best avoided if using multiple medications.

NARCISSUS (ABSOLUTE), *Narcissus poeticus* (Plant Family: Amaryllidaceae)

Type of plant: Perennial bulbous herb with long leaves and white flowers with orange centers trimmed in red
Part used: Flowering heads
Method of extraction: Solvent extraction
Data: It takes 500 kilograms of narcissus flowers to produce 300 grams of absolute, making it one of the most expensive floral fragrances. It grows wild in well-drained and rocky habitats. Narcissus has been a popular ingredient in perfumery since ancient Roman times. The word comes from the Greek *narkao*, meaning "to be made numb."
Principal places of production: France, Holland, Egypt, Morocco
When buying look for: A viscous, golden brown to dark-orange or green liquid with an intense, sweet, warm, floral aroma
Therapeutic properties: Antispasmodic, hypnotic, nervine, sedative, soporific
Therapeutic uses: Stress, tension, anxiety, insomnia, muscular spasm, aches and pain, nervousness, inability to relax, troubled minds
Blends well with: Bergamot, black pepper,

cananga, cardamom, carnation, cinnamon leaf, cistus, clove bud, geranium, ginger, ho wood, immortelle, jasmine, lavandin, lavender, lemon, lemongrass, lime, mandarin, mimosa, orange (sweet), petitgrain, rose maroc, rosewood, spearmint, tangerine, tuberose, vanilla, ylang ylang, yuzu
Precautionary advice: May cause headaches in susceptible people. Best avoided during pregnancy and while breast-feeding.

NEEM (MARGOSA OIL), *Azadirachta indica, Melia azadirachta* (Plant Family: Meliaceae)

Type of plant: Evergreen tree growing to 60 feet high, with long leaves and fragrant white flowers
Part used: Pulp of fruit and seeds
Method of extraction: Expression
Data: The neem tree is economically important in India, where it's used for everything from acne to fevers. All parts of the tree are used medicinally — the bark, leaves, flowers, and seeds. The essential oil is used particularly for skin diseases and to deter lice and parasites; the small branches are used to make toothpicks; and the leaves are pressed between the pages of books to deter mites and used in grain stores to deter insects and pests.
Principal place of production: India
When buying look for: A viscous, light-brown to dark-brown oil that often needs heat to transform into a usable liquid, with a highly tenacious odor.
Therapeutic properties: Analgesic, anthelmintic, antibacterial, antifungal, anti-inflammatory, antiviral, insecticide, pesticide, sedative
Therapeutic uses: Psoriasis, eczema, parasitic skin infection, ringworm, scabies, ulceration, bacterial skin infection, scalp infection, dandruff, head lice, acne, sores, pimples, insect bites, insect stings
Blends well with: Intense citrus essential oils such as lemon and bergamot, or camphorous essential oils such as rosemary and sweet birch

Precautions for use: May cause irritation on sensitive skin. Best avoided during pregnancy and while breast-feeding.

NEROLI, *Citrus aurantium*
(Plant Family: Rutaceae)

Type of plant: Thorny evergreen tree ranging in size from 10 to 30 feet in height with evergreen leaves, waxy white flowers with tufts of yellow stamens, and small orange fruits
Part used: Blossom
Method of extraction: Steam distillation
Data: The fragrant flowers of the bitter orange tree are nestled in the leaves and must be carefully hand-picked early in the morning. It takes 220 pounds of flowers to produce 2½ fluid ounces of neroli oil. Highly prized in perfumery. The name *neroli* was given to the fragrance of orange blossom after it was made fashionable in the seventeenth century by the Princess of Nerola in Italy. Neroli blossom was traditionally used by brides to decorate their hair, as it was associated with purity and marital fidelity. The bitter orange tree, also known as *Seville orange*, is cultivated for making marmalade and for bitter orange essential oil, which is used in food manufacture and perfumery. The essential oil from the leaves, twigs, and small unripe fruits is called *petitgrain*.
Principal places of production: Tunisia, Morocco, Italy, France, Egypt
When buying look for: A pale-yellow to golden-yellow liquid that turns darker with age, with a highly radiant, light, sweet, floral aroma
Therapeutic properties: Antidepressant, anti-infectious, antimicrobial, antiseptic, calmative, carminative, cicatrizing, circulatory, cytophylactic, regenerative, restorative, sedative, spasmolytic, tonic
Therapeutic uses: Insomnia, convalescence, indigestion, abdominal spasm, intestinal cramp, stress and related conditions, scar tissue, scarring,

skin regenerating, acne, problematic skin, stretch marks, menopausal anxieties, insomnia, sleep disorders, nervousness, depression, tension, emotional exhaustion
Blends well with: Bergamot, black pepper, cananga, cardamom, chamomile roman, clary sage, frankincense, geranium, jasmine, lavender, lemon, magnolia leaf, mandarin, orange (sweet), petitgrain, rose otto, rosewood, sandalwood, tangerine, ylang ylang
Precautionary advice: No contraindications known. GRAS status.

NIAOULI, *Melaleuca quinquenervia*
(Plant Family: Myrtaceae)

Type of plant: Tree growing to 60 feet high with a peeling white bark and fluffy white "bottle-brush" flowers
Part used: Leaves and twigs
Method of extraction: Steam distillation
Data: Because there are so many closely related species, this plant is sometimes referred to as *true niaouli* to avoid confusion. Native to New Caledonia — an island group in the southwest Pacific — as well as Australia and Madagascar. The leaves and twigs are often harvested from wild-growing niaouli trees. Wherever it grows, the tree has long been used in indigenous medicine. Due to the invasive root system, the trees can cause major environmental problems because even when felled they continue to grow from the stumps.
Principal places of production: Madagascar, Tasmania, Australia, New Caledonia
When buying look for: A colorless to pale-yellow liquid with an intense, fresh, balsamic, camphorous aroma
Therapeutic properties: Analgesic, antibacterial, anticatarrhal, antifungal, antiseptic, antiviral, balsamic, decongestant, expectorant, pectoral, tonic, vulnerary

Therapeutic uses: Bronchitis, respiratory tract disorders, influenza, sinus congestion, sore throat, catarrh, cough, colds, uterine infection, rheumatism, muscular injury, rashes, pimples, acne, herpes, wounds, cuts and grazes; insect repellent

Blends well with: Basil linalol, black pepper, cajuput, cedarwood, chamomile german, chamomile roman, cypress, eucalyptus lemon, eucalyptus radiata, fragonia, frankincense, geranium, ginger, lavender, lavender (spike), lemon, lemongrass, manuka, marjoram (sweet), myrrh, ravensara, ravintsara, rosemary, sage (Greek), tea tree

Precautionary advice: No contraindications known

NUTMEG, *Myristica fragrans*
(Plant Family: Myristicaceae)

Type of plant: Small evergreen tree growing to around 50 feet high with small, bell-shaped, waxy, creamy-colored flowers and large fruits

Part used: Nut/fruit

Method of extraction: Steam distillation

Data: Native to the Moluccas Islands in Indonesia, the nutmeg has a long history of use. Wars were fought over access to nutmeg, with the Portuguese trying to keep its source a secret until it was discovered by the Dutch, and then the British, who introduced the plant to the Caribbean, where it is now widely grown. The tree produces nuts after 9 years and is fully productive after 20 years. The fruit opens to reveal a single nut/seed, recognized as nutmeg, around which is a red filamentous material, mace, which is itself distilled into an essential oil. Nutmeg is now distributed around the world and plays an important part in cuisine from the Americas to Asia.

Principal places of production: Indonesia, Grenada, Sri Lanka

When buying look for: A colorless to pale-yellow liquid with a warm, sweet, rich, spicy aroma

Therapeutic properties: Analgesic, anti-infectious, antiseptic, calmative, carminative, digestive, nervine, sedative, spasmolytic

Therapeutic uses: Gastrointestinal spasm, nausea, upset stomach, rheumatism, arthritis, muscular aches and pains, muscular injury, menstrual cramp, insomnia, restlessness, nervousness, tension

Blends well with: Basil linalol, bay (West Indian), bergamot, cananga, cardamom, carnation, clary sage, coriander seed, galbanum, geranium, ginger, grapefruit, jasmine, lavandin, lemon, lemongrass, lime, mandarin, marjoram (sweet), may chang, neroli, orange (sweet), petitgrain, rose absolute, ylang ylang

Precautionary advice: Best avoided during pregnancy and while breast-feeding. GRAS status.

ORANGE, SWEET, *Citrus sinensis*, *C. aurantium var. sinensis*
(Plant Family: Rutaceae)

Type of plant: Tree growing to around 25 feet high with dark-green leaves, fragrant white flowers, and large, bright, round orange fruits

Part used: Rind of fruit

Method of extraction: Cold-pressed, steam distillation

Data: While the bitter orange came west from China, the sweet orange originated in India, from where it was brought to Europe by Portuguese sailors, who further carried it to South America, where Jesuit priests were growing sweet orange trees extensively as early as 1549. Today, Brazil is a major supplier of sweet orange essential oil. The oil contains vitamins, minerals, and enzymes and is widely used in the food, drinks, and confectionery industry, as well as in perfumery.

Principal places of production: Brazil, United States, Italy, Spain, Israel, Argentina

When buying look for: A yellow to orange liquid with a fresh, sweet, fruity, citrus aroma.

While sweet orange is derived from *Citrus sinensis*, bitter orange essential oil is distilled from *Citrus aurantium* and has a yellowish-green to yellow-orange color with a slightly more sweet and sour, woody, citrus aroma.

Therapeutic properties: Antibacterial, antiseptic, calmative, cholagogue, depurative, diuretic, sedative, stimulant, stomachic, tonic

Therapeutic uses: Nervous anxiety, constipation, intestinal spasm, fluid retention, detoxifying, cellulite, insomnia, depression, anxiety and stress-related conditions, tension, convalescence

Blends well with: Basil linalol, bay (West Indian), bay laurel, bergamot, black pepper, cananga, cardamom, chamomile german, chamomile maroc, chamomile roman, clary sage, clove bud, coriander seed, cypress, fennel (sweet), frankincense, geranium, ginger, grapefruit, jasmine, juniper berry, lavandin, lavender, lemon, lime, linden blossom, mandarin, marjoram (sweet), may chang, mimosa, myrtle, neroli, nutmeg, patchouli, petitgrain, pine, rose absolute, rosemary, rose otto, rosewood, sandalwood, spearmint, spikenard, thyme linalol, valerian, vetiver, ylang ylang

Precautionary advice: No contraindications known. GRAS status.

OREGANO, *Origanum vulgare*
(Plant Family: Lamiaceae/Labiatae)

Type of plant: Perennial herb with fragrant leaves and reddish hairy stalks, bearing at their tip clusters of small pink flowers

Part used: Whole plant including flowers

Method of extraction: Steam distillation

Data: Distillation takes place immediately after harvesting, just as the flowers start to bloom. Native to southern and central Europe, oregano is now grown worldwide. The herb had been used medicinally for many centuries before the first-century Roman medic Pliny sung its praises

in his book *Natural History*. Oregano is used extensively in Mediterranean cooking, and, indeed, no self-respecting pizza would be without it. The plant is much favored by bees.

Principal places of production: France, Morocco, Egypt, Turkey, Italy, Spain

When buying look for: A colorless to pale-yellow or pale-reddish-brown liquid with an intense, herbaceous, slightly medicinal-like aroma

Therapeutic properties: Analgesic, anthelmintic, antibacterial, antifungal, antiseptic, antiviral, expectorant, rubefacient, stimulant

Therapeutic uses: Viral infection, bacterial infection, respiratory tract infection, muscular pain

Blends well with: Bergamot, cedarwood, cinnamon leaf, cypress, eucalyptus peppermint, eucalyptus radiata, fragonia, frankincense, grapefruit, ho wood, hyssop decumbens, juniper berry, lavender, lavender (spike), lemon, lemongrass, lime, manuka, marjoram (sweet), may chang, myrtle, peppermint, ravensara, ravintsara, rosemary, tea tree, thyme linalol

Precautionary advice: May cause skin sensitivity; a skin patch test is advisable. Avoid during pregnancy and while breast-feeding. Best avoided if using multiple medications. GRAS status.

OREGANO, GREEK, *Origanum heracleoticum, O. vulgaris hirtum*
(Plant Family: Lamiaceae/Labiatae)

Type of plant: Hardy perennial herb with silver-haired leaves with purple undersides

Part used: Flowering tops

Method of extraction: Steam distillation

Data: The botanical names here relate to the same species, the *hirtum* name often being used instead of *heracleoticum*. In Greek, this herb species is known as the best for cooking as it has a very flavorsome, pungent, and even spicy taste.

Principal places of production: France, Greece, Turkey

When buying look for: A pale-yellow to dark-yellow liquid with a peppery, herbaceous, green, camphorous-like aroma

Therapeutic properties: Analgesic, anthelmintic, antibacterial, antifungal, anti-infectious, antiseptic, antiviral, immunostimulant, stimulant

Therapeutic uses: Viral infection, bacterial infection, parasitic infection, respiratory tract infection, gastrointestinal infection, bronchitis, catarrh, colds, influenza, rheumatism, muscular pain, acne, abscesses

Blends well with: Bergamot, cedarwood, cypress, eucalyptus peppermint, eucalyptus radiata, grapefruit, ho wood, hyssop decumbens, juniper berry, lavender, lavender (spike), marjoram (sweet), may chang, myrtle, peppermint, ravensara, rosemary, tea tree, thyme linalol

Precautionary advice: May cause irritation on highly sensitive skins; a patch test is advisable. Best avoided during pregnancy and while breastfeeding. GRAS status.

PALMAROSA, *Cymbopogon martinii*
(Plant Family: Poaceae)

Type of plant: Tall grass-like plant growing in dense tufts of long, thin, fragrant leaves and small yellow flowers

Part used: Leaves

Method of extraction: Steam distillation

Data: The long-leafed grass is harvested before its flowers bloom and left for a week to optimize the yield of essential oil before distillation. Previously called *Turkish geranium oil* or *East Indian geranium oil*, although the aroma is naturally more a lemony-rose than a geranium. If palmarosa oil is shaken with gum arabic solution and left in the sun, it becomes lighter in color and has a more rose-like aroma and is used to adulterate rose essential oil. Palmarosa is indigenous to India and Nepal, where it's still collected from wild-grown plants. It's called *Rosha oil* in Ayurvedic medicine.

Principal places of production: Nepal, India, Brazil, Central America

When buying look for: A pale-yellow to green-tinged yellow liquid and a lemony floral aroma with a faint woody note. The subspecies *var. sofia* is the source of gingergrass oil, which should not be confused with palmarosa oil.

Therapeutic properties: Antibacterial, antifungal, anti-infectious, antiseptic, antiviral, cicatrizing, cytophylactic, digestive, immunostimulant, insect deterrent, vulnerary

Therapeutic uses: Sinusitis, excess mucus, cystitis, urinary tract infection, gastrointestinal disorders, scarring, wounds, acne, pimples, boils, fungal infection, general fatigue, muscular aches, overexercised muscles, stress, irritability, restlessness, insect bites and stings

Blends well with: Bergamot, cajuput, cedarwood, chamomile german, chamomile roman, cinnamon leaf, citronella, clary sage, coriander seed, cypress, eucalyptus radiata, frankincense, geranium, ginger, grapefruit, ho wood, immortelle, lavender, lavender (spike), lemon, lemongrass, manuka, may chang, patchouli, plai, rose absolute, rosemary, tangerine, tarragon, tea tree, sandalwood, ylang ylang

Precautionary advice: Best avoided during pregnancy. GRAS status.

PATCHOULI, *Pogostemon cablin*
(Plant Family: Lamiaceae/Labiatae)

Type of plant: Perennial evergreen shrub growing to 3 feet high with large, velvety, highly fragrant leaves and spikes of purple flowers

Part used: Young leaves and stems

Method of extraction: Steam distillation

Data: Some patchouli leaves are distilled fresh; others are left in a pile in the shade so slight fermentation can take place, breaking down the secretory cell walls before distillation. Patchouli leaves used to be placed between the valuable paisley-designed pashmina scarves the British brought back from colonial India in the nineteenth century. Fakes could be identified because they didn't have the characteristic patchouli aroma.

Principal places of production: India, Indonesia, Malaysia, Madagascar, China

When buying look for: Mature oil: a viscous, dark-yellow to reddish-brown liquid with a rich, earthy, sweet, smoky aroma. The younger oil: a dark-yellow liquid with a rich, sweet, lighter aroma.

Therapeutic properties: Antidepressant, antifungal, anti-infectious, anti-inflammatory, antimicrobial, antiseptic, astringent, calmative, cicatrizing, cytophylactic, nervine

Therapeutic uses: Fungal infection, parasitic skin infection, ringworm, scabies, mites, scalp infection, problematic skin conditions, sores, abscess, cuts, grazes, insect repellent, insect bites and stings, premenstrual syndrome, depression, moodiness, irritability

Blends well with: Amyris, bergamot, black pepper, cananga, cardamom, cedarwood, chamomile maroc, clary sage, copaiba, frankincense, geranium, ginger, jasmine, lemon, lemongrass, mandarin, myrrh, orange (sweet), palmarosa, rose absolute, sandalwood, tangerine, ylang ylang

Precautionary advice: No contraindications known

PEPPERMINT, *Mentha piperita*
(Plant Family: Lamiaceae/Labiatae)

Type of plant: Perennial plant with small, highly aromatic leaves and spikes of small pinkish-mauve flowers

Part used: Fresh or partially dried plant

Method of extraction: Steam distillation

Data: According to Greek mythology, the genus *Mentha* takes its name from a nymph named Minthe. She had an affair with the god of the underworld, Hades, whose jealous wife, Persephone, turned Minthe into a nondescript plant and trod her into the ground. But then Hades turned the plant into an herb that people would appreciate and value until the end of time. In the United States, cultivation of peppermint began in 1855, and today the U.S. is one of the main producers of peppermint essential oil, particularly in the states of Washington, Oregon, and Idaho.

Principal places of production: United States, India, China, England, Italy, Russia

When buying look for: A colorless to pale-yellow liquid with a fresh, green, minty aroma and a faint peppery note

Therapeutic properties: Analgesic, antibacterial, anti-infectious, anti-inflammatory, antiseptic, antispasmodic, antiviral, carminative, cholagogue, circulatory, decongestant, digestive, stimulant, stomachic, tonic

Therapeutic uses: Headache, migraine, digestive problems, nausea, colic, gastrointestinal disorder, flatulence, colitis, diverticulitis, Crohn's disease, irritable bowel syndrome, sinus congestion, sinusitis, muscular aches and pains, muscular injury, muscular spasm, sciatica, sprains, rheumatism, menstrual cramp, neuralgia, acne, pimples, mental exhaustion, tension, physical exhaustion, fatigue, apathy

Blends well with: Angelica seed, basil linalol, bay laurel, bergamot, cananga, chamomile german, clove bud, cypress, eucalyptus lemon, eucalyptus radiata, geranium, grapefruit, ho wood, juniper berry, lavender, lavender (spike), lemon, lemongrass, lime, marjoram (sweet), myrtle, niaouli, orange (sweet), oregano, petitgrain, pine, ravensara, ravintsara, rosemary, spruce (black), tangerine, tarragon, tea tree, thyme linalol, tuberose, ylang ylang

Precautionary advice: Avoid during pregnancy

and while breast-feeding. Avoid using undiluted in baths and showers. GRAS status.

PETITGRAIN, *Citrus aurantium*
(Plant Family: Rutaceae)

Type of plant: Thorny evergreen tree ranging in height from 10 to 30 feet with evergreen leaves, waxy white flowers with tufts of yellow stamens, and small orange fruits

Part used: Leaves, twigs, and small, unripe green fruits

Method of extraction: Steam distillation

Data: There are records showing that petitgrain was being distilled from the bitter orange tree in 1694, and it was one of the first ingredients to be used in eau de cologne. The oil is distilled from the leaves, twigs, and tiny green fruit buds of the bitter orange tree. Some petitgrains are produced from a hybrid of the orange trees *C. aurantium* and *C. sinensis* — in Paraguay, for example. Although some petitgrain oils are distilled from the leaves of various other citrus trees such as mandarin, tangerine, lemon, grapefruit, lime, and bergamot, the therapeutic properties ascribed here are only for the petitgrain derived from the bitter orange tree (*Citrus aurantium*).

Principal places of production: Spain, Italy, France, Egypt, Brazil, Paraguay

When buying look for: A colorless to pale-yellow liquid with a green, woody, citrus, floral aroma

Therapeutic properties: Antidepressant, anti-inflammatory, antiseptic, antispasmodic, calmative, cicatrizing, cytophylactic, nervine, relaxant, sedative, tonic

Therapeutic uses: Stress-related conditions, nervous spasm, muscular spasm, general aches, hypertension, nervous asthma, insomnia, depression, general debility, stress, tension, irritability

Blends well with: Bergamot, black pepper, cananga, cardamom, cedarwood, chamomile roman, clary sage, coriander seed, cypress, frankincense, geranium, ginger, grapefruit, jasmine, lavender, lemon, linden blossom, marjoram (sweet), mimosa, myrtle, neroli, nutmeg, orange (sweet), patchouli, rose absolute, rosemary, rose otto, rosewood, sandalwood, vetiver, ylang ylang

Precautionary advice: No contraindications known. GRAS status.

PIMENTO BERRY, *Pimenta dioica*
(Plant Family: Myrtaceae)

Type of plant: Evergreen tree growing to 40 feet high with fragrant bark and twigs, fragrant leathery leaves, berries, and flowers

Part used: Berries

Method of extraction: Steam distillation

Data: Although the fragrant leaves are also made into an essential oil, it's the pimento berry essential oil that's used throughout this book. The berries are collected when they're green by climbing the tree and breaking off branches. It's forbidden to prune using machetes because the metal reacts with tannic acid in the tree and can lead to its demise. The branches are then threshed to release the berries, which are dried in the sun for up to 10 days, crushed, and then distilled. Native to the Caribbean and Central America, pimento berry is commonly known as Jamaican allspice because it smells like a combination of other common spices.

Principal places of production: Jamaica, Cuba, Réunion, India

When buying look for: A pale-yellow to dark-yellow or light-brown liquid with a sweet, soft, warm, spicy, clove-type aroma. The oil is sometimes sold as allspice essential oil.

Therapeutic properties: Analgesic, antifungal, anti-infectious, antimicrobial, antioxidant, antiseptic, rubefacient, stimulant

Therapeutic uses: Rheumatism, arthritis, aches and pain, muscular spasm, muscular strains, numbness, cold limbs, bronchial infection, coughs, chills, influenza, digestive problems, constipation, upset stomach, stomachache, coldness, tension

Blends well with: Benzoin, black pepper, cananga, cardamom, carnation, chamomile maroc, citronella, fennel (sweet), galbanum, geranium, lemon, lemongrass, mandarin, may chang, nutmeg, orange (sweet), rose absolute, tangerine, ylang ylang

Precautionary advice: Avoid if using multiple medications. May cause irritation on sensitive skin or skin prone to allergic reaction; a skin patch test is advisable. Best avoided during pregnancy and while breast-feeding.

PINE, *Pinus sylvestris* (Plant Family: Pinaceae)

Type of plant: Long-living tree reaching 130 feet with slightly orange-red bark when young, with bluish-green evergreen needles and male and female cones

Part used: Needles on branches

Method of extraction: Steam distillation

Data: Also known as *Scots pine*. The oil is used in some medication and men's toiletries. Pinecones are the source of edible pine kernels. Pines are full of flammable resin, and the branches have been used as torches by native people over a huge area — from the United States to Europe, to China. Pines are extensively cultivated for wood, cellulose, tar, pitch, turpentine, and essential oils.

Principal places of production: Scotland, Austria, France, United States, Russia

When buying look for: A colorless to pale-yellow liquid with a crisp, clean, resinous, balsamic aroma reminiscent of pine forest

Therapeutic properties: Anti-infectious, antimicrobial, antiseptic, balsamic, decongestant, diuretic, expectorant, pectoral, tonic

Therapeutic uses: Rheumatism, muscular pain,

muscular injury, muscular fatigue, fatigued and heavy legs, gout, bronchial infection, sinus congestion, general debility, fatigue, mental and nervous exhaustion

Blends well with: Bergamot, cajuput, cardamom, cedarwood, chamomile german, chamomile roman, copaiba, cypress, eucalyptus radiata, fir, juniper berry, lavandin, lavender, lavender (spike), lemon, marjoram (sweet), niaouli, peppermint, ravensara, rosemary, spruce, tea tree, thyme linalol

Precautionary advice: May cause irritation on highly sensitive skin or skin prone to allergic reaction; a skin patch test is advisable. Best avoided by those with respiratory problems.

PLAI, *Zingiber cassumunar, Z. montanum* (Plant Family: Zingiberaceae)

Type of plant: Flowering plant with tuberous root with long fleshy fibers and large glossy leaves

Part used: Rhizome

Method of extraction: Steam distillation

Data: The name *plai* is the Thai word for this plant. The plant is widely used in the traditional medicine systems of Southeast Asia, including in Thailand, Laos, and Cambodia. Plai is of the same botanical family as ginger — although having different properties — and is a relative of galangal.

Principal places of production: Thailand, India, Indonesia

When buying look for: A pale-yellow liquid with a fresh, herbaceous, spicy, slightly green aroma

Therapeutic properties: Analgesic, antibacterial, anti-inflammatory, antineuralgic, antispasmodic, calmative, carminative, diuretic, stimulant, tonic

Therapeutic uses: Arthritis, joint pain, muscle pain, muscular injury, torn ligaments, muscular

spasm, tendonitis, swelling, menstrual cramp, abdominal spasm, colitis, diverticulosis
Blends well with: Basil linalol, bergamot, black pepper, cardamom, chamomile roman, clary sage, elemi, eucalyptus radiata, geranium, ginger, hyssop decumbens, immortelle, juniper berry, lavender, marjoram (sweet), peppermint, pimento berry, sage (Greek), spearmint
Precautionary advice: No contraindications known

RAVENSARA, *Ravensara aromatica* (Plant Family: Lauraceae)

Type of plant: Large, flowering evergreen tree with fragrant bark and dark, aromatic stems and fragrant, glossy leaves
Part used: Leaves
Method of extraction: Steam distillation
Data: Native to Madagascar but now cultivated elsewhere, this tree produces seeds that are used as a spice known as Madagascan nutmeg, which is used in cooking and in medicines. The dark, smooth evergreen leaves are distilled to produce the oil. Used predominantly by clinical aromatherapists, although now widely available.
Principal places of production: Madagascar, Australia
When buying look for: A colorless to slightly yellow-tinged liquid with a fresh, slightly spicy, camphorous, woody aroma
Therapeutic properties: Antibacterial, anti-infectious, antiseptic, antiviral, expectorant, immunostimulant, stimulant
Therapeutic uses: Colds, influenza, bacterial infection, viral infection, herpes, shingles, bronchial infection, bronchitis, respiratory tract infection, rhinitis, sinusitis, muscular pain, muscular fatigue, chronic fatigue
Blends well with: Bergamot, black pepper, cedarwood, cinnamon leaf, cypress, eucalyptus

peppermint, eucalyptus radiata, fragonia, frankincense, geranium, ginger, grapefruit, ho wood, hyssop decumbens, juniper berry, lavandin, lavender, lemon, lemongrass, mandarin, manuka, myrtle, palmarosa, ravintsara, rosemary, spearmint, tangerine, thyme linalol
Precautionary advice: Best avoided during pregnancy and while breast-feeding.

RAVINTSARA, *Cinnamomum camphora* *ct. cineole* (Plant Family: Lauraceae)

Type of plant: Broadleaf evergreen tree growing to 100 feet with rough bark, glossy, fragrant leaves, a profusion of white flowers, and black berries
Part used: Leaves
Method of extraction: Steam distillation
Data: The large, glossy, leathery leaves are hand picked and distilled within a day. Ravintsara was introduced into Madagascar in the mid-twentieth century from Taiwan. It now grows wild in the rain forests of Madagascar or is cultivated. Despite the botanical name of *Cinnamomum camphora*, the essential oil from Madagascar has very little camphor within it, instead having a high percentage of 1,8-cineol, between 40% and 65%. Ravintsara has the same botanical name as ho wood, but ho wood oil is completely different, having a very low percentage of 1,8-cineol and instead having a very high percentage of linalool.
Principal place of production: Madagascar
When buying look for: A colorless to pale-yellow liquid with a strongly herbaceous aroma. Although the aroma is quite similar to saro essential oil, the two have different properties.
Therapeutic properties: Anthelmintic, antibacterial, anticatarrhal, antifungal, anti-infectious, antiseptic, antiviral, expectorant, immunostimulant, mucolytic

Therapeutic uses: Bronchitis, bronchial congestion, colds, sinusitis, rhinitis, excess mucus, laryngitis, viral respiratory infection, viral infection, herpes, shingles, general fatigue

Blends well with: Bay laurel, bergamot, black pepper, cardamom, cedarwood, cypress, eucalyptus radiata, fragonia, frankincense, geranium, ginger, ho wood, hyssop decumbens, lavender, lavender (spike), lemon, manuka, myrtle, niaouli, oregano, palmarosa, ravensara, rosemary, tea tree, thyme linalol

Precautionary advice: Best avoided during pregnancy and while breast-feeding.

ROSALINA (SWAMP PAPERBARK),
Melaleuca ericifolia (Plant Family: Myrtaceae)

Type of plant: Tree growing between 10 and 25 feet high with pale, papery bark, short, needle-like leaves, and scented, creamy-white bottle-brush flowers

Part used: Leaves

Method of extraction: Steam distillation

Data: Native to southeastern Australia and northwest Tasmania, this plant grows well near water, hence its name. It can grow into a tree, although is often pruned into a tall shrub for easier cultivation. As the shoots rise from the roots into thickets, the plant is often used as natural fencing. Rosalina is from the same botanical family as tea tree and is sometimes called lavender tea tree because it seems to have the properties of tea tree yet is calming, like lavender, and sweeter-smelling. Aboriginal people use the leaves and bark in their medicine.

Principal place of production: Australia

When buying look for: A colorless to pale-yellow liquid with a soft, herbaceous, woody, floral-type aroma

Therapeutic properties: Analgesic, antibacterial, anti-infectious, antimicrobial, antiseptic, antispasmodic, antiviral, calmative, expectorant, immunostimulant, nervine, pectoral

Therapeutic uses: Respiratory tract infection, sinusitis, sinus headache, coughs, colds, restlessness, nervousness, irritability, acne, pimples, insect bites

Blends well with: Basil linalol, benzoin, black pepper, cajuput, cedarwood, chamomile roman, elemi, fragonia, frankincense, geranium, grapefruit, lavandin, lavender, marjoram (sweet), rosemary, spikenard, thyme linalol, valerian, vetiver

Precautionary advice: No contraindications known

ROSE ABSOLUTE (ROSE DE MAI),
Rosa centifolia (Plant Family: Rosaceae)

Type of plant: A deciduous bush with thorny stems growing to 6 feet high with large fragrant pink flowers that have very many petals

Part used: Fresh flower heads

Method of extraction: Steam distillation, solvent extraction

Data: The name of this rose, *centifolia*, refers to its many petals (*folia*), perhaps not quite a century (a hundred), but more than other varieties. The essential oil is first extracted into a form known as a concrete, then further extraction produces the absolute. The picking season is between April and June, but a few days in May are the optimum time, hence the name *May rose.* The flower heads have to be picked very early in the morning to retain their fragrance, and it takes approximately 6 tons of flower heads to produce 1 pound of rose absolute. Only *Rosa centifolia* and *Rosa damascena* are grown for rose fragrance, with *centifolia* being more heady and seductive than *damascena*, which is more subtle and delicate.

Principal places of production: Morocco, Turkey, France, China

When buying look for: A reddish-orange liquid of medium viscosity with a deep, soft, honey-spicy, intense rose aroma

Therapeutic properties: Antidepressant, antiseptic, antispasmodic, astringent, calmative, cicatrizing, cytophylactic, hypnotic, nervine, sedative, tonic

Therapeutic uses: Infertility, menstrual problems, endometriosis, dysmenorrhea, menstrual cramp, abdominal cramp, circulatory problems, depression, anxiety, tension, phobias, nervous tension, stress-related conditions, scarring

Blends well with: Basil linalol, benzoin, bergamot, black pepper, cardamom, carnation, chamomile roman, clary sage, clove bud, coriander seed, fennel (sweet), frankincense, geranium, ginger, jasmine, lemon, linden blossom, mandarin, may chang, neroli, orange (sweet), palmarosa, patchouli, rosewood, sandalwood, tangerine, ylang ylang

Precautionary advice: No contraindications known

ROSEMARY, *Rosmarinus officinalis*
(Plant Family: Lamiaceae/Labiatae)

Type of plant: Dense bush of thin branches with spike-like green leaves with grayish undersides and blue flowers

Part used: Leaves, twigs, and flowers

Method of extraction: Steam distillation

Data: Rosemary has been used throughout known history, and it appears in all old herbals. It has long been recognized as a plant that can enhance memory. Historically, in Europe, rosemary was widely used at weddings and funerals, while in law courts the herb was placed in the prisoner's dock as a preventative against "jail fever."

Principal places of production: France, Spain, Morocco, Tunisia

When buying look for: A colorless to pale-yellow, slightly green-tinged liquid with a fresh camphor-like, green, woody, herbaceous aroma

Therapeutic properties: Analgesic, antimicrobial, antiseptic, antispasmodic, carminative, cicatrizing, decongestant, depurative, diuretic, immunostimulant, restorative, spasmolytic, stomachic, stimulant

Therapeutic uses: Muscular aches and pain, rheumatism, arthritis, muscular weakness, muscular injury, headache, migraine, gastric upset, abdominal spasm, respiratory conditions, sinus congestion, fluid retention, heavy legs, edema, cellulite, detoxifying, memory enhancement, general debility, acne, pimples, boils, abscesses, dandruff, hair loss

Blends well with: Basil linalol, basil tulsi, chamomile german, chamomile roman, cistus, citronella, coriander seed, cypress, elemi, eucalyptus lemon, eucalyptus radiata, geranium, greenland moss, hyssop decumbens, immortelle, juniper berry, lavandin, lavender, lavender (spike), lemon, lemongrass, mandarin, marjoram (sweet), niaouli, peppermint, petitgrain, ravensara, ravintsara, saro, spearmint, spruce, tangerine, tarragon, thyme linalol, turmeric, ylang ylang

Precautionary advice: Best avoided during pregnancy. GRAS status.

ROSE OTTO (BULGARIAN ROSE/ TURKISH ROSE), *Rosa damascena*
(Plant Family: Rosaceae)

Type of plant: A deciduous bush with thorny stems growing to 6 feet with fragrant pink flowers

Part used: Fresh flower heads

Method of extraction: Steam distillation

Data: Eighty percent of *Rosa damascena* essential oil comes from the Kazanlak Valley in Bulgaria, where rose growing was introduced in the seventeenth century. This knowledge may have come from the Persians, who are known to have been distilling rose in Shiraz (present-day Iran) since 1612. Writings of the Persian intellectual Ibn Sīnā (Avicenna) described rose distillation as early as the eleventh century, possibly to produce rose water, along with a small amount of oil. It takes literally millions of rose petals to produce just a few fluid ounces of this highly prized essential oil. The roses are hand-picked very early in the morning, and the roses are distilled immediately. Harvesting is between May and June, when the air in the valley is redolent with the aroma of rose and the distilleries are working night and day to process the roses while they still retain their essential oil.

Principal places of production: Bulgaria, Turkey, Iran

When buying look for: A colorless to pale-yellow-tinged liquid with a soft, deep, slightly lemony rose aroma with a faint spice note. It crystallizes at low temperatures, becoming liquid with warmth.

Therapeutic properties: Antidepressant, anti-infectious, antiseptic, astringent, calmative, cicatrizing, circulatory, cytophylactic, emmenagogue, emollient, sedative, spasmolytic, tonic

Therapeutic uses: Female reproductive problems, infertility, menstrual irregularity, endometriosis, dysmenorrhea, menstrual cramp, abdominal cramp, circulatory conditions, acne, skin dehydration, scarring, premature aging, depression, anxiety, emotional anxiety, nervous tension, stress-related conditions

Blends well with: Benzoin, bergamot, black pepper, cananga, carrot seed, chamomile roman, cistus, clary sage, fennel (sweet), frankincense, geranium, jasmine, lavender, lemon, linden blossom, magnolia flower, mandarin, melissa, neroli, orange (sweet), sandalwood

Precautionary advice: No contraindications known. GRAS status.

ROSEWOOD (BOIS DE ROSE),
Aniba rosaeodora (Plant Family: Lauraceae)

Type of plant: Evergreen tree growing to 120 feet high with thick feathery leaves and red flowers and fruits

Part used: Sawdust and wood chippings

Method of extraction: Steam distillation

Data: This South American rain forest tree is endangered and now under protection, with only sustainable sources allowed to be harvested. The heartwood of this laurel-family tree was once much prized for furniture production and instrument making. The essential oil is distilled from sawdust and wood chippings created by wood working. The wood is said to have an aroma similar to the rose flower, hence the name. The essential oil is used in perfumery and cosmetics.

Principal places of production: Brazil, Central America, Peru

When buying look for: A colorless to pale-yellow liquid with a warm, slightly spicy, sweet, floral, woody aroma

Therapeutic properties: Analgesic, anthelmintic, antifungal, antimicrobial, antiseptic, antiviral, calmative, cytophylactic, insect deterrent, spasmolytic, stimulant, tonic

Therapeutic uses: Bronchial infection, tonsillitis, cough, stress headache, convalescence, acne, eczema, psoriasis, scarring, insect bites and stings, nervousness, depression, anxiety, stress-related conditions; tonic

Blends well with: Bergamot, cananga, cardamom, cedarwood, chamomile roman, clary sage, frankincense, galbanum, geranium, ho wood, immortelle, jasmine, lavandin, lavender, lemon, linden blossom, magnolia leaf, marjoram (sweet), myrtle, narcissus, neroli, nutmeg, orange (sweet), petitgrain, rose absolute, rose otto, sandalwood, tuberose, ylang ylang, yuzu

Precautionary advice: No contraindications known. GRAS status.

SAGE, *Salvia officinalis*
(Plant Family: Lamiaceae/Labiatae)

Type of plant: Perennial herb with small, gray-silver leaves and erect stems bearing spikes of purple flowers

Part used: Leaves and flowers

Method of extraction: Steam distillation

Data: Another herb with a long history of use. The word *salvia* translates from Latin as "alive," "save," or "be in good health," and from the ancient Romans onward many European cultures regarded sage as an essential herb for anyone to have growing nearby so it could be used for medicinal purposes. The term *officinalis* refers to the *officina* in monasteries, where the healing herbs were stored. All the classic herbals of history recommended the herb salvia for a variety of purposes, including improving women's fertility. Today sage leaves are perhaps best known as an ingredient in cooking.

Principal places of production: Spain, France, Italy, Croatia, Albania, China

When buying look for: A colorless to pale-yellow liquid with an intense herbaceous, camphorous aroma

Therapeutic properties: Antibacterial, anti-inflammatory, antiseptic, antispasmodic, antiviral, astringent, cholagogue, cicatrizing, digestive, diuretic, emmenagogue, expectorant, mucolytic, stomachic, tonic

Therapeutic uses: Arthritis, rheumatism, cold limbs, numbness, bronchitis, catarrh, sinusitis, influenza, muscular aches and pain, muscular injury, tendonitis, painful joints, menstrual pain, menstrual cramp, menopausal symptoms, hot flashes, excess perspiration, varicose congestion, heavy and tired legs

Blends well with: Basil linalol, bergamot, chamomile german, chamomile roman, clary sage, cypress, geranium, lavender, lemon, lemongrass, marjoram (sweet), myrtle, niaouli, orange (sweet), ravensara, rose absolute, thyme linalol

Precautionary advice: Must be used with care and well diluted. Avoid prolonged use. Do not use if subject to seizures, epilepsy, and high blood pressure. Avoid all types of use during pregnancy and while breast-feeding. Best avoided if on multiple medications. GRAS status.

SAGE, GREEK, *Salvia fruticosa, S. triloba* (Plant Family: Lamiaceae/Labiatae)

Type of plant: Bushy perennial herb growing up to 3 feet high with hairy leaves and stems and with pinkish-purple flowers

Part used: Leaves and flowering tops

Method of extraction: Steam distillation

Data: The young leaves are chosen to be distilled. The plant grows on dry, rocky hillsides all around the Mediterranean, including on the Greek island of Crete. Greek sage was considered sacred by the ancient Greeks, who dedicated it to their god Zeus.

Principal places of production: Greece, Turkey

When buying look for: A colorless to pale-yellow liquid with a warm, fresh, herbaceous, slightly resinous aroma

Therapeutic properties: Anti-inflammatory, antimicrobial, antiseptic, antispasmodic, astringent, digestive, sedative, stomachic, tonic

Therapeutic uses: Muscular aches and pain, muscular injury, painful joints, headache, stomachache, stomach upset, sore throat, menstrual cramp, nervousness, mental fatigue, emotional exhaustion, memory loss, acne, pimples

Blends well with: Basil linalol, bergamot, chamomile german, chamomile roman, cistus, clary sage, cypress, eucalyptus lemon, geranium lavandin, lavender, lemon, lemongrass, marjoram (sweet), may chang, myrtle, niaouli, orange (sweet), rose absolute, rosemary, spikenard, thyme linalol, valerian, vetiver

Precautionary advice: Use with care, well diluted. Avoid prolonged use. Avoid during pregnancy and while breast-feeding. GRAS status.

*ayurvedic med
says headaches
see notes*

SANDALWOOD, *Santalum album*
(Plant Family: Santalaceae)

Type of plant: Small tree growing to 30 feet in height with bark that can be red, brown, or black, with long leaves, small red flowers, and small black fruits
Part used: Chipped heartwood and root
Method of extraction: Steam distillation
Data: Known as *East Indian sandalwood* or *white sandalwood* because the heartwood is sometimes white. The tree is harvested when mature at 30–40 years by uprooting it during the rainy season. Production in the traditional growing area of Mysore Province is strictly controlled by the Indian government, which maintains a sustainable growth policy. The sandalwood tree is parasitic in that as a sapling it gathers water and nutrients from the roots of host plants, yet this relationship does not cause damage to the host. Sandalwood has been used in incense, as a perfume, and in medicine for thousands of years. The trees can live for 100 years, and when more abundant they were used to build ever-fragrant temples and carved religious sculptures.
Principal places of production: India, Indonesia
When buying look for: A pale-yellow, slightly viscous liquid maturing into a darker yellow, with a soft, rich, sweet, warm, woody aroma
Therapeutic properties: Antidepressant, anti-inflammatory, antiseptic, antispasmodic, astringent, calmative, cicatrizing, diuretic, emollient, nervine, pectoral, restorative, sedative, tonic
Therapeutic uses: Coughs, sore throat, heavy legs, swelling, urinary infection, cystitis, vaginal infection, scarring, insomnia, anxiety, nervous tension, nervous exhaustion, depression
Blends well with: Benzoin, cananga, cardamom, chamomile roman, clary sage, coriander seed, frankincense, geranium, ginger lily root, jasmine, juniper berry, lavender, lemon, linden blossom,

mandarin, neroli, orange (sweet), palmarosa, patchouli, petitgrain, rose absolute, rose otto, rosewood, spikenard, tuberose, valerian, ylang ylang
Precautionary advice: No contraindications known

SANDALWOOD, PACIFIC,
Santalum austrocaledonicum
(Plant Family: Santalaceae)

Type of plant: Small parasitic tree with dark grayish bark and pale wood
Part used: Chipped heartwood and roots
Method of extraction: Steam distillation
Data: Known as *New Caledonian sandalwood*, grown on the island groups of New Caledonia and Vanuatu, to the northeast of Australia in the South Pacific Ocean. As it takes a minimum of 20 years before the wood is considered mature, strict conservation and replanting are necessary to ensure species preservation. Other plants of the *Santalum* genus produce an oil that's similar in smell, such as the Australian *Santalum spicatum* (or *Fusanus spicatus*).

Some essential oils sometimes sold as sandalwood come from the same plant family — such as the African *Osyris tenuifolia* — or from unrelated plant families, such as *Rutaceae* — for example, the West Indian *Amyris balsamifera*. Neither of these can be considered sandalwood or substituted for it for therapeutic purposes.
Principal places of production: New Caledonia, Vanuatu
When buying look for: A pale-yellow, slightly viscous liquid with a soft, sweet, woody, balsamic, slightly spicy aroma
Therapeutic properties: Antiseptic, antispasmodic, calmative, emollient, expectorant, sedative
Therapeutic uses: Insomnia, stress, uterine spasm, depression, nervous anxiety

Blends well with: Benzoin, black pepper, cananga, cardamom chamomile roman, coriander seed, cypress, frankincense, geranium, ginger lily root, jasmine, juniper berry, lavender, lemon, mandarin, neroli, nutmeg, orange (sweet), palmarosa, petitgrain, rose absolute, saro, spikenard, tangerine, valerian, ylang ylang
Precautionary advice: No contraindications known

SARO (MANDRAVASAROTRA), *Cinnamosma fragrans* (Plant Family: Canellaceae)

Type of plant: Evergreen tree growing up to 20 feet high with long, oval-shaped, glossy, fragrant leaves, small yellow flowers that bud directly from the branches, and seed-bearing fruits
Part used: Leaves
Method of extraction: Steam distillation
Data: This tree grows largely on the western side of the large island of Madagascar and is used in traditional medicine. Its many health benefits are reflected in the names given to it locally, such as the "tree that keeps illness away" or "overcomes all difficulties." Along with its uses for specific conditions, saro is used as a general tonic as well as having an antipoison effect.
Principal place of production: Madagascar
When buying look for: A colorless to pale-yellow liquid with a warm, green, medicinal, slightly lemony, floral aroma
Therapeutic properties: Analgesic, antifungal, anti-infectious, antimicrobial, antiparasitic, antiseptic, antispasmodic, antiviral, expectorant, immunostimulant, mucolytic, restorative
Therapeutic uses: Bronchitis, catarrh, coughs, colds, influenza, sinusitis, muscular pain, muscular injury, cellulite, wounds, abscesses, physical exhaustion
Blends well with: Cinnamon leaf, clove bud, cypress, eucalyptus lemon, eucalyptus radiata, fragonia, frankincense, geranium, ginger, grapefruit, juniper berry, lavandin, lemongrass, lime, myrtle, patchouli, thyme linalol, turmeric
Precautionary advice: Best avoided during pregnancy

SAVORY, SUMMER, *Satureja hortensis* (Plant Family: Lamiaceae/Labiatae)

Type of plant: A hardy annual herb growing to 1 foot high with a central stem off which extend 10 or so branches bearing long, slim leaves, at the axis of which are small pinkish-white flowers and small brown fruits
Part used: Leaves and flowering tops
Method of extraction: Steam distillation
Data: The word *savory* is said to derive from the Latin *satyrus*, meaning "satyr," a mythological part-human creature notorious for lasciviousness. In other words, savory is an aphrodisiac. It was not only for this use that the Mediterranean herb savory was listed in all pharmacopeias since Roman times, as it is a versatile and useful medicinal herb as well as a culinary and perfumery ingredient.
Principal places of production: Hungary, Spain, France, United States
When buying look for: Pale-yellow to pale-orange-tinged oil with a fresh, slightly spicy, medicinal, herbaceous aroma. Not to be confused with winter savory (*Satureja montana*).
Therapeutic properties: Anthelmintic, antifungal, anti-infectious, antimicrobial, astringent, carminative
Therapeutic uses: Bronchial infection, catarrh, bronchitis, influenza, respiratory viral infection, muscular aches and pains, fungal infection, insect bites
Blends well with: Basil linalol, basil tulsi, bergamot, carrot seed, chamomile german, eucalyptus radiata, ho wood, lavandin, lavender, lemon, niaouli, oregano, palmarosa, spearmint, thyme linalol, turmeric, valerian, yarrow

Precautionary advice: Can cause skin irritation; a skin patch test is advisable. Avoid during pregnancy and while breast-feeding. Best avoided if using multiple medications. GRAS status.

SAVORY, WINTER, *Satureja montana*
(Plant Family: Lamiaceae/Labiatae)

Type of plant: A perennial herb growing to 3 feet high with branches growing vertically, small, long, slim leaves, and dense spikes of small whitish-purple flowers

Part used: Plant including flowers

Method of extraction: Steam distillation

Data: Also known as *mountain savory*, the plant grows well in hilly and mountainous terrain, growing on rocky soil and even between the stones of walls. Used as a culinary herb throughout the Mediterranean.

Principal places of production: Albania, Croatia, Turkey, Spain, Morocco, Russia

When buying look for: A pale-yellow liquid with a strong herbaceous, medicinal-type aroma

Therapeutic properties: Anthelmintic, antibacterial, antifungal, anti-infectious, antiparasitic, antiviral, immunostimulant, tonic

Therapeutic uses: Viral infection, respiratory infection, bronchitis, rheumatism, skeletal aches and pains, muscular pain, digestive problems, wounds, abscesses

Blends well with: Basil linalol, bergamot, chamomile german, chamomile roman, eucalyptus peppermint, eucalyptus radiata, ho wood, lavandin, lavender, lemon, niaouli, oregano, palmarosa, peppermint, sage (Greek), spearmint, thyme linalol, turmeric, valerian, yarrow

Precautionary advice: Can cause skin irritation; a skin patch test is advisable. Avoid during pregnancy and while breast-feeding. Best avoided if using multiple medications. GRAS status.

SPEARMINT, *Mentha spicata*
(Plant Family: Lamiaceae/Labiatae)

Type of plant: A fast-growing herb with fragrant green leaves and flower spikes bearing small white, pink, or purple flowers

Part used: Leaves

Method of extraction: Steam distillation

Data: The plant material is distilled after having been partially dried. The mint has underground suckers that provide new shoots and constant expansion of new growth. Native to Europe, spearmint is now grown extensively in the United States, where it's the essential oil most used in the flavoring industry, particularly in candy, chewing gum, toothpaste, and oral hygiene products.

Principal places of production: United States, China, Hungary, Spain, Russia, India

When buying look for: Colorless to pale-yellow-tinged liquid with a soft, sweet, herbaceous, mint aroma

Therapeutic properties: Antiseptic, calmative, decongestant, digestive, nervine, restorative, spasmolytic, stimulant, stomachic

Therapeutic uses: Colic, dyspepsia, nausea, flatulence, digestive upset, stomachache, neuralgia, lumbago, muscular ache, nervous migraine, nervous fatigue

Blends well with: Angelica seed, bergamot, black pepper, cananga, cardamom, chamomile roman, cypress, eucalyptus lemon, eucalyptus peppermint, eucalyptus radiata, frankincense, geranium, lavender, lemon, mandarin, marjoram (sweet), niaouli, nutmeg, orange (sweet), petitgrain, pine, ravintsara, rosemary, tangerine, tea tree, thyme linalol, tuberose, ylang ylang

Precautionary advice: No contraindications known. GRAS status.

SPIKENARD, *Nardostachys jatamansi* (Plant Family: Valerianaceae)

Type of plant: Flowering plant growing to 2 feet high with around three stems atop, which are clusters of pinkish-mauve, bell-shaped flowers
Part used: Roots
Method of extraction: Steam distillation
Data: Some essential oils have a very long history, and spikenard is one. It's mentioned in the Bible and was often referred to as *nard* in ancient times. It comes from the root of a perennial herb that is related to valerian, and it is often used as a sedative. In India today it is a common ingredient in Ayurvedic medicinal oils. The essential oil is very pungent, and only very few drops are used in blends.
Principal places of production: India, Nepal
When buying look for: A deep yellow to rich amber green-tinged liquid with a deep, earthy, slightly root-like, musky, spicy aroma
Therapeutic properties: Analgesic, antibacterial, anti-infectious, anti-inflammatory, antiseptic, calmative, depurative, nervine, regenerative, restorative, sedative, soporific, spasmolytic
Therapeutic uses: Insomnia, menstrual problems, muscular spasm, muscular contractions, neuralgia, sciatica, bodily congestion, detoxifying, aging skin, physical tension, stress-related conditions, anxiety, nervous tension; soothing, calming
Blends well with: Bergamot, cananga, cedarwood, chamomile german, chamomile roman, coriander seed, cypress, frankincense, galbanum, geranium, immortelle, jasmine, juniper berry, lavender, lemon, lemongrass, linden blossom, mandarin, marjoram (sweet), mimosa, neroli, palmarosa, patchouli, petitgrain, rose absolute, rose otto, tangerine, valerian, vetiver, ylang ylang

Precautionary advice: No contraindications known

SPRUCE, *Picea abies* (Plant Family: Pinaceae)

Type of plant: Evergreen conifer tree growing to 180 feet high with dark-green needles and male and female cones
Part used: Twigs and needles
Method of extraction: Steam distillation
Data: Native to Russia, northern Europe, Scandinavia, and the Alps, this tree can live up to 1,000 years. The tree is fast growing and widely used as a raw material to make paper. The tree is often used at Christmas, especially when large trees are required for public spaces.
Principal places of production: United States, Canada
When buying look for: A colorless to pale-yellow liquid with a fresh, green, coniferous aroma
Therapeutic properties: Antibacterial, antifungal, anti-inflammatory, antispasmodic, antitussive, expectorant, tonic
Therapeutic uses: Bronchitis, respiratory problems, physical fatigue, mental exhaustion, rheumatism, general aches and pains, acne, anxiety, stress
Blends well with: Bay laurel, camphor (white), cedarwood, chamomile german, cypress, frankincense, geranium, lavandin, lavender, lavender (spike), lemon, manuka, niaouli, orange (sweet), peppermint, pine, ravintsara, rosemary, sage (Greek), spearmint, tea tree, thyme linalol, vetiver, yarrow
Precautionary advice: May cause irritation on sensitive skins; a skin patch test is advisable. Best avoided during pregnancy.

SPRUCE, BLACK, *Picea mariana*
(Plant Family: Pinaceae)

Type of plant: Slow-growing evergreen conifer tree growing to 60 feet with blue-green needles and small purplish seed cones
Part used: Twigs and needles
Method of extraction: Steam distillation
Data: Native throughout Canada. The branches exude an edible gum — the source of spruce gum, the original American chewing gum first sold commercially in the early 1800s. It was introduced to the colonists by people of the First Nations, who also showed how the gum could be used to heal wounds. They also used the needles to make spruce beer, which can be alcoholic or nonalcoholic, to alleviate scurvy during the long winter months when fruits weren't available.
Principal place of production: Canada
When buying look for: A colorless to yellow-tinged liquid with a sweet, fresh, woody, resinous, fruity, green aroma
Therapeutic properties: Anthelmintic, analgesic, antibacterial, antifungal, anti-inflammatory, antispasmodic, diuretic, expectorant, insect deterrent, pectoral
Therapeutic uses: Bronchial infection, catarrh, sinus congestion, arthritis, rheumatism, gout, overexercised muscles, stiff joints, muscular strain, tendonitis, cellulite
Blends well with: Bay laurel, camphor (white), cedarwood, chamomile german, cypress, geranium, lavandin, lavender, lavender (spike), lemon, niaouli, orange (sweet), peppermint, pine, ravintsara, rosemary, spearmint, tea tree, thyme linalol, yarrow
Precautionary advice: May cause irritation on highly sensitive skins; a skin patch test is advisable. Best avoided during pregnancy.

TAGETES, *Tagetes minuta, T. glandulifera*
(Plant Family: Asteraceae/Compositae)

Type of plant: Fast-growing annual plant growing up to 2 feet high, depending on the species, with smallish yellow to orange flowers
Part used: Flowers
Method of extraction: Steam distillation
Data: There are over 50 varieties of the genus *Tagates*. Native to South America, tagetes is now grown all over the world as a decorative flower, sometimes called *African* or *Mexican marigold*. Shamans in Mexico used the plant to induce visions. Extract of tagetes is added to chicken feed to make the egg yolks yellow, and it is used in fish farming to improve the color of trout, salmon, and shrimp. The essential oil distilled from various tagetes species has long been used in perfumery and in the food and beverage industries.
Principal places of production: Egypt, France, Brazil, Argentina
When buying look for: A yellow to orange liquid with a fruity green, slightly floral aroma. Not to be confused with calendula oil, *Calendula officinalis*, which is sometimes called *true marigold*.
Therapeutic properties: Antifungal, antimicrobial, antiparasitic, antiseptic, insect deterrent
Therapeutic uses: Athlete's foot, corns, calluses, bunions, parasitic infestations, resistant fungal infections
Blends well with: Benzoin, bergamot, chamomile german, chamomile roman, citronella, clary sage, geranium, grapefruit, lavandin, lavender, lemon, may chang, tangerine
Precautionary advice: Photosensitizer; do not apply to the skin prior to sun exposure. May cause irritation on sensitive skin; a skin patch test is advisable. Avoid during pregnancy.

TANGERINE, *Citrus reticulata, C. nobilis*
(Plant Family: Rutaceae)

Type of plant: Small evergreen tree with dark-green leaves, fragrant creamy-white flowers, and small orange-colored fruit
Part used: Fruit rind
Method of extraction: Cold expression
Data: The fruit is harvested before fully ripe so the rind can remain attached to the body of the fruit during the extraction process. Tangerine is larger and darker in color than mandarin. Although the fruit and aromas of tangerine and mandarin can easily be confused, their essential oils have slightly different therapeutic properties. Originally from China, tangerine is closely related to mandarin. The name *tangerine* comes from the fact that the fruit was widely grown around Tangiers, a port town in Morocco.
Principal places of production: China, United States, Mexico, Spain, Japan, Argentina, Brazil
When buying look for: A dark orangey-yellow to orange liquid with a fresh, fruity, bright, citrus aroma typical of the fruit
Therapeutic properties: Antiseptic, antispasmodic, cytophylactic, depurative, digestive, sedative, stomachic, tonic
Therapeutic uses: Stress-induced insomnia, nervous exhaustion, mild muscular spasm, cellulite, digestive problems, detoxifying, flatulence, constipation, bodily congestion, tired all the time, irritability, generally dispirited, overly anxious
Blends well with: Basil linalol, bergamot, black pepper, cananga, caraway seed, cardamom, carrot seed, chamomile german, chamomile maroc, chamomile roman, clary sage, clove bud, fennel (sweet), frankincense, geranium, immortelle, jasmine, juniper berry, linden blossom, marjoram (sweet), mimosa, neroli, patchouli, petitgrain, rose absolute, rosemary, sandalwood, ylang ylang

Precautionary advice: No contraindications known. GRAS status.

TARRAGON, *Artemisia dracunculus*
(Plant Family: Asteraceae/Compositae)

Type of plant: Perennial herb growing to 3 feet in height with a central stalk off which are branches with long, thin, bright-green leaves. Depending on the subspecies, there may be clusters of tiny green-yellow flowers.
Part used: Leaves and stems
Method of extraction: Steam distillation
Data: Tarragon is best known as a culinary herb. Tarragon essential oil is used in perfumery and for fragrancing detergents. To grow French tarragon, keep in mind that fertile seeds are not available so propagation is carried out by root separation. When purchasing essential oils, the botanical name is important to confirm because there are some *Artemisia* genus plants and oils that need to be avoided. Look for the botanical name above and avoid Russian tarragon, which has a very similar name — *Artemisia dracunculoides*.
Principal places of production: France, Hungary, Russia, Germany
When buying look for: A colorless to pale-yellow liquid that may have a slight green hint, with a fresh, herbaceous, slightly earthy, aniseed-like aroma
Therapeutic properties: Anti-inflammatory, antispasmodic, carminative, stomachic, tonic
Therapeutic uses: Dyspepsia, flatulence, indigestion, intestinal spasm, gastrointestinal problems, constipation, nausea, muscular cramp, muscular spasm, rheumatism, abdominal congestion and swelling
Blends well with: Basil linalol, black pepper, caraway seed, cardamom, coriander seed, cypress, ho wood, juniper berry, lavandin, lemon,

mandarin, marjoram (sweet), niaouli, rosemary, tea tree, vetiver

Precautionary advice: Avoid if using multiple medications. Avoid prolonged use. May cause irritation on highly sensitive skins; a skin patch test is advisable. Avoid during pregnancy and while breast-feeding. GRAS status.

TEA TREE, *Melaleuca alternifolia*
(Plant Family: Myrtaceae)

Type of plant: Bushy tree with long branches and twigs, small narrow leaves, and white cotton-puff flowers

Part used: Leaves and branches

Method of extraction: Steam distillation

Data: Native to Australia but now grown commercially elsewhere. The Aboriginal people of Australia have used the medicinal properties of tea tree for untold millennia. Findings of its medicinal properties were first presented to the scientific community by an Australian government scientist, Dr. A. R. Penfold, in 1923. Tea tree oil was so valued by the 1940s that cutters and producers were exempted from military service during the Second World War until sufficient supplies were available to provide all military personnel with a personal supply in their first aid kits.

Principal places of production: Australia, Tasmania, Kenya

When buying look for: Colorless to pale-yellow liquid with a strongly medicinal, slightly spicy, camphorous aroma

Therapeutic properties: Anthelmintic, antibacterial, antifungal, antiseptic, antiviral, decongestant, immunostimulant, vulnerary

Therapeutic uses: Bacterial skin infection, parasitic skin infection, respiratory tract infection, sinusitis, rhinitis, laryngitis, bronchitis, wounds, ulceration, pimples, acne, abscesses, head and body lice, fungal infection, athlete's foot, warts, verrucas

Blends well with: Bergamot, black pepper, chamomile german, chamomile roman, elemi, eucalyptus lemon, eucalyptus radiata, fragonia, geranium, ho wood, lavandin, lavender, lavender (spike), lemon, manuka, orange (sweet), palmarosa, peppermint, ravensara, rosemary, tangerine

Precautionary advice: May cause irritation; a skin patch test is advisable.

THYME LINALOL, *Thymus vulgaris ct. linalool*
(Plant Family: Lamiaceae/Labiatae)

Type of plant: Bushy perennial evergreen dwarf shrub with branches of woody stems, growing up to 1 foot in height with small, dark-green, oval leaves and white-through-purple flowers

Part used: Flowering tops

Method of extraction: Steam distillation

Data: Native to southern Europe, thyme is well known as a culinary herb. It was used medicinally by the Greeks and the Romans. The king who united much of western Europe into the kingdom of Francia in the early eighth century, Charlemagne, issued instructions to his estate managers that thyme must be grown in all gardens. He no doubt recognized the remarkable healing properties of thyme, which are the subject of intense scientific research today. Different types of thyme essential oil are used in aromatherapy, and although all are distilled from *Thymus vulgaris*, they're distinguished from one another by their chemical constituents, having, for example, a larger proportion of geraniol or thujanol. The thyme used throughout this book is the chemotype *linalool*.

Principal places of production: France, Morocco, Turkey, Spain

When buying look for: Colorless to pale-yellow liquid with a soft, sweet, herbaceous aroma

Therapeutic properties: Analgesic, antibacterial, antifungal, anti-infectious, antiputrescent, antiseptic, antispasmodic, antiviral, expectorant, immunostimulant, pectoral, restorative, stimulant, tonic, vermifuge

Therapeutic uses: Influenza, coughs, colds, bronchitis, sinusitis, rhinitis, laryngitis, sore throat, bronchial chest infection, mucous congestion, viral and bacterial skin infections, circulatory problems, cold limbs, numbness, muscular pain, muscular debility, tendonitis, arthritis, rheumatism, general debility, chronic fatigue, acne, warts, verrucas, lethargy, inability to concentrate

Blends well with: Basil linalol, basil tulsi, bergamot, black pepper, cedarwood, chamomile german, chamomile roman, clary sage, cypress, elemi, eucalyptus lemon, eucalyptus radiata, fragonia, geranium, ginger, grapefruit, ho wood, lavandin, lavender, lemon, manuka, marjoram (sweet), mastic, niaouli, orange (sweet), oregano, palmarosa, peppermint, plai, ravensara, ravintsara, rosalina, rosemary, rosewood, spearmint, tangerine

Precautionary advice: No contraindications known. GRAS status.

TUBEROSE (ABSOLUTE), *Polianthes tuberosa* (Plant Family: Asparagaceae)

Type of plant: Perennial bulbous plant with tall, straight stems on top of which are highly fragrant, creamy-white, star-shaped flowers

Part used: Flowers

Method of extraction: CO_2 and solvent extraction, enfleurage

Data: Tuberose is a night-flowering plant pollinated by moths. Despite the name, it's not related to rose and derives its name from its tuberous root. Native to Mexico and Central America, the flower has been adopted in Hawaii, where the highly fragrant flowers are used as personal decoration, and in India, where garlands are offered to images of gods and goddesses. It's said that the plant was brought to France in the sixteenth century by a missionary who then cultivated it in a monastery garden. The fragrance of tuberose is so intense it became a mainstay of the French perfume industry as it developed in Grasse, Provence.

Principal places of production: India, France, Egypt, Madagascar, Morocco

When buying look for: Viscous, deep yellow to golden amber-brown liquid with a creamy, deeply intense floral aroma and a very faint spicy, minty note

Therapeutic properties: Antidepressant, antimicrobial, calmative, carminative, hypnotic, relaxant, sedative, spasmodic, stimulant

Therapeutic uses: Muscular spasm, stress-induced conditions, physical tension, insomnia, nervousness, restlessness, irritability, anxiety, depression

Blends well with: Amyris, balsam de Peru, benzoin, bergamot, black pepper, cananga, cistus, clove bud, coriander seed, frankincense, galbanum, geranium, ginger, grapefruit, jasmine, lavender, lemon, linden blossom, mandarin, mimosa, narcissus, orange (sweet), patchouli, peppermint, petitgrain, rose absolute, rose otto, sandalwood, spearmint, tangerine, vanilla, ylang ylang

Precautionary advice: May cause irritation on sensitive skins; a skin patch test is advisable. Best avoided during pregnancy and while breast-feeding. GRAS status.

TURMERIC, *Curcuma longa* (Plant Family: Zingiberaceae)

Type of plant: Tall perennial herb with very long and wide leaves, yellow to white flowers, and clusters of bright-orange rhizomes

Part used: Rhizomes

Method of extraction: Steam distillation

Data: Turmeric was one of the spices made available to the Western world through the vast trading links of the ancient Arabs. The essential oil is distilled from the fresh rhizomes. As a spice, the rhizomes are either used fresh, or boiled and then dried in the sun or in ovens before being ground to a powder. Turmeric is used in Indian Ayurvedic medicine and traditional Chinese medicine, as well as being widely used in cooking.

Principal places of production: India, Indonesia

When buying look for: A yellow to dark-orange liquid with a fresh, earthy, rooty, warm, slightly spicy aroma

Therapeutic properties: Analgesic, anti-inflammatory, antimicrobial, antispasmodic, cholagogue, digestive, restorative, stimulant, stomachic, tonic

Therapeutic uses: Gastrointestinal conditions, indigestion, dyspepsia, stomach cramp, intestinal spasm, general aches and pains, rheumatism, rheumatoid arthritis

Blends well with: Basil tulsi, black pepper, cajuput, caraway seed, cardamom, carrot seed, chamomile german, cinnamon leaf, clove bud, copaiba, coriander seed, davana, geranium, ginger, greenland moss, lemon, lemongrass, mandarin, nutmeg, orange (sweet), rose absolute, sandalwood, saro, tangerine, ylang ylang

Precautionary advice: Avoid prolonged use. May cause irritation on sensitive skins; a skin patch test is advisable. Best avoided during pregnancy. Best avoided if using multiple medications. GRAS status.

VALERIAN, *Valeriana officinalis*
(Plant Family: Valerianaceae)

Type of plant: A tall herb growing to 5 feet in height, with dark leaves and long stems with flower heads comprising many small white flowers with a pink tinge

Part used: Roots

Method of extraction: Steam distillation

Data: Valerian roots are quite thick, and when removed from the ground they appear as bundles of rope. This is an herb that was once considered magical, probably because of its hypnotic properties. There are many different varieties of valerian in the world, all of which appear to be sedative to some degree. Valerian is used in homeopathic as well as in herbal medicine.

Principal places of production: France, Croatia, Hungary, China, India

When buying look for: A pale-yellow to dark-yellow liquid with a warm, musty, earthy, balsamic aroma

Therapeutic properties: Antimicrobial, antispasmodic, calmative, depurative, diuretic, hypnotic, nervine, sedative, soporific, stomachic

Therapeutic uses: Gastrointestinal infections, insomnia, nervousness, stress, tension, tension headache, stress-induced migraine, muscular spasm, cramps, restlessness, inability to relax, restless leg, trembling disorders, pimples, acne, problematic skin

Blends well with: Amyris, basil linalol, bergamot, cananga, cedarwood, chamomile german, chamomile roman, clary sage, coriander seed, geranium, ginger lily root, hop, ho wood, jasmine, juniper berry, lavender, linden blossom, magnolia flower, magnolia leaf, mandarin, orange (sweet), petitgrain, rose absolute, sandalwood, spikenard, tangerine, vetiver, ylang ylang

Precautionary advice: Avoid if taking sedatives or antidepressant medication. Best avoided during pregnancy and while breast-feeding.

VANILLA (ABSOLUTE), *Vanilla plantifolia*
(Plant Family: Orchidaceae)

Type of plant: A climbing vine that can grow to 80 feet long but is pruned well back, with orchid flowers that produce the fruit, known as pods, which are 6–7 inches long

Part used: Bean pod

Method of extraction: Solvent and CO_2 extraction

Data: The now ubiquitous vanilla started life in a very specific area of eastern Mexico, looked over by the Totonaco tribal people and pollinated by a tiny bee called the melipona bee. But the Aztecs invaded, and they in turn were invaded by the Spanish conquistadors in 1520, led by Hernán Cortés. The Aztec leader Moctezuma offered Cortés a nice drink of cacao beans and vanilla, but Cortés proceeded to trash the entire civilization and steal their gold. Everyone in Europe wanted the vanilla he brought back, but without the little bee, all plants taken away remained sterile. Hundreds of years passed. Eventually people realized they would have to hand-pollinate the flowers, on the one day they open, and the vanilla industry was born. Today, the best quality vanilla still comes from Mexico, and also from Madagascar and nearby islands. The unripe green fruit pods are put through a fermentative process to develop the familiar vanilla fragrance and become the pliable black cured pods that we recognize as natural vanilla.

Principal places of production: Réunion, Comoro Islands, Madagascar, Mexico, Tahiti, India

When buying look for: A dark-brown, very sticky, viscous liquid with a warm, rich, sweet balsamic, vanilla aroma. The classic vanilla aroma is released when the essential oil is diluted.

Therapeutic properties: Antidepressant, balsamic, calmative, sedative, stimulant

Therapeutic uses: Stress-induced conditions, nervous anxiety, nervousness, insomnia and restlessness, unexplained painful limbs, nervous stomach, nausea, inability to relax

Blends well with: Amyris, balsam de Peru, bay (West Indian), benzoin, cananga, cardamom, cedarwood, chamomile maroc, chamomile roman, cinnamon leaf, clove bud, frankincense, geranium, ginger, ginger lily (white), ginger lily root, jasmine, lemon, lime, linden blossom, magnolia leaf, mandarin, mimosa, narcissus, neroli, nutmeg, orange (sweet), rose absolute, rose otto, rosewood, sandalwood, tangerine, ylang ylang

Precautionary advice: May cause irritation on highly sensitive skin; a patch test is advisable. GRAS status.

VETIVER, *Vetiveria zizanoides* (Plant Family: Poaceae)

Type of plant: Perennial grass with stiff, thin leaves growing up to 5 feet high, with fragrant roots that can grow over 8 feet in length

Part used: Roots

Method of extraction: Steam distillation

Data: Harvesting takes place every year and a half. First, the grass is cut low to the ground — this will be woven into floor mats, screens, and fans that deter insects. Then the roots are dug up, washed, and dried in the shade before distillation. The roots are extremely numerous, and the plant is very hardy and useful in preventing soil erosion. Small pieces of root are placed between stored clothing to deter insects. This is a very pungent essential oil, and it can easily overpower other essential oils in a blend.

Principal places of production: Réunion, Comoro Islands, Madagascar, Indonesia, Haiti, India, Sri Lanka, Paraguay

When buying look for: Viscous, golden brown to amber-brown liquid with a deep, earthy, green, rooty aroma

Therapeutic properties: Antimicrobial, antiseptic, antispasmodic, depurative, nervine, restorative, sedative, tonic

Therapeutic uses: Stress-induced conditions, nervous tension, stress-related menstrual problems, muscular spasm, muscular pain, menstrual cramp, premenstrual syndrome, restlessness, workaholism, physical exhaustion, irritability, depression

Blends well with: Amyris, bergamot, black pepper, cardamom, citronella, clary sage, coriander seed, eucalyptus lemon, geranium, ginger, grapefruit, ho wood, lavandin, lavender, lemongrass, mandarin, may chang, orange (sweet), peppermint, petitgrain, sandalwood, spikenard, tangerine, valerian, yuzu

Precautionary advice: No contraindications known

VIOLET LEAF (ABSOLUTE), *Viola odorata* (Plant Family: Violaceae)

Type of plant: Small perennial plant with dark-green, heart-shaped leaves and small, deep-violet flowers

Part used: Leaves

Method of extraction: Solvent and CO_2 extraction

Data: The leaves are mentioned in old European herbals, recommended for a wide range of conditions, including bad breath, urinary tract infections, aches and pains, skin rashes, and bruising. The methods they used were infused oils and poultices. Violet pastilles were once a common European candy for sweetening breath, while violet flowers are still crystallized for cake and confectionery decoration. Violet syrups were once widely used in Europe as a throat salve, but today gourmet violet syrups are more likely to be found in floral-flavored cocktails.

Principal places of production: Egypt, France, Italy, Greece

When buying look for: A dark-green, viscous liquid with a green, earthy, mossy, floral aroma

Therapeutic properties: Analgesic, antiseptic, astringent, cytophylactic, diuretic, emollient, soporific, stimulant

Therapeutic uses: Rheumatic conditions, fluid retention, edema, cellulite, stress-induced acne,

prematurely aged skin, bruising, sore skin, nervous exhaustion; skin care and perfumery

Blends well with: Benzoin, bergamot, cedarwood, chamomile german, clary sage, clove bud, galbanum, geranium, ho wood, jasmine, lemon, linden blossom, mandarin, may chang, melissa, mimosa, myrtle, neroli, orange (sweet), petitgrain, rose absolute, rose otto, rosewood, spikenard

Precautionary advice: No contraindications known

YARROW, *Achillea millefolium* (Plant Family: Asteraceae/Compositae)

Type of plant: Common perennial meadow herb growing over 2 feet high with feathery leaves and erect stems on which are heads of tiny white or pink flowers

Part used: Leaves and flowering tops

Method of extraction: Steam distillation

Data: The name *Achillea* comes from the ancient Greek myth of Achilles, who when wounded in battle was treated with yarrow by the goddess Aphrodite. This is more than myth though, because yarrow was still being used by soldiers in the field during the First World War to dress wounds, both to stem bleeding and to prevent infection. And even today herbalists refer to yarrow as "soldier's wound wort," "staunchwort," and "nosebleed plant." Yarrow is used in some pharmaceutical products for skin conditions, due to its anti-inflammatory agent, azulene, which gives the oil its characteristic blue color. The long, wood-like, dried stems of the yarrow plant continue to be used as the most traditionally correct tool for casting the *I Ching*, a mode of prophesy in China.

Principal places of production: Hungary, Bulgaria, Germany, France, China

When buying look for: A deep-dark-blue liquid with an herbaceous, fruity aroma

Therapeutic properties: Anti-inflammatory, antiseptic, antispasmodic, astringent, carminative, cicatrizing, circulatory, expectorant, restorative
Therapeutic uses: Rheumatism, arthritis, inflamed or injured muscles, muscular cramp, menstrual cramp, scarring, acne
Blends well with: Cedarwood, chamomile german, chamomile roman, cypress, geranium, ho wood, juniper berry, lavender, marjoram (sweet), niaouli, orange (sweet), palmarosa, rosemary, rosewood, tea tree
Precautionary advice: Avoid use if on multiple medications. May cause irritation on highly sensitive skins; a skin patch test is advisable.

YLANG YLANG, *Cananga odorata*
(Plant Family: Annonaceae)

Type of plant: A tree of around 60 feet in height with drooping branches carrying clusters of large, golden yellow, star-shaped flowers
Part used: Flowers
Method of extraction: Steam distillation
Data: Cultivated trees are often cut back to 6 feet so the flowers can easily be reached. Harvesting takes place year round, with each flower hand-picked only when its maturity is signaled by a red tinge at its base. The flowers are picked very early in the morning and distilled immediately. Ylang ylang was native to southeast Asia but is now cultivated in other tropical or subtropical areas, particularly on the island of Nosy Bé and the Comoro Islands, north of Madagascar, and Réunion, to the east, which approaching sailors called "the perfumed isles." The essential oil has a reputation as an aphrodisiac and has long been a component in some of the most expensive perfumes.

Some flowers are processed by fractional steam distillation, resulting in oils of different densities, classed as grades: extra, first, second, and third. Extra grade is produced after two

hours of distillation, whereas grade three is the result of up to 20 hours of distillation. The fragrance intensity is strongest in the extra oil, reducing with each grade to third. Complete essential oil results from a single distillation process, which can take up to 10 hours. The essential oil of cananga is produced, usually in Asia, from a tree of the same genus and species as ylang ylang but a different variety. It has an aroma similar to ylang ylang but not as floral, but it is sometimes sold as ylang ylang.

Principal places of production: Nosy Bé, Réunion, Comoro Islands, Madagascar, Indonesia
When buying look for: Pale-yellow to deeper-yellow liquid with a rich, sweet, soft, floral aroma
Therapeutic properties: Antidepressant, antiphlogistic, antiseptic, antispasmodic, calmative, circulatory, hypotensive, nervine, sedative, tonic
Therapeutic uses: Hypertension, circulatory conditions, muscular cramp, menstrual cramp, intestinal spasm, insomnia, nervous tension, stress, nervousness, physical exhaustion, chronic fatigue, depression
Blends well with: Amyris, basil, bay (West Indian), bay laurel, benzoin, bergamot, black pepper, cananga, cinnamon leaf, clove bud, coriander seed, eucalyptus lemon, frankincense, galbanum, ginger, ginger lily root, grapefruit, ho wood, jasmine, lavender, lemon, linden blossom, magnolia flower, magnolia leaf, mandarin, may chang, neroli, orange (sweet), palmarosa, patchouli, petitgrain, rose maroc, rose otto, rosewood, sandalwood, spikenard, tangerine, tuberose, vetiver, yuzu
Precautionary advice: May cause irritation on highly sensitive skin; a skin patch test is advisable. GRAS status.

YUZU, *Citrus junos* (Plant Family: Rutaceae)

Type of plant: Small, thorny evergreen tree with dark, glossy leaves, creamy-white flowers, and large green or yellow fruit with an uneven surface

Part used: Fruit rind

Method of extraction: Cold pressed

Data: The tree is extensively grown in Japan, where it was introduced over 1,000 years ago. Yuzu is very cold-hardy and is therefore grown in areas too cold for other citrus fruits. In Japan and Korea the rind, juice, and fruit are used as flavoring, especially in vinegars, soups, seafood dishes, sauces, pickles, salads, cakes, candy, and both alcoholic and nonalcoholic drinks. In Japan, the yuzu fruit is added to bathwater, especially during the winter solstice, to ward off infections and bring a prosperity of health. Different parts of the yuzu fruit are used in beauty preparations, including the seeds, rind, and essential oil.

Principal places of production: Japan, Korea

When buying look for: A green-tinged yellow to deeper green-yellow liquid with a warm, sweet, slightly green, uniquely citrus aroma

Therapeutic properties: Analgesic, antibacterial, anti-infectious, antiseptic, calmative, diuretic, nervine, sedative, stimulant, tonic

Therapeutic uses: Nervous stomach cramp, cellulite, neuralgia, influenza, colds, convalescence, stress-induced skin conditions, devitalized skin, nervous tension, nervous exhaustion, chronic fatigue; general tonic

Blends well with: Basil linalol, bay (West Indian), black pepper, cananga, clary sage, clove bud, frankincense, geranium, ginger, ginger lily root, grapefruit, jasmine, lavender, magnolia leaf, may chang, orange (sweet), palmarosa, patchouli, petitgrain, rose absolute, vetiver, ylang ylang

Precautionary advice: May cause irritation on highly sensitive skin; a skin patch test is advisable.

Safety Information

Essential oils are natural and, when chosen and used correctly, safe. But they are also powerful, and deserve respect. All essential oil users should be aware of the following precautions, so please take the time to read all through this short chapter.

When using essential oils there are a few basic rules to remember:

- Keep essential oils and blends in lidded, dark-glass bottles or in aluminum containers.
- Always ensure the bottle top or the container lid is secure to avoid spillage.
- Store essential oils in a cool, dark place, away from light and heat.
- Keep all essential oils and blends out of reach of children and pets.
- Wash hands thoroughly before and after using diluted or undiluted essential oils.
- Avoid all contact with the eyes — if essential oil accidentally gets into the eye, immediately wash the eye as best as you can and seek medical assistance.
- Don't apply essential oils directly to the eyes, up the nose, in the ears, or to genital areas.
- If a large amount of undiluted essential oil is accidentally ingested, drink milk or another fatty substance, and contact your local poison unit for advice.

- Never apply undiluted essential oil over large areas of the body, unless under the direction of a professional therapist.
- Those prone to sensitivities or allergic reactions to fragrance ingredients should conduct a skin test before use.

Skin Irritation

Some essential oils contain components that have the potential to cause skin irritation in people who are susceptible to having skin reactions generally or allergic reactions to fragrances. If you have sensitive skin, carry out a patch test before using any essential oil. Dilute the essential oil you intend to use in a small amount of carrier oil and apply to the inner elbow area. Leave for 24 hours to see if there's been a reaction. Try to always buy organic essential oils and carrier oils.

Essential oils in common use but with the potential to cause skin irritation in susceptible people include basil, basil tulsi, bay laurel, sweet birch, white camphor, clove bud, lemon verbena, melissa, opopanax, bitter orange (not to be confused with sweet orange), oregano, Peru balsam, pimento leaf, tagetes, tea tree, thyme, and wintergreen. However, *any* essential oil or fragrance ingredient has the potential to cause skin irritation, depending on the individual person and on the particular essential oil being used, the condition under which the plant material was grown including pesticide use, the way in which it was extracted, the storage period, and so on.

Allergic Reaction

When blending essential oils and carrier oils for someone else — someone who, perhaps, you don't know well — find out first if they have any allergies. Peanut oil (groundnut or arachis) is not generally used in aromatherapy practice precisely because it could inadvertently be used on a person who is allergic to peanuts. But people are allergic to other nuts, to wheat, and to all kinds of things. So just be aware of this factor when choosing both carrier oils and essential oils.

Photosensitivity

An increased skin reaction to the ultraviolet rays of sunlight is known as *photosensitivity*. It can be brought about by certain medications, including antibiotics. Essential oils whose constituents contain a percentage of furocoumarins such as bergapten may cause photosensitization if applied to the skin before exposure to direct sunlight. Bergamot has the highest percentage of furocoumarins, and because of this some bergamot essential oils have been processed to remove the furocoumarin content and are known as "FCF" — furocoumarin-free. Other oils that cause photosensitivity are grapefruit, angelica root, and tagetes (a type of marigold). When tested, lemon verbena essential oils elicit different results, showing that each essential oil needs to be considered on its own merits. The citrus oils are sometimes considered photosensitizing although their furocoumarin content varies considerably, with mandarin's being practically zero.

If using one of the potentially photosensitizing essential oils in a body oil or spray, cover up the area where the oil has been applied before going out in sunlight or using a sunbed, and be aware that the effect may last up to 12 hours. Try to avoid photosensitizing essential oils in face preparations that are used during the day.

Flammability

Most essential oils are flammable. For this reason, they're kept away from naked flames and any heat sources, including sunny windowsills and anywhere else that receives direct sunlight. Keeping essential oils in a cool, dark place away from heat and light also preserves their quality. Candle diffusers are designed to separate the fragrance, whether natural essential oil or synthetic fragrance, away from the flame of the candle. Electronic diffusers designed to use water and essential oil should have safety features in place to prevent the electric components from coming into contact with the water.

Phytoestrogens

A few essential oils are said to have phytoestrogenic properties, by which it's meant that they elicit a response in the body similar to that caused by the hormone estrogen. The three essential oils in common use most often attributed with these effects are sweet fennel, sage, and clary sage. The plants from which these essential oils are extracted have a long history of being used for female reproductive problems, and the essential oils have been successfully used for many female conditions. However, although there is very little evidence of contrary effects, a certain degree of circumspection needs to be taken in regard to these essential oils, most specifically by anyone with estrogen-sensitive conditions, at least until more definitive information becomes available.

Pregnancy and Lactation

When a woman is pregnant, unless otherwise directed by a professional, it's best to use the minimum quantities of essential oils and avoid all use during the first trimester.

The number of essential oils suitable for women to use while pregnant or lactating is limited. Please see the "Pregnancy" section in chapter 8, "A Woman's Natural Choice," for a list of essential oils that can be used during those times (see pages 224–225).

Essential Oils to Be Avoided

Essential oils are produced for a wide variety of industrial, agricultural, and commercial reasons and are available for all these purposes, as well as for aromatherapy use. Some degree of care, therefore, needs to be taken when purchasing essential oils to ensure they're suitable for use by the home practitioner.

Although knowing the botanical name of an essential oil is helpful, it's not a foolproof method of distinguishing between essential oils. For example, tangerine and mandarin, which are not dissimilar in their effects, have the same botanical name, *Citrus reticulata*. But three essential oils are made from the orange tree *Citrus aurantium* and have entirely different uses: neroli is made from the flowers, petitgrain is made from the leaves and twigs, and bitter orange is made from the fruit. And, while bitter orange essential oil is not used in aromatherapy, sweet orange is. Sweet orange is *Citrus sinensis* but it is often described as *Citrus aurantium var.* [variety] *sinensis*. A good supplier should clarify in the labeling whether the orange being sold is sweet or bitter, but when purchasing essential oils, have all the information to hand — the common name and the botanical name — and don't suppose that because it nearly sounds right, it is! Care needs to be taken with the common name as well as with the botanical.

For example, sweet and bitter fennel essential oils have the same botanical name, *Foeniculum vulgare*, but sweet fennel is used in aromatherapy, and bitter fennel is not. Precision is important when using essential oils for therapeutic purposes.

The names of some of the essential oils listed below might seem very familiar, but they're not generally recommended for use by home practitioners. Others on the list have been deemed "best avoided" by a variety of regulators, including those of the cosmetic industry.

ESSENTIAL OILS TO BE AVOIDED
Boldo leaf (*Peumus boldus*)
Buchu (*Agathosma betulina*)
Cade (*Juniperus oxycedrus*)
Calamus (*Acorus calamus*)
Camphor, yellow/brown (*Cinnamomum camphora*)
Cassia (*Cinnamomum cassia*)
Cinnamon bark (*Cinnamomum zeylanicum, C. verum*)
Costus (*Saussurea lappa*)
Croton (*Croton tiglium*)
Elecampane (*Inula helenium*)
Fennel, bitter (*Foeniculum vulgare*)
Fig leaf (*Ficus carica*)
Horseradish (*Cochlearia armoracia, Armoracia rusticina*)
Huon pine (*Dacrydium franklinii*)
Jaborandi leaf (*Pilocarpus jaborandi*)
Lavender sage (*Salvia lavandulifolia*)
Mugwort (*Artemisia vulgaris, A. arborescens*)
Mustard (*Brassica nigra, B. negra*)
Oakmoss (*Evernia prunastri*)
Pennyroyal (*Mentha pulegium*)
Pine, dwarf; or Pumilio (*Pinus mugo*)
Rue (*Ruta montana*)
Sassafras (*Sassafras albidum / Ocotea cymbarum*)
Savin (*Juniperus sabina*)
Southernwood (*Artemisia abrotanum*)
Tansy (*Tanacetum vulgare*)
Thuja (*Thuja occidentalis khell / Thuja plicata*)
Wormseed (*Chenopodium ambrosioides*)
Wormwood (*Artemisia absinthium*)

$$\bigodot{1}$$

The Chemistry of Essential Oils

There's nothing simple about essential oil chemistry. Each essential oil contains dozens, and in some cases hundreds, of natural phytochemicals. The variation in the chemical composition of an essential oil, for example *Lavandula angustifolia*, will depend on where the lavender plant was grown, the altitude of that location, the soil it was grown in, the climatic conditions at the time of growing, the time of harvesting, and the specific method of steam distillation, including the temperature used. Despite all these variations, a lavender oil is expected to contain, among its main constituents, linalool, linalyl acetate, lavandulyl acetate, b-caryophyllene, and terpinen-4-ol. The term *eucalyptus* is meaningless in terms of essential oil phytochemistry because there are so many varieties, with hugely varying chemical compositions. For example, *Eucalyptus globulus* might contain between 60% and 90% of 1,8-cineol, while *Eucalyptus dives* (eucalyptus peppermint) may contain less than 2%.

Gas chromatography and mass spectrometry (GC/MS) are the main methods of analyzing essential oils. After they are run for a couple of hours, the smaller elements show up on the printout, and the whole essential oil is revealed as a highly complex composition. Depending on the age and sophistication of the analyzing machinery, and the length of time it's allowed to run, more elements can be revealed. To most producers and suppliers these smaller elements are something of an irrelevance — they can sell the product so long as they can prove the essential oil contains the expected main chemicals in the right proportions. Sometimes the trace elements account for well under 0.01% of the whole, and might include unidentifiable components. To young chemists looking to make a name for themselves, these tiny trace elements represent a chance to explore new phytochemicals and give us a fuller picture about what's actually going on.

As well as their chemical constituents, essential oils are classified in terms of their specific gravity, refractive index, and optical rotation. An isomer can be either dextrorotatory, prefixed with the symbol (+); or it can be laevorotatory and prefixed with the symbol (-). Chiral compounds have asymmetric carbon atoms occurring as enantiomers — they have two or more optical isomers. If negative, the aroma is like a mint, and if positive, it smells like caraway. The structure of the two is the same, except they are mirror images of one another. The dextrorotatory and laevorotatory aspects of the phytochemicals that compose an essential oil are hugely important, and if adulteration is taking place by the addition of substances with a different optical rotation from what is expected, it can be detected. If synthetic chemicals are being added, they have none of the vibrancy of natural components and the ratio between dextrorotatory and laevorotatory molecules is flat and bland at 50:50.

Essential oils contain several main types of components including alcohols, aldehydes, coumarins, esters, ethers, ketones, monoterpenes, oxides, and phenols. Under the general heading of "alcohols" there are phytochemicals, including linalool, citronellol, and geraniol; while eugenol, thymol, and carvacrol are types of phenol. A certain amount is known about the therapeutic action of some of these components, in terms of both the larger groupings and the individual constituents. For example, the phenols have been shown to have antimicrobial action, while citronellol, which is an alcohol, has been shown to have sedative properties, and when found in citronella oil, for example, it is known to deter insects.

Because essential oils are comprised of so many phytochemicals, it can't be said that the main component by volume, or even the two or three most prevalent constituents, account for an essential oil's particular therapeutic characteristics. It's all the constituents working in synergistic harmony that makes an essential oil what it is, not just a few particular chemicals within it. Think of it in terms of a cake that's composed of flour, sugar, water, eggs, and a trace amount — a drop — of vanilla essence for flavoring. Altogether, they make something delicious, but when they're sitting on the counter as individual components, none of them on their own look or taste like a cake.

Nevertheless, it's interesting to know some of the main chemicals found in essential oils and the therapeutic properties attributed to them. When looking for an essential oil to do a particular job — to fight inflammation, say — a chemist might look for one that contains particular esters or sesquiterpenes. And if a research lab was looking for an essential oil that's sedative, perhaps in the hope of identifying a new product or use that could be patented, they might look for those containing large amounts of certain types of aldehydes or coumarins. But the focus on just one phytochemical within an essential oil is just a part of the story, and it's a complex story at that. The profusion of constituents within an essential oil accounts for the fact that one single essential oil has a multitude of therapeutic applications and can be used for many conditions, not only for the actions its major components might suggest.

Within the groups below are many phytochemicals. For example, aldehydes include a great number besides citronellal, citral, and vanillin.

TABLE 23. PHYTOCHEMICALS IN ESSENTIAL OILS

PHYTOCHEMICAL GROUP	PROPERTIES
ALDEHYDES	Antibacterial, antiviral, antifungal, immunostimulant, anti-inflammatory, calming, relaxing, sedative, nerve tonic, uplifting
COUMARINS	Calming, sedative, hypotensive, antispasmodic; can cause photosensitivity in UV light
ESTERS	Antifungal, analgesic, antispasmodic, anti-inflammatory, sedative, calming, relaxing, hypotensive, balancing, general tonic
ETHERS	Anti-infectious, antispasmodic, sedative, analgesic, balancing
KETONES	Antibacterial, antiviral, antifungal, antiparasitic, cicatrisive, mucolytic, expectorant, decongestant, immunostimulant, analgesic
LACTONES	Calming, relaxing, febrifuge, mucolytic, expectorant, antiparasitic, immunostimulant
MONOTERPENES	Antibacterial, antiviral, antiseptic, analgesic, respiratory decongestant, expectorant, general tonic, immunostimulant
MONOTERPENOLS	Antibacterial, antifungal, antiseptic, immunostimulant, tonic, stimulant, balancing
OXIDES	Antifungal, respiratory decongestant, expectorant, analgesic, antispasmodic
PHENOLS	Antibacterial, antiviral, antifungal, antiparasitic, analgesic, antispasmodic, immunostimulant, general tonic, stimulant; can be irritant to mucous membrane and skin
SESQUITERPENES	Antibacterial, antiseptic, calming, anti-inflammatory, stimulant, hypotensive, blood and lymph decongestant, antiallergenic
SESQUITERPENOLS	Anti-infectious, anti-inflammatory, vascular tonic, immunotonic, stimulant, balancing

anticholagogue not in dictionary or on internet

must mean does not promote evacuation of bile from gall bladder + ducts

2

Glossary of Therapeutic Properties

Analgesic: reduces pain sensation

Anthelmintic: repels intestinal parasites

Antibacterial: prevents bacterial growth

Anticatarrhal: effective against catarrh

Anticoagulant: reduces blood clotting

Antidepressant: alleviates depression

Antifungal: prevents fungal growth

Anti-infectious: prevents uptake of infection

Anti-inflammatory: alleviates inflammation

Antimicrobial: prevents microorganism growth

Antioxidant: inhibits oxidation

Antiphlogistic: acts against inflammation and fever

Antiputrescent: acts against putrefaction

Antirheumatic: relieves symptoms associated with rheumatic conditions

Antisclerotic: prevents hardening of cells and tissues

Antiseborrheic: relieves excessive secretion of sebum

Antiseptic: destroys microbes and prevents their development

Antispasmodic: prevents or relieves spasms, convulsions, or contractions

Antisudorific: prevents sweating

Antitoxic: able to neutralize toxins

Antitussive: relieves coughs

Antivenomous: used against the effects of venom

Antiviral: prevents viral growth

Aphrodisiac: increases sexual desire

Astringent: contracts or tightens tissues

Balsamic: soothes sore throats, coughs, etc.

Calmative: sedative, calming agent

Carminative: relieves flatulence, easing abdominal pain and bloating

Cholagogue: promotes the evacuation of bile from gall bladder and ducts

Cicatrizing: promotes the formation of scar tissue, thus healing

Circulatory: promotes flow of blood and lymph

Cytophylactic: promotes cell turnover, thus healing

Decongestant: reduces congestion such as mucus

Deodorant: masks or removes unpleasant smell

Depurative: cleanser, detoxifier

Diaphoretic: promotes perspiration

Digestive: helps in the digestion of food

Disinfectant: helps fight the spread of germs

Diuretic: promotes the removal of excess water from the body

Emmenagogue: induces or regularizes menstruation

Emollient: soothes and softens skin

Expectorant: promotes removal of mucus from the body

Febrifuge: an antifebrile (antifever) agent

Galactagogue: induces the flow of breastmilk

Hemostatic: arrests blood flow

Hepatic: acts on the liver

Hypertensive: raises blood pressure

Hypnotic: sedative effect

Hypotensive: lowers blood pressure

Immunostimulant: stimulates the action of the immune system

Laxative: assists in bowel elimination

Mucolytic: breaks down mucus

Nervine: acts on nerves; relieves nervous disorders

Pectoral: beneficial for diseases or conditions of the chest and respiratory system

Regenerative: tends to regenerate

Restorative: strengthens and revives the body's systems

Rubefacient: a counterirritant producing redness of the skin

Sedative: relaxes psychological and physical activity

Soporific: induces, or tends to induce, sleep

Spasmolytic: eases smooth muscle spasm

Stimulant: increases overall function of the body

Stomachic: good for the stomach; gastric tonic, digestive aid

Sudorific: promotes perspiration

Thermogenic: stimulates heat production

Tonic: invigorates, refreshes, restores the body and bodily functions

Vasodilatory: promotes dilation of blood vessels

Vermifuge: expels intestinal worms

Vulnerary: heals wounds and sores by external application

Acknowledgments

The writing of this book has involved a profound personal journey and may never have been finished without the encouragement of some very special people.

A sincere thank-you goes to Julia Stonehouse for her invaluable assistance and confidence in this book, and her unwavering belief in my work and the healing power of essential oils.

Georgia Hughes, Editorial Director at New World Library, for her incredible patience and understanding, and Kristen Cashman, Managing Editor, for her hard work and commitment.

My family for giving me the motivation and precious time to write.
And the unseen hand that guides me in all I do.

Bibliography

Alberts, Bruce, Alexander Johnson, Julian Lewis, David Morgan, Martin Raff, Keith Roberts, and Peter Walter. *Molecular Biology of the Cell*. 6th ed. New York: Garland Science, 2014.

Baker, Richard T., and Henry G. Smith. *Research on the Eucalypts: Especially in Regard to Their Essential Oils*. Sydney: Government of the State of New South Wales, 1902.

Balz, Rodolphe. *Les Huiles Essentielles et Comment les Utiliser*. Paris: Lib. Commerce International, 1986.

Bardeau, Fabrice. *La Médecine Aromatique*. Paris: Robert Laffont, 1976.

Beckstrom-Sternberg, Stephen M., and James A. Duke. *CRC Handbook of Medicinal Mints (Aromathematics): Phytochemicals and Biological Activities*. Boca Raton, FL: CRC Press, 1996.

Belaiche, P. *Traits de Phytothérapie et d'Aromathérapie (Treatise on Phytotherapy and Aromatherapy)*. 3 vols. Paris: Librairie Maloine, 1979.

Bernadet, Marcel. *La Phyto-aromathérapie Pratique*. Saint-Jean-de-Braye, France: Editions Dangles, 1983.

Franchomme, P., and D. Pénoël. *L'Aromathérapie Exactement*. Limoges, France: Roger Jollois Editeur, 1990.

Gattefosse, R. M. *Antiseptiques Essentials*. Paris: Desforges, Girardot & Cie., 1931.

Hay, Robert K. M., and Peter G. Waterman, eds. *Volatile Oil Crops: Their Biology, Biochemistry and Production*. Harlow, UK: Longman Scientific and Technical, 1993.

Linskens, H. F., and J. F. Jackson, eds. *Essential Oils and Waxes*. Berlin: Springer-Verlag, 1991.

Moncrieff, R. W. *Odour Preferences*. London: Grampian Press, 1966.

Piesse, G. W. Septimus. *The Art of Perfumery*. London: Longman, Brown, Green, 1856.

Rimmel, Eugene. *The Book of Perfumes*. London: Chapman and Hall, 1867.

Tierno, Philip M. *The Secret Life of Germs: What They Are, Why We Need Them, and How We Can Protect Ourselves against Them*. New York: Atria, 2004.

Tisserand, Robert, and Rodney Young. *Essential Oil Safety: A Guide for Health Care Professionals*. 2nd ed. Edinburgh: Churchill Livingstone/Elsevier, 2013.

Uphof, J. C. Th. *Dictionary of Economic Plants*. Lehre, Germany: J. Cramer, 1968.

Valnet, J., C. Duraffourd, and J. C. Lapraz. *Une Médecine Nouvelle: Phytothérapie et Aromathérapie*. Paris: Presses de la Renaissance, 1978.

Van Toller, George Dodd. *Perfumery*. London: Chapman and Hall, 1988.

Worwood, Valerie Ann. *Aromatherapy for the Beauty Therapist*. London: Thompson Learning, 2001.

———. *Aromatherapy for the Healthy Child*. Novato, CA: New World Library 2000.

———. *Aromatherapy for the Soul*. Novato, CA: New World Library, 2006.

———. *Aromatics*. London: Pan Books, 1987.

———. *Essential Aromatherapy*. Novato, CA: New World Library, 2003.

———. *The Fragrant Mind*. London: Doubleday, 1995.

———. *Scents and Scentuality*. Novato, CA: New World Library, 1999.

Worwood, Valerie Ann, and Julia Stonehouse. *The Endometriosis Natural Treatment Program*. Novato, CA: New World Library, 2007.

Index

health, 253–54; for lymphedema, 327; for massage, 180, 264, 311, 413, 415; for menopause, 209–10; for mindfulness, 111; for moodiness/mood swings, 108; for multiple sclerosis, 346; for muscle tone, 301; for muscular fatigue, 348; for ovarian cysts, 197; for paralysis, 175; for PCOS, 199; for penis pain, 247; in perfumes, 453–55; for PMS and PMDD, 205–6; for positivity, 112; for prostate cancer, 330–31; for PVCS, 212; in room sprays, 62; for rosacea, 378; for running/walking/jogging, 298; for scalp eczema/psoriasis, 398; for skin care, 381t, 421t; in skin care oils, 368; for spasticity, 177–78; for spina bifida, 172; in spiritual practice, 441; for swollen ankles and feet, 265; for tenosynovitis, 80; therapeutic uses/properties of, 549t, 596; for toning/slimming, 422t; for vaginal infections/inflammation, 219, 221; for varicose veins, 200

kanuka: defensive properties of, 53t; for infections, 57, 63; for pneumonia, 275
ketones, 639t
kiwi seed, 365, 367–68, 373
knee-cartilage injury, 309
knee synovitis (water on the knee), 310
Kräuterbuch (Lonitzer), 6
kukui, 393, 518

labdanum. *See* cistus
Labrador tea. *See* Greenland moss
lactation, 635
lactic acid, 131
lactones, 639t
lacunar infarction, 337. *See also* stroke
laevorotatory vs. dextrorotatory phyto-chemicals, 637–38
lamb: Garlic Lamb, 466; Minced Beef or Lamb, 467
laryngitis, 45
laurel, 384t
laurel, bay, 570; for cellulite, 414; defensive properties of, 52t, 67, 427; for exhaustion, 243; in facial sprays and tonics, 363; for hair loss, 255; in hair oils, 388; for infections, 57, 63; for moodiness/mood swings, 108; Red Meat Marinade, 464; for skin care,

382–83t; for stress, 98; therapeutic uses/properties of, 536t, 570
lavandin, 597; for animals, 491; for ankle sprain, 305; for focus and concen-tration, 114; for foot care, 299; for hangovers, 475; for hemorrhoids, 252; as insect/pest repellent, 491; for massage, 305; for muscle tone, 301; for pelvic pain, 211; for running/walking/jogging, 298; for sprains/strains, 305; therapeutic uses/properties of, 549t, 597
lavender, 597–98; for abrasions, 32, 135, 150–51; for abscesses, 32; for aches/pains, 153; for Achilles tendinitis, 304; for acne, 375–77; for ADHD, 188–89; for aging skin, 370, 372; in air freshener, 3; for air quality, 67; for Alzheimer's disease, 280; for anal fissures, 32; for androgen decline, 244; for anger, 188; for animals, 479–81, 483–85, 488–93; for ankle/heel contu-sion, 305; antiseptic cooling/calming by, 169; for anxiety, 88t, 101–2, 189, 279t; for apathy/helplessness, 88t; for arms, 416; for arthritis, 181–82, 284–87, 484; for asthma, 159; for athlete's foot, 166; for atrophic vaginitis, 220; for autism, 185–86; for babies, 144; for bacillary dysentery, 127; for back pain, 79; Baked Egg Custards, 467; for balanitis, 248; for the bathroom, 433; in baths, 63, 139, 196, 229, 407, 409–10; for beards, 259; for bee stings, 160; for bereavement, 109; for bites, 45, 130–35; for blackheads, 374; for bleeding, 33; for bleeding nose, 33; for blemishes, 374; for blisters, 33–35, 300–301; in body oils, 63, 124, 195, 215, 264; in body splashes/spritzers, 406; for boils, 34; for breast abscess, 194, 237; for breast cancer, 329–30; for breast contusion, 306; for breast soreness, 193, 236; for breathing difficulties, 272; for bron-chitis, 157–58; for bruises, 34, 135, 151, 305, 307; for bumps, 135; for burnout, 93; for burns, 3, 34–35, 77–78, 151; for bursitis, 83; for buttock contusion, 306; for carpal tunnel syndrome, 309; for cerebral palsy, 178–79; for cervical cancer, 328–29; for CFS, 347; for chapped skin, 36; chemical

composition of, 637; for chest muscle strain, 306; for chicken pox (varicella), 163; for chilblains, 36; for childbirth, 232–33; for circulation, 263–64; for cleansing, 354–55; for club foot, 183; for colds, 37, 149–50; for cold sores, 36; as a companion crop, 504; for con-valescence, 38; for COPD, 343; cost of, 2, 10; for coughs, 38; for cramps, 229; for cuts and burns, 28; for cuts and wounds, 39, 135–36, 150–51, 483; for cystitis, 195–96; for dandruff, 397; defensive properties of, 3, 28, 51, 53t, 56, 130, 313, 426; for dental abscess, 39; for depression, 88t, 103, 105, 107; for diabetes mellitus, 180; for diaper rash, 146; for diarrhea, 39–40; for dieters, 412; for disk injury, 305; on dressings for cuts, 64; for drug abuse, 170; for dry, flaky skin, 135; for dysmenorrhea, 207; for earache, 40–41, 157; for ear in-fection, 41; for edema, 230; for elbow contusion, 307; for endometriosis, 214–15; for exhaustion/fatigue, 41, 61, 135, 230, 242–43, 323; for exposure to heat, 135; for face contusion, 307; in face masks, 359; in facial sprays and tonics, 362–63; for facial steaming, 361–62; for fainting, 41; for feet, 420; for fevers, 126, 135, 154–55; for fibrocystic breast conditions, 194; for fibrositis, 41–42; for finger sprain, 308; for flu, 44; for flying, 120–22; for food poisoning, 127; in foot baths, 293; for foot care, 300–301; for fractures, 135; for fretful babies, 147; for ganglion, 81; for gap-year travel, 122; in gels, 62; for genital herpes, 59–60; for gout, 288; for groin strain, 308; for hair, afro-textured, 393; for hair, dry, 389–90; for hair, falling, 395; for hair, fragile, 392; for hair, normal, 388; for hair, oily, 391; for hair loss, 255–56, 396; in hair oils, 387–88; in hallways, 425; for hamstring injury, 311; for hands, 416; for hangovers, 475–76; for hay fever, 42; for headaches, 3, 43, 61, 68, 89t, 135, 279t, 324; for head injury, 309; for head lice, 168–69; for heart care, 335; for heat exhaustion/heat-stroke/sunstroke, 124–25, 135–36; for hemorrhoids, 252, 293; for high

About the Author

Valerie Ann Worwood is a consultant clinical aromatherapist and author with a doctorate in complementary medicine, and has been Chairperson and Chair of Research for the International Federation of Aromatherapists. As well as her involvement in essential oil research, she has acted as a consultant and expert on the clinical use of essential oils internationally. Valerie is the innovator of Aroma-Genera® and the Mother Essences®, the aroma-psychology system for personality and emotional well-being, which she has taught in the United Kingdom, the United States, Canada, and China. Valerie continues in clinical essential oil practice, as well as lecturing and holding workshops around the world. Her work with essential oils has taken her down many diverse aromatic pathways — from designing skin care and spa products and treatments for international companies to creating essential oil blends for artisan chocolatiers. Valerie Ann Worwood's first book was published in 1987, and since then she has authored many titles that have been translated into fifteen languages.

www.valerieworwood.com

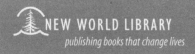